TRENDS IN IMMUNOLABELLED AND RELATED TECHNIQUES

Edited by **Eltayb Abuelzein**

Trends in Immunolabelled and Related Techniques
Edited by Eltayb Abuelzein

Published by InTech

Janeza Trdine 9, 51000 Rijeka, Croatia

Publishing Process Manager Maja Bozicevic

Technical Editor Teodora Smiljanic

Cover Designer InTech Design Team

Additional hard copies can be obtained from orders@intechopen.com

Trends in Immunolabelled and Related Techniques, Edited by Eltayb Abuelzein
p. cm.
ISBN 978-953-51-0570-1

For EU product safety concerns:
IN TECH d.o.o., Prolaz Marije Krucifikse Kozulić 3, 51000 Rijeka, Croatia,
info@intechopen.com or visit our website at intechopen.com.

Meet the editor

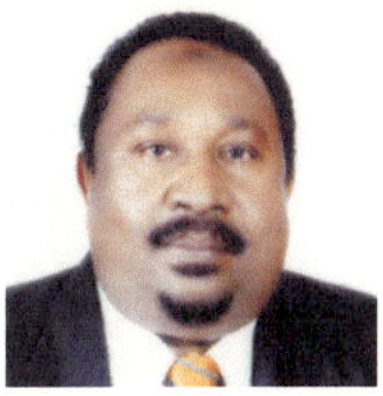

Professor Eltayb Abuelzein has graduated from the University of Khartoum, Sudan, with the B.V.Sc. in Veterinary Medicine. He obtained his Master's and Ph.D. degrees in virology from the University of Reading, Britain. He also got a Post-Doctoral Fellowship (FIAEA), in Immunolabelled Techniques & Arbovirology , the World Reference Laboratory, Pirbright Britain. Since 1975 he has been engaged in active research, technological developments and teaching in several Universities in Sudan and Saudi Arabia. He acted as a Consultant to the International Atomic Energy Agency (IAEA) in Immunolabelled Techniques. He is an Editor and reviewer for a number of Scientific Journals including the International Journal "Tropical Animal Health & Production", Britain. Published 123 peer reviewed papers in reputable scientific journals and 60 peer reviewed articles in conferences. He was the first to develop the ELISA technique in Foot and mouth disease (FMD) Virus Research. Quoted in the highly reputed international scientific journal "Nature". Contributed in the Book: "Immunoassay in the 80's", 1981, ATP publishing Co., London. Made first records of several viral diseases of great international significance. Presently, Chair Professor of Viral Haemorrhagic Fevers, King Abdulaziz University, Saudi Arabia.

Contents

Preface

"Trends in Immunolabelled and Related Techniques" is intended to present new concepts in immunolabelled techniques (IMLT) and to encourage more research on some already existing highly versatile ones, which seems to have been overlooked for a while.

Since their early developments IMLT have found their way with great success in biological scientific research. The pace of their progress over the years was great. For instance, the developments in ELISA since its discovery in the early seventies of the last century were immense. It was extensively utilized with great success in laboratory diagnosis and research in the medical field, veterinary medicine, agricultural sciences, biotechnology and in many fields of research where it could be applied.

This book encompasses two sections. One focuses on emerging immunolabelled methods such as: 'utility of one step immunoassays, an immune chromatographic method', 'non-competitive immunoassays', 'ultra sensitive ELISA', 'modified ELISA', 'new views in evaluation of the detection limits in immunoassay methods' and 'multiplex immunoassays'.

The other section includes overviews on important immunoassay methods which are of special value in specific areas of research, such as: 'utilization of *Staphylococcus aureus* Protein 'A' and *Streptococcus Spps.* Protein 'G' in immunolabelled techniques', 'general concepts in immunoassay systems' and 'the use of bead-based multiplex immunoassay systems'.

The book is most useful for researchers and postgraduate students, in all fields where immunolabelled techniques are applied.

I would like to acknowledge the kind help and support of Ms. Maja Bozicevic, the Publishing Process Manager of the book, whose continuous devotion and patience led to success of production of this book. I would also like to acknowledge the authors who participated by writing the chapters and those who in many ways helped in preparing this book.

Prof. Eltayb Abuelzein
Chair Professor, The Chair of Viral Haemorrhagic Fevers, King Abdulaziz University,
Saudi Arabia

Section 1

Emerging Uni-and-Multiplex Immunolabeled Methods

1

Utility of One Step Immunoassay in Detecting False Negativity in Routine Blood Bank Screening of Infectious Diseases

Kafil Akhtar
Department of Pathology, Jawaharlal Nehru Medical College, Aligarh Muslim University, India

1. Introduction

Immunoassays are chemical tests used to detect or quantify a specific substance, the analyte, in a blood or body fluid sample, using an immunological reaction. Immunoassays for antibodies produced in viral hepatitis and HIV are commonly used to identify patients with these diseases.(Bishop et al., 2001). The commonly used immunoassay methods for detection of infectious diseases are immunoprecipitation, which measures the quantity of precipitate formed after the reagent antibody (precipitin) has been incubated with the sample and reacted with its respective antigen to form an insoluble aggregate, and enzyme immunoassay in the form of enzyme-linked immunosorbent assay (ELISA). The basic principle of these assays is the specificity of the antibody-antigen reaction.(Burtis & Ashwood,2001).

Though being very specific and sensitive, immunoassays are easy to perform which has contributed to it's widespread use and tremendous success.(Henry,2001). Their high specificity results from the use of antibodies and purified antigens as reagents. An antibody is a protein (immunoglobulin) produced by B-lymphocytes (immune cells) in response to stimulation by an antigen. Immunoassays measure the formation of antibody-antigen complexes and detect them via an indicator reaction. High sensitivity is achieved by using an indicator system (e.g., enzyme label) that results in amplification of the measured product.

The purpose of an immunoassay is to measure (or, in a qualitative assay, to detect) an analyte. Immunoassay is the method of choice for measuring analytes normally present at very low concentrations that cannot be determined accurately by other less expensive tests. (Wallach,2000). Immunoassays for antibodies produced in viral hepatitis, HIV, and syphilis are commonly used to identify patients with these diseases. Although immunoassays are both highly sensitive and specific, false positive and negative results may occur. False-negative results may be caused by improper sample storage, reagent deterioration, improper washing technique or prozone effect. False-positive results have been reported for samples containing small fibrin strands that adhere to the solid phase matrix or due to substances in the blood or urine that cross-react or bind to the antibody used in the test. (Wild, 2000).

Large quantities of antigen in an immunoassay system impair antigen-antibody binding, resulting in low antigen determination. This is called the 'high dose hook effect'. The first description of the prozone effect in the literature was made by Miles et al.,1974. Large quantities of antigen in an immunoassay system impair antigen-antibody binding, resulting in low antigen determination. This is called the prozone or high dose hook effect, which describes the inhibition of immune complex formation by excess antigen concentrations. The prozone or high-dose hook effect, documented to cause false-negative assay results >50 years ago, still remains a problem in one-step immunometric assays. (Brensing,1989; Haller et al,1992;Landsteiner,1946). To detect the prozone effect, samples are often tested undiluted and after dilution. (Saryan et al,1989). If the result on dilution is higher than for the undiluted sample, then the undiluted sample most likely exhibited the prozone effect. Unfortunately, this approach increases labour and reagent costs for assays that may only rarely encounter extremely high analyte concentrations.

2. Material and methods

The present study was performed on voluntary blood donors at our transfusion centre. Hepacard device (J Mitra Laboratory Systems-India) for detection of hepatitis B surface antigen was labelled with patient's identification number. Blood was collected by venipuncture and allowed to clot naturally and completely. Subsequently serum was separated from the clot with the help of a clot retractor. Then 70 μl of donors serum was added into the inbuilt sample well of the hepacard device containing the coated antibodies, using a calibrated dropper and allowed to react for 20 minutes. Results were read thereafter in the form of visually detectable pink control and test lines.

3. Observations

The hepacard device when read after 20 minutes showed only one distinct pink test line and no control line. Serial dilutions (1:10,1: 20) of the donors serum sample was performed in normal saline and the test was re-run with serum samples of each dilution step-wise. Serum sample with 1: 10 dilution showed a control and faint pink test line.(Figure 1). This faint pink test line intensified to a broad pink band when the test was performed with 1: 20 diluted serum sample of the donor.(Figure 2). So to overcome the prozone effect, which

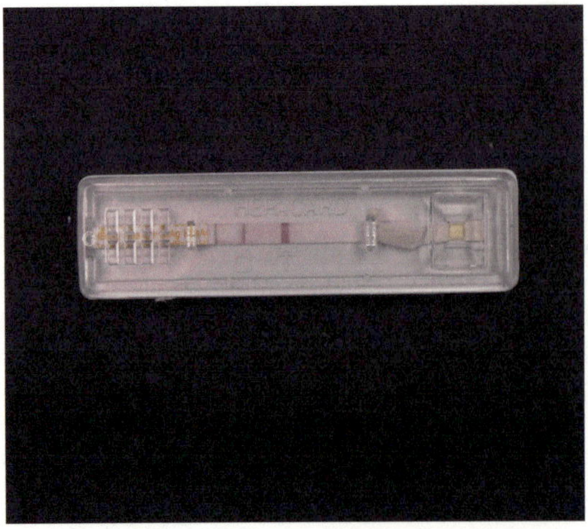

Fig. 1. Depicting faint pink test line

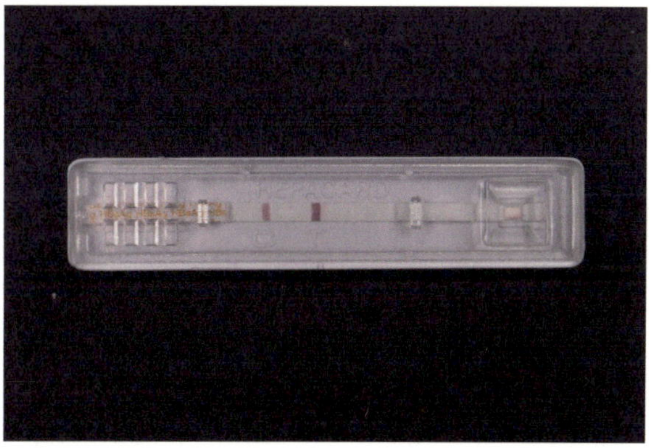

Fig. 2. Depicting broad pink test line

describes the inhibition of immune complex formation by excess antigen concentrations, the donors serum sample was serially diluted. In our case, a 1:10 dilution did not show a prominent pink line but a higher dilution of 1:20 was tried to get a broad pink band.

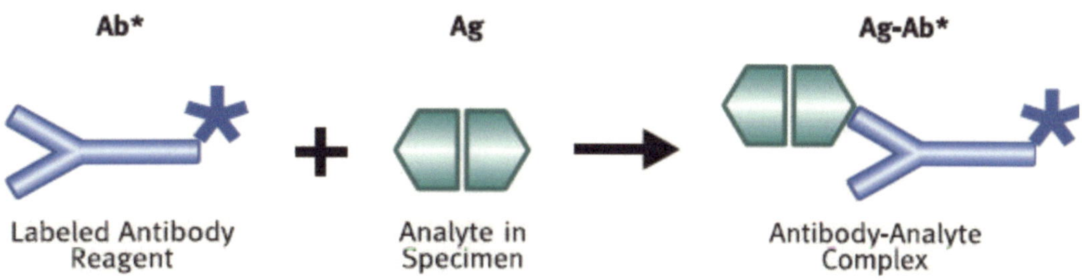

Fig. 3. Schematic diagram showing antigen-antibody reaction in the hepacard device.

4. Discussion

The intensity of an antigen-antibody interaction depends primarily on the relative proportion of the antigen and the antibody. A relative excess of either will impair adequate immune complex formation. (Stites et al, 1997). This is called the 'high dose hook effect' or the 'prozone phenomenon'. This has been classically described in serological tests for diagnosis of brucellosis. (Young ,1995). In addition to hormonal assays, the high dose hook effect has also been demonstrated in immune-based techniques used in the measurements of CA 125, IgE and prostrate specific antigen. (Wolf,1989; St-Jean et al, 1996). All immunoassays are based on antigen antibody interactions. The high dose hook effect often interferes with the assay result. The goal in the immunoassay in screening of infectious diseases should be to minimize erroneous results; so as not to endanger patient health and the blood supply. Reporting of an erroneous result can have serious medical implications, and sample pooling is a simple method for detecting falsely low concentrations attributable to the prozone effect. Although this screening approach increases reagent costs by 10% and involves additional labour to prepare and analyze pools, it is considerably more cost-effective than analyzing all samples undiluted and after dilution, which doubles reagent costs.

The prozone or (high-dose) hook effect, still remains a problem in one-step immunometric assays (Pesce,1993; Vaidya et al,1988; Zweig & Csako, 1990), immunoturbidimetric assays (Jury et al,1990), and immunonephelometric assays (Van Lente,1997) for immunoglobulins. To detect the prozone effect, samples are often tested undiluted and after dilution. (Saryan et al,1989).If the result on dilution is higher than for the undiluted sample, then the undiluted sample most likely exhibited the prozone effect. Unfortunately, this approach increases labor and reagent costs for assays that may only rarely encounter extremely high analyte concentrations. An alternative approach involves pooling patient samples and measuring the pool and a 10-fold dilution of the pool. (Cole et al,1993). If one or more of the samples in the pool is falsely low because of the prozone effect, then the results from the undiluted and diluted pools (after correcting for the 10-fold dilution) will differ significantly.(Cole et al,1993). Other approaches to eliminate the prozone effect include using two-step immunoassays that have a wash step between the addition of sample and labeled antibody (Vaidya et al,1988), and the use of neural network classifier systems that analyze reaction kinetics.(Papik et al,1999).

Serum immunoglobulins can be markedly increased in patients presenting with large myeloma tumor burdens and may lead to falsely low results in nephelometric assays. (Van Lente,1997). Anthony W. Butch, 2000 combined 50-μL aliquots from each of 10 samples used to dilute each sample 10-fold in order to eliminate any prozone effect. The concentrations of IgG, IgA, and IgM in the pool were measured using a nephelometer (BNII; Dade Behring, Inc.) and compared with the mean values when all samples in the pool were analyzed (calculated value). When the two values for an immunoglobulin differed by a specified quantity, all samples in the pool were reanalyzed after a 10-fold dilution.

Anthony W. Butch, 2000 further stated that criteria for detecting the prozone effect are based on data obtained from routine samples during a 10-day period. Measured immunoglobulin concentrations for 27 pools (10 samples per pool) were compared with the mean values of samples in the pools. The range of values for the measured serum pools and the differences between the measured pool value and the value derived from the mean of individually measured samples in the pool (calculated value) for each immunoglobulin were as follows: IgG, range 10.20-32.50 g/L, mean difference 4.6%, SD 4.1%; IgA, range 0.31-17.90 g/L, mean difference 12.6%, SD 8.6%; and IgM, range 0.27-5.96 g/L, mean difference 13.2%, SD 8.2%. The small SD indicated that none of the samples exhibited the prozone effect. A percentage difference less than the mean plus 2 SD was considered acceptable and was determined to be 15% for IgG, 30% for IgA, and 30% for IgM. Large differences were considered suggestive of a prozone effect. (Anthony W. Butch, 2000).

The ability of this approach to identify samples exhibiting the prozone effect during routine analysis was further evaluated by Anthony W. Butch, 2000 during a 6-month period. Approximately 750 samples/month were received, and 460 pools were analyzed. Ten samples from five different myeloma patients were identified as being falsely low because of the prozone effect. Four samples were from patients with IgA myeloma, and one was from a patient with IgG myeloma. The discrepancy between the measured and calculated pool was 62-88% (initial difference). When the sample generating the erroneous value was identified and the "correct" result (obtained after dilution) was used in the calculation, the difference between the measured and calculated pool was within the established limits of 30% for IgA and 15% for IgG (corrected difference). The falsely low values differed from the actual results by as much as 11-fold for IgA and 40-fold for IgG. The prozone effect was not restricted to IgA and IgG because samples exhibiting this phenomenon were also identified, when measuring IgM. (Anthony W. Butch, 2000).

A 2% incidence (1 of 46 pools) for the prozone effect when measuring immunoglobulins may be higher at institutions not specializing in the treatment of multiple myeloma. However, the incidence of multiple myeloma over the age of 25 is 30 per 100 000 (Cooper & Lawton,1987), and most laboratories will eventually encounter a sample exhibiting the prozone effect when measuring immunoglobulins by nephelometry.(Van Lente,1997). Reporting of an erroneous result can have serious medical implications, and sample pooling is a simple method for detecting falsely low concentrations attributable to the prozone effect. Although this screening approach increases reagent costs by 10% and involves additional labor to prepare and analyze pools, it is considerably more cost-effective than analyzing all samples undiluted and after dilution, which doubles reagent costs. Furthermore, this simple prozone detection method can be adapted to other nephelometric assays with the potential for erroneous results from antigen excess. (Anthony W. Butch, 2000).

The one-step sandwich immunoassay is increasingly replacing the traditional two-step immunoassay due to obvious advantages such as assay speed. However, the one-step sandwich immunoassay suffers from the 'hook' effect irrespective of the analyte characteristics. The 'hook' effect is dependent primarily on the analyte concentration. Three different model analytes, human growth hormone (hGH), the dimeric form of hGH (D-hGH, having a discrete number of repeating epitopes) and ferritin (multiple epitopes) having different immunological properties have been employed in studies of the one-step sandwich immunoassay. The characteristics of each of the model analytes offer new insights into general guidelines for assay procedures. These guidelines permit rapid optimization of assay conditions for an immunoassay without a prior knowledge of the immunological characteristics of the antibody or antigen. Both experimental and theoretical data show several instances where high capacity solid-phase antibodies can effectively shift the 'hook' to relatively higher analyte concentrations. The effect of the concentration of labeled antibody on assay response was examined theoretically. (Fernando & Wilson, 1992; Uotila et al, 1981)

Lebeouf et al, 2005 described a case of a 41-yr-old man with metastatic medullary thyroid carcinoma. Despite extensive disease in the neck as well as metastatic lesions in the liver, his serum calcitonin, measured with a commercial one-step immunoradiometric assay, was only minimally elevated (244 ng/liter). After serial dilutions, a nonlinear relationship became evident, suggesting the presence of a "hook effect." Treatment of the serum with heterophilic blocking reagent revealed no change. Calcitonin was then measured with a different immunoradiometric assay and revealed a much higher level. Similar discrepancies were found in different samples from various patients when analyzed with different calcitonin immunoassays. They concluded that clinicians following patients with cancer and using tumor markers need to be aware of the phenomena such as the hook effect, because a low calcitonin result could give false reassurance to both the patient and the clinician and could dramatically change the prognosis of the patient (Lebeouf et al, 2005 ;Quayle & Moley ,2005).

Unnikrishnan et al,2001 have reported that large quantities of antigen in an immunoassay system impair antigen-antibody binding, resulting in low antigen determination, a phenomenon known as 'high dose hook effect' in a patient with a large macroprolactinoma. In this patient, the correct estimate of serum prolactin (PRL) was obtained only after appropriate dilution of serum. They suggested that in order to avoid the high dose hook effect, the serum PRL be estimated in appropriate dilution in all patients with large pituitary tumours. This is particularly important when the clinical suspicion of high PRL is strong, as in women with amenorrhoea-galactorrhoea and men with long standing hypogonadism. They further suggested that in order to accurately estimate PRL in patients with large pituitary tumours, PRL should be assayed in 1:100, 1:200 or even higher dilutions of serum in order to get an accurate estimate of serum PRL.

Miles et al,1974 and Miles & Hales,1968 have stated that a high dose hook effect is observed, if too much free hemoglobin that is not bound to the gold-labeled antibody reaches the test result region. In this case the antibody immobilized at the test result region becomes saturated with free hemoglobin. This prevents the binding of the hemoglobin complexed with the gold-labeled antibody, thus interfering with the formation of the test result line. The test result appears negative in spite of the presence of hemoglobin in the sample. The high dose hook effect can be avoided using the color of the sample as a guide. The visual detectable color caused by hemoglobin vanishes between 10^{-3} and 10^{-4} dilution. At this concentration range, there is no danger of a high dose hook effect. In contrast, samples that are clearly colored due to hemoglobin are likely to cause false negative results because of the high dose hook effect. Good results are obtained when the extract has a "straw" color. They suggested that if one is concerned, that a negative result is from High Dose Hook Effect, then a simple remedy is to dilute the extract and re-run the sample. (Miles et al,1974;Miles & Hales,1968). Immunoassay is an *in vitro* procedure, and is therefore not associated with complications. When blood is collected, slight bleeding into the skin and subsequent bruising may occur. The patient may become lightheaded or queasy from the sight of blood.

4.1 Immunoassays and forensic science

Forensic toxicology encompasses the determination of the presence and concentration of drugs, other xenobiotics and their metabolites in physiological fluids and organs and the interpretation of these findings as they may have impact on legal issues. These include medical examiner investigations, driving under the influence of drugs/alcohol and other transportation accident investigations, workplace pre-employment, random and for-cause drug testing and judicial monitoring of arrestees and parolees. For the most part, forensic toxicologists use commercial immunoassays directed primarily towards abused drugs. Commercial immunoassays developed for therapeutic monitoring of other drugs, veterinary drugs and pesticides, as well as immunoassays developed in research laboratories for specialized studies, may find a role in the forensic toxicology laboratory for specialized cases. While most commercial immunoassays have been developed for a urine matrix, they have been applied by forensic toxicologists to other matrices, including blood, hair, saliva, sweat, tissue homogenates, blood stains and most other physiological samples that may be of value in the investigation. The non urine matrix usually is much more complex in its composition. Sample pretreatments that range from simple deproteinations to multistep extractions to remove matrix components and/or concentrate the sample are often required. The heterogenous RIAs and ELISAs usually require less rigorous, if any, pretreatments. (Bell, 2006; Moody, 2006).

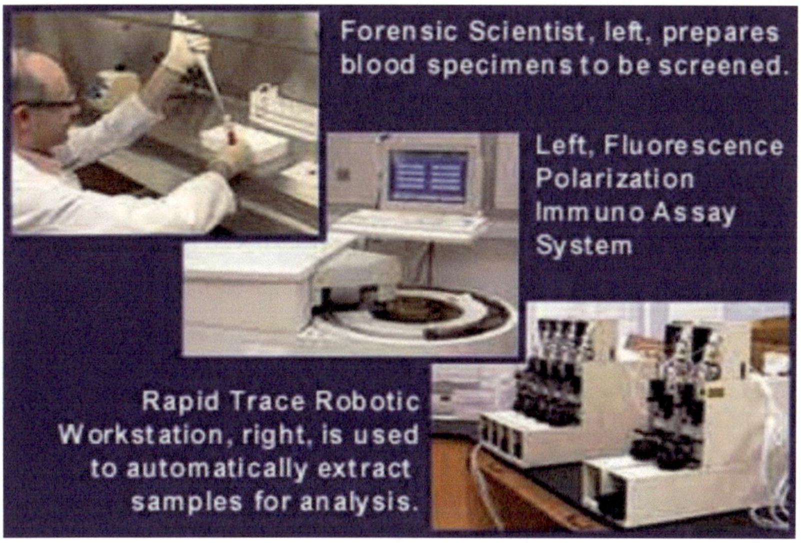

Fig. 4. Rapid trace robotic workstation used in forensic lab.

4.2 Types of Immunoassay

4.2.1 Enzyme Immunoassay (EIA)

Enzymes occur naturally and catalyze biochemical reactions. Enzymes are cheap, readily available, have a long shelf life, easily adaptable to automation and automation is relatively inexpensive. The techniques pose no health hazards, little reagent enzyme necessary, can be used for qualitative or quantitative assays. The test tubes are filled with the antigen solution (e.g., blood/serum) to be assayed. Any antigen molecules present bind to the immobilized antibody molecules. The antibody-enzyme conjugate is added to the reaction mixture. The antibody part of the conjugate binds to any antigen molecules that were bound previously, creating an antibody-antigen-antibody "sandwich". After washing away any unbound conjugate, the substrate solution is added. After a set interval, the reaction is stopped (e.g., by adding 1 N NaOH) and the concentration of colored product formed is measured in a spectrophotometer. The intensity of color is proportional to the concentration of bound antigen. (Bosch et al, 1975; Engvall & Perlmann,1971; Schuurs & Van Weemen, 1980; Van Weemen & Schuurs,1971).

4.2.2 Rapid Immunoassays

Membrane based cassettes are rapid, easy to perform and give reproducible results. Membrane coated with antigen or antibody produces color reaction. Designed to be of single use and are disposable. Different types of rapid tests are membrane based enzyme immuno-assay, particle agglutination assay and immunochromatography

4.2.3 Immunochromatography

Test sample is applied to the sample well, from where it migrates forward. Sample dissolves labeled antigen or antibody to which it binds, and migrates further towards detection zone, where it will bind to immobilized antigen or antibody. Finally color change occurs.

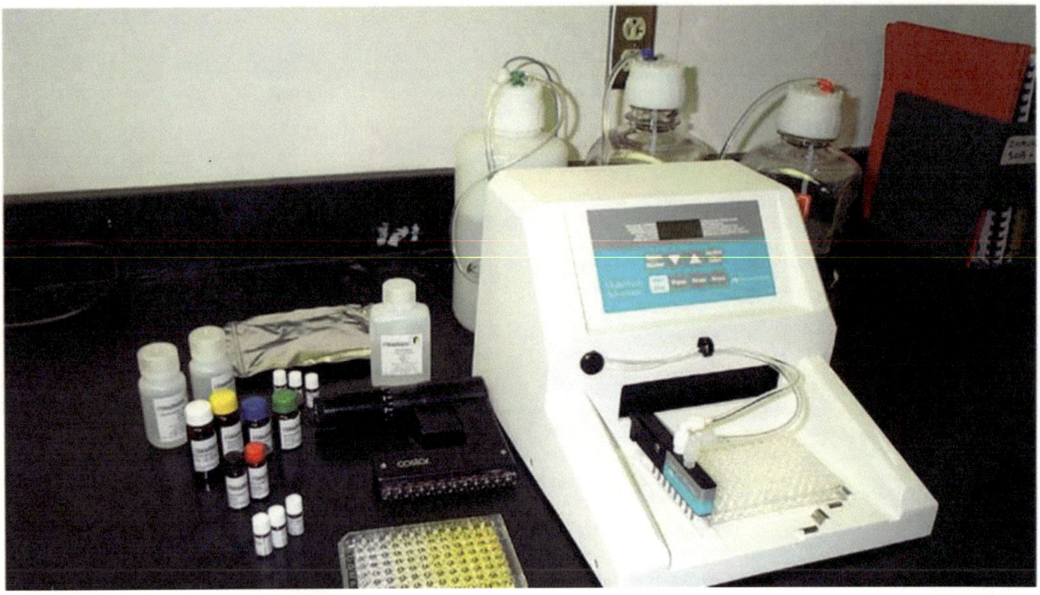

Fig. 5. Workstation of enzyme Immunoassay.

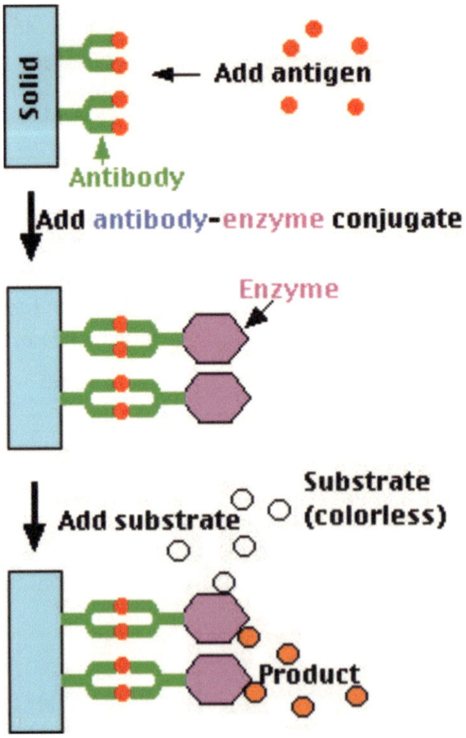

Fig. 6. Schematic diagram of EIA

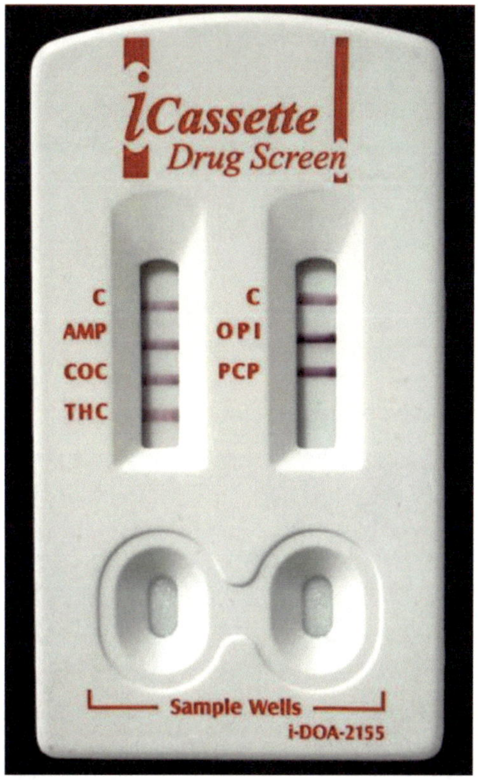

Fig. 7. Depicting Immunochromatography cassette

4.2.4 Chemiluminescent Immunoassays

The process of chemiluminescence occurs when energy in the form of light is released from matter during a chemical reaction. Large number of molecules capable of chemiluminescence are luminal, acridium esters, ruthenium derivatives, and nitrophenyl oxalates. Uses sodium hydroxide as a catalyst. Light emission ranges from quick burst or flash to light which remains for a longer time. Different types of instruments are required based on emission.

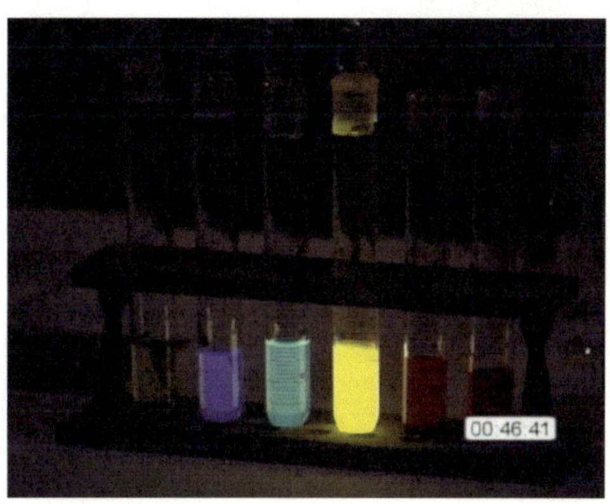

Fig. 8. Test colors in different samples

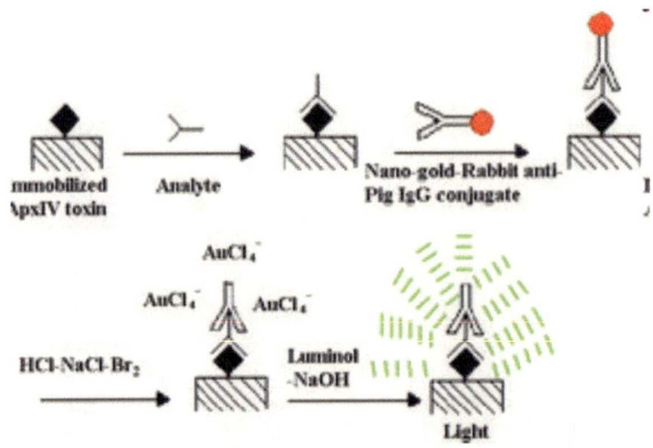

Fig. 9. Schematic diagram of chemi-luminescent Immunoassay.

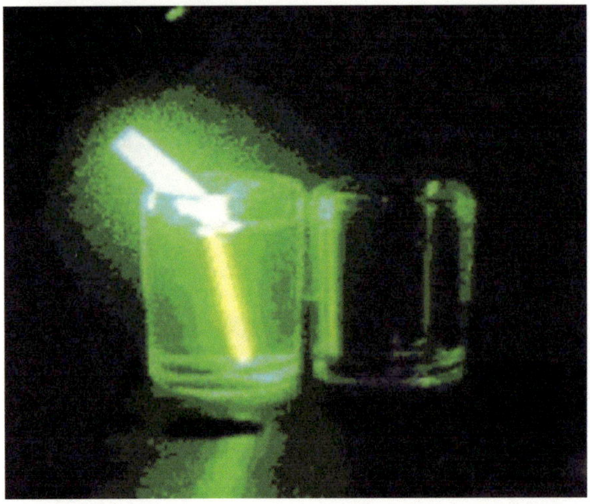

Fig. 10. Showing effect of fluorescein.

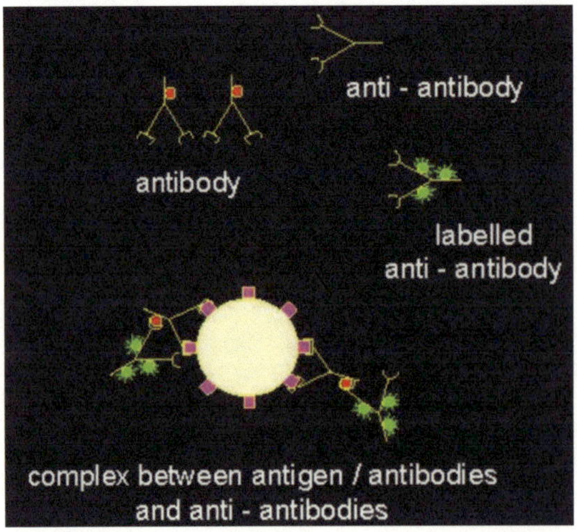

Fig. 11. Depicting antigen-antibody complex

4.2.5 Fluorescent Immunoassay

Two most commonly used markers that have ability to absorb energy and emit light are fluorescein - green and tetramethylrhodamine - red. In direct immunofluorescence, tagged antibody added to unknown antigen are fixed to the slide. If patient's antigen is present, then fluorescence is seen. Complex must form for fluorescence to occur.(Avrameas & Uriel, 1966).

4.2.6 Radioimmunassay (RIA)

Radioimmunoassay (RIA) involves the separation of a protein (from a mixture) using the specificity of antibody - antigen binding and quantitation using radioactivity. RIA was first described in 1960 for measurement of endogenous plasma insulin by Solomon Berson and Rosalyn Yalow of the Veterans Administration Hospital in New York (1). It is a sensitive technique used to measure small concentrations of antigens which is an example of competitive binding. Uses radioactive Iodine 125 (I^{125}) as label which competes with patient for sites. High radioactivity with small amount of patient's sample is required. Radioimmunoassay is widely-used because of its great sensitivity. Using antibodies of high affinity, it is possible to detect a few picograms (10^{-12} g) of antigen in the tube. (Catt & Tregear, 1967; Wide & Porath, 1966).

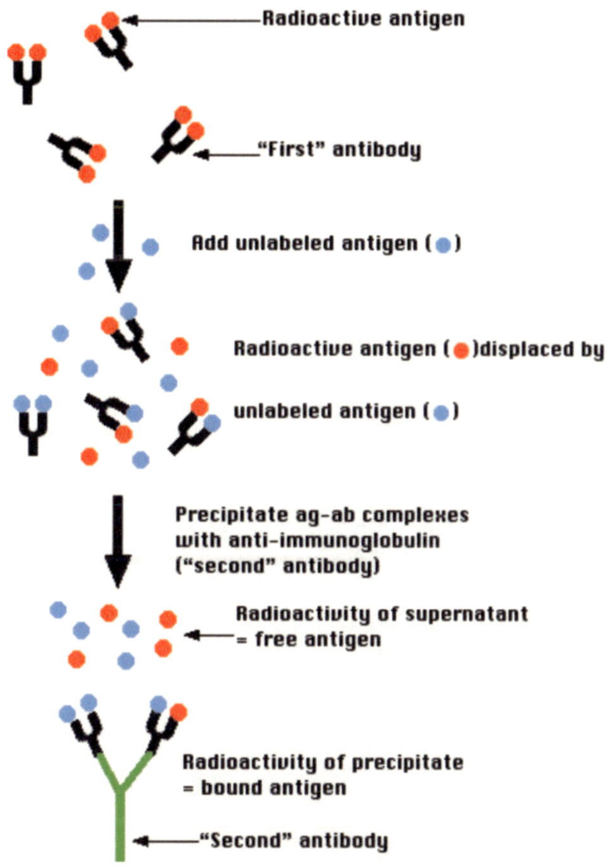

Fig. 12. Flow diagram of the process of radioimmunoassay.

The future of immunoassay lies in human toxicology, like hepatotoxicity, neurotoxicity and chemical carcinogenesis, drug discovery and food and water microbiology.

5. Conclusion

Transfusion practitioners following voluntary blood donors need to be aware of phenomena such as the 'high dose hook effect' or prozone effect, because it could give false reassurance to both the patient and the doctor. Future developments of serological assays should include monoclonal antibodies that recognize epidemiologically relevant surface antigen mutants with nucleic acid amplification techniques as an alternative to screening of blood donors, so as to reduce the false-negative results in commercial assays.

6. References

Anthony W. Butch.(2000). Dilution Protocols for Detection of Hook Effects/Prozone Phenomenon. *Clinical Chemistry*.46:1719-1720.

Avrameas S and Uriel J.(1966). Méthode de marquage d'antigènes et d'anticorps avec des enzymes et son application en immunodiffusion. *Acad Sci Hebd Seances Acad Sci* 262:2543-2545.

Bell, Suzanne (2006). Forensic Chemistry. Upper Saddle River, New Jersey: Pearson Prentice Hall.

Bishop M.L, Duben-Engelkirk JL, Fody P.(2001) Clinical Chemistry Principles, Procedures, Correlations. 4th ed. Lippincott, Williams, and Wilkins.

Bosch AMG, van Hell H, Brands JAM, van Weemen BK, Schuurs AHWM.(1975). Methods for the determination of total estrogens (TE) and human placental lactogen (HPL) in plasma of pregnant women by enzyme-immunoassay. *Clin Chem* 21:1009-1012.

Brensing AK, Dahlmann N, Entzian W, Bidlingmaier F, Klingmuler D.(1989). Underestimation of LH and FSH hormone concentrations in a patient with a gonadotropin secreting tumor: the high dose "hook effect" as a methodological and clinical problem. *Horm Metab Res* 21:697-698.

Burtis, C.A., and E. R. Ashwood.(2001). Tietz Fundamentals of Clinical Chemistry. 5th ed. Philadelphia: W.B. Saunders.

Catt K and Tregear GW. (1967).Solid-phase radioimmunoassay in antibody-coated tubes. *Science* 158:1570-1572.

Cole TG, Johnson D, Eveland BJ, Nahm MH.(1993). Cost-effective method for detection of "hook effect" in tumor marker immuometric assays. *Clin Chem* 39:695-696.

Cooper MD, Lawton AR. Disorders of the immune system.(1987). In: Braunwald E, Isselbacher KJ, Petersdorf RG, Wilson JD, Martin JB, Fauci AS, eds. Harrison's principles of internal medicine. New York: McGraw-Hill,1396–1403.

Engvall E and Perlmann P.(1971). Enzyme-linked immunosorbent assay (ELISA). Quantitative assay of immunoglobulin G. *Immunochemistry* 8:871-874.

Fernando SA and Wilson GS.(1992).Studies of the 'hook' effect in the one-step sandwich immunoassay. *Immunol Methods*.6;151:47-66.

Haller BL, Fuller KA, Brown WS, Koenig JW, Evelend BJ, Scott MG.(1992). Two automated prolactin immunoassays evaluated with demonstration of a high-dose "hook effect" in one. *Clin Chem* 38:437-438.

Henry, J. B.(2001). Clinical Diagnosis and Management by Laboratory Methods. 20th ed. Philadelphia: W. B. Saunders.

Jury DR, Mikkelsen DJ, Dunn PJ.(1990).Prozone effect and the turbidimetric measurement of albumin in urine. *Clin Chem* 36:1518-1519.

Landsteiner K.(1946).The specificity of serological reactions, Harvard University Press Cambridge, MA. 240-252.

Leboeuf R, Marie-France Langlois, Marc Martin, Charaf E. Ahnadi, Guy D. Fink.(2005)"Hook Effect" in Calcitonin Immunoradiometric Assay in Patients with Metastatic Medullary Thyroid Carcinoma: Case Report and Review of the Literature. *Annal Biochem*.65: 20-25.

Miles LEM, Hales CN.(1968). Labelled antibodies and immunological assay systems. *Nature* 219:186-189.

Miles LE, Lipschitz DA, Bieber CP, Cook JD.(1974). Measurement of serum ferritin by a 2-site immunoradiometric assay. *Anal Biochem* 61:209–224.

Moody, David E. (2006).Immunoassay in Forensic Toxicology. *Encyclopedia of Analytical Chemistry*.26,34-43.

Papik K, Molnar B, Fedorcsak P, Schaefer R, Lang F, Sreter L, et al.(1999).Automated prozone effect detection in ferritin homogeneous immunoassays using neural network classifiers. *Clin Chem Lab Med* 37:471-476.

Pesce MA.(1993). "High-dose hook effect" with the Centocar CA 125 assay. *Clin Chem* 39:1347-1351.

Petakov MS, Damjanovic SS, Nikolic-Durovic MM, Dragojlovic ZL, Obradovic S, Gilgorovic MS, et al.(1998). Pituitary adenomas secreting large amounts of prolactin may give false low values in immunoradiometric assays. The hook effect. *J Endocrinol Invest* 21:184-188

Porstmann T and Kiessig ST.(1992). Enzyme immunoassay techniques. An overview. *Immunol Methods* 24;150(1):5-21.

Quayle FJ and Moley JF(2005). Medullary thyroid carcinoma: including MEN 2A and MEN 2B syndromes. *J Surg Oncol 89*:122–129

Saryan JA, Garrett PE, Kurtz SR. (1989).Failure to detect extremely high levels of serum IgE with an immunoradiometric assay. *Ann Allergy* 63:322-324.

Schuurs AHWM, van Weemen BK.(1980). Enzyme-immunoassay: a powerful analytical too. *J Immunoassay* 1980;1:229-249.

Stites DP, Channing Rodgers RP, Folds JD.(1997).Clinical laboratory methods for detection of antigens and antibodies. In : Medical immunology 9th ed. Stites DP, Terr AI, Parslow TG (Eds.). Appleton and Lange, Connecticut. 211-253.

St-Jean, Blain F, Comtois R.(1996). High prolaction levels may be missed by immunoradiometric assay in patients with macroprolactinomas. *Clin Endocrinol*. 44: 305-309.

Unnikrishnan AG, Rajaratnam S, Seshadri MS, KanagasapabathyS, Stephen C.(2001) .The 'hook effect' on serum prolactin estimation in a patient with macroprolactinoma. *Neurol India*. 49:78-80.

Uotila M, Ruoslathi E, Envall E.(1981). Two-site sandwich enzyme immunoassay with monoclonal antibodies to human alphafetoprotein. *J Immunol Methods* 42:11-15.

Vaidya HC, Wolf BA, Garrett N, Catalona WJ, Clayman RV, Nahm H.(1988). Extremely high values of prostate-specific antigen in patients with adenocarcinoma of the prostate; demonstration of the "hook effect". *Clin Chem* 34:2175-2177.

Van Lente F. Light scattering immunoassays. Rose NR de Macario EC Folds JD Lane HC Nakamura RM. (1997). Manual of clinical laboratory immunology, 5th ed,ASM Press Washington, DC. pp 13-19.

Van Weemen BK, Schuurs AH.(1971). Immunoassay using antigen-enzyme conjugates. *FEBS Letts* 15:232-236.

Van der Waart M, Snelting A, Cichy J, Wolters G, Schuurs AHWM.(1978).Enzyme-immunoassay in diagnosis of hepatitis with emphasis on the detection of "e" antigen (HbeAg). *J Med Virol* 3:43-49

Wallach, Jacques.(2000). Interpretation of Diagnostic Tests. 7th ed. Philadelphia: Lippincott Williams & Wilkens, pp 34-45.

Wild, D. (2000). Immunoassay Handbook. 2nd ed. London: Nature Publishing Group. Zweig MH, Csako G.(1990). High-dose hook effect in a two site IRMA for measuring thyrotropin. *Ann Clin Biochem* 27:494-495.

Wide L and Porath J. (1966). Radioimmunoassay of proteins with the use of Sephadex-coupled antibodies. *Biochem Biophys Acta* 30:257-260.

Wolters G, Kuijpers LPC, Kacaki J, Schuurs AHWM. (1976).Enzyme-immunoassay for HbsAg. *Lancet* 2:690-692.

Wolf BA, Garret MC, Nahm MH. (1989).The hook effect : High concentrations of the prostrate specific antigen giving artefactually low values on one step immunoassay. *N Eng J Med* 320 : 1755-1756.

Yalow RS, Berson SA.(1960). Immunoassay of endogenous plasma insulin in man. Clin Invest 39:1157-1175.

Young EJ.(1995). Brucella species. In: Principles and practice of infectious disease (4th ed) . Churchill Livingstone, New York, 2053-2057.

2

Assays for Assessing the Compatibility of Therapeutic Proteins with Flexible Drug Containers

Shawn F. Bairstow and Sarah E. Lee
Baxter Healthcare Corporation, USA

1. Introduction

Biotherapeutics are among the fastest-growing segments of the pharmaceutical market. The packaging requirements for these therapeutics can be unique, primarily due to the multitude of factors that can influence the stability and overall potency of each particular therapeutic. Additionally, packaging has become a prominent concern in the healthcare industry due to the prevalence of medication errors, hospital acquired infections and potential for injury to the healthcare worker. The ability to provide these therapies in ready to use (RTU) containers would provide several advantages to both patients and clinicians: the RTU systems are closed containers, which minimize the risk of hospital-acquired infections; there are no reconstitution or admixture steps required, which minimize the risk of medication errors and healthcare worker exposure; and the RTU systems save time for the clinicians. However, the decision about drug formulation and packaging often needs to be made early in development when supplies of the drug are scarce.

Many of the biotherapeutics sold today are monoclonal antibodies. This circumstance lends itself well to the development of immunoassays for assessment of the activity of the particular therapeutic antibody. ELISA (enzyme-linked immunosorbent assay), also known as EIA (enzyme immunoassay), based assays are the most common approach for development of an immunoassay. This methodology has been extensively reviewed elsewhere (Wild 2001; Lequin 2005). These assays are usually performed in 96-well plates, but advances in automated liquid handling and spectrophotometric and fluorescent plate readers provide for formats as large as 1536 wells. The assays are typically structured in three basic formats, depending on the design of the assay. These include: 1) antibody capture assays, or solid-phase coated with antigen; 2) antigen capture assays, or solid phase coated with antibody; and 3) sandwich assays, which leverage an antibody pair, with one antibody coating the solid phase and the other binding the antigen in solution. The choice of assay format is primarily dictated by the analyte to be detected. In cases where the analyte is a small molecule that is either intrinsically fluorescent or has a distinct absorption spectrum, an antigen capture assay might be most applicable. Alternatively, if an antibody pair is available for an analyte, the sandwich ELISA is most commonly used. Since biotherapeutics are often antibodies themselves, this poses more of a challenge and usually an antibody capture assay is most appropriate.

Traditional ELISA/EIA assays are only a subset of potential immunoassay applications. These plate-based assays can also be leveraged in a competitive format, to allow for comparison of a standard to a test article directly in a binding reaction (as opposed to interpolation from the response curve of a known standard in a traditional ELISA). Competitive binding reactions can also be utilized in non-plate assay systems as well. Cell-based assays, using the same direct binding or competitive binding principles, can be used to assess the binding of antibodies or ligands to cell surface receptors. Often these assays provide a more physiological approach to the assessment of the bioactivity of the therapeutic. However, this technique usually requires chemical modification of the antibody or ligand to include a fluorescent tag or radioisotope for detection, as the traditional ELISA colorimetric signal generation via horseradish peroxidase (HRP) is usually not feasible with these types of assays. Alternative signal generation methods have been developed, such as electrochemiluminescence detection (Meso Scale Discovery), which provides a much greater dynamic range and sensitivity compared to HRP based signals (Zhao *et al.* 2004). Fluorescent bead-based technologies, such as those developed by Luminex and PerkinElmer's AlphaScreen® are also alternatives to standard solid phase ELISAs (Kellar *et al.* 2006; Eglen *et al.* 2008). These are analogous to ELISA sandwich assays, but use suspended beads as the solid phase in the assay, rather than the plate surface. A caveat to bead-based assays and electrochemiluminescence, however, is the requirement for specialized equipment to perform the detection step. Nevertheless, there are multiple approaches and assay formats that can be used in developing an immunoassay for the characterization of a specific biotherapeutic.

This study focuses on the development and use of biological assays for assessing the compatibility of therapeutic proteins with flexible drug containers, including the development of in-house immunoassays for two therapeutic antibodies, cetuximab and rituximab. Cetuximab (marketed under the trade name Erbitux®) is a humanized chimeric mouse monoclonal antibody directed against the epidermal growth factor receptor (EGFR). It was approved by the United States Food and Drug Administration (FDA) for the treatment of metastatic colorectal cancer in 2004, and also has indications for the treatment of head and neck squamous cell carcinomas. Binding of cetuximab to the soluble extracellular portion of EGFR (sEGFR) has been previously demonstrated *in vitro* and the crystal for the centuximab-sEGFR complex has been solved (Li *et al.* 2005). Additionally, it has recently been shown that cetuximab is ineffective in patients with K-ras mutations, providing an effective screening tool for oncology patients (Ramos *et al.* 2008). Rituximab (marketed under the trade name Rituxan®) is also a humanized chimeric mouse monoclonal antibody, but it is directed against the CD20 cell surface protein. CD20 is a transmembrane phosphoprotein expressed on the surface of the B-cells of the immune system (Perosa *et al.* 2005). Rituximab is used medicinally for the treatment of non-Hodgkin's lymphomas (i.e. various B-cell leukemias and lymphomas) (Sacchi *et al.* 2001).

Both of these antibodies are used prevalently in their respective oncology settings, and therefore were good candidates to evaluate as model proteins. Here we present data from the development of two immunoassays along with the subsequent use of the immunoassays to support a full protein-container compatibility study.

2. Materials and methods

2.1 Cetuximab immunoassay

A recombinantly expressed sEGFR domain is commercially available (Fitzgerald Industries International) and we developed an antibody capture ELISA using this domain. Microtiter plates (Costar® high-bind 8-well strips) were coated overnight at 4 °C with 100 µL/well of 1 µg/mL sEGFR reconstituted in 200 mM Na_2CO_3, pH 9.6. The coating solution was subsequently discarded and the plate was washed once with PBS-T (Phosphate Buffered Saline with 0.5% Tween® 20). The plates were then blocked with 200 µL/well of PBS-1% BSA (bovine serum albumin), sealed and stored at 4 °C until use. BSA only control plates were prepared by blocking uncoated plate strips with PBS-1% BSA as above. The required number of plate strips were removed from storage at 4 °C and allowed to reach room temperature prior to use. Dilutions of cetuximab (from the 2 mg/mL formulation concentration) were prepared in a range of 1:10-1:4096000 by serial dilution with PBS-0.5% BSA. The plate strips were washed three times with PBS-T. The dilutions were then added to the strips, in duplicate or triplicate, at 100 µL/well. The strips were then sealed and incubated at room temperature for one hour. During the incubation, a 1:5000 dilution of goat anti-human IgG-HRP secondary antibody (Sigma) was prepared in PBS-0.5% BSA by serial dilution. The strips were then washed three times with PBS-T and 100 µL/well of 1:5000 secondary antibody was added. The strips were sealed and incubated for 1 hr at room temperature. The o-Phenylenediamine (OPD) substrate (Sigma) was then prepared by adding one OPD tablet and one buffer tablet to 20 mL of water. The strips were washed three times with PBS-T and 100 or 200 µL/well of OPD substrate was added. The strips were incubated 10 min at room temperature and the reaction was quenched with 50 µL/well of 1M H_2SO_4. The plate was then read on a plate reader at 490 nm. The cetuximab standard curves were fit using a four parameter nonlinear regression model.

Competition reactions using unbound sEGFR were also performed. A standard curve was prepared using serial dilutions of cetuximab ranging from 1:5000-1:320000 in PBS-0.5% BSA. A vial of lyophilized sEGFR (25 µg) was reconstituted at 100 ng/mL with water. Additional sEGFR stocks were prepared by serial dilution with PBS over a range of 20-0.0064 ng/µL. Competition reactions were prepared by combining 10 µL of sEGFR with 90 µL of cetuximab (diluted 1:50000 with PBS-0.5% BSA) for each concentration of sEGFR tested. The reactions were incubated for 10 min at room temperature. The entire volume of each reaction and the cetuximab standards were then used in the cetuximab ELISA procedure described above.

2.2 Rituximab immunoassay

Rituximab was labeled with fluorescein isothiocyanate (FITC; Sigma). Rituximab (0.7 mL @ ~2.8 mg/mL) was labeled with 20 µL of 10 mg/mL FITC at room temperature for 2.25 hrs. The free FITC was removed via gel filtration with an EconoPac DG10 (BioRad) using Tris Buffered Saline (TBS) as the mobile phase. The pooled antibody had a concentration of 1.22 mg/mL with an F/P ratio of 10.4. Rituximab was diluted serially with PBS-1% FBS (fetal bovine serum) to generate various dilutions. A 1:5000 stock of fluorescein labeled rituximab (FITC-rituximab) was prepared by serial dilution with PBS-1% FBS (fetal bovine serum) for the competition assay. Whole blood was drawn from the same donor in heparin-coated vacutainers (BD) prior to each experiment. The competition experiments for each dilution of unlabeled rituximab were then prepared by combining 100 µL of whole blood with 10 µL of diluted unlabeled rituximab and 20 µL of diluted FITC-Rituximab. The reactions were vortexed and incubated at room temperature for 30 min in the dark. All reactions were vortexed again after the incubation and 2 mL of 1x lysis solution (BD) was added to each tube. The reactions were then incubated for 15 min at room temperature in the dark and spun down for 5 min at 3550 RPM. The supernatants were decanted and the cell pellets were washed with 2 mL of PBS-1% FBS. After spinning down the cells again as above, the supernatants were decanted and the cells were resuspended in 500 µL of PBS-1% FBS prior to analysis by flow cytometry on a BD FACScan cytometer. A forward-scatter and side-scatter gate was established to isolate the lymphocyte population, and the mean fluorescent intensity value for this gate was calculated for each competition reaction. A standard curve was generated by serial dilution of a control rituximab sample in the competition reaction described above. The resulting standard curve was then used to interpolate the effective concentration value of the rituximab test samples.

2.3 Assessment of flexible container compatibility

Flexible film pouches were constructed using plastic film material and filled with 2 mL of antibody solution (cetuximab was formulated at 2 mg/mL and rituximab was formulated at 10 mg/mL). Glass vials were also filled in the same manner to serve as controls. The containers were sealed in a laminar flow hood, using a bench-top impulse sealer for the pouches. After filling, the units were stored at the temperatures listed in Tables 2 and 3. Samples were removed from storage at the time points indicated and the contents of the pouches were analyzed. This analysis included standard physical and chemical testing, and running a bioassay to determine the activity of the protein (as described above for cetuximab and rituximab).

Container	Testing Schedule				
	Temp. (°C)	2 week	4 week	8 week	16 week
Film 1	5			X	2X
	25		X	X	X
	40	X	X	X	X
Film 2	5			X	2X
	25		X	X	X
	40	X	X	X	X
Glass Control	5			X	2X
	25		X	X	X
	40	X	X	X	X

Table 1. Testing Matrix for Cetuximab Samples

		Testing Schedule					
Container	Temp. (°C)	0 days	3 days	1 week	2 weeks	4 weeks	8 weeks
Film 1	5	X			X	X	X
	25			X	X	X	X
	40		X	X	X	X	
Film 2	5	X			X	X	X
	25			X	X	X	X
	40		X	X	X	X	
Film 3	5	X			X	X	X
	25			X	X	X	X
	40		X	X	X	X	
Film 4	5	X			X	X	X
	25			X	X	X	X
	40		X	X	X	X	
Glass Control	5	X				X	X

Table 2. Testing Matrix for Rituximab Samples

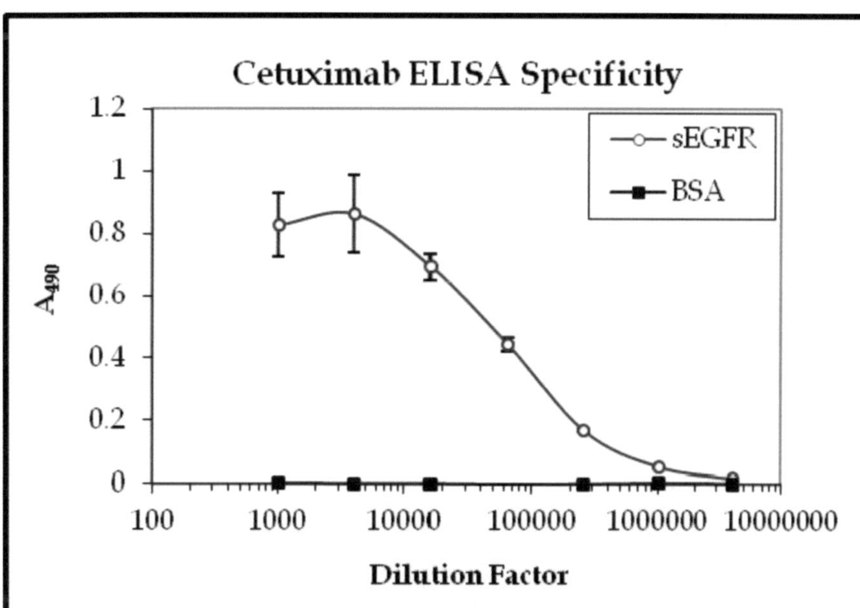

Fig. 1. Specificity of the cetuximab for sEGFR versus BSA

3. Results and discussion

3.1 Cetuximab immunoassay development

An immunoassay was developed for cetuximab, using commercially available sEGFR as the bound antigen for antibody capture. As shown in Figure 1, cetuximab has a specific response to sEGFR-coated strips with minimal background binding to BSA-only coated strips. A typical sigmoidal response was observed over a dilution range of 1:1000-1:4096000 of cetuximab.

The precision of the cetuximab ELISA was then examined over three independent experiments. Quadruplicate 1:50000 cetuximab dilutions (serially diluted with PBS-0.5% BSA) were prepared and analyzed in each experiment. The dilutions of the cetuximab standards were also varied across these experiments to determine the optimal range of concentrations for maximum linear response. All standards were run in triplicate and all test samples (1:50000 replicate dilutions) were run in duplicate. The optimal range for the cetuximab standard curve was ~1:5000-1:2000000 (typical standard curve is shown in Figure 2). The standards also had well-to-well CVs < 15% in all three experiments. The cetuximab standard curves were fit as described in the procedure and the concentrations were calculated for the 1:50000 diluted samples. The intraexperimental replicate variance (%CV) for the quadruplicate 1:50000 dilutions ranged from 8.6-12.8%. Additionally, the interexperimental variance (%CV) for the average calculated concentration for the 1:50000 diluted cetuximab samples from the three experiments was 14.2%. The average concentration across the three experiments, 39.6 ng/mL, was very near the expected value of 40 ng/mL for a 1:50000 dilution of the neat cetuximab formulated at 2 mg/mL.

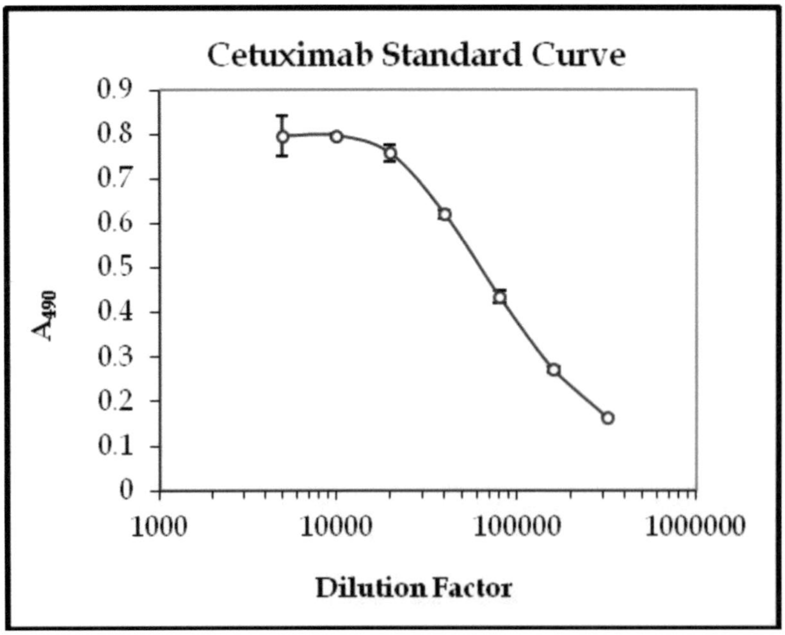

Fig. 2. Typical cetuximab standard curve for the sEGFR based ELISA

A competition experiment was also performed using free sEGFR in the ELISA assay as described in the Materials and Methods section. As shown in Figure 3, the percentage of cetuximab bound dropped to less than 5% with 10 ng/µL of free sEGFR and the observed IC_{50} was between 1-2 ng/µL or 12.5-25 nM. This result is comparable to the published Kd of 2.3 ± 0.5 nM for cetuximab binding to sEGFR via Biacore (Li *et al.* 2005).

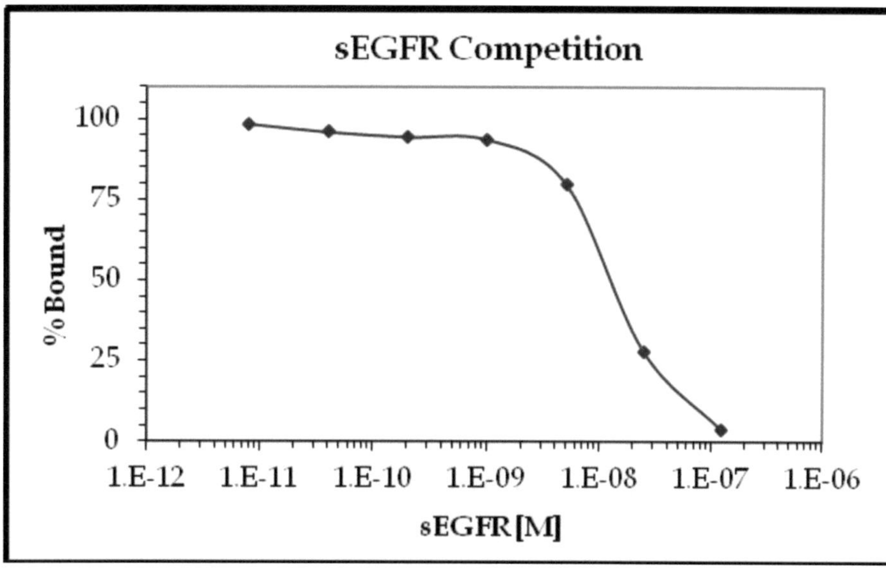

Fig. 3. Competition experiment using sEGFR titrated into the sEGFR ELISA

Cetuximab had a consistent response towards sEGFR in this ELISA based assay with minimal background binding to BSA. Across three independent experiments, the intraexperimental and interexperimental CVs were all < 15%, which is typical for most ELISA based assays. Additionally, free sEGFR was able to completely inhibit binding to the sEGFR coated plates and the observed Kd for sEGFR was similar to published results. Overall, the assay appeared to be adequate to serve as a bioassay for cetuximab.

3.2 Cetuximab container compatibility

Test articles were prepared consisting of pouches made of plastic films filled with cetuximab protein formulation (2 mL fill at 2 mg/mL). Additionally, glass vials were filled with cetuximab (2 mL fill) to serve as controls. The sampling time points and incubation conditions are summarized in Table 1.

The binding activity of cetuximab was monitored over the course of the study using the ELISA assay described here. The results are shown in Figures 4A-C, where the error bars represent plus or minus one standard deviation from the mean of triplicate assays of a single sample. The glass controls were used to normalize the ELISA data and these results were all well within the range of the assay variance (<15% CV). The physical and chemical test data (S. E. Lee, *et al.*, in preparation) showed that cetuximab solution held in plastic containers behaved similarly to cetuximab solution held in glass vials. These data suggest that cetuximab solution is compatible with both Film 1 as well as Film 2.

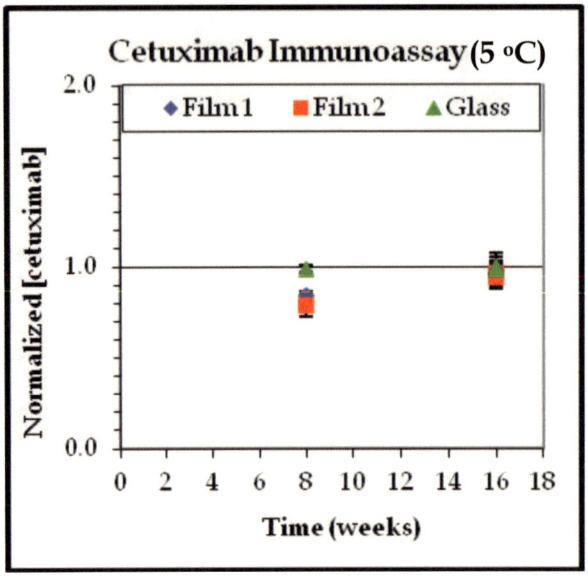

Fig. 4A. Immunoassay results for the various cetuximab test articles at 5 °C

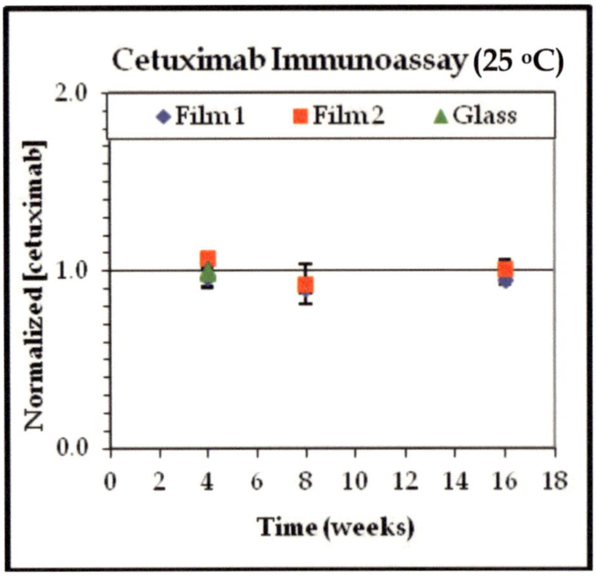

Fig. 4B. Immunoassay results for the various cetuximab test articles at 25 °C

3.3 Rituximab immunoassay development

Since CD20 extracellular domain was not commercially available for the development of an ELISA-based assay, a cell-based immunoassay was developed to evaluate the binding of rituximab to the CD20 cell surface receptor on B-cells. This assay format has the advantage of observing the direct binding of rituximab to the CD20 receptors on B-cells in the more physiological context of whole blood (as compared to ELISA-based approaches). Whole blood

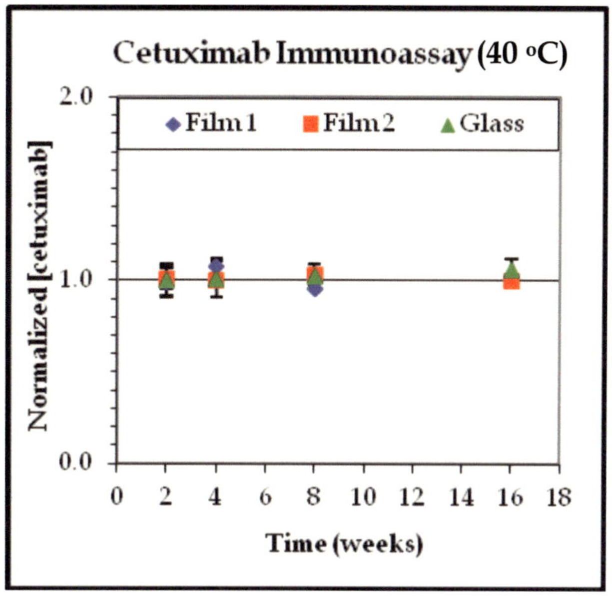

Fig. 4C. Immunoassay results for the various cetuximab test articles at 40 °C

was drawn from the same single donor at each time point throughout the study to serve as the source of B-cells. A competitive assay format was utilized for the immunoassay by titrating an unlabeled rituximab antibody standard against a constant concentration of FITC-labeled rituximab. A typical competitive response curve is shown in Figure 5, using a 1:5000 dilution of the FITC-rituximab. At each testing time point (as described in Table 2) a competitive standard curve was established based on the observed mean fluorescence intensity (MFI) for each dilution of the rituximab standard. The test articles were each diluted 1:2000 (to fall approximately at the midpoint of the standard curve) and the observed MFI value for each test article was used to interpolate a concentration value relative to the rituximab standard.

3.4 Rituximab container compatibility

To generate the samples for this study, rituximab solution was pipetted into pouches made from four different flexible films and then the pouches were sealed using a heat sealer. Care was taken to avoid dripping protein solution into the area where the final seal was formed. The sealed pouches were incubated at either 5 °C, 25 °C, or 40 °C, as indicated in Table 2. Glass controls were maintained at 5 °C for the duration of the study. Samples were removed from storage and the contents of the pouches were analyzed to determine the physical and chemical stability of the formulation and running an immunoassay to determine the activity of the protein.

Rituximab binding activity was assayed using the whole blood competitive binding immunoassay described here. The data shown here have been corrected using the apparent protein concentrations determined from SEC-MALLS data (S. E. Lee, *et al.*, in preparation). These data indicate that there is little decrease in binding activity over the course of the study and that there is no significant differentiation among the four film types tested in this study (Figures 6A-C). There was day-to-day variation in the normalized concentrations of the test samples, which is likely inherent to the competition assay used. At most time points,

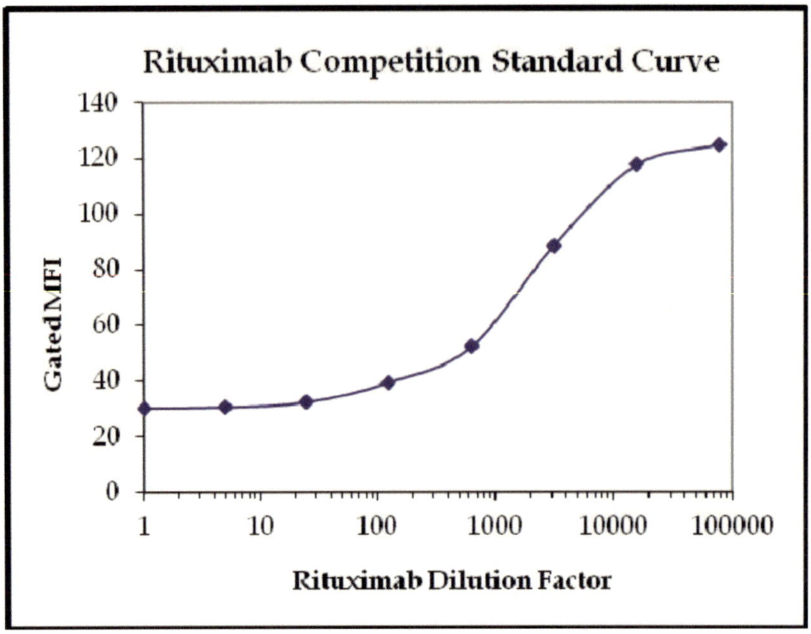

Fig. 5. Typical standard curve for the rituximab competitive cell binding immunoassay

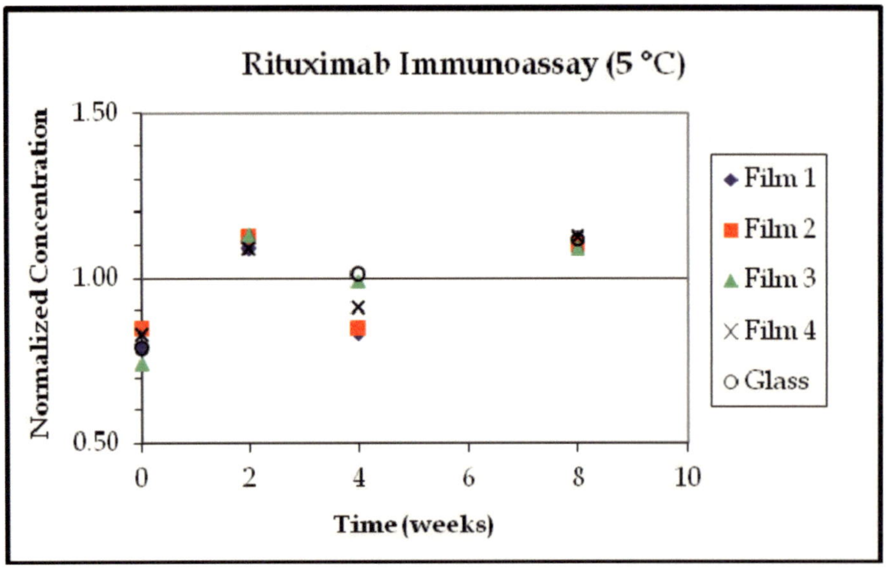

Fig. 6A. Immunoassay results for rituximab test articles at 5 °C (results normalized to the 5 °C glass controls)

all films were clustered in terms of effective concentration and the average effective concentration varied approximately ± 10% from normal for the 5 °C and 25 °C storage conditions. This was not the case for the 40 °C storage condition, as other samples from the same testing interval had higher effective concentrations. These data indicate a slight downward trend in bioactivity in the samples stored at 40 °C for 4 weeks.

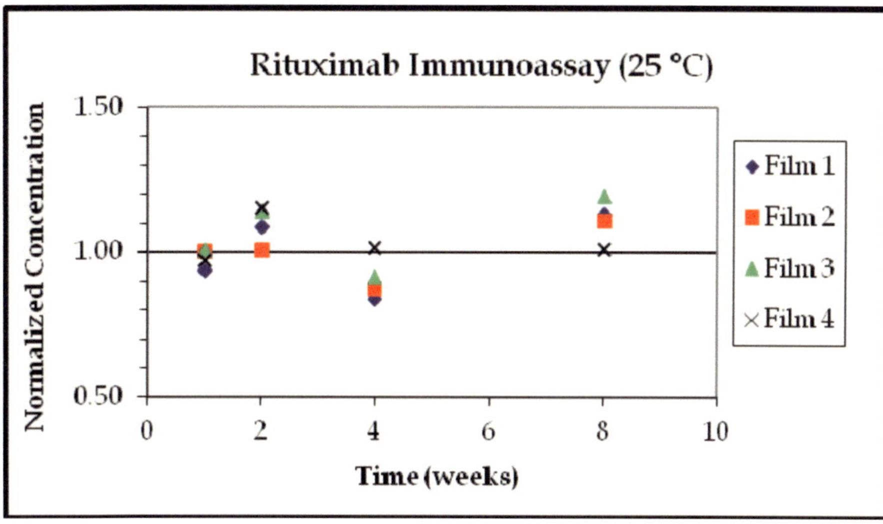

Fig. 6B. Immunoassay results for rituximab test articles at 25 °C (results normalized to the 5 °C glass controls)

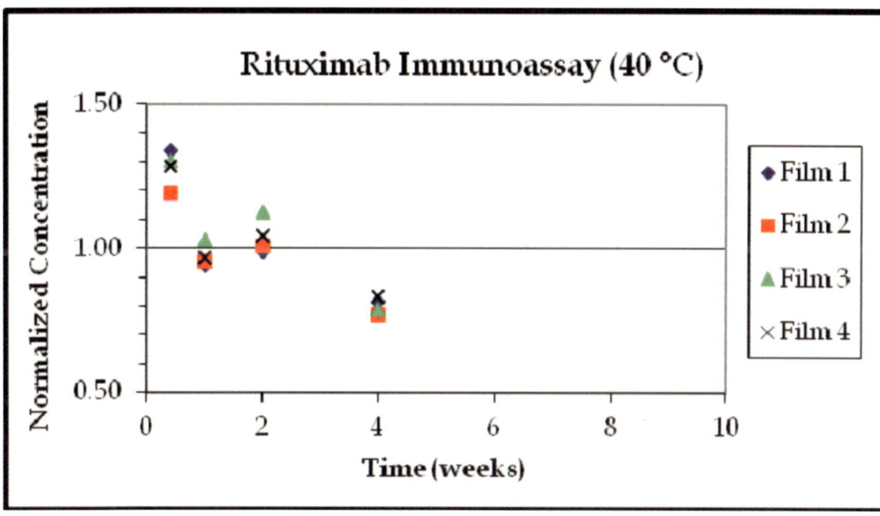

Fig. 6C. Immunoassay results for rituximab test articles at 40 °C (results normalized to the 5 °C glass controls)

The results of this study show that Rituximab solution is compatible with all four film types tested. Bioactivity assays confirm that the protein behaves similarly in all four film types over the course of the study, despite a slight decrease in activity upon storage for 4 weeks at 40 °C.

4. Conclusion

The primary aim of this study was to develop and implement protein-specific immunoassays to support the evaluation of the compatibility of two protein biotherapeutics with plastic RTU prototype containers. Here we have demonstrated, through the use of in-house developed immunoassays and standard chemical and chromatographic techniques, that flexible plastic containers can have equivalent performance to standard glass vials. This observation was true both in terms of the observed binding activities and the physical and chemical data collected (S. E. Lee, *et al.*, in preparation) for the two monoclonal antibodies tested, cetuximab and rituximab. Establishing this compatibility is essential to enabling a shift to this type of container system in the healthcare sector. Flexible plastic RTU containers provide a more convenient format for dosing to the patient, they can reduce medication errors by providing a ready to infuse format and also pose a lower risk of injury to both healthcare workers and patients. As the number of commercialized biotherapeutics increases, the need for these types of container systems becomes readily apparent. The methodology used in these studies can be used as a guideline for compatibility evaluations of other types of therapeutic proteins. As more types of biotherapeutic products make their way to market, there will be an increasing need for biological assays to assess their potency. The work described here illustrates the importance of using specifically tailored immunoassays to assess the activity of biotherapeutics selected for use as model proteins.

5. Acknowledgment

The authors would like to acknowledge Matthew Fonk for his assistance with sample pouch fabrication.

6. References

Eglen, R. M., T. Reisine, P. Roby, N. Rouleau, C. Illy, R. Bosse and M. Bielefeld (2008) The use of AlphaScreen technology in HTS: current status. *Curr Chem Genomics*. 1, 2-10.

Kellar, K. L., A. J. Mahmutovic and K. Bandyopadhyay (2006) Multiplexed microsphere-based flow cytometric immunoassays. *Curr Protoc Cytom*. Chapter 13, Unit13 1.

Lequin, R. M. (2005) Enzyme immunoassay (EIA)/enzyme-linked immunosorbent assay (ELISA). *Clin Chem*. 51, 2415-8.

Lee, S. E., Bairstow, S. F., Chaubal, M. V. (in preparation) Compatibility of Therapeutic Proteins with Flexible Containers.

Li, S., K. R. Schmitz, P. D. Jeffrey, J. J. Wiltzius, P. Kussie and K. M. Ferguson (2005) Structural basis for inhibition of the epidermal growth factor receptor by cetuximab. *Cancer Cell*. 7, 301-11.

Perosa, F., E. Favoino, M. A. Caragnano, M. Prete and F. Dammacco (2005) CD20: A target antigen for immunotherapy of autoimmune diseases. *Autoimmunity Reviews*. 4, 526-531.

Ramos, F. J., T. Macarulla, J. Capdevila, E. Elez and J. Tabernero (2008) Understanding the predictive role of K-ras for epidermal growth factor receptor-targeted therapies in colorectal cancer. *Clin Colorectal Cancer*. 7 Suppl 2, S52-7.

Sacchi, S., M. Federico, G. Dastoli, C. Fiorani, G. Vinci, V. Clo and B. Casolari (2001) Treatment of B-cell non-Hodgkin's lymphoma with anti CD 20 monoclonal antibody Rituximab. *Crit Rev Oncol Hematol*. 37, 13-25.

Wild, D. (2001) *The Immunoassay handbook*, 2nd ed., Nature Pub. Group, London

Zhao, X., T. You, H. Qiu, J. Yan, X. Yang and E. Wang (2004) Electrochemiluminescence detection with integrated indium tin oxide electrode on electrophoretic microchip for direct bioanalysis of lincomycin in the urine. *J Chromatogr B Analyt Technol Biomed Life Sci*. 810, 137-42.

3

Evaluation of an Immuno-Chromatographic Detection System for Shiga Toxins and the *E. coli* O157 Antigen

Ylanna Burgos and Lothar Beutin*
National Reference Laboratory for Escherichia coli, Unit 41: Microbial Toxins, Federal Institute for Risk Assessment (Bundesinstitut für Riskobewertung BfR), Berlin, Germany

1. Introduction

The production of Shiga toxins (Verotoxins) is a characteristic trait of some strains of *Escherichia coli*. Shiga toxin-producing *Escherichia coli* (STEC), also called Verotoxin-producing *E. coli* (VTEC), were first described by Konowalchuk et al. in 1977 by their cytotoxic activity on African green monkey kidney (Vero) cells (Konowalchuk et al. 1977). STEC of serotype O157:H7 were linked to cases of Haemorrhagic Colitis (HC) and to the consumption of STEC- contaminated meat of bovine origin for the first time in 1982 (Karmali et al. 2010; Riley et al. 1983). Since 1982, hundreds of outbreaks of disease caused by STEC O157 and non-O157 strains have been reported in different countries and geographical regions of the world. A growing number of genetic variants of Shiga toxins 1 + 2 (Stx1 and Stx2) were identified and today more than 400 serotypes of *E. coli* strains isolated from human patients were found associated with Stx production (Scheutz and Strockbine 2005).

Some STEC serogroups such as O157, O26, O103, O111 and O145 were most frequently associated with outbreaks and with Haemorrhagic Colitis and Haemolytic Uraemic Syndrome (HUS) in human patients worldwide. Accordingly, these strains were designated as Enterohaemorrhagic *E. coli* (EHEC) (Nataro and Kaper 1998). Classical EHEC belonging to these serotypes are responsible for more than 80% of HUS cases in Europe and in the United States (Brooks et al. 2005; Eblen 2007; EFSA 2007; Karmali et al. 2003). As EHEC O157 was reported to be the most frequent and virulent EHEC type a number of diagnostic tools (indicator media, O157 antigen detection kits, specific O157 enrichment media and O157-specific PCRs) have been developed for its specific identification (Frank et al. 2011). However, the recent outbreak of Enteroaggregative Haemorrhagic *E. coli* (EAHEC) *E. coli* O104:H4 in Germany indicates that serotypes other than O157 can suddenly become the most highly virulent human pathogens (Frank et al. 2011).

Healthy dairy and beef cattle are recognized as a major natural reservoir of EHEC and other STEC strains. There are more than 100 serotypes of STEC which have been also isolated

* Corresponding Author

from other animals such as sheep, pigs, goats, deer, horses, dogs and birds (Gyles 2007). Humans become infected most frequently by consuming STEC-contaminated food of different kinds, but also waterborne infections and the direct transmission from STEC-excreting animals or humans are frequent (Caprioli et al. 2005). By contrast, humans but not animals were identified as the reservoir for the newly emerging EAHEC O104:H4 strain (ECDC et al. 2011). Studies have shown that STEC infections are more frequent in the warmer months and that the serotypes that are implicated may vary from country to country (Beutin 2006; Gyles 2007).

2. Genetic and functional diversity of Shiga toxins

The Shiga toxin family consists of two major groups, Shiga toxin 1 (Stx1) and Shiga toxin 2 (Stx2). Shiga toxins are composed of two subunits. The active toxin subunit A (N-glycosidase 32-KDa) is linked to five B-subunits as a pentamer (7.7-kDa monomers). The toxin subunit B is responsible for binding the toxin to GB3 or GB4 receptors on the eukaryotic cells. Stx1 and Stx2 are immunologically not cross-reactive and show themselves to be 55% different in their amino acid sequences (Muthing et al. 2009). A number of genetic variants were identified within the Stx1 and the Stx2 toxin families (Burk et al. 2003; Leung et al. 2003; Muthing et al. 2009). The variants differ in the amino-acid substitutions in their StxA and StxB subunits, which can have an influence on their toxicity and receptor-binding specificity (Muthing et al. 2009). The Stx1 group has been divided into the subtypes Stx1, Stx1a, Stx1c and Stx1d (Burk et al. 2003) (Figure 1).

Stx1 is produced by some species of *Shigella* (Scheutz and Strockbine 2005). Stx1a is frequently found in STEC from cattle and in food of bovine origin (Martin and Beutin 2011) and it is found in major EHEC strains causing HC and HUS in humans. Stx1c was found to be associated with non-bloody diarrhoea in humans and is frequent in STEC from goats, sheep and red deer (Friedrich et al. 2003; Martin and Beutin 2011).

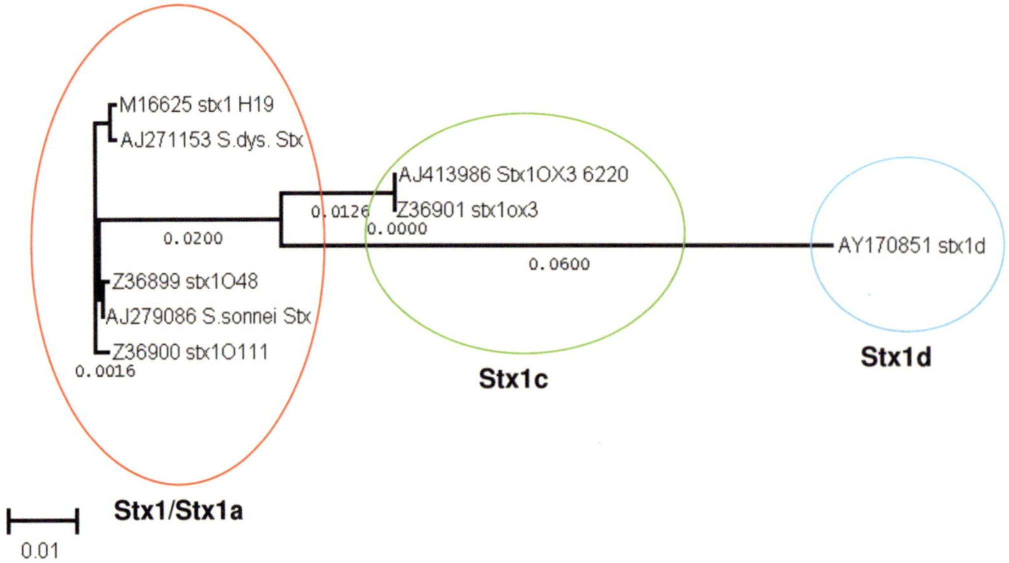

Fig. 1. Genetic distances within the group of Stx1 family toxins

The Stx2 branch splits into the subgroups Stx2a, Stx2b, Stx2c, Stx2d, Stx2e, Stx2f and Stx2g (Persson et al. 2007) (Figure 2).

The infection of humans with STEC-producing toxin variants Stx2a, Stx2c and Stx2d-(activatable) was associated with an increased risk of developing HC and HUS, while STEC-producing Stx1c, Stx2b and Stx2f were found to be more associated with uncomplicated cases of diarrhoea or with asymptomatic infections (Friedrich et al. 2002; Persson et al. 2007). Stx1d- and Stx2g-producing STEC have been isolated from animals and food but the possible role of these toxins in human disease needs to be confirmed (Beutin et al. 2007a; Kuczius et al. 2004; Miko et al. 2009). Humans are rarely infected with Stx2e-producing strains (Friedrich et al. 2002). STEC-producing Stx2e are linked to pigs as a hosts and are agents of oedema disease in pigs. Aside from Stx2e, these strains frequently produce heat-stable and heat-labile enterotoxins and Stx2e has not been shown to play a role as a virulence marker for humans (Beutin et al. 2008).

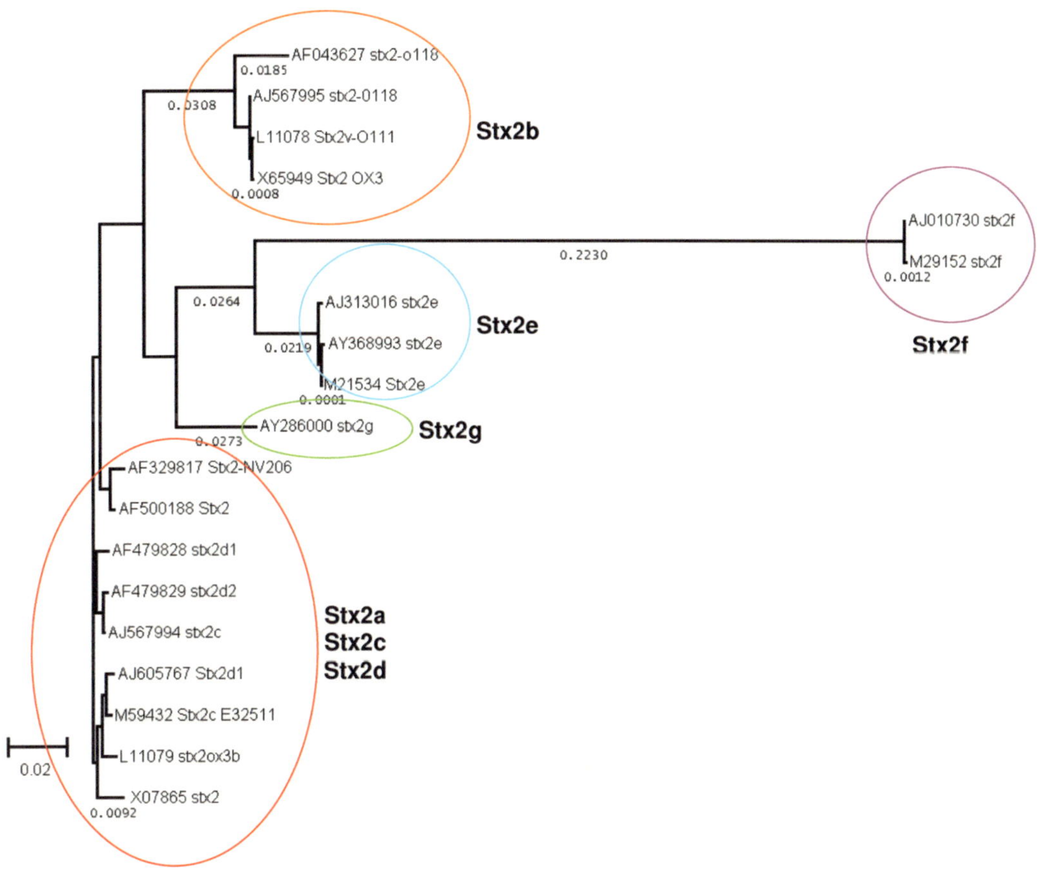

Fig. 2. Genetic distances within the group of Stx2 family toxins

The Shiga toxin genes are encoded by lambdoid bacteriophages which are integrated into the bacterial chromosome by lysogenization where they remain present as prophages (Schmidt 2001). Some kinds of physico-chemical stress can trigger a cascade reaction called bacterial "SOS response" leading to the transcription of the prophage genome, resulting in the production of both Shiga toxins and phage particles. The release of phages by bacterial lysis leads to the infection of new *E.coli* hosts and the generation of new STEC strains (Herold et al. 2004).

3. Diagnosis of STEC by detection of Shiga toxins

A number of indicator media for the identification of some STEC strains and types have been developed, as well as immunological, genetic and cell culture toxicity assays for Stx-detection. The detection of Shiga toxins is the only way to identify all members of the STEC group which consists of strains with different phenotypes and serotypes (Bettelheim and Beutin 2003). The Vero cell toxicity assay (VCA) is used as a gold standard for detection of Stx production as it is the most sensitive. However, its specificity must be confirmed in neutralization assays with antisera directed against Stx. As the VCA is laborious, time-consuming and demands a specifically designed laboratory and specially trained personnel there is a need for STEC detection systems which are rapid, reliable, standardized and easy to employ. Almost all STEC testing methods screen for Stx production with commercial serological assays or the presence of *stx*-genes is detected using PCR or DNA-hybridization assays (Paton and Paton 2003).

Some STEC strains that were identified by *stx*-specific PCR failed to show serological reactivity in immunological detection systems for Stx (Beutin et al. 2007; Beutin et al. 2008). The lack of an Stx phenotype (serologically or cytotoxic) in a strain that tests positive when using *stx*-specific PCR may have several causes such as defective *stx*-genes, the absence of Stx expression, or the amount of Stx produced being below the detectable level of the given serological or cytological assay. Commercially-obtainable serological assays (EIA, RPLA) for Stx were found to vary greatly in their sensitivity (Bettelheim and Beutin 2003; Beutin et al. 2007; Beutin et al. 2010; Beutin et al. 1996; Beutin et al. 2002; Beutin et al. 2008; Feng et al. 2011; Jahn et al. 2008; Willford et al. 2009), and some STEC strains were found to produce low amounts of Stx, that were not detectable by tissue culture or serological tests. Previous work showed that about 1% of strains that carry *stx*-genes showed no production of Stx in the VCA as a gold standard (Beutin et al. 2007). A lack of Stx expression or low expression was found to be more frequent among certain *stx*-subtypes such as stx_{2b}, stx_{2e} and stx_{2g} (Beutin et al. 2007; Beutin et al. 2007a; Beutin et al. 2008). Another possible cause of these discrepancies between the presence of *stx*-genes and the absence of Stx production may be caused by the specificity of anti-Stx antibodies or *stx* PCR primers used for the identification of the various Stx subtypes (Feng et al. 2011).

Efforts to find reliable, specific and rapid methods for the detection of STEC have been increased over the last decades. Media containing inducing agents such as mTSB with Mitomycin C were used to trigger Stx production by bacteria for detection (Beutin et al. 2008; Klie et al. 1997; Shimizu et al. 2009). Some antibiotics such as trimethoprim-sulfamethoxazole and ciprofloxacin were found to enhance Stx production by bacteria and may increase the risk of HUS when used as therapeutic agents in human infections with STEC (McGannon et al. 2010; Wong et al. 2000).

The detection of STEC can cause problems if food or clinical, animal and environmental samples that contain a mixture of different microorganisms are examined. Specific enrichment media are used for the recovery of injured STEC strains, which are often present in food and environmental samples. The bacteria may be stressed during the processing and storage of food. The enrichment procedure provides an optimal growth medium and a period of time that can be effectively used, allowing the resuscitation of the bacterial cells (Hussein and Bollinger 2008). The detection of stressed STEC from samples depends largely on the choice of the cultivation media and conditions. Non-selective media such as buffered peptone water were found to be advantageous for the resuscitation of damaged STEC from various samples (Hussein and Bollinger 2008; Jahn and Beutin 2009).

Stx detection kits such as enzyme-linked immunoassays (EIA) have been commercialized and are widely used as standardized assays in diagnostic laboratories. The evaluation of commercially available diagnostic test kits for Stx by *E. coli* reference laboratories has been shown to be valuable for the assessment of their specificity and sensitivity. In this work, we have evaluated an immuno-chromatographic lateral flow test for the detection of Shiga toxins and the *E. coli* O157 antigen which recently came on the market.

4. Principle of the immuno-chromatographic lateral flow test system and test procedure

The introduction of immuno-chromatographic lateral flow test systems has made Stx detection even quicker and simpler to perform than with the classical ELISA test. A specific photometer (ELISA-reader) is not necessary and the results are recorded by eye after 15 minutes. A new development allowing the simultaneous detection of Stx-production and of the O157 antigen (as the most important EHEC type) is the commercially available "RIDA Quick" test (RIDA® QUICK Verotoxin/O157 Combi, R-biopharm AG, Darmstadt, Germany).

The assay is bound to a plastic stick which is introduced with its absorbent end into the liquid sample containing Stx and O157 LPS as antigens. The principle of this assay is a single-step immuno-chromatographic lateral-flow test, where specific antibodies directed towards both target antigens are attached to red (Shiga toxin-specific) or green (O157-specific) latex particles. Other specific antibodies against the two antigens are firmly attached to the membrane.

Modified Tryptic Soy Broth (mTSB) containing Mitomycin C (Klie et al. 1997) is inoculated with the test strain or sample and incubated at 37°C for 18 to 24 hours for the production of Shiga toxin. Mitomycin C serves as an enhancer to stimulate Stx-production and release in the culture fluid. After growth, the sample is centrifuged (1500g for 15 minutes) and 1 ml of the supernatant fluid is diluted 1:1 with a sample buffer (part of the test system). The mixture is used directly for the test. The RIDA-QUICK test stick is placed into the test sample and the reaction occurs by the lateral flow of specific antibodies bound to coloured latex particles. Antibodies bind themselves to specific antigens (Stx and/or O157 LPS) if present in the sample and the antigen-antibody complex flows via the membrane to specific collection bands where they are fixed by immobilized, specific antibodies. A green (O157 LPS) and/or red (Stx) band becomes visible if these antigens are present in the sample. The test does not differentiate between Stx1 and Stx2. A blue band is always shown as a control. The coloured bands become visible after 15 minutes and the strength of the reaction is rated between 0 (not visible) and 4+ (maximum colour development), according to colour intensity (Figure 3). A description is provided by the producer and the assay was performed accordingly (http://www.r-biopharm.de/).

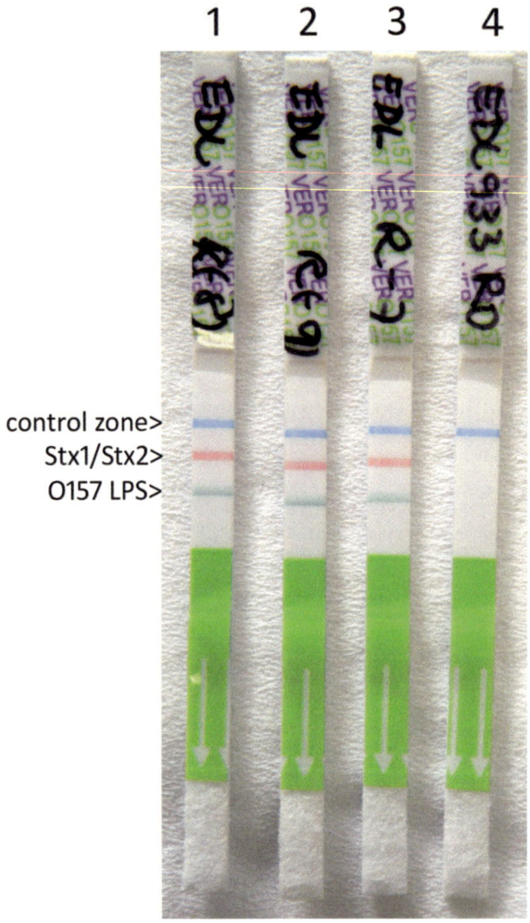

Fig. 3. Detection of Stx production and the O157 antigen from enrichment cultures of salad samples inoculated with different quantities of EHEC O157 strain EDL933.

5. Results

5.1 Evaluation of the RIDA®QUICK Verotoxin/O157 Combi (Rida Quick) test with *Shigella* and *E. coli* reference strains

We have evaluated the RIDA Quick test for its sensitivity and specificity with all the known variants of Stx1 and Stx2. For the evaluation, we employed STEC references strains for the different Stx-types and subtypes together with STEC isolates from food and other sources that were previously characterized at the NRL-*E.coli* at the BfR (Beutin et al. 2007a; Miko et al. 2009). The RIDA Quick was compared for its sensitivity and specificity with the Ridascreen® Verotoxin enzyme immunoassay (R-Biopharm, Darmstadt, Germany), and Stx-specific ELISA which was evaluated previously (Beutin et al. 2007). The Vero cell toxicity test was used as a gold-standard for toxin activity.

In total, two strains of *Shigella dysenteriae* and *S. sonnei* (Stx1) and 18 *E. coli*-producing toxins of the Stx1 family (Stx1 (n=2), Stx1a (n=9), Stx1c (n=5) and Stx1d (n=4) were tested. The RIDA Quick detected all strains of the Stx1 family (sensitivity of 100%). All the reactions were 4+, except for Stx1d strains showing reaction intensities between 1+ and 3+. Similar results were obtained with the Ridascreen-Stx-EIA (Beutin et al. 2007, this work).

Fifty-five strains were tested as representatives of the Stx2 family. The results were very good for the Stx2a (12/12 positive) and Stx2c (6/6 positive). Stx2b, formerly called Stx2d non-activatable (Pierard et al. 1998) was detected in 8 of 9 strains tested (88.9 %). The mucus-activatable Stx2d (Melton-Celsa et al. 2002) was detected in 5 of 7 positive strains (71.4 %). The Stx2e variant was detected in only 3 of 11 Stx2e strains (27.3%) and Stx2g in only 1 of 4 positive strains (25%). The Stx2f variant was not detected in any of the six Stx2f-producing strains that were tested. Thirty-three strains producing multiple types of Stx strain were all detected. Four Stx-negative strains were used as controls and false positive reactions were not recorded (Table 1). The results obtained with the Rida Screen Verotoxin ELISA were identical to those obtained with the RIDA Quick Test for Stx-detection (Table 1).

			Numbers of strains testing positive for Stx	
numbers of strains	**bacterial species**	**Stx type**	**by *stx*-PCR and Verocellassay**	**by Rida Sccreen and by Rida Quick (%)**
1	*S. dysenteriae*	Stx1	1 (100)	1 (100)
1	*S. sonnei*	Stx1	1 (100)	1 (100)
9	*E. coli*	Stx1a	9 (100)	9 (100)
5	*E. coli*	Stx1c	5 (100)	5 (100)
4	*E. coli*	Stx1d	4 (100)	4 (100)
12	*E .coli*	Stx2a	12 (100)	12 (100)
6	*E. coli*	Stx2c	6 (100)	6 (100)
9	*E. coli*	Stx2b	9 (100)	8 (88.9)
7	*E. coli*	Stx2d	7 (100)	5 (71.4)
11	*E. coli*	Stx2e	11 (100)	3 (27.3)
4	*E. coli*	Stx2g	4 (100)	1 (25.0)
6	*E. coli*	Stx2f	6 (100)	0 (0)
33	*E. coli*	multiple	33 (100)	33 (100)
4	*E. coli*	none	0 (0)	0 (0)

Table 1. Types of Stx tested and their percentages detected by Rida Screen Verotoxin Elisa and Immuno-chromotographic RIDA quick.

5.2 Detection of the O157 antigen

The specificity of the assay for the *E. coli* O157 antigen was tested with 134 strains belonging to 45 different O-antigen groups of *E. coli*, including 17 *E. coli* O157 strains. The RIDA Quick assay detected all *E. coli* O157 strains tested, irrespective of whether these were STEC or not. Strains belonging to the non-O157 serogroups did not react for the O157 antigen in the Rida Quick assay indicating a specificity of 100%.

5.3 Detection of Stx- and the O157 antigens from EHEC-contaminated food samples

The sensitivity of the Rida Quick test for detection of Stx and the O157 antigen was analyzed for food samples spiked with different amounts of EHEC strains. Twenty-five-gram portions of retailed ready-to-eat salads were inoculated with different amounts (<10, 10-100, 100-1000 cfu) with different concentrations of EHEC reference strains belonging to serogroups O26, O103, O111, O145, O157 (Table 2).

		Numbers of EHEC per 25g salad sample inoculated							
		none		≤10		10-100		100-1000	
EHEC-serotype	Stx-Type	Rida screen[a]	Rida-Quick	Rida-Screen	Rida-Quick	Rida-Screen	Rida-Quick	Rida-Screen	Rida-Quick
O157:H7[b]	Stx1a + Stx2a	0.015	-	3.448	4+	9.992	4+	9.992	4+
O26:H11	Stx1a	0.001	-	0.727	3+	2.655	4+	9.993	4+
O103:H2	Stx1a	0.015	-	9.983	4+	9.983	4+	9.983	4+
O145:H28	Stx2a	0.003	-	2.932	4+	3.475	4+	3.402	4+
O111:H8	Stx1a	0.001	-	3.269	4+	3.303	4+	9.995	4+
O118:H16	Stx2a	0.007	-	9.986	3+	9.986	4+	9.986	4+
O121:H19	Stx2a	0.007	-	2.911	4+	3.479	4+	3.278	4+

a) Extinction values at OD450 nm for the Rida Screen were calculated as described previously (Beutin et al. 2007) b) the O157 antigen was detected as 4+ in all concentrations with the Rida-Quick test

Table 2. Detection of Shiga toxins produced by EHEC strains from spiked ready-to-eat salad samples.

Spiked and unspiked control 25 g salad samples were each homogenized in 225 ml BRILA-Broth and the homogenates were grown aerobically for six hours at 37°C for EHEC enrichment (Tzschoppe 2010). After, 1 ml of BRILA broth enrichment culture was inoculated into 5ml of mTSB + Mitomycin (Klie et al. 1997) and incubated at 37°C for a further 18 hours. The mTSB+ Mitomycin C cultures were examined for the presence of Stx and O157 antigens with the Rida Screen and the Rida Quick assay. Unspiked salad samples were taken as negative controls. In all the spiked salad samples tested we detected positive reactions (Table 2). No false positive reaction was found. The results obtained with O157:H7-inoculated salad samples are shown in Figure 3.

6. Discussion

The RIDA Quick was found suitable for the routine screening of bacterial isolates and for the detection of all Stx subtypes tested, except for Stx2f. All other Stx-variants were easily detectable with this assay. Negative Stx detection results obtained for some Stx2b, Stx2d, Stx2e and Stx2g strains are probably due to the poor Stx production, which is below the detectable level for the serological assays.

The results obtained with the Rida Screen Verotoxin ELISA were identical to those obtained with the RIDA Quick Test for Stx-detection (Table 1). As both tests are from the same producer, it is possible that the antibodies used for Stx detection are the same in both assays.

All Stx types except Stx2f were detectable with the RIDA Quick assay and the Rida Screen ELISA. Stx2f is genetically the most distant from all other toxins of the stx2 group (Persson et al. 2007; Schmidt et al. 2000). It is therefore possible that the Stx2-specific antibody used for the RIDA Quick and the RidaScreen assay does not react with the Stx2f variant toxin. The nucleotide sequence of Stx2f is sufficiently divergent (Fig. 2) that it is not detected by many Stx2-specific PCR primers (Schmidt et al. 2000), nor in Real time Stx- detection kits for Stx2 (Beutin et al. 2009). Some Stx2b, Stx2d, Stx2e and Stx2g strains did not produce enough toxins to be detectable by both Rida Screen and RIDA Quick (Beutin et al. 2007; Beutin et al. 2007a; Beutin et al. 2008). The Stx types Stx1, Stx2a and Stx2c that are associated with typical EHEC strains (Nataro and Kaper 1998) were detected in all the tested strains.

The first results with EHEC inoculated food samples indicate that the RIDA Quick assay is suitable for the screening of food samples such as ready-to-eat salads. These kinds of vegetable food samples are characterized by their high level of contamination (10^6-10^7 cfu / g) with *Pseudomonas* and *Enterobacteriaceae* from their own natural flora (Klepzig et al. 1999; Tzschoppe 2010). Low numbers (<10 cfu / 25g) of EHEC were still detectable in these inoculated food samples after enrichment (Fig. 3). The choice of enrichment medium and procedure was found to be important. The presence of an enhancer (Mitomycin C) in the growth medium is needed for the best results (data not shown). Further tests on food samples contaminated naturally with STEC / EHEC are needed to evaluate the suitability of the Rida Quick assay for the routine examination of food samples.

7. References

Bettelheim, K.A. and Beutin, L. (2003) Rapid laboratory identification and characterization of verocytotoxigenic (Shiga toxin producing) *Escherichia coli* (VTEC/STEC). *Journal of Applied Microbiology* 95, 205-217.

Beutin, L., Steinruck, H., Krause, G., Steege K., Haby, S., Hultsch, G. and Appel B. (2007) Comparative evaluation of the Ridascreen((R)) Verotoxin enzyme immunoassay for detection of Shiga-toxin producing strains of *Escherichia coli* (STEC) from food and other sources. *J. Appl. Microbiol.* 102, 630-639.

Beutin, L., Martin, A., Krause, G., Steege, K., Haby, S., Pries, K., Albrecht, N., Miko, A. and Jahn, S. (2010) Ergebnisse, Schlussfolgerungen und Empfehlungen aus zwei Ringversuchen zum Nachweis und zur Isolierung von Shiga (Vero) Toxin bildenden *Escherichia coli* (STEC) aus Hackfleischproben [Results, conclusions, and recommendations of two ring trials for the detection and isolation of shiga (Vero) toxin producing *Escherichia coli* (STEC) from minced beef samples]. *Journal für Verbraucherschutz und Lebensmittelsicherheit* 5, 21-34.

Beutin, L. (2006) Emerging Enterohaemorrhagic *Escherichia coli*, Causes and Effects of the Rise of a Human Pathogen. *J. Vet. Med. B Infect. Dis. Vet. Public Health* 53, 299-305.

Beutin, L., Jahn, S. and Fach, P. (2009) Evaluation of the 'GeneDisc' real-time PCR system for detection of enterohaemorrhagic *Escherichia coli* (EHEC) O26, O103, O111, O145 and O157 strains according to their virulence markers and their O- and H-antigen-associated genes. *J Appl Microbiol* 106, 1122-1132.

Beutin, L., Kruger, U., Krause, G., Miko, A., Martin, A. and Strauch, E. (2008) Evaluation of major types of Shiga toxin 2e producing *Escherichia coli* present in food, pigs and in the environment as potential pathogens for humans. *Appl Environ Microbiol*. 74: 4806–4816.

Beutin, L., Miko, A., Krause, G., Pries, K., Haby, S., Steege, K. and Albrecht, N. (2007a) Identification of human-pathogenic strains of Shiga toxin-producing *Escherichia coli* from food by a combination of serotyping and molecular typing of Shiga toxin genes. *Appl Environ Microbiol* 73, 4769-4775.

Beutin, L., Zimmermann, S. and Gleier, K. (1996) Rapid detection and isolation of Shiga-like toxin (verocytotoxin)-producing *Escherichia coli* by direct testing of individual enterohemolytic colonies from washed sheep blood agar plates in the VTEC-RPLA assay. *Journal of Clinical Microbiology* 34, 2812-2814.

Beutin, L., Zimmermann, S. and Gleier, K. (2002) Evaluation of the VTEC-screen "Seiken" test for detection of different types of Shiga toxin (verotoxin)-producing *Escherichia coli* (STEC) in human stool samples. *Diagnostic Microbiology and Infectious Disease* 42, 1-8.

Brooks, J.T., Sowers, E.G., Wells, J.G., Greene,K.D., Griffin, P.M., Hoekstra, R.M. and Strockbine, N.A. (2005) Non-O157 Shiga toxin-producing *Escherichia coli* infections in the United States, 1983-2002. *The Journal of Infectious Diseases* 192, 1422-1429.

Burk, C., Dietrich, R., Acar, G., Moravek, M., Bulte, M. and Martlbauer, E. (2003) Identification and characterization of a new variant of Shiga toxin 1 in *Escherichia coli* ONT:H19 of bovine origin. *Journal of Clinical Microbiology* 41, 2106-2112.

Caprioli, A., Morabito, S., Brugère, H. and Oswald, E. (2005) Enterohaemorrhagic *Escherichia coli*: emerging issues on virulence and modes of transmission. *Vet. Res.* 36, 289-311.

Eblen, D. R. (2007) Public Health Importance of non-O157 Shiga-Toxin producing *Escherichia coli* (non-O157 STEC) in the US food supply. ed. United States Department of Agriculture pp. 1-48.

ECDC, EFSA (2011) Shiga toxin/verotoxin-producing *Escherichia coli* in humans, food and animals in the EU/EEA, with special reference to the German outbreak strain STEC O104. ed. ECDC and EFSA. http://www.efsa.europa.eu/en/supporting/doc/166e.pdf

EFSA. (2007) Scientific opinion of the panel on biological hazards on a request from EFSA on monitoring of verotoxigenic *Escherichia coli* (VTEC) and identification of human pathogenic types. *The EFSA Journal* 579, 1-61.

Feng, P.C., Jinneman, K., Scheutz, F. and Monday, S.R. (2011) Specificity of PCR and Serological Assays in the Detection of *Escherichia coli* Shiga Toxin Subtypes. *Appl Environ Microbiol* 77, 6699-6702.

Frank, C., Faber, M., Askar, M., Bernard, H., Fruth, A., Gilsdorf, A., Hohle, M., Karch, H., Krause, G., Prager, R., Spode, A., Stark, K. and Werber, D. (2011) Large and ongoing outbreak of haemolytic uraemic syndrome, Germany, May 2011. *Euro. Surveill* 16.

Friedrich, A.W., Bielaszewska, M., Zhang, W.L., Pulz, M., Kuczius, T., Ammon, A. and Karch, H. (2002) *Escherichia coli* harboring Shiga toxin 2 gene variants: frequency and association with clinical symptoms. *J. Infect. Dis.* 185, 74-84.

Friedrich, A.W., Borell, J., Bielaszewska, M., Fruth, A., Tschape, H. and Karch, H. (2003) Shiga toxin 1c-producing *Escherichia coli* strains: phenotypic and genetic characterization and association with human disease. *Journal of Clinical Microbiology* 41, 2448-2453.

Gyles, C.L. (2007) Shiga toxin-producing *Escherichia coli*: an overview. *J Anim Sci* 85, E45-E62.

Herold, S., Karch, H. and Schmidt, H. (2004) Shiga toxin-encoding bacteriophages--genomes in motion. *Int J Med Microbiol* 294, 115-121.

Hussein, H.S. and Bollinger, L.M. (2008) Influence of selective media on successful detection of Shiga toxin-producing *Escherichia coli* in food, fecal, and environmental samples. *Foodborne. Pathog. Dis* 5, 227-244.

Jahn, S. and Beutin, L. (2009) Evaluation Of The "GeneDisc" Real-Time PCR System For Detection Of Major EHEC Type Strains From different Food matrices (minced meat, "Mettwurst", salami and raw milk). Buenos Aires, Argentina: VTEC 2009. Book of Abstracts

Jahn, S., Weber, H. and Beutin, L. (2008) Comparison of enzyme immunoassay and quantitiver real time PCR as proof of Shigatoxin producing *Escherichia coli* (STEC) in mincemeat. *Journal fur Verbraucherschutz und Lebensmittelsicherheit-Journal of Consumer Protection and Food Safety* 3, 385-395.

Karmali, M.A., Gannon, V. and Sargeant, J.M. (2010) Verocytotoxin-producing *Escherichia coli* (VTEC). *Vet Microbiol* 140, 360-370.

Karmali, M.A., Mascarenhas, M., Shen, S., Ziebell, K., Johnson, S., Reid-Smith, R., Isaac-Renton, J., Clark, C., Rahn, K. and Kaper, J.B. (2003) Association of Genomic O Island 122 of *Escherichia coli* EDL 933 with Verocytotoxin-Producing *Escherichia coli* Seropathotypes That Are Linked to Epidemic and/or Serious Disease. *Journal of Clinical Microbiology* 41, 4930-4940.

Klepzig, I., Teufel, P., Schott, W. and Hildebrandt, G. (1999) Auswirkungen einer Unterbrechung der Kühlkette auf die mikrobiologische Beschaffenheit von vorzerkleinerten Mischsalaten. *Archiv für Lebensmittelhygiene* 50, 95-104.

Klie, H., Timm, M., Richter, H., Gallien, P., Perlberg, K.W. and Steinruck, H. (1997) [Detection and occurrence of verotoxin-forming and/or shigatoxin producing *Escherichia coli* (VTEC and/or STEC) in milk]. *Berl Munch. Tierarztl. Wochenschr* 110, 337-341.

Konowalchuk, J., Speirs, J.I. and Stavric, S. (1977) Vero response to a cytotoxin of *Escherichia coli*. *Infect Immun* 18, 775-779.

Kuczius, T., Bielaszewska, M., Friedrich, A.W. and Zhang, W. (2004) A rapid method for the discrimination of genes encoding classical Shiga toxin (Stx) 1 and its variants, Stx1c and Stx1d, in *Escherichia coli*. *Mol Nutr Food Res* 48, 515-521.

Leung, P.H.M., Peiris, J.S.M., Ng, W.W.S., Robins-Browne, R.M., Bettelheim, K.A. and Yam, W.C. (2003) A Newly Discovered Verotoxin Variant, VT2g, Produced by Bovine Verocytotoxigenic *Escherichia coli*. *Applied and Environmental Microbiology* 69, 7549-7553.

Martin, A. and Beutin, L. (2011) Characteristics of Shiga toxin-producing *Escherichia coli* from meat and milk products of different origins and association with food producing animals as main contamination sources. *Int J Food Microbiol* 146, 99-104.

McGannon, C.M., Fuller, C.A. and Weiss, A.A. (2010) Different classes of antibiotics differentially influence shiga toxin production. *Antimicrobial Agents and Chemotherapy* 54, 3790-3798.

Melton-Celsa, A.R., Kokai-Kun, J.F. and O'Brien, A.D. (2002) Activation of Shiga toxin type 2d (Stx2d) by elastase involves cleavage of the C-terminal two amino acids of the A2 peptide in the context of the appropriate B pentamer. *Mol. Microbiol* 43, 207-215.

Miko, A., Pries, K., Haby, S., Steege, K., Albrecht, N., Krause, G. and Beutin, L. (2009) Assessment of Shiga toxin-producing *Escherichia coli* isolates from wildlife meat as potential pathogens for humans. *Appl Environ Microbiol* 75, 6462-6470.

Muthing, J., Schweppe, C.H., Karch, H. and Friedrich, A.W. (2009) Shiga toxins, glycosphingolipid diversity, and endothelial cell injury. *Thromb Haemost.* 101, 252-264.

Nataro, J.P. and Kaper, J.B. (1998) Diarrheagenic *Escherichia coli. Clinical Microbiology Reviews* 11, 142ff.

Paton, J.C. and Paton, A.W. (2003) Methods for detection of STEC in humans. An overview. *Methods Mol Med* 73, 9-26.

Persson, S., Olsen, K.E., Ethelberg, S. and Scheutz, F. (2007) Subtyping method for *Escherichia coli* shiga toxin (verocytotoxin) 2 variants and correlations to clinical manifestations. *J Clin Microbiol* 45, 2020-2024.

Pierard, D., Muyldermans, G., Moriau, L., Stevens, D. and Lauwers, S. (1998) Identification of new verocytotoxin type 2 variant B-subunit genes in human and animal *Escherichia coli* isolates. *J Clin Microbiol* 36, 3317-3322.

Riley, L.W., Remis, R.S., Helgerson, S.D., McGee, H.B., Wells, J.G., Davis, B.R., Hebert, R.J., Olcott, E.S., Johnson, L.M., Hargrett, N.T., Blake, P.A. and Cohen, M.L. (1983) Hemorrhagic Colitis Associated with A Rare Escherichia-Coli Serotype. *New England Journal of Medicine* 308, 681-685.

Scheutz, F. and Strockbine, N. A. (2005) Genus I. Escherichia. In *Bergey's Manual of Systematic Bacteriology* ed. Garrity,G.M., Brenner,D.J., Krieg,N.R. and Staley,J.T. pp. 607-624. Springer.

Schmidt, H., Scheef, J., Morabito, S., Caprioli, A., Wieler, L.H. and Karch, H. (2000) A new Shiga toxin 2 variant (Stx2f) from *Escherichia coli* isolated from pigeons. *Applied and Environmental Microbiology* 66, 1205-1208.

Schmidt, H. (2001) Shiga-toxin-converting bacteriophages. *Research in Microbiology* 152, 687-695.

Shimizu, T., Ohta, Y. and Noda, M. (2009) Shiga toxin 2 is specifically released from bacterial cells by two different mechanisms. *Infect Immun.* 77, 2813-2823.

Tzschoppe, M. (2010) Untersuchungen zur Kontamination von pflanzlichen, für den Rohverzehr vorgesehenen, Lebensmitteln mit pathogenen, insbesondere Shiga-Toxin-bildenden *Escherichia coli.* pp. 1-119. Diploma-Thesis: Beuth Hochschule für Technik, Federal Institute for Risk Assessment, Berlin, Germany.

Willford, J., Mills, K. and Goodridge, L.D. (2009) Evaluation of three commercially available enzyme-linked immunosorbent assay kits for detection of Shiga toxin. *J Food Prot* 72, 741-747.

Wong, C.S., Jelacic, S., Habeeb, R.L., Watkins, S.L. and Tarr, P.I. (2000) The risk of the hemolytic-uremic syndrome after antibiotic treatment of *Escherichia coli* O157:H7 infections. *N Engl. J Med* 342, 1930-1936.

4

Use of Antibodies in Immunocytochemistry

Hakkı Dalçık[1,*] and Cannur Dalçık[2]
[1]*Kocaeli University, School of Medicine, Department of Histology and Embryology,*
[2]*Kocaeli University, School of Medicine, Department of Anatomy,*
Turkey

1. Introduction

Immunostaining can be used to pinpont the subcellular localization of a protein antigen, to follow its changing position as cells respond to stumuli, or to compare its position to other proteins in the same cell. Using these methods one can follow an antigen's distribution during development, mark the location of a particular cell type in a multicellular in vivo setting, or determine the presence of an antigen in a diseased tissue. The protocoles normally require multiple steps over several days as well as extensive knowledge of architecture of the tissues been studied. These procedures demand methods to preserve the structure of tissues, which unfortunately are often damaging to antigens.

The important propeties of the antibodies are; they specifically bind to a particular protein or molecule, that are called antigens. This binding property keeps the antibody binding unaltered in the physiological conditions. Also, any other noval antibodies could be made to other interested molecules. These are the crucial properties of the antibodies that are used in immunocytochemistry. An antigen is defined as a substance that can be bound by an antibody molecule through its antigen-binding sites, also called epitopes or antigenic determinants. Treatment of tissues with chemical fixatives and detergents can change the reactivity of proteins to antibodies because the exposure of epitopes to these chemicals can change the chemical and physical nature of the molecules in the epitope region. Many substances can, and are known to be antigenic, for example: proteins; nucleic acids: DNA, RNA; carbohydrates or sugar groups; lipids; small chemical groups; peptides (10-15 amino acids long). Thus antibodies can bind almost any repertoire of antigens, including chemicals and things B-cells have never encountered before.

Development, characterization and manufacturing of antibodies has made tremendous progress in using the antibodies in many research, diagnostic, and therapeutic areas. However, it has been emphasized that antibodies both monoclonal and polyclonal remain the primary site in the vast majority of research and dianostic applications (Leduc and Connolly., 1955). New types of antibodies, recombinant and synthetic, have been developed and validated. Recombinated antibodies can be produced in transgenic mice (He et al., 2002), also using bacteriophage (Hoogenboom and Chames., 2000) high quantities of high-affinity antibodies can be produced. Synthetic antibodies (diabodies, triabodies, tetrabodies)

* Corresponding Author

are generated using chemical or biological cross-linking to produce di-, tri-, and tetrameric multivalent conjugates exhibiting enhanced specifity and functional activity (Tomlinson and Holliger., 2000). There are some investigations on antibodies that have been made to replace amino acids by other biological molecules to ctreate chemical diversity and produce nucleic acid-based molecules forming specific binding to target antigens (Proske et al., 2005).

Antibodies are the responsible proteins that hold the key step in immunocytochemistry. Antibodies have been used as research reagents for many years. Technology has improved and created new techniques and enhanced their value in immunocytochemistry. Antibody is tagged with a visible label. The visual marker which may be a fluorescent dye, colloidal metal, hapten, nanocrystal, radioactive marker or the more commonly in the light microscopic field, an enzyme. Experimental samples ranging from frozen sections, cell culture/suspension, to whole tissue samples have been used. Ideally, maximal signal strength along with minimal background is required to give optimal antigen demonstration.

There are multiple ways of performing immunological stains on tissues, some of which include the direct method of staining, where the antibody is bound directly onto the antigen on a cell with a fluorescent or colored dye bound directly to the antibody. Another method includes the indirect method where the antigen is reacted with a primary antibody which binds directly. This is followed by a secondary antibody which binds to the primary antibody. Next, a tertiary reagent is applied, which binds to the secondary antibody, with an enzymatic end. When the quarternary reagent is applied, the enzymatic end of the tertiary reagent converts the substrate into a chromogen (DAB; Diaminobenzadine or others), which stains the cell, usually a brown color.

In the immunocytochemical application, since there are many different staining methods, the investigator should know how to optimize the staining method when the sataining fails. Fore example; there may be other methods that although using the same primary antibody concentrations, the degree of the staining intensity may be increased due to the method.

Recommendations of the optimal dilutions of the primary antibody should be aquired. When the sataining does not work the investigators should have the basic nowledge to deal with the sepisific problem. In, particular, tissue fixation and tissue processing can have inportant effect on the antigenicity of the protein by changing the conformation of the epitope, therefore, creating non-specific background. Specificity of the antibodies needs to be tested in control experiments to avoid non-specific staining due to nonspecific binding to tissue components or binding to other proteins that share similar epitopes.

2. Antibody molecules

The antibodies, or immunoglobulins (Igs) are a group of glycoproteins present in the serum and tissue fluids. They are produced when the host's lymphoid cells come into contact with immunogenic foreign molecules called antigens, and they bind specifically to the antigen which induced their formation.

Each antibody molecule consists of four polypeptides– two heavy chains and two light chains joined to form a "Y" shaped molecule. Antibodies are further classified into multiple classes or isotypes. Five distinct classes of immunoglobulin molecule are recognized in most higher mamals, namely IgG, IgA, IgM, IgD and IgE (Table 1). These differ from each other in size, charge, amino acid composition and carbohydrate content. In addition to the differences between classes the immunoglobulins within each class are also very heterogeneous.

IgG;	Is the major immunoglobulin in normal human serum accounting for 70-75% of the total immunoglobulin pool. It is distributed evenly between the intra- and extravascular pools, is the major antibody of secondary immune responses and the exclusive anti-toxin class.
IgA;	Represents 15-20% of the human serum immunoglobulin pool. In man more than 80% of IgA occurs as the basic four chain monomer but in most mammals the IgA in serum is mainly plymeric and occurs mostly as a dimer. It is the predominant immunoglobulin in sero-mucous secretions such as saliva, tracheobronchial secretions, colostrum, milk, and genito-urinary secretions.
IgM;	Accounts for about 10% of the immunoglobulin pool. The molecule has a pentameric structure.This protein is largely confined to the intravascular pool and is the predominant "early" antibody frequently directed against antigenically complex infectious organisms.
IgD;	Accounts for less than 1% of the total plasma immunoglubulin but it is known to be present in large quantities on the membrane of many circulating B lymphocytes. It is involved in initial immune response
IgE;	Though a trace serum protein, is found on the surface membrane of basophils and mast cells in all individuals. This class may play a role in active immunity to parasites and commonly associated with immediate hypersensitivity reactions.

Table 1. Ig classes

Essentially each immunoglobulin molecule is bifunctional; one region of the molecule is concerned with binding to antigen while a different region mediates binding of the immunoglobulin to host tissues. IgG isotype is the immunoglobulin that is used in immunocytochemistry because it is generated in high quatities and its binding property is more consistent. Knowledge of the IgG structure (Fig. 1), is important in order to understand the mechanisms of the antibody and antigen reactions. The basic structure of IgG and all other immunoglobulin molecules is a unit consisting of two identical light polypeptide chains (variable region) and two identical heavy polypeptide chains (constant region) linked together by disulphide bonds.

The class and subclass of an immunoglobulin molecule is determined by its heavy chain type. Thus the four IgG subclasses (IgG1, IgG2, IgG3 and IgG4) have heavy chains called $\gamma1$, $\gamma2$, $\gamma3$, and $\gamma4$ which differ only slightly although all are recognizable γ heavy chains. The differences between the various subclasses within an immunoglobulin class are less than the differences between the different classes; thus IgG1 is more closely related to IgG2, 3, or 4 than to IgA, IgM, IgD or IgE. The amino acid sequence in the tips of the "Y" varies greatly among different antibodies. This variable region, composed of 110-130 amino acids, give the

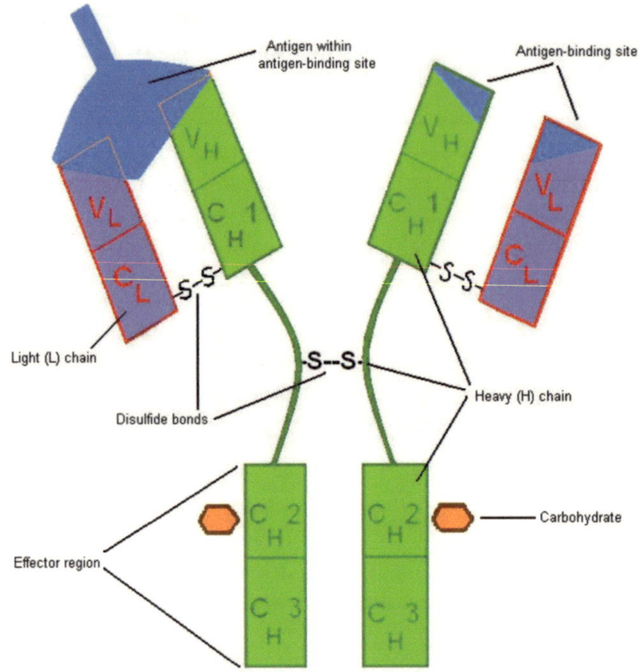

Fig. 1. The antibody. An IgG antibody has a single constant region (C) and the variable region. The constant region containing light (C_L) and heavy chain (C_H) with the fragment crystallizable (Fc) region (effector region). The variable region contains the the antigen binding site. The small protein, only in the variable region, is known as the light chain; the large protein that is part of the constant and variable region is the heavy chain. The IgG can be digested by the protease enzyme, papain, into an Fc end (constant end) and a Fab end (variable end).

antibody its specificity for binding antigen. The variable region includes the ends of the light and heavy chains. When the primary amino acid structure of a large number of light and heavy polypeptide chains is examined it is found that the variability between their V domains is not distributed evenly throughout the length of these regions. Some short polypeptide segments are termed hypervariable regions. It is now generally accepted that such hypervariable regions are involved directly in the formation of the antigen binding site. Hypervariable regions are sometimes referred to as Complementarity Determining Regions (CDR) and the intervening peptide segments as Framework Regions (FR). In both light and heavy chain three hypervariable regions exist - HV 1, 2 and 3. Four FR regions which have more stable amino acids sequences separate the HV regions. Treating the antibody with a protease can cleave this region, producing fragment antigen binding (Fab) that include the variable ends of an antibody. The constant region contains species specific sequences and the Fc portion that binds an Fc receptor, which is found on circulating white cells, macrophages, and natural killer cells. The Fc portion also has species-specific sites that are unique to the animal species in which the antibody was generated. Thus, generation of an antibody against IgG from rabbit will result in antibodies that bind the constant region from rabbit IgG only and not, for example, from mouse IgG.

Antibodies or IgG molecules are generated to other IgG molecules by injecting purified IgG molecules from one species into another species. In the case of mouse IgG injected into rabbit, it will produce rabbit anti-mouse IgG antibodies. Antibodies made against an IgG will only bind to the constant region or Fab region of the IgG. The variable end of the antibody contains the unique epitope-binding regions that give each antibody its specificity (Fig. 1). This variable region is the fraction antigen binding (Fab) portion. The unique configuration of the Fab specifically binds the epitope. When an antigen is injected into a rabbit, the resulting antibodies against the antigen have Fab portions that are unique to the antigen, but the rest of the IgG is similar to other IgG molecules. Each IgG antibody has two Fab ends, which can bind to two identical epitopes at the same time. The advantage of this bivalent epitope binding is that it can amplify the epitope detection.

An antigen is a protein, peptide, or molecule used to cause an immune response in an animal. The animal responds by making antibodies to individual epitopes or antigenic determinant region located on the antigen. An individual antigen has multiple epitopes that can generate antibodies. An epitope can be an amino acid sequence on a denatured peptide or a several sequences on the surface of a folded protein. Animals frequently generate multiple antibodies to the same epitope. Also, an epitope on one protein might also exist on a different, unrelated protein because it has the same sequence or the same surface configuration.

3. Producing antibodies

When the macrophage engulf the bacteria, proteins (antigens) from the bacteria are broken down into short peptide chains and those peptides are then presented on the macrophage membrane attached to special molecules referred to as Major Histocompatibility Complex Class II (MHC II). Bacterial peptides are similarly processed and displayed on MHC II molecules on the surface of B lymphocytes. When a T lymphocyte determines the same peptide on the macrophage and on the B cell, the T cell stimulates the B cells. The stimulated B cell undergoes repeated cell divisions, enlargement and differentiation to form a clone of antibody producing plasma cells. Therefore, by recognizing a specific antigen, clonal expansion and differentiation of B cells to the plasma cells are acquired and all these cells start to produce the same specific antibody to only a single epitope. Epitopes are regions on an antigen that an antibody can bind to, and are also known as antigenic determinants. Epitopes can be: conformational; in which the antibody recognizes the secondary structure of the molecule, linear; in which the antibody binds to the determinant in both the denatured protein and the native protein; neoantigenic, which is an epitope which is not present in the native protein but becomes an epitope after the protein is cleaved by a protease.

3.1 Polyclonal antibodies

Polyclonal antibodies are multiple clones of antibodies produced to different epitopes of the antigen. In Fig. 2, the serum from an immunized rabbit contains antibodies from many clones of B-cells. In the rabbit serum, the different clones of antibodies have multivalent property, consisting of antibodies that bind to several regions (epitopes) of the antigen molecule, providing a strong dectecting capacity. This feature is important in that it gives high levels of staining for a single antigen. However, shared epitopes on different proteins can label multiple proteins which can cause false evaluation, and it is referred to as cross-reactivity.

Polyclonal antibodies depend on a living animal thus if the animal dye no more antibody of that specific type can be produced. In addition, when a new animal is immunized with the same antigen, the exact epitopes generating antibodies will be different. An immunocytochemical study using a polyclonal antibody to detect IGF-I protein is demonstrated in Figure 3.

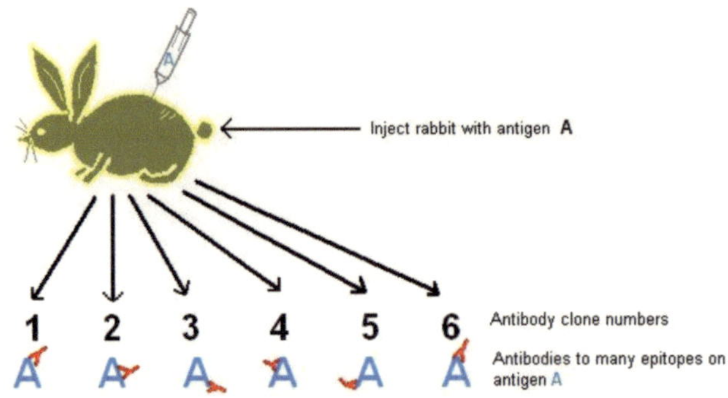

Fig. 2. Schematic representation of the production of polyclonal antibodies. Polyclonal antibody preparations are usually a mixture of different specific antibodies known as "antibody clones"which all recognize the same antigen (A). The specificity difference means the antibodies bind to different epitopes on the antigen with different strength. The blood serum that is obtained from the rabbit that contains polyclonal antibodies is known as "antiserum".

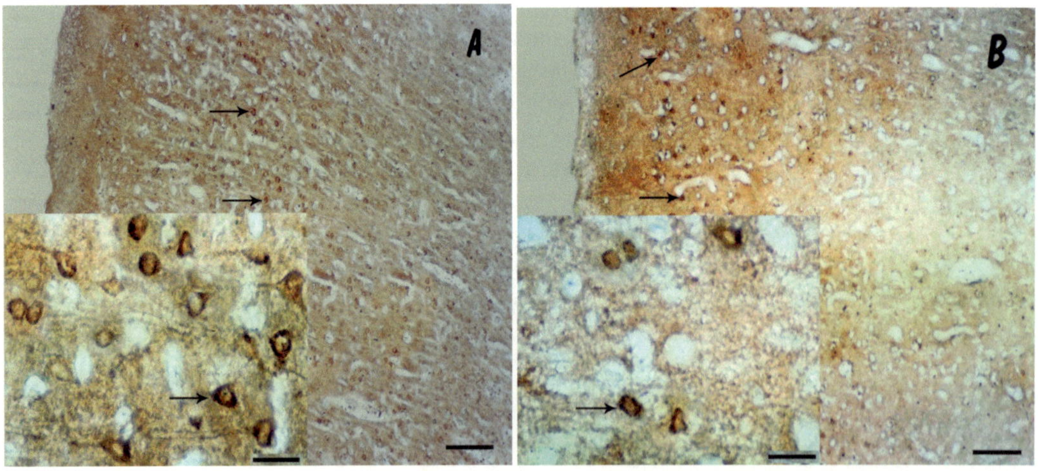

Fig. 3. Photomicrographs of IGF-I immunoreactivity in the cortex. In the present immunostaining antihuman IGF-I polyclonal antibody is used to detect the IGF-I protein in various areas in the cortex. In the present study the siginificant decrease in density of IGF-I immunoreactive neurons in ethanol treated (B) compared to the control (A) rats. At a higher magnification neuronal processes are evident (inset). (Dalçik et al., 2009).

3.2 Monoclonal antibodies

Monoclonal antibodies, originally from one mouse, contain a single antibody from one clone of B-cells to a single epitope on the antigen. This procedure was first described by Cesar Milstein, (Milstein et al., 1979; Milstein C., 1980). The antibodies are produced in mice (Fig. 4), and when antibodies are produced, the spleen of the immunized mouse is removed. Then the spleen cells are dissociated. These spleen cells so-called the B-cells are fused with mouse myeloma cells in culture. The fusion process allows the hybrid cells to continue to proliferate. Each cell produces only one type of antibody. The procedure consists of screening the culture fluid from various clones for antibody via RIA, ELISA, or immunocytochemistry (Ritter M.A., 1986). One mouse spleen can give many different antibodies to different epitopes on the same antigen molecule. Antibodies spesific to fragments of the molecules could be produced in this way and, the culture can be stored until further production is required. Rabbit and mice monoclonal antibodies are available than other animals because good rabbit and mice myeloma cell lines are available.

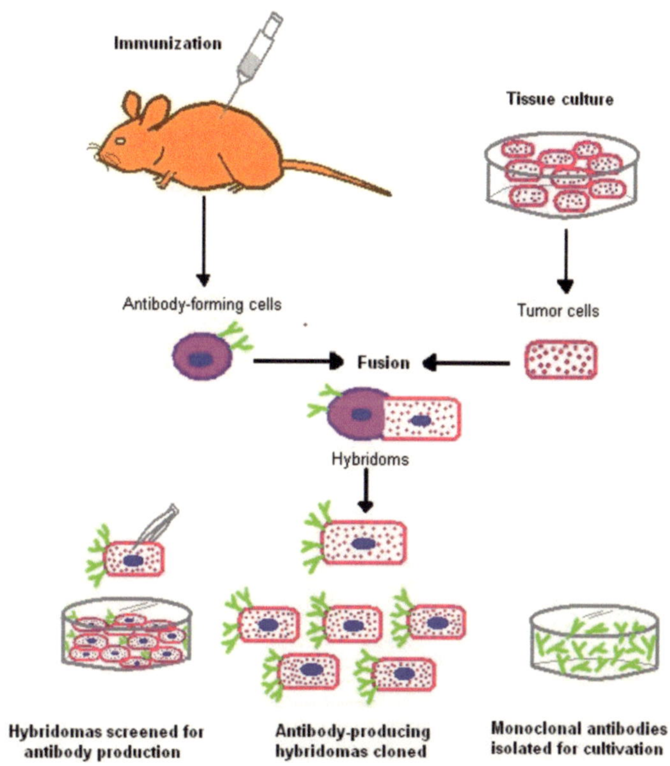

Fig. 4. Monoclonal Antibody production is the process by which large quantities of antibodies are produced. A mouse is immunized by injection of an antigen to stimulate the production of antibodies targeted against that particular antigen. The antibody forming cells are isolated from the mouse's spleen. Monoclonal antibodies are produced by fusing single antibody-forming cells to tumor cells grown in culture. The resulting cell is called a hybridoma. Each hybridoma produces relatively large quantities of identical antibody molecules. By allowing the hybridoma to multiply in culture, it is possible to produce a population of cells, each of which produces identical antibody molecules. These antibodies are called "monoclonal antibodies" because they are produced by the identical cloned antibody producing cell.

The advantage of monoclonal antibodies compared to polyclonal antibodies is their absolute specificity for a single epitope on the antigen molecule, and different clones of antibodies can be generated to different epitopes on the same antigen. Therefore, since the cross-reactivity is very much decreased the immunostaining can be clean without any artifacts on the slide. However, if the monoclonal antibody happens to bind to an antigenic sequence that is shared by other substance then in this case cross-reactivity will occur in the usage of monoclonal antibodies. Since the monoclonal antibodies bound to only one site on the molecule its binding results in weaker staining. In addition, since the specific sequence of the epitope may be altered with the fixation this may also cause no staining compared to the polyclonal antibodies because in polyclonal antiserum there are several regions (epitopes) in the antigen that the antibody can bind, if one region gets altered the others can be available. Therefore, in many cases frozen materials are been used rather than fixed paraffin sections. If using paraffin sections it may be wise to use many different antibodies spesific to different regions of the same antigen molecule to get better results.

Although much work is required to generate monoclonal antibodies, with the aid of cultured hybridoma cells it can be generated indistinctly. However, polyclonal preparations are generally easier and less expensive to generate than monoclonal antibodies, and they can withstand greater variations in temperature and pH. An immunocytochemical study using a monoclonal antibody to detect IGF-I protein is depicted in Figure 5.

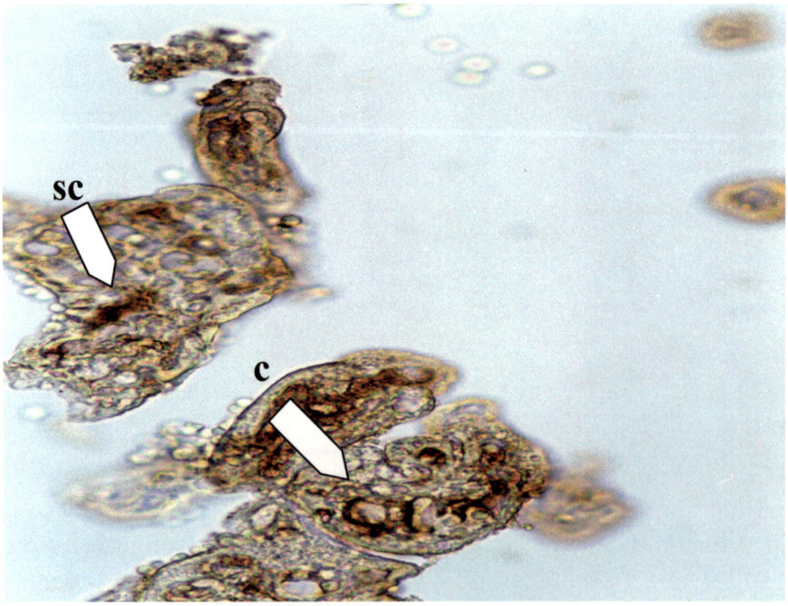

Fig. 5. Photomicrograph showing IGF-I immunoreactivity from the placenta of the intrauterine growth retarded placental villus. In the present immunostaining anti-human IGF-I monoclonal antibody is used to detect the IGF-I protein in various areas in the placental villi. IGF-I immunoreactivity is observed in the stromal cells (sc) and capillary endothelial cells (Dalçik et al., 2001).

4. Selection of the antibody

In the immunocytochemical applications the desired antibody used, is referred to as the "primary antibody". There is also a "secondary antibody" to detect and bind to the primary antibody. The secondary antibodies usually have tag to make the primary-secondary antibody complex visible under the microscope. In order to detect a protein for example IGF-I protein in human tissue with anti-human rabbit polyclonal or anti-human mouse monoclonal antibody, it is appropriate to use an anti-rabbit secondary or anti-mouse secondary antibodies. This is followed by using either a horseradish peroxidase (HRP)-DAB (Fig. 4,5) or alkaline phosphatase-Vector Red reagents to produce a color in order to detect the localization of the desired antigen. Other colorimetric detection systems are also commercially available.

Blocking reagents are used during the immunostaining procedure to avoid the problem of detecting endogenous immunoglobulins that are detected by the secondary antibody, in order to reduce the background staining. On the other hand, in the immunofluorescence technique the secondary antibodies are chemically conjugated with a fluorescent dye such as fluorescein isothiocyanate (FITC). There are two types of immunofluorescence staining methods; direct immunofluorescence staining and indirect immunofluorescence staining. In the direct immunofluorescence staining, the primary antibody is labelled with fluorescence dye and in the indirect immunofluorescence staining (Fig. 6) the secondary antibody is labelled with the fluorochrome (FITC or Texas Red). Immunofluorescence staining can be performed on cells that are fixed on slides and also tissue sections and these can be examined under a fluorescence microscope.

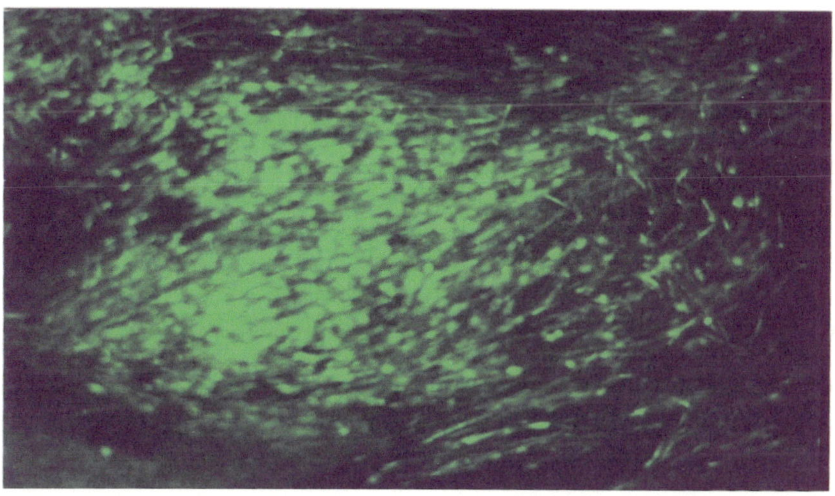

Fig. 6. Photomicrograph showing nestin immunoreactivity from a 9 day old embryonic stem cells. In the present study mouse anti-nestin monoclonal antibody is used to detect the nestin protein which are the primary marker for the neuronal differentiation, and anti-mouse IgM FITC is used for secondary antibody (Tas et al., 2007).

5. Handling of the antibody

Commonly the antibodies are commercially available. There are many companies that manufacture and sell antibodies. For example, antibodies may be sold in the form of hybridoma tissue culture supernatant, ascites fluid or crude serum.

It is important to get a good and efficeint antibody. Before obtaining the primary antibody, relevant work that has been done by other investigators should be examined thoroughly. In addition, recommendations from collegues that have used the antibody in their previous study is a good way to obtain a reliable antibody. After purchasing the antibody, one should read the product information and instructions in the datasheets provided by the supplier. The company supplies the antiserum in a liquid or powder form. Antibodies in powder form are liyophilized and transfered at room temperature. Antibodies in liquid form are transfered in ice packages.

Antibodies should be stored as indicated by the vendor or supplier. When receiving the powder or liquid form of the antibody to prepare the stock solution it should be diluted and saved as small aliquots in microcentrifuge tubes at -20 ^{0}C or -70 ^{0}C. The aliquots should not be less than 10μl. When using the antiserum the antibody should be thawed, the left over antibodies should not be freezed again, repeated freezing and thawing is not recommended since these processes destroy the stability of the antibody. Damage can be reduced by adding glycerol to the solution. Extreme pH, and high salt environments can also damage the structure of the antibody. However, in some cases the antibodies are supplied as "ready to use" form. In this case, without diluting the antiserum it is applied directly on the tissue sections.

When using the antibody it is note worthy to keep in mind that the antiserum can be contaminated by bacteria. The manufacturer supplies the antibody with a preserver substance such as sodium azide (NaN_3). If there is a bacteria contamination it will be wise to discard the antibody and not use it, because the antiserum will create significant amount of background staining.

A good antibody should have high affinity (binding strength) for its antigen. Therefore, they are not washed off the sections during the immunocytochemical staining. In addition, the concentration of the antibody is important to get clean appeareance of the tissue. A high dilution means decreased population of antibodies is present in the used antiserum and that unwanted antibodies are removed. Therefore, unwanted reactions are discarded. A low dilution means; increased population of antibodies is present in the used antiserum. The optimum dilution is required to get a better binding and staining, also to get low background staining (maksimum signal to noise ratio). High dilutions of the antibody are advantageous because they allow the total use of the available antibodies. If monoclonal antibodies are used in the immunocytochemical procedure, since the primary antibody is specific to the antigen, it is likely that unwanted reactions are absent, and therefore, the dilution in many cases becomes less important. Polyclonal antibodies come in as whole serum or as purified antibodies and an antibody concentration is given as μg/ml. The initial dilution of the monoclonal antibodies obtained via the hybridoma technology should be between 1:5-1:100. The secondary antibody used in the immunocytochemistry should be used at the optimum dilution such as; 1:200. The dilution propotion differ according to the type of tissue used and according to the tissue sections either paraffin or frozen section. The dilution is usually made commonly by phosphate buffered saline (PBS) solution. In order to obtain the working dilution (for example; 1:1000) the stock antibody is removed from the refrigerator, first 1:100 diluted solution is prepared than in the second step the solution is further diluted 10 times and 1:1000 working solution is prepared. The incubation period of the antibody with the tissue section in the antiserum can provide important information for the binding charecteristics of the antibody. Frequently, the incubation period of the antibody with the sections at 37 ^{0}C is between 30 min. to 2 hour, at room temperature is 1-6 hour, at +4 ^{0}C is 6-24 hour.

The methods where the antibody is used other than immunocytochemsitry (ICC) are; immunfluorescence (IF), western blot (WB), immunoblot (IB), immunoprecipitation (IP) and ELISA.

6. Control application of the antibody

It is important to make control studies in the immunocytochemistry procedures to make sure that the staining is specific. When the antibody targets a certain protein, the antibody should be unique to that particular protein. Before performing the study, other related protein family in the cell that may have homologous peptide sequence should be evaluated by identifing their aminoasid sequence. Because these proteins may cross react with the antibody and therefore, nonspecific binding and background staining may occur. The antibody specificity is best determined by immunoblot and or immunoprecipitation. The specificity of the method is best determined by preabsorption/preincubation control (Swaab et al., 1977; Willingham., 1999), negative control, replacing the primary antibody with serum, and a positive control, using the antibody with cells known to contain the protein. In the preabsorption control, the antibody is mixed with the desired antigen (protein or peptide) before it is delivered to the sections. The goal of this process is to eliminate the binding of the antibody to the target protein. Therefore, when the antibody-protein complex at appropriate concentrations is applied to the tissue section, and if there is no staining then we can conclude that the antibody used is specific to that particular protein. We should also remember that the antibody can bind to any epitope of a protein that has the right conformation. Therefore, the competitive blocking experiment may produce a false data because, many peptides may bind nonspecifically to formalin-fixed tissues and can increase the immunostaining. Another test for antibody sensitivity and specificity is performing immunocytochemistry on negative control.

7. Conclusion

Immunocytochemistry is a technique that is used for staining cells or tissues using antibodies against target antigens or proteins. It is common to use unlabelled first antibody also referred to as the primary antibody, and then use the second antibody also referred to as secondary antibody directed against the first (anti-IgG). This secondary antibody is conjugated either with enzymes for colorimetric reactions, or fluorochromes, or gold particles (for EM) to visulaize the location of the antigen.

In order to get best of the immunocytochemical technique the antibody used should have specificity, ability to reach and bind to the antigen. On the other hand, in the target antigen or protein epitope alterations can occur, and therefore weak staining will be visualized. The antibodies should be carefully selected. Search for specific antibodies and related protocols from the literture is necessary. Since monoclonal antibodies recognize single epitope they have greater specificty. However, polyclonal antibodies recognize multiple epitopes, and have increased risk of binding non-specific molecules with similar epitope. Thus, significant staining variations could occur according to different batches. Once receiving the antibody before using it in the immunocytochemical procedure, it should be tested at higher and lower concentrations in order to define the best dilution to study.

8. References

Dalçik, C.; Yildirim, G.K. & Dalçik, H. (2009). The effects of ethanol on insulin-like growth factor-I immunoreactive neurons in the central nervous system. Saudi Medical Journal, Vol.30, No.8, 995-1000, ISSN: 0379-5284

Dalçik, H.; Yardımoğlu, M.; Vural, B.; Dalçik C.; Filiz, S.; Gonca, S.; Köktürk, S. & Ceylan, S. (2001). Expression of insulin-like growth factor in the placenta of intrauterine growth-retarded human fetuses. Acta Histochemica, Vol.103, No.2, 195-207, ISSN: 0065-1281

He, Y.; Honnen, W. J.; Krachmarov, C.P.; Burkhart, M.; Kayman, S.C.; Corvalan, J. & Pinter, A. (2002). Efficient isolation of noval human monoclonal antibodies with neutralizing activity against HIV-1 from transgenic mice expressing human Ig loci. Journal of Immunology, Vol.169, No.1, 595-605, ISSN: 0022-1767

Hoogenboom, H.R.; & Chames, P. (2000). Natural designer binding sites made by phage display technology. Immunology Today, Vol.21, No.8, 371-378, ISSN: 0167-5699

Leduc, E.H. & Connolly, J.M. (1955). Studies of antibody production. A method for the histochemical demonstration of specific antibody and its application to a study of the hyperimmune rabbit. Journal of Experimental Medicine, Vol.102, No.1, 49-50, ISSN:0022-1007

Milstein, C.; Galfre, G.; Secher, D.S.; & Springer, T. (1979). Monoclonal antibodies and cell surface antigens. Cell Biology International Reports, Vol.3, No.1, 1-16, ISSN: 0309-1651

Milstein, C. (1980). Monoclonal antibodies. Scientific American, Vol.243, No.4, 66-74, ISSN: 0036-8733

Proske, D.; Blank, M.; Buhmann, R. & Resch, A. (2005) Aptamers-basic research, drug development, and clinical applications. Applied Microbiology and Biotechnology, Vol. 69, No.4, 367-374, ISSN: 0175-7598

Ritter, M.A. (1986). Raising and testing monoclonal antibodies for immunocytochemistry. In: Immunocytochemstry, Modern Methods and Applications, J.M. Polak & S. Van Noorden, (Ed.), 13-25, John Wright and Sons, Bristol, ISBN: 978-0-89603-813-4

Swaab, D.F.; Pool, C.W. & Van Leeuwen, F.W. (1977). Can specificity ever be proven in immunocytochemical staining? The Journal Histochemistry & Cytochemistry, Vol.25, No.5, 388–390, ISSN:0022-1554

Tas, A.; Arat, S. & Dalcik, H. (2007). Comparative investigation of spontaneous and retinoik acid-induced differentiation of embryonic stem cells. Clinical Dermatology: retinoids and other treatment, Vol.23, No.2, 24-26, ISSN: 1879-1131

Tomlinson, I. & Holliger, P. (2000). Methods for generating multivalent and bispecific antibody fragments. Methods In Enzymology, 326, 461-479, ISSN: 0076-6879

Willingham, M.C. (1999) Conditional epitopes: is your antibody always specific? The Journal Histochemistry & Cytochemistry, Vol.47, No.10, 1233-1236, ISSN: 0022-1554

5

Recent Progress in Noncompetitive Hapten Immunoassays: A Review

Mingtao Fan[1] and Jiang He[2]
[1]*College of Food Science and Engineering, Northwest A&F University,*
[2]*College of Life Science, Hunan University of Arts and Science,*
China P.R.

1. Introduction

Detection of small molecules (hapten molecules), such as food contaminants, environmental pollutants, disease factors, drugs and so on, is an area with great significance. Immunoassay, as a simple, rapid and cost-effective detection system, is widely used for the detection of low molecular weight analytes in varied matrix. However, the number of commercial available immunoassay kits for hapten molecules is still limited, this might be partly due to the poor performance such as sensitivity of these immunoassays which can not fulfill the actual requirement. Traditionally, detection of small molecules in solution must employ competitive immunoassay formats, either with immobilized antibody or with immobilized coating conjugate. However, theoretical study has demonstrated that competitive immunoassays are inferior to noncompetitive immunoassays in terms of sensitivity, precision, kinetics and working range of analyte (Jackson and Ekins, 1986). Hence, there is a trend now to develop noncompetitive immunoassay systems for hapten molecules assay.

Although sandwich immunoassay is widely applied to noncompetitive assay of antigen concentration, it has a fundamental limit that the antigen to be measured must be large enough to have at least two epitopes to be captured. Hence, it can not be used to measure low molecular weight compounds. During the last two decades, researchers in related fields have made great efforts to overcome this drawback, and some novel immunoassay systems that can noncompetitively detect small molecules have been established. These new formats are based on chemical modification to the analytes, unconventional antibodies (anti-idiotype antibody, anti-metatype antibody or antibody fragment), special separation steps (capillary electrophoresis, affinity column or membrane), or other elegant tricks. In this paper, an overview of the recent development and application of these elegant approaches was presented.

2. Noncompetitive immunoassays based on chemical modification to the analytes

2.1 Ishikawa's method

As stated, it is due to hapten molecules with just one epitope that can not simultaneously be bound by two antibodies, so traditional sandwich immunoassay can not be implemented. An ingenious scheme, developed by Ishikawa's group in 1990, introduces a molecule of biotin into the analyte prior to the assay, and then the biotinylated analyte can simultaneously be bound by anti-analyte antibody and avidin. According to this principle, a novel and sensitivity noncompetitive (two-site) enzyme immunoassay for haptens is described and exemplified by L-Thyroxine (T4) detection initially (Tanaka et al. 1990). The principle of this method is outlined in Figure 1. Briefly, samples (or standards) are firstly biotinylated, and then these biotinylated samples are purified by anti-analyte antibody coated polystyrene balls. Secondly, the samples are mixed with labeled anti-analyte antibody and transferred onto a solid phase coated with avidin. Finally, signal can be directly measured after a washing step. The signal strength is directly proportional to the analyte concentration as traditional noncompetitive immunoassay.

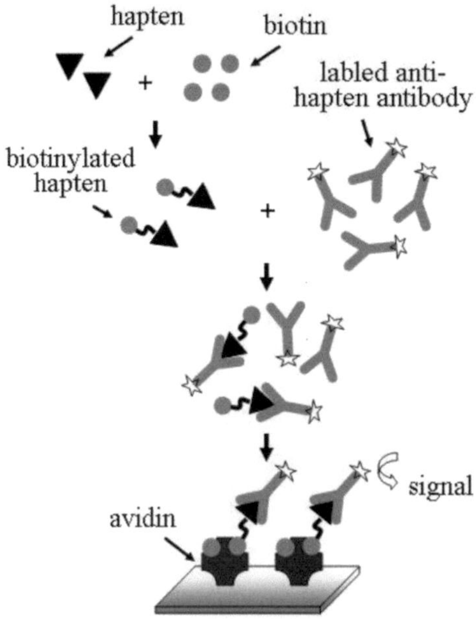

Fig. 1. Principle of Ishikawa's method. Step 1: biotinylation of the analyte and affinity purification; Step 2: formation of antibody/antigen complex; Step 3: captured by immobilized avidin.

This method has been successfully applied to several analytes bearing a primary amino group, which can react with the biotin. The sensitivity of this technique is nearly 10 attomoles for small peptides like angiotensin I (Ishikawa et al. 1990) or arginine vasopressin (Hashida et al. 1991). However, the biotinylated reaction and affinity purification procedures are complicated and time consuming. Due to this weakness, this method is not popularized to the detection of other hapten molecules.

2.2 Solid phase immobilized epitope-immunoassay (SPIE-IA)

The solid phase immobilized epitope-immunoassay (SPIE-IA) method for measuring hapten molecules in noncompetitive format was firstly described by Pradelles et al. in 1994 and its principle is outlined in Figure 2. The method involves a critical cross-linking and epitope release step. Briefly, the analyte is firstly captured by solid phase immobilized antibody, and then covalently cross-linked with corresponding antibody molecules by homobifunctional reagent (glutaraldehyde or disuccinimidyl suberate). After a dissociating treatment (HCl or methanol) of the analyte/antibody complex to release the epitope from the antibody binding site, the presence of analyte on the solid phase is detected using a labeled antibody. This procedure involves the use of excess reagents (capture and tracer antibodies) to insure the efficiency of analyte/antibody complexes formation and generates calibration curves in which the signal is directly proportional to the analyte concentration, as in conventional sandwich immunoassays (Pradelles et al. 1994).

Like Ishikawa's method, SPIE-IA was firstly applied to the measurement of analytes bearing a primary amino group excluded from the epitope site. But a prederivatization step before performing the SPIE-IA can be applied to introduce amino group to molecules that lack this function group. As in the work of Etienne et al.(1996), in order to develop a SPIE-IA system for thyroliberin, the thytoliberin and biological samples were prederivatized by diazotized 2(4-amino-phenyl)ethyl amine, and then operated as the initial approach. With the aim of extending the procedure to haptens devoid of an amine moiety, new strategies of cross-linking have been developed. For example, in another work of Etienne et al. (1995) the capacity of thyroxine to be photoactivated directly by UV treatment was utilized and resulting in covalent cross-linking with its binding protein. SPIE-IA involving direct cross-linking of hapten by UV irradiation was then named as Photo-SPIE-IA, and it was also successfully applied to the detection of 17ß-estradiol (Buscarlet et al. 1999). More recently, new SPIE-IA procedure (named SPIE-Rad) using the free radical species produced by the Fenton-like reactions during the cross-linking step has been developed and also successfully applied to the detection of 17β-estradiol (Buscarlet et al. 2001)

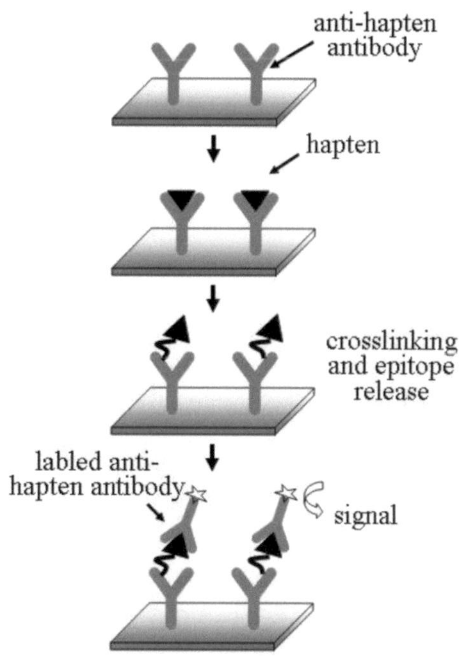

Fig. 2. Principle of SPIE-IA. Step 1: immobilization of analyte on an anti-analyte antibody-coated plate; Step 2: cross-linking of the analyte with solid-phase antibody and then dissociate the analyte/antibody complex; Step 3: analyte is revealed by labeled antibody.

As for the sensitivity, good results have been obtained by this method for various small analytes (<2500 Da) (Pradelles et al., 1994; Volland et al., 1994; Ezan et al., 1995; Volland et al., 1999). In each case, the sensitivity was enhanced (10–300 folds) when compared to the corresponding competitive immunoassay performed using the same antibody. For example, limit of detection of angiotensin II is close to 0.5 and 45pM with SPIE-IA and competitive assay, respectively (Volland et al., 1999). Moreover, the precision of SPIE-IA is equivalent to that of conventional immunoassays. Although, satisfactory performance was obtained from the published SPIE-IA, it is still very difficult to be applied to every hapten molecules.The UV irradiation approach appears limit due to the need for an irradiation device and the limited number of available irradiation wavelengths. In addition, UV irradiation has some deleterious effects by degrading the immunological complex more or less rapidly, depending on the wavelength and the energy used. The SPIE-Rad protocol might work efficiently to assay different molecules, but lots of parameters need to be optimized.

3. Noncompetitive immunoassays based on unconventional antibody

3.1 Anti-idiotype antibody based noncompetitive immunoassay (Idiometric assay)

Anti-idiotype antibody (AId or Ab2), refering to an antibody raised against the variable region of an original antibody (Ab1), is one of the most important concepts on "immune network theory". Jerne et al. (1982) have classified anti-idiotype antibodies according to the location of the idiotype recognization in their early report, and two main types of anti-idiotype antibodies have been distinguished: alphatype (α-AId) and betatype (β-AId). By definition, α-AId recognizes an epitope within the framework of the variable region of the primary antibody, but is not sensitive to the presence or absence of the analyte at the binding site. While, β-AId compete with the antigen for an epitope at the binding site， i.e. the former will bind to the primary antibody in the presence of the antigen, whereas the latter will not. In addition, the α-AId will not bind to the β-AId/Ab1 complex because of steric hindrance. Based on the properties of α-AId and β-AId, Barnard and Kohen (1990) described an original noncompetitive immunoassay (denoted "idiometric assay") for small molecules in 1990, and typified by the measurement of estradiol in serum. The general principle of this method is outlined in Figure 3. After coating wells with anti-hapten antibody (Ab1), test samples (or standard analytes) are added, and then β-AId is used to block the binding sites that are not occupied by hapten molecules on the Ab1. At last, by adding labeled α-AId, the amount of haptens can be detected.

Since the establishment of this method, Barnard's group has applied it to the detection of estradiol (Barnard & Kohen, 1990; Barnard et al., 1991; Mares et al., 1995) and progesterone (Barnard et al., 1995a) in serum and Estrone-3 Glucuronide (Barnard et al., 1995b) in urine， Kobayashi et al. have applied it to the detection of UDCA 7-NAG (a bile acid metabolite) (Kobayashi et al., 2000; Kobayashi et al., 2003 a) and 11-deoxycortisol (Kobayashi et al. 2003 b). More recently, Niwa et al. (2009) established a noncompetitive-type ELISA for cortisol based on idiometric assay model. This assay had an approximately threefold higher sensitivity (detection limit: 90 pg cortisol) than a competitive ELISA using the same anti-cortisol antibody and had practical specificity for providing reasonable determination of normal urinary cortisol levels.

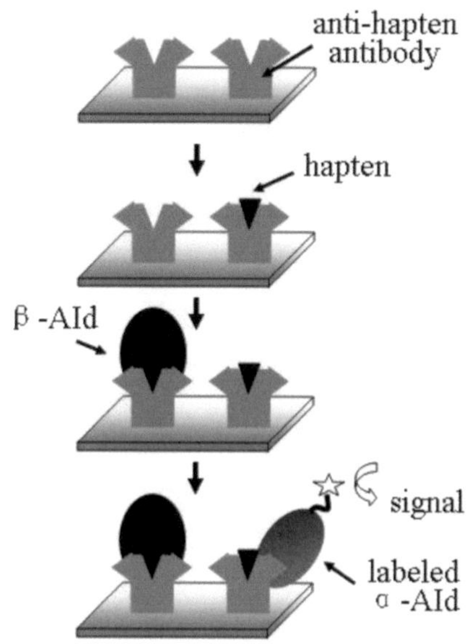

Fig. 3. Principle of idiometric assay. Step 1: capture the analyte by anti-analyte antibody (Ab1)-coated plate; Step 2: blocking the unoccupied binding site on Ab1 by β-AId; Step 3: analyte is revealed labeled α-AId.

Although good performances have been obtained, the idiometric assay requires the sequential addition of the three antibody reagents (capture antibody, α-AId and β-AId). The production of capture antibody is nothing special, but the production and identification of anti-idiotype antibody are very complicated. The difficulties inherent in anti-idiotype antibody generation, especially in producing an array of different AId, from which the most suited ones could be chosen, largely restrict the application of idiometric assay.

3.2 Anti-metatype antibody based noncompetitive immunoassay

The term "metatype" was initially proposed by Voss et al. (1988) for the immunological definition of the liganded active site to distinguish it from idiotype (non-liganded). Therefore, the anti-metatype antibodies recognize the antibody/antigen complex but exhibit very low or no affinity for the antibody or the antigen alone. This remarkable property was cleverly utilized by Self et al. (1994) to develop noncompetitive immunoassay for small molecules, and exemplified by digoxin detection. In this case, the analyte is captured by the specific antibody, and formatted a second epitope for anti-metatype antibody reorganization. If labeled anti-metatype antibody is applied, a detect signal directly proportional to the analyte concentration can be obtained (Figure 4).

Self et al. (1994) showed that this noncompetitive immunoassay system provides a high-performance assay for digoxin in serum samples, being conveniently simple (immobilized primary antibody binds digoxin and then labeled secondary antibody so that when excess unbound label is washed away the immunometric readout reflects the digoxin concentration), rapid (incubation time 1-10 min), sensitive (detection limit 30 ng/L), precise (3-4% within-run CV, 1-8% total CV), and free from interference from digoxin-like immunoreactive factors. In addition, satisfactory results were also obtained by Towbin et al.

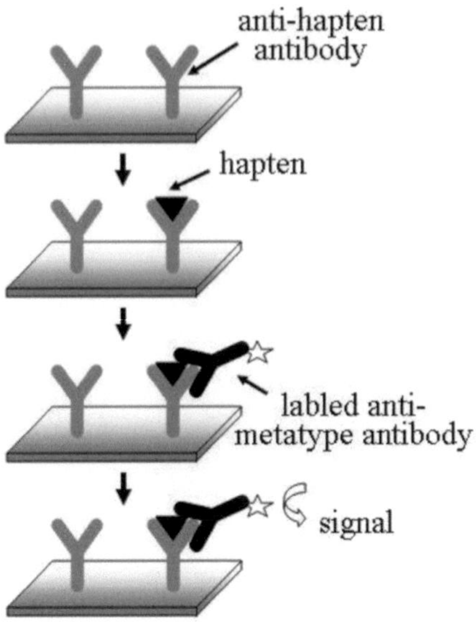

Fig. 4. Principle of anti-metatype antibody based noncompetitive immunoassay. Step 1: capture the analyte by anti-analyte antibody (Ab1)-coated plate; Step 2: labeled anti-metatpye antibody was added for specifically bind to the analyte/antibody complex; Step 3: signal formation.

(1995) and Nagata et al. (1999) for the detection of haptens angiotensin II and microcystin respectively. However, as per the idiometric assay, the difficulties of anti-metatype antibody production are main barriers for the widely application of this method. Such an anti-metatype antibody can seldom be generated by the conventional antibody production methods, consequently, the information now available concerning the strategy for its production is very limited.

3.3 Open sandwich immunoassay (OSIA)

A new kind of noncompetitive immunoassay, named "open sandwich immunoassay (OSIA)", has been described by Ueda et al. in 1996, and successfully applied to detect hen egg lysozyme (Ueda et al. 1996). This assay is based on the observation that for some antibodies, the association of separated VH and VL chains from the variable domain of antibody is strongly favored in the presence of antigen. The general principle of this method is outlined in Figure 5. Briefly, the VL fragment was immobilized on plate, and then the VL plate was incubated with VH fragment together with antigen. If labeled VH fragment is used, the signal can be directly measured after a washing step; otherwise a labeled second antibody is applied. After Ueda's work, this method was extended to hapten molecules detection and new formats such as homogeneous assays were also developed. These homogeneous assay systems are either based on enzymatic complementation (Ueda et al. 2003) or resonance energy transfer (fluorescence (Ueda et al. 1999; Arai et al. 2000; Wei et al. 2006) or bioluminescence (Arai et al. 2001)).

Up to now, the OSIA system has been successfully applied in the detection of hapten molecules such as gibberellin (Lee et al., 2008), benzaldehyde (Shirasu et al., 2009), zearalenone

(Suzuki et al., 2007), 4-hydroxy-3-nitrophenylacetyl (Yokozeki et al. 2002), the carboxyl-terminal peptide of human osteocalcin (BGP) (Lim et al. 2007), bisphenol A (Sakata et al. 2009), and 11-Deoxycortisol (Ihara et al., 2009). This novel immunoassay system could be done in a shorter period of time than using a conventional sandwich assay, due to the omission of an incubation/washing cycle. And in the homogeneous format OSIA, the washing steps can even completely be avoided. Also, the assay was found to be compatible with traditional competitive immunoassay, similar or a lower detection limit as well as wider working range could be attained. However, the preparation of the reagents is complex and time consuming (production and selection of monoclonal antibodies; preparation of DNA fragments encoding VH and VL, construction, production and purification of fusion proteins). Moreover, the principle of this assay, based on differential interactions between separated VH and VL chains in the presence or absence of the antigen, requires a strong antibody selection since only some antibodies meet these criteria. For these reasons, it is still difficult to apply this method widely at present.

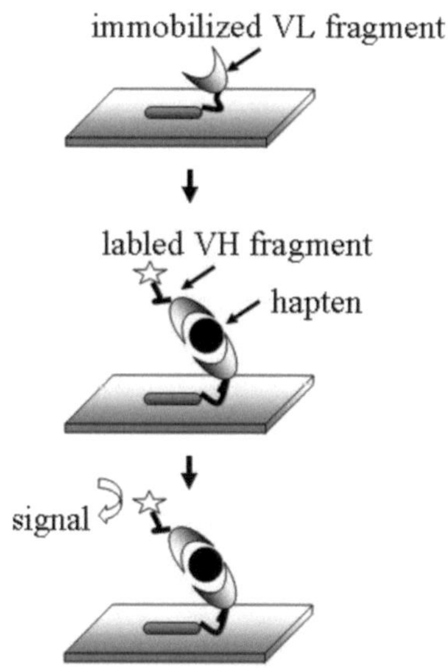

Fig. 5. Principle of the initial OSIA. Step 1: immobilization of VL fragment; Step 2: incubation of labeled VH fragment with analyte; Step 3: measurement of signal.

4. Noncompetitive immunoassay based on special separation steps

4.1 Flow injection immunoassay (FIIA)

Flow injection analysis (FIA) is developed in response to the need for automated analysis, in which a sample is injected into a continuous flow of a carrier solution mixed with other continuously flowing solutions before reaching a detector. FIA-based immunoassays were developed in the early 1980s. After that, Freytag et al. (1984) applied this flow injection immunoassay (FIIA) system to noncompetitive detection of hapten molecules and also exemplified by digoxin detection. This novel approach involves reaction of the sample with an excess of enzyme-labeled antibody. And this mixture is then passed through an affinity column containing immobilized antigen. The excess unreacted antibody is captured in the column and only Ab-Ag complex is contained in eluate. At last, substrate is added and the concentration of the original antigen is related to the signal produced by the product of the enzymatic reaction (Figure 6). As it is developed, chemiluminescence and fluorescence labels are also applied to the FIIA system for further simplifying its operation. In addition, delicate modifications of this approach have been proposed by other groups. For example, Rabbany et al. used an activated porous membrane to immobilize antibody, then the labeled antigen was applied to saturating the binding sites. After which, target analyte is passed through the membrane, and the displacement of labeled antigen is monitored downstream.

This method has been successfully applied to the detection of numerous hapten molecules and satisfactory sensitivity have been obtained: 10pM for thyroxine (Arefyev et al., 1990); 20 pM for α-(difluoromethyl) ornithine (Gunaratna et al., 1993) and 40pM for digoxigenin (Lovgren et al., 1997). The most inviting advantage of this method is the ability to realize automatic detection. For example, a semi-automated flow-through immunoassay system consisting of an amperometric immunosensor and reagent flow arrangements has been developed by Wilkins's group (Abdel-Hamid et al., 1998). However, during the development of different assays, numerous parameters must be optimized. For instance, the column capacity, related to the immobilized analyte density and column dimensions, must allow removal of all excess free labeled antibody; and the residence time of the sample in the column, related to the flow rate and column dimensions, should be suitable for total binding of free labeled antibody but not so long as to risk the dissociation of the antibody and immobilized analyte (Volland et al., 2004).

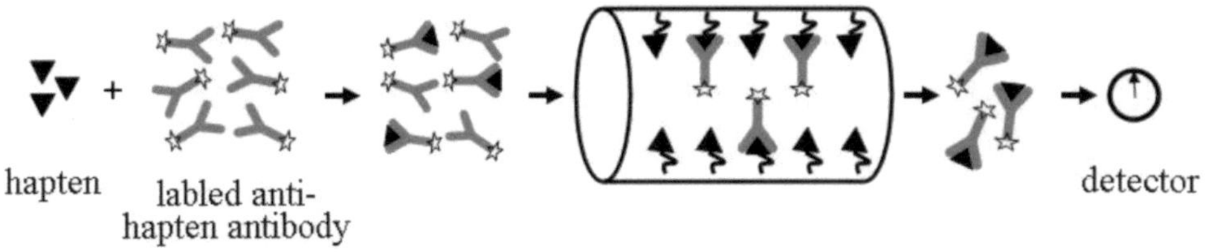

Fig. 6. Principle of FIIA. Step 1: Analyte is mixed with excess labeled antibody; Step 2: Separation of complex antibodies from free antibodies; Step 3: Signal measurement.

4.2 Affinity probe capillary electrophoresis (APCE)

A similar method, which relies on the high separating effect of capillary electrophoresis, was recently emerged for noncompetitive immunoassay of hapten molecules. This method is named as affinity probe capillary electrophoresis (APCE) and first described by Shimura and Karger (1994) using capillary isoelectric focusing for human growth hormone assay and further applied to small analytes by Hafner et al. (2000). In this case, the immune complex is separated from excess labeled antibody since the complexation of the antigen with the antibody induces small changes of electrophoretic behavior of the labeled antibody.

The performances of this method are good, with a limit of detection of 5 pM for human growth hormone (Shimura and Karger, 1994) and 10pM for digoxin (Hafner et al. 2000), respectively. However, the correct separation appears difficult for some neutral analytes and the use of a charged analogue of the analyte is necessary to differentiate the complex from the unbound antibody. In addition, this technique only analyzes one sample at a time, thus limiting its potential application to routine assay of numerous samples (Volland et al., 2004).

5. Noncompetitive immunoassays based on other principles

More recently, Tozzi's group (2002) have invented a new noncompetitive immunoassay system with blocking of unoccupied specific binding sites on sold phase and exemplified this strategy by cortisol detection. This method is based on the use of a "blocking reagent", which is able to bind to antibody sites not occupied by the analyte in a stronger way than the analyte itself. When a labeled analyte is added it substitutes the analyte in the antibody complex, but not the blocking reagent. Generally, this method includes the following steps: initially the analyte is bound to a specific binding partner, after which the unoccupied binding sites of the binding partner are inactivated by a blocker. Then, the bound analyte is dissociated from the binding partner and replaced by a labeled marker, after which the bound labeled marker is determined (Figure 7). The signal from the bound labeled marker is directly proportional to the initial amount of analyte in the sample.

As to the performance of this method, results of Anfossi et al. (2002) showed that the 3σ limit of detection (LOD, 0.2 nmol/L) obtained by the above method was 10 times lower than that obtained by the corresponding ELISA, and recoveries in saliva samples ranged from 80 to 120%. And recently, Acharya and Dhar (2008) have developed a novel broad-specific noncompetitive immunoassay for aflatoxins detection by the blocking & replacement method. In this work, an AFB1-protein conjugate was used as blocking reagent, and the limit of detection was 0.1 μg/L. Generally speaking, the key point of this method is to find an effective blocking reagent.

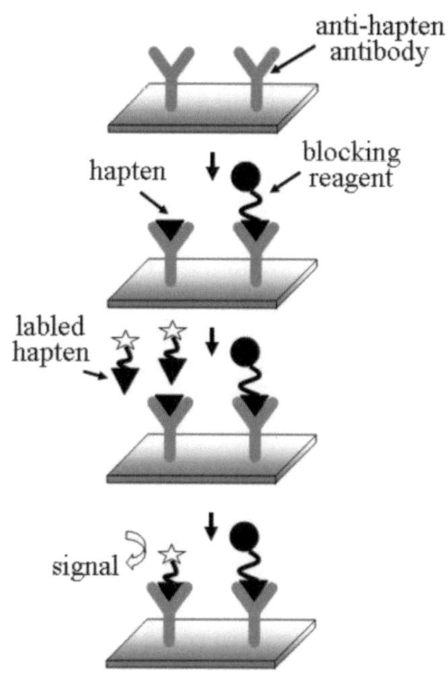

Fig. 7. Principle of the blocking & replacement method. Step 1: the analyte is bound to a immobilized specific binding partner and then blocking reagent is applied to inactivate the unoccupied binding sites; Step 2: labeled analyte is applied to replace the bound analyte; Step 3: signal is developed and measured.

6. Conclusion

From the literature and research finding above and others not concluded in this paper, a question might be put forward, which method is the best one that can be widely applied to most of the hapten molecules, it is not easy to answer this question, the answer may depend on what kind of analyte measured and the purpose of the analysis, but a comparative analysis of these methods could help researchers to choose the most suitable one for their purpose.

The methods based on chemical modification to the analytes need an extra step to immobilize the target, apart from this step, it is very complicated and hard to standardize, whether it will work as we expect is a problem. X-ray analysis of hapten-antibody complexes have indicated that small molecules are buried deep in the binding site with surface areas of 200-400 $Å^2$ (Arevalo et al., 1993; Xu et al., 1999). Hence, although a model study have indicated that molecules constituting of two epitopes of only 300 $Å^2$ separated by a spacer as small as 5 Å may be bound by two antibodies (Quinton et al., 2010), a optimization process of the spacer between biotin and analytes in Ishikawa's method or between captured antibody and analytes in SPIE-IA is required. Otherwise, these methods may not work as per the principle.

As to the methods based on unconventional antibody, the difficulties to prepare and identify these unusual antibodies are limitations for their wide application. However, once these specific antibodies have been prepared, these methods can easily be standardized. The recently developed phage display technology is a powerful and reliable technique for generating antibodies, and has successfully been applied to the preparation of anti-idiotype antibody (Goletz et al., 2002; Zhang et al., 2002; Raats et al., 2003;Coelho et al., 2004; Tometta et al., 2007) and anti-metatype antibody (Kim et al., 2009; Kim et al., 2010). Also, a phage display technology-based "split-Fv system" has recently been developed to rapidly evaluate and select antibody variable region (Fv) fragments that are suitable to open sandwich immunoassay (Aburatani et al., 2003). Along with the further improvement of the phage display technology, it will become the conventional method for the preparation of these unconventional antibodies, and then promote the wide application of idiometric assay, anti-metatype antibody based immunoassay and open-sandwich immunoassay in the future.

The methods based on special separation steps need extra equipment, but their greatest strength is the easiness to realize automatic detection. Along with the development of relevant separation technologies, this kind of method will become the choice for developing immunosensor to hapten molecules detection.

As to the method based on "blocking reagent", although various blocking reagents have been utilized in the published work, the available information concerning the strategy for their selection and the principle for their work is very limited. Hence, this type of noncompetitive immunoassay appears hard to wide application, unless a general preparation method and the inherent principle of the blocking reagent was available.

7. References

Abdel-Hamid, I., Atanasov, P., Ghindilis, A.L., Wilkins, E., 1998. Development of a flow-through immunoassay system. Sens. Actuators, B. 49(3): 202–210.

Aburatani, T., Sakamoto, K., Masuda, K., Nishi, K., Ohkawa, H., Nagamune, T., Ueda, H., 2003. A general method to select antibody fragments suitable for noncompetitive detection of monovalent antigens. Anal. Chem. 75(16): 4057–4064.

Acharya, D., Dhar, T.K., 2008. A novel broad-specific noncompetitive immunoassay and its application in the determination of total aflatoxins. Anal. Chim. Acta. 630(1): 82–90.

Anfossi, L., Tozzi, C., Giovannoli, C., Baggiani, C., Giraudi, G., 2002. Development of a noncompetitive immunoassay for cortisol and its application to the analysis of saliva. Anal. Chim. Acta. 468(2): 315–321.

Arai, R., Ueda, H., Tsumoto, K., Mahoney, W.C., Kumagai, I., Nagamune, T., 2000. Fluorolabeling of antibody variable domains with green fluorescent protein variants: application to an energy transfer-based homogeneous immunoassay. Protein Eng. Des. Sel. 13(5): 369–376.

Arai, R., Nakagawa, H., Tsumoto, K., Mahoney, W., Kumagai, I., Ueda, H., 2001. Demonstration of a homogeneous noncompetitive immunoassay based on bioluminescence resonance energy transfer. Anal. Biochem. 289(1): 77–81.

Arefyev, A., Vlasenko, S.B., Eremin, A.P., Osipov, A.P., Egorov, A.M., 1990. Flow-injection enzyme immunoassay of haptens with enhanced chemiluminescence detection. Anal. Chim. Acta 237(2): 285–289.

Arevalo, J.H., Taussig, M.J., Wilson, I.A., 1993. Molecular basis of cross-reactivity and the limits of antibody-antigen complementarity. Nature. 365(6449): 859–863.

Barnard, G., Kohen, F., 1990. Idiometric assay: noncompetitive immunoassay for small molecules typified by the measurement of estradiol in serum. Clin. Chem. 36(11): 1945–1950.

Barnard, G., Karsiliyan, H., Kohen, F., 1991. Idiometric assay, the 3rd way - a noncompetitive immunoassay for small molecules. Am J Obstet Gynecol, 165(2): 1997–2000.

Barnard, G., Osher, J., Lichter, S., Gayer, B., Deboever, J., Limor, R., 1995a. The measurement of progesterone in serum by a noncompetitive idiometric assay. Steroids. 60(12): 824–829.

Barnard, G., Amirzaltsman, Y., Lichter, S., Gayer, B., Kohen, F., 1995b. The measurement of estrone-3 glucuronide in urine by noncompetitive idiometric assay. J Steroid Biochem. 55(1): 107–114.

Buscarlet, L., Grassi, J., Créminon, C., Pradelles, P., 1999. Cross-linking of 17 β-estradiol to monoclonal antibodies by direct UV irradiation: application to an enzyme immunometric assay. Anal. Chem. 71(5): 1002–1008.

Buscarlet, L., Volland, H., Dupret-Carruel, J., Jolivet, M., Grassi, J., Creminon, C., Taran, F., Pradelles, P., 2001. Use of free radical chemistry in an immunometric assay for 17 beta-estradiol. Clin. Chem. 47(1): 102–109.

Coelho, M., Gauthier, P., Pugniere, M., Roquet, F., Pelegrin, A., Navarro-Teulon, I., 2004. Isolation and characterisation of a human anti-idiotypic scFv used as a surrogate tumour antigen to elicit an anti-HER-2/neu humoral response in mice. Br. J. Cancer. 90(10): 2032–2041.

Etienne, E., Creminon, C., Lamourette, P., Grassi, J., Pradelles, P., 1995. Enzyme immunometric assay for L-thyroxine using direct ultraviolet irradiation. Anal. Biochem. 225(1): 34–38.

Etienne, E., Creminon, C., Grassi, J., Grouselle, D., Roland, J., Pradelles, P., 1996. Enzyme immunometric assay of thyroliberin (TRH). J. Immunol. Methods. 198(1): 79–85.

Ezan, E., Tarrade, T., Cazenave, C., Ardouin, T., Genet, R., Grassi, J., Grognet, J.M., Pradelles, P., 1995. Immunometric assay of BN 52080, a heptapeptide C-terminal analogue of sorbin. Peptides 16(3): 449–455.

Freytag, J.W., Lau, H.P., Wadsley, J.J., 1984. Affinity-column-mediated immunoenzymometric assays: influence of affinity-column ligand and valency of antibody-enzyme conjugates. Clin. Chem. 30(9): 1494–1498.

Goletz, S., Christensen, P.A., Kristensen, P., Blohm, D., Tomlinson, I., Winter, G., Karsten, U., 2002. Selection of large diversities of antiidiotypic antibody fragments by phage display. J. Mol. Biol. 315(5): 1087–1097.

Gunaratna, P.C., Wilson, G.S., 1993. Noncompetitive flow injection immunoassay for a hapten, α-(difluoromethyl) ornithine. Anal. Chem. 65(9): 1152–1157.

Hafner, F.T., Kautz, R.A., Iverson, B.L., Tim, R.C., Karger, B.L., 2000. Noncompetitive immunoassay of small analytes at the femtomolar level by affinity probe capillary electrophoresis: direct analysis of digoxin using a uniform-labeled scFv immunoreagent. Anal. Chem. 72(23): 5779–5786.

Hashida, S., Tanaka, K., Yamamoto, N., Uno, T., Yamaguchi, K., Ishikawa, E., 1991. Novel and sensitive noncompetitive enzyme immunoassay (hetero-two-site enzyme immunoassay) for arginine vasopressin in plasma. Anal. Lett. 24(7): 1109–1123.

Ihara, M., Suzuki, T., Kobayashi, N., Goto, J., Ueda, H., 2009. Open-sandwich enzyme immunoassay for one-step noncompetitive detection of corticosteroid 11-deoxycortisol. Anal Chem. 81(20): 8298–8304.

Ishikawa, E., Tanaka, K., Hashida, S., 1990. Novel and sensitive noncompetitive (two-site) immunoassay for haptens with emphasis on peptides. Clin. Biochem. 23(5): 445–453.

Jackson, T.M., Ekins, R.P., 1986. Theoretical limitations on immunoassay sensitivity. J. Immunol. Methods. 87(1): 13–20.

Jerne, N.K., Roland, J., Cazenave, P.A., 1982. Recurrent idiotypes and internal images. EMBO J. 1(2):243–247.

Kim, H.J., Ahn, K.C., González-Techera, A., González-Sapienza, G.G., Gee, S.J., Hammocka, B.D., 2009. Magnetic bead-based phage anti-immunocomplex assay (PHAIA) for the detection of the urinary biomarker 3-phenoxybenzoic acid to assess human exposure to pyrethroid insecticides. Anal. Biochem. 386(1): 45–52.

Kim, H.J., Rossotti, M.A., Ahn, K.C., González-Sapienza, G.G., Gee, S.J., Musker, R., Hammock, B.D., 2010. Development of a noncompetitive phage anti-immunocomplex assay for brominated diphenyl ether 47. Anal. Biochem. 401(1): 38–46.

Kobayashi, N., Oiwa, H., Kubota, K., Sakoda, S., Goto, J., 2000. Monoclonal antibodies generated against an affinity-labeled immune complex of an anti-bile acid metabolite antibody: an approach to noncompetitive hapten immunoassays based on anti-idiotype or anti-metatype antibodies. J. Immunol. Methods. 245(1-2): 95–108.

Kobayashi, N., Kubota, K., Oiwa, H., Goto, J., Niwa, T., Kobayashi, K., 2003a. Idiotype-antiidiotype-based noncompetitive enzyme-linked immunosorbent assay of ursodeoxycholic acid 7-N-acetylglucosaminides in human urine with subfemtomole range sensitivity. J. Immunol. Methods. 272(1-2): 1–10.

Kobayashi, N., Shibusawa, K., Kubota, K., Hasegawa, N., Sun, P., Niwa, T., 2003b. Monoclonal anti-idiotype antibodies recognizing the variable high-affinity antibody against 11-deoxycortisol. Production, characterization and application to a sensitive noncompetitive immunoassay. J. Immunol. Methods. 274(1-2): 63–75.

Kobayashi, N., Iwakami, K., Kotoshiba, S., Niwa, T., Kato, Y., Mano, N., 2006. Immunoenzymometric assay for a small molecule, 11-deoxycortisol, with attomole-range sensitivity employing a scFv-enzyme fusion protein and anti-idiotype antibodies. Anal. Chem. 78(7): 2244–2253.

Lee, Y., Asami, T., Yamaguchi, I., Ueda, H., Suzuki, Y., 2008. A new gibberellin detection system in living cells based on antibody V-H/V-L interaction. Biochem. Biophys. Res. Commun. 376(1): 134–138.

Lim, S.L., Ichinose, H., Shinoda, T., Ueda, H., 2007. Noncompetitive detection of low molecular weight peptides by open sandwich immunoassay. Anal. Chem. 79(16): 6193-6200.

Lovgren, U., Kronkvist, K., Backstrom, B., Edholm, L.E., Johansson, G., 1997. Design of non-competitive flow injection enzyme immunoassays for determination of haptens. Application to digoxigenin. J. Immunol. Methods. 208(2): 159–168.

Mares, A., Deboever, J., Osher, J., Quiroga, S., Barnard, G., Kohen, F., 1995. A direct noncompetitive idiometric enzyme-Immunoassay for serum estradiol. J. Immunol. Methods. 181(1): 83–90.

Nagata, S., Tsutsumi, T., Yoshida, F., Ueno, Y., 1999. A new type sandwich immunoassay for microcystin: production of monoclonal antibodies specific to the immune complex formed by microcystin and an anti-microcystin monoclonal antibody. Nat. Toxins. 7(2): 49–55.

Niwa, T., Kobayashi, T., Sun, P., Goto, J., Oyama, H., Kobayashi, N., 2009. An enzyme-linked immunometric assay for cortisol based on idiotype-anti-idiotype reactions. Anal. Chim. Acta. 638(1): 94–100.

Pradelles, P., Grassi, J., Creminon, C., Boutten, B., Mamas, S., 1994. Immunometric assay of low molecular weight haptens containing primary amino groups. Anal. Chem. 66(1): 16–22.

Quinton, J., Charruault, L., Nevers, M.C., Volland, H., Dognon, J.P., Cre´minon, C., Taran, F., 2010. Toward the limits of sandwich immunoassay of very low molecular weight molecules. Anal. Chem. 82(6): 2536–2540.

Raats, J., van Bree, N., van Woezik, J., Pruijn, G., 2003. Generating recombinant anti-idiotypic antibodies for the detection of haptens in solution. J. Immunoassay Immunochem. 24(2): 115–146.

Sakata, T., Ihara, M., Makino, I., Miyahara, Y., Ueda, H., 2009. Open sandwich-based immuno-transistor for label-free and noncompetitive detection of low molecular weight antigen. Anal Chem. 81(18): 7532–7537.

Self, C.H., Dessi, J.L., Winger, L.A., 1994. High-performance assays of small molecules: enhanced sensitivity, rapidity, and convenience demonstrated with a noncompetitive immunometric anti-immune complex assay system for digoxin. Clin. Chem. 40(11): 2035–2041.

Shirasu, N., Onodera, T., Nagatomo, K., Shimohigashi, Y., Toko, K., Matsumoto, K., 2009. Noncompetitive immunodetection of benzaldehyde by open sandwich ELISA. Anal. Sci. 25(9): 1095–1100.

Shimura, K., Karger, B.L., 1994. Affinity probe capillary electrophoresis: Analysis of recombinant human growth hormone with a fluorescent-labeled antibody fragment. Anal. Chem. 66(1): 9–15.

Suzuki, T., Munakata, Y., Morita, K., Shinoda, T., Ueda, H., 2007. Sensitive detection of estrogenic mycotoxin zearalenone by open sandwich immunoassay. Anal. Sci. 23(1): 65–70.

Tanaka, K., Kohno, T., Hashida, S., Ishikawa, E., 1990. Novel and sensitive noncompetitive (two-site) enzyme immunoassay for haptens with amino groups. J. Clin. Lab. Anal. 4(3): 208-212.

Tometta, M., Fisher, D., O'Neil, K., Geng, D., Schantz, A., Brigham-Burke, M., Lombardo, D., Fink, D., Knight, D., Sweet, R., Tsui, P., 2007. Isolation of human anti-idiotypic antibodies by phage display for clinical immune response assays. J. Immunol. Methods. 328(1-2): 34–44.

Towbin, H., Motz, J., Oroszlan, P., Zingel, O., 1995. Sandwich immunoassay for the hapten angiotensin II. A novel assay principle based on antibodies against immune complexes. J. Immunol. Methods. 181(2): 167–176.

Tozzi, C., Anfossi, L., Baggiani, C., Giraudi, G., 2002. New immunochemical approach to low-molecular-mass analytes determination. Talanta 57(1): 203–212.

Ueda, H., Tsumoto, K., Kubota, K., Suzuki, E., Nagamune, T., Nishimura, H., 1996. Open sandwich ELISA: A novel immunoassay based on the interchain interaction of antibody variable region. Nat. Biotechnol. 14(12): 1714–1718.

Ueda, H., Kubota, K., Wang, Y., Tsumoto, K., Mahoney, W., Kumagai, I., 1999. Homogeneous noncompetitive immunoassay based on the energy transfer between fluorolabeled antibody variable domains (open sandwich fluoroimmunoassay). Biotechniques 27(4): 738–742.

Ueda, H., Yokozeki, T., Arai, R., Tsumoto, K., Kumagai, I., Nagamune, T., 2003. An optimized homogeneous noncompetitive immunoassay based on the antigen-driven enzymatic complementation. J. Immunol. Methods. 279(1-2): 209–218.

Volland, H., Vulliez, L.N., Mamas, S., Grassi, J., Creminon, C., Ezan, E., Pradelles, P., 1994. Enzyme immunometric assay for leukotriene C4. J. Immunol. Methods 175(1): 97–105.

Volland, H., Pradelles, P., Ronco, P., Azizi, M., Simon, D., Creminon, C., Grassi, J., 1999. A solid-phase immobilized epitope immunoassay (SPIE-IA) permitting very sensitive and specific measurement of angiotensin II in plasma. J. Immunol. Methods 228(1-2): 37–47.

Volland, H., Pradelles, P., Taran, F., Buscarlet, L., Creminon, C., 2004. Recent developments for SPIE-IA, a new sandwich immunoassay format for very small molecules. J. Pharm. Biomed. Anal. 34(4): 737–752

Voss Jr., E.W., Miklasz, S.D., Petrossian, A., Dombrink-Kurtzman, M.A., 1988. Polyclonal antibodies specific for liganded active site (metatype) of a high affinity anti-hapten monoclonal antibody. Mol. Immunol. 25(8): 751–759.

Wei, O.D., Lee, M., Yu, X., Lee, E.K., Seong, G.H., Choo, J., 2006. Development of an open sandwich fluoroimmunoassay based on fluorescence resonance energy transfer. Anal. Biochem. 358(1): 31–37.

Xu, J., Deng, Q., Chen, J., Houk, K.N., Bartek, J., Hilvert, D., Wilson, I.A., 1999. Evolution of shape complementarity and catalytic efficiency from a primordial antibody template. Science. 286(5448): 2345–2348.

Yokozeki, T., Ueda, H., Arai, R., Mahoney, W., Nagamune, T., 2002. A homogeneous noncompetitive immunoassay for the detection of small haptens. Anal. Chem. 74(11): 2500–2504.

Zhang, W., Frank, M.B., Reichlin, M., 2002. Production and characterization of human monoclonal anti-idiotype antibodies to anti-dsDNA antibodies. Lupus 11(6): 362–369.

6

Immunoassay in Toxicology Diagnosis

Ewa Gomolka
Jagiellonian University, Medical College, Department of Toxicology and Environmental Disease, Laboratory of Analytical Toxicology and Drug Monitoring, Krakow, Poland

1. Introduction

Immunoassays are useful laboratory methods for clinical and forensic toxicology diagnostics. The methods are fast, sensitive, accurate and let determine poisons concentrations in different kinds of biological fluids. There are blood and urine or alternative: saliva, sweat and hair. The choice of the sample depends on the purpose of analysis. In acute poisoning the blood or serum poison concentration is important, but when the diagnosis is made more than 24 h post-ingestion, the urine sample should be collected and analyzed. The urine toxicology analysis let confirm the poison's ingestion. Alternative samples are more and more common, but they are used usually in forensic toxicology, in medical toxicology the results of hair or sweat determination are useful in the history of drugs overdosing or abusing research. Toxicological diagnostics is consequence, enables to make distinction if observed patient's symptoms are correlated to poisoning or other reasons. Fast quantitative measurement is important for poisoning confirmation, prognosis and decisions about specific treatment. All emergency rooms and poisoning treatment centers should have full access to such diagnostics. The most important immunoassay determinations are: the most often (e.g. alcohol, benzodiazepines, drugs of abuse) and the decision making ones (e.g. acetaminophen, phenobarbital, digoxin, amanitines).

The attributes of toxicological tests differ depending on the purpose of determination. When poisoning cause is to be identified - specificity is most important, to distinguish the poison from other exogenous or endogenous substances. When screening is made to check patient's abstinence - sensitivity of the test is most important. The sensitivity is usually set as a cut-off value - the concentration, above which the result is reported as positive. When test is used for therapeutic drug monitoring (TDM) purpose - test precision is most important, to follow changes of drug concentration in a narrow, therapeutic range. The most important points of toxicological tests are presented in Table 1.

The immunoassay method should be selected after consulting it's advantages and disadvantages. The choice of immunoassays is wide. There are simple qualitative cassettes or bar-tests and more accurate apparatus for semi-quantitative and quantitative measurements. They differ with sensitivity, cut-off values, kind of tested sample, result interpretation. All of them have some limitations and sometimes need confirmation by reference method.

Test	Indication	Preselection or Suspicion	Probability	Test Attribute	Example
Poisoning Diagnostics	Finding a Poisoning Cause	No	Moderate	Specificity	Looking for a poison
Screening	Checking	Yes	Low	Sensitivity	Abstinence Checking
Therapeutic Drug Monitoring	Monitoring Concentration Changes	Yes	High	Precision	Therapy

Table 1. Toxicological tests and their attributes

Aspects concerned with pre-analytical, analytical and post-analytical phases are important in a diagnosis process. The laboratory staff must know all immunoassay limitations and watch out for false results. The immunoassay methods became commonplace and toxicology diagnostics is performed in laboratories, where there are no reference and confirmation methods. Low cost and easy-automation encourage to start toxicology determinations in many clinical laboratories. Sometimes there are no toxicology specialists in the laboratories. Sometimes results interpretation cannot be performed properly without confirmation.

There are some analytical problems connected with toxicology diagnosis, especially when it is performed by immunoassay. One of the most important problem is result verification and creation result report. Immunoassay is not quite reliable. Analyst is responsible for false results, even when the misinterpretation is caused by limitation of immunoassay method. Some proceedings should be considered, for example, what to do when the result is doubtful and how to perform confirmation.

Most toxicology laboratories have access to reference methods and can confirm uncertain results. Analyst performing toxicology immunoassay in general laboratory should know all limitations of used method, know how to prepare reports, when to confirm results, how to store and transport sample for confirmation.

2. Immunoassays in toxicology

Acute intoxicated patient should be diagnosed as soon as possible. The biological samples are usually collected from poisoned patients in emergency rooms or in toxicology department. The collection time should be noted, because it influences the result interpretation. Medical laboratories usually use automatic immunoanalysers with methods: enzyme multiplied immunoassay technique (EMIT), fluorescent polarization immunoassay (FPIA), microparticle enzyme immunoassay (MEIA), cloned enzyme donor immunoassay (CEDIA), kinetic interaction of microparticles in solution (KIMS). They are useful for blood or serum therapeutic drug monitoring. They are also useful for serum and urine determinations of ethanol, medicines, drugs of abuse and other toxins. Other common immunoassays are cassette or strip rapid tests. Such tests are dedicated for urine or saliva determinations of drugs of abuse (amphetamines, barbiturates, benzodiazepines, cannabnoids, cocaine, ecstasy, methadone, opiates, phencyclidine, tricyclic antidepressants). Their sensitivity is usually set on a level appropriate for workers control or abstinence control of patients participating in drug substitution treatment.

Immunoassay methods do not enable to determine all poisons, drugs or biomarkers of exposition. In order to measure all of them, other methods are needed. There are spectrometry methods: ultraviolet/visible spectrometry, atomic absorption spectrometry (AAS); chromatography methods: thin layer chromatography (TLC), gas chromatography (GC), high performance liquid chromatography (HPLC) and chemical tests. They are complements to immunoassays, and they are used for confirmation positive immunoassay results. Examples of methods and determined substances in clinical and forensic toxicology are showed in Table 2.

Immunoassay	Chromatography	Spectrometry
RIA CEDIA EIA / EMIT ELISA FIA / FPIA, DELFIA KIMS MEIA POC (casette/strip rapid test)	TLC, HPTLC GC HPLC GC/MS LC/MS	Colorimetry Spectrophotometry UV Spectrophotometry VIS Spectrophotometry IR AAS AES
Amanitine Ethanol Drugs of abuse Therapeutic Drug Monitoring	Ethanol and other alcohols (Methanol, Ethylene Glycol, Izopropanol) Solvents Drugs of abuse Designer Drugs Medicines and metabolites Natural Toxins (e.g. Atropine, Scopolamine) Pesticides	Solvents Alcohols Medicines Pesticides Metals and Metalloids Biomarkers of exposition to chemical compounds (Carboxyhemoglobine COHb, Methemoglobine MetHb, Blood Acetycholinoesteraze activity AChE)

RIA - Radioimmunoassay, CEDIA - Cloned Enzyme Donor Immunoassay, EIA / EMIT - Enzyme-Immunoassay / Enzyme Multiplied Immunoassay Technique, ELISA - Enzyme-Linked Immunosorbent Assay, FIA / FPIA - Fluorescence Immunoassay / Fluorescence Polarization Immunoassay, KIMS - Kinetic Interaction of Microparticles in Solution, MEIA - Microparticle Enzyme Immunoassay, POC - Point of Care
TLC, HPTLC - Thin Layer Chromatography, GC - Gas Chromatography, HPLC - High Performance Liquid Chromatography, GC/MS - Gas Chromatography with Mass Spectrometry, LC/MS - Liquid Chromatography with Mass Spectrometry

Table 2. Examples of laboratory methods and determined substances in toxicology

3. Pre-analytical aspects of immunoassay in toxicology

3.1 Collecting samples for immunoassay in toxicology diagnostics

Homogenous methods, in which a sample is added to mixture of reagents, immunological reaction goes between analyte and antibody in homogenous solution, (e.g. EMIT, FPIA, CEDIA, KIMS). They are useful for diagnostics of acute poisoned patients performed in blood, serum and urine. Heterogeneous methods, in which a sample is added to reaction vessels with antibodies immobilized on the bottom (e.g. ELISA) can be used for forensic determinations of drugs in previous mentioned samples and in alternative samples (hair, sweat, saliva) after sample preparation. Rapid tests are usually dedicated for urine or saliva determinations. Drugs of abuse and some medicines are measured qualitative or semi-quantitative; TDM needs quantitative determinations (Table 3).

Qualitative tests (cassettes, strips)	Semi-quantitative tests	Quantitative tests
Urine or Saliva	Urine or Serum	Serum or Whole Blood
Acetaminophen Amphetamine Barbiturates Benzodiazepines Buprenorphine Cannabinoids (THC) Cocaine EDDP (methadone metabolite) Ecstasy (MDMA) Ethanol LSD Methadone Metamphetamine Morphine Opiates Phencyclidine (PCP) Tramal Tricyclic antidepressants	Amanitine Amphetamine/Metamphetam ine Barbiturates Benzodiazepines Cannabinoids (THC) Cocaine Ecstasy (MDMA) LSD Tricyclic antidepressants	Acetaminophen Amikacine Carbamazepine Cyclosporine Digoxin Ethanol Gentamycine Lidocaine Phenobarbital Phenytoine Salicylates Teophylline Tobramycine Tricyclic antidepressants Valproic Acid Vancomycine

Table 3. Some substances determined by qualitative, semi-quantitative and quantitative immunoassays in different biological samples

Each kind of sample has a different detection time. The pharmacokinetics parameters of analyzed substances also influence the results interpretation. The detection window is the period of time when the substance can be detected in the sample. Blood, serum and saliva have a narrow detection window (1-24 h). Urine has a wider one (2-7 days) and hair has the widest one (several months). The detection window depends on the kind of collected sample, the kind of determined drug and the frequency of the drug ingestion (Table 4). Sometimes the detection time is prolonged, for example marihuana metabolites can be detected in urine for one to three weeks, depending on the size and frequency of marihuana ingestion. When the sample is collected in time out of the detection window (too early or too late) the result is negative in spite of visible patients symptoms connected with drug ingestion.

Collecting samples for therapeutic drug monitoring is different. Before starting TDM, the steady state of drug should be achieved. Depending on drug biological half time, the steady state is achieved in time from several hours to several days (Table 11).

Substance	Detection window	
	Occasionally	Chronic
Amphetamine derivatives	48 h	Up to 7 days
Barbiturates	Short acting: 24 h Long acting: 2-3 weeks	
Benzodiazepines	Short acting: 24 h Long acting : 3 days	
Cocaine	2-3 days	Up to 7 days
Methadone	2-3 days	1-2 weeks
Opiates	2-3 days	Up to 7 days
THC (Marijuana)	once: to 4 days occasionally: to 10 days passive exposition: not detected	4-6 weeks

Table 4. Urine detection window for drugs of abuse

The assay tests and reagents are dedicated for different kinds of samples. Every kind of sample contains specific background and it is not allowed to analyze serum using urine or saliva tests and vice versa.

The choice of the kind of sample depends on the purpose of determination. Blood and serum samples contain ingested substances. Urine samples contain mainly their metabolites. When acute poisoning diagnostics is made, the blood or serum samples are chosen. The blood and serum concentrations correlate with ingested dose of drug, correlate with poisoning symptoms and sometimes, give information about predictable poisoning effects. The diagnosis is useful when the physician wants to make decision about specific treatment with antidote or extracorporeal elimination. But when the time from drug ingestion to diagnosis is too long (longer than five biological halftimes) collecting the blood for poisoning diagnosis can be useless. The blood or serum results will be negative and urine sample should be collected. The urine concentration does not correlate the poisoning symptoms and does not have prediction value. But the urine presence of drug and it's metabolites confirms the patient has ingested the drug and the observed symptoms are connected with the poisoning.

Urine samples are collected when abstinence of patients and workers is analyzed. When the abstinence is checked, the urine adulteration or cheating is possible. Table 5 presents some possible urine cheating and ways of their recognition. Probably there are not all possible ways of cheating samples, that's why the best way of avoiding cheating is control the patients during collecting urine samples. Despite some disadvantages, the urine is quite good kind of sample for abstinence control. Urine is collected non-invasive and has a wide detection window. The most important differences between urine and blood (serum) samples are showed in Table 6.

Tests for urine determination of drugs of abuse and medicines have sensitivity on different levels. Laboratories should have tests with different cut-off levels. Cut-off levels in acute poisoning diagnosis should be the lowest, in patients of substitution therapy can be higher, in workers control can be the highest. High cut-off level means lower sensitivity and reduction of questionable or "false positive" results (caused by substances present in food or supplements). Cut-off concentrations dedicated for qualitative urine and saliva drugs of abuse determination are showed in Table 7 and Table 8.

Adulteration	Recognition
Dilution	Evaluation of urine colour, temperature, creatinine concentration, density
Glutaric alhehyde	Urine strip test
Nitrates	Urine adulteration strip test
Soup, Bleach etc.	Evaluation of pH, look (foam), colour, fragrance
Acid, Alkali	Evaluation of pH, Urine adulteration strip test
Peroxides	Urine adulteration strip test
Vitamines, medicines	Chromatography analysis

Table 5. Urine adulteration and it's recognition

	Urine	Blood (serum)
Detection window	Wide (days, weeks)	Narrow (hours)
Concentration levels	High	Low
Analytes	Metabolites and toxins	Toxins
Correlation to intoxication symptoms	No	Yes
Cut off values	High	Low
pH influence	Yes	Yes
Adulteration risk	Yes	No
Cost	Low	High

Table 6. Differences between urine and blood (serum) samples

Analyte	cut-off concentration ng/ml
Amphetamine	1000, 500
Barbiturates	300
Benzodiazepines	200, 300
Cannabinoids (THC)	50
Cocaine	300
Extasy (MDMA)	1000, 500
Methadone	300
Methamphetamine	1000, 500
Opiates	300, 2000
Phencyclidyne (PCP)	25
Tricyclic antidepressants	1000

Table 7. Cut-off concentrations dedicated for urine drugs of abuse determination by immunoassay

Analyte	cut-off concentration ng/ml	detection window
Amphetamine	50	10 min - 72 h
Cannabinoids (THC)	12	10 min - 72 h
Cocaine	20	10 min - 24 h
Methamphetamine	50	10 min - 72 h
Opiates	40	10 min - 72 h
Phencyclidyne (PCP)	10	10 min - 72 h

Table 8. Cut-off concentrations and detection windows for saliva drugs of abuse determination by immunoassay

4. Analytical aspects of immunoassay in toxicology

Immunoassay reagents are usually dedicated to closed auto-sampler systems, in which analyst's errors are minimized. Anyway, some aspects are important, and no automatic system can solve them. For example in situation of acute poisoned patient, when the measured poison concentration is out of calibration range. The necessity of sample dilution cause some manual manipulation. The diluent is usually distilled water or saline. Sometimes reagent kit contains a special diluent dedicated for a sample and analyte.

Cassette or strip immunotests are performed manually. Cassette is a device in which a sample is dropped into a special reservoir, strip is usually drown into liquid sample. Usually they are simple to do, but some errors are possible when the laboratory staff is unqualified. Too much or too little sample amount used for the test, inadequate reading time and invalid reading are possible. The factors can cause false test result. When the laboratory staff is experienced the error factors are reduced. Both cassette and strip contain a control bar placed in a distance from reading area. The control bar is getting colour when sample reaches the control area. It shows if the test is performed correctly. Laboratory staff must realize, the control bar is not a quality control. Quality assurance is realized only when controls samples (with known concentrations of measured substances) are analyzed.

4.1 Quality controls in immunoassay in toxicology

All laboratories are obliged to keep internal and external quality control (EQC) systems. They are dedicated for the analyzed kind of sample (biological matrix), and the proper levels of analytes concentrations. Usually three levels of internal quality controls (low, medium and high) are performed. They let asses precision of the method on tree controlled levels. Precision is graphical illustrated as control charts (for example Levey-Jennings charts).

External quality controls let verify accuracy of the method. Laboratories participating in EQC programme get certificate of quality assurance which is necessary in laboratory accreditation procedure.

4.2 Immunoassay sensitivity and specificity

Sensitivity reflects the lowest concentration giving positive result. Some immunoassays are useful for determination of a group of substances, for example benzodiazepines, barbiturates, amphetamines or opiates. The substances derivatives influence the results depending on their sensitivity. Some of the derivatives have higher, and some have lower sensitivity, so they produce different results. For example 3,4-methylendioxymethamphetamine (MDMA) usually is not detected in immunoassays dedicated to amphetamines measurements because MDMA cross react when it's concentration in sample is nine times higher than amphetamine. We name the result "false negative".

Specificity is a property enabling to distinguish measured drug from other compounds. The drug metabolites, it's derivatives and other unknown compounds can interact the immunoassay reagents and produce elevated or "false positive" results. For example in therapeutic drug monitoring the physician is interested in the blood or serum concentration of the drug ingested by patient. But the result usually is elevated by the drug metabolites.

Another example of interfering substance is codeine, which cross react in morphine and opiates tests and produce positive results. We name them "false positive". The interfering substances can be medicines, supplements, drug components or endogenous compounds (for example DLIS - digoxin like immunoreactive substances). Other examples of interferences in immunoassays are showed in Table 9.

Analyzed compound or group	Interfering substance
Amphetamines	Fenfluramine, Ephedrine
Opiates (Morphine)	Codeine
Benzodiazepines	Oxaprozin
Cannabinoids	Niflumic Acid
Tricyclic Antidepressants	Carbamazepine, Phenotiazines
Digoxin	DLIS

Table 9. Examples of interferences in immunoassay

The positive results should be confirmed by specific chromatography methods. The confirmation is obligatory in forensic toxicology. Forensic toxicology use immunoassays as initial screening analysis; all the positive results must be confirmed by chromatography methods coupled with mass detection (GC/MS, LC/MS). The confirmation is optional in clinical toxicology. Most clinical laboratories do not have an access to time consuming and expensive chromatography methods.

5. Comparison of immunoassay and chromatography methods in some toxicology diagnostics

5.1 Alcohol determination

Alcohol is the most often abused drug and one of the most often cause of hospitalization in toxicology departments. Immunological methods became common in measurement of ethanol about 20 years ago. The methods are automated and reliable, they replaced manual Widmark's method and are comparable to gas chromatography and breathanalysis. Their sensitivity is usually less than 0,05 g/l. Interferences of non consumable alcohols (e.g. methanol, ethylene glycol, isopropanol) is insignificant (less than 1 %). The only interfering alcohol can be n-butanol (18,5 %), but n-butanol is rather not present in any home products, and intoxication with the compound is hardly likely.

Correlation of alcohol results obtained by immunoassay and gas chromatography is acceptable. The only disadvantage of alcohol immunoassay test is a relatively narrow linearity range. In heavy drinkers blood the alcohol concentration can be higher than 3 g/l. When the linearity range is not wide enough, the sample dilution is needed.

The attention should be drown to collection of blood sample for alcohol measurement. Blood can be contaminated when alcohol solution is used during draw blood.

Interpretation of blood and serum alcohol concentration should mind that serum alcohol concentration is higher than whole blood alcohol concentration. The difference is correlated to the concentration and can be calculated: blood alcohol concentration = serum alcohol concentration / 1,2. When serum ethanol concentration is not higher than 1 g/l, the difference is up to 0,16 g/l. Higher ethanol concentration implicate higher difference between serum and blood concentration.

5.2 Benzodiazepines determination

Benzodiazepines are often abused drugs. They are also used as date-rape drugs. The immunological methods measure concentration of benzodiazepines as a group of substances with basic shell of benzodiazepines rings. There are several known benzodiazepines and their metabolites that influence the immunoassay dedicated to this group of drugs. The interpretation of serum or urine benzodiazepines concentration result is not easy. They have different doses, applications, acting times and therapeutic ranges. Their affinities to immunoassay reagent are also different. In addition the immunoassay result is correlated to the sum of ingested benzodiazepines and their metabolites in biological sample. Some drugs (e.g. lorazepam, chlordiazepoxide) cross react with low efficiency. Other cross react with high efficiency (e.g. diazepam, oxazepam, alprazolam). The comparison of EMIT and HPLC showed, that benzodiazepines can produce results higher (alprazolam, diazepam), equel (nordiazepam) and lower (estazolam) than real drug concentration.

5.3 Carbamazepine determination

Carbamazepine is a common anticonvulsive drug. There are indications to measure carbamazepine concentration during therapy. Therapeutic drug monitoring make therapy safe, reduce risk of too low or too high dosage, and side effects. Immunoassay enables to control the blood carbamazepine concentration.

Comparison of EMIT and HPLC method showed differences in measured carbamazepine concentrations. EMIT results reflects sum of carbamazepine and it's metabolites concentrations. HPLC is a method enabling to separate carbamazepine and it's metabolites and quantify them separately.

The carbamazepine results interpretation should provide for the method. Anyway immunoassay is a good method for therapeutic drug monitoring, when the blood samples are collected in a drug stationary phase and minimum drug concentration is measured (blood sample is collected before ingestion a dose).

Carbamazepine determination by immunoassay in acute poisoning does not let distinguish intoxication phase. Carbamazepine metabolites concentrations are low in absorption phase, later the equilibrium between drug and their metabolites concentration is established. Finally, in the elimination phase, carbamazepine metabolites concentrations are the highest. Immunoassays do not let demonstrate the changes, the result just reflects the sum of drug and it's metabolites.

5.4 Tricyclic antidepressants determination

Tricyclic antidepressants (TCA) are the group of drugs used in psychiatric treatment. They are often abused by patients addicted to drugs of abuse. The drugs are toxic in elevated doses, but the correlation between serum TCA concentration and poisoning symptoms is rather weak. The serum TCA concentrations can be referred to ingested dose when analyst knows the name of drug. Table 11 shows variations among TCA therapeutic ranges.

The TCA concentration measured by immunoassay can be influenced by other substances. For example carbamazepine and some phenotiazines are common medicines elevating TCA immunoassay results (Table 9).

Substance	Volume of distribution	Elimination half-life
Amphetamines	3-33 L/kg	10-30 h Excretion pH dependent
Barbiturates (Phenobarbital)	0,7-1,5 L/kg	48-288 h
Benzodiazepines (Diazepam)	0,5-5 L/kg	20-40 h
Cannabis	10 L/kg	20-30 h
Cocaine	1,2-1,9 L/kg	0,5-1,5 h
LSD		3-4 h
Methadone	1-8 L/kg	15-55 h
Opiates (Morphine)	3-4 L/kg	1-7 h

Table 10. Pharmacokinetics parameters of drugs of abuse

6. Post-analytical aspects of immunoassay in toxicology

When the results are obtained, the staff must decide how to prepare the report. Quantitative blood and serum results seem to be easy interpreted. But for full interpretation the physician needs to know some more information, for example elimination half-life, volume of distribution. The pharmacokinetic parameters of some drugs of abuse are showed in Table 10. Other data also influence the results interpretation: poisoning circumstances, information about the dose of ingested compound, time from exposition or ingestion to collecting blood or urine sample, treatment started in ambulance.

Drug	Time to achieve steady state	Elimination half life	Protein binding	Usual sampling time	Usual therapeutic range
Acetaminophen	5-20 h	1-4 h	20-30 %	1 h	10-20 mg/l
Carbamazepine	2-6 days	6-25 h	65-80 %	before next dose (Cmin)	4-11 mg/l
Ethosuximide	5-15 days	30-60 h (adults) 20-56 h (children)	0 %	before next dose (Cmin)	40-100 mg/l
Phenobarbital	10-25 days (adults and adolescents) 8-20 days (infants and children)	50-150 h (adults) 40-130 h (infants and children) 60-200 h (newborns)	50 %	before next dose (Cmin)	10-40 mg/l
Phenytoin	2-6 h	20-30 h	92 %	before next dose (Cmin)	10-20 mg/l (adults and children) 6-14 mg/l (neonates)
Primidone	2-4 days	4-22 h	≤ 35 %	before next dose (Cmin)	5-15 mg/l
Valproic Acid	2-4 days	6-17 h (adults) 5-15 h (infants and children) 15-60 h (newborns)	90 %	before next dose (Cmin)	50-100 mg/l
Theophylline	2-3 days (adults) 1-2 days (children) 1-5 days (infants) 120 h (newborns)	3-12 h (adults non smokers) 4 h (adults smokers) 2-10 h (children) 3-14 h (infants) 24-30 h (newborns)	55-65 %	4-6 h after infusion beginning (max) 4-8 h after oral administration (Cmax) before infusion or next dose (Cmin)	8-20 mg/l (asthma) 6-11 mg/l (neonatal apnea)
Digoxin	5-7 days	20-50 h (adults) 12-24 h (children) 18-33 h (infants) 35-42 h (neonates)	20 %	8-24 h after administration	0,8-2,0 ng/ml

Drug	Time to achieve steady state	Elimination half life	Protein binding	Usual sampling time	Usual therapeutic range
Tricyclic Antidepressants					
Amitryptyline	3-8 days	17-40 h	90 %	before next dose (Cmin)	120-250 ng/ml
Clomipramine	7-14 days	19-37 h	90-98 %		Up to 700 ng/ml
Desipramine	2,5-11 days	12-54 h	75-90 %		125-300 ng/ml
Doxepin	9 days	8-25 h	68-85 %		150-250 ng/ml
Imipramine	2-5 days	6-28 h	63-96 %		150-250 ng/ml
Nortryptyline	4-20 days	18-56 h	87-93 %		50-150 ng/ml
Trimipramine	3-8 days	16-40 h	93-97 %		70-250 ng/ml
Antibiotics					
Amikacin	2,5-15 h (adults < 30 years) 7,5-75 h (adults > 30 years) 2,5-12,5 h (children) 10-45 h (neonates)	0,5-3 h (adults < 30 years) 1,5-15 h (adults > 30 years) 0,5-2,5 h (children) 2-9 h (neonates)	≤ 10 %	0,5-1 h after infusion (Cmax) before next dose (Cmin)	20-30 mg/l (Cmax) < 5 mg/l (Cmin)
Gentamycin					5-10 mg/l (Cmax) < 2 mg/l (Cmin)
Netilmicin					5-12 mg/l (Cmax) < 3 mg/l (Cmin)
Tobramycin					5-10 mg/l (Cmax) < 2 mg/l (Cmin)
Streptomycin	10-15 h	2-3 h	30 %	1-2 h after IM dose (Cmax) before next dose (Cmin)	15-40 mg/l (Cmax) < 5 mg/l (Cmin)
Vancomycin	20-30 h	4-10 h (adults) 2-3 h (children) 6-10 h (neonates)	30-55 %	1 h after infusion (Cmax) before next dose (Cmin)	20-40 mg/l (Cmax) 5-10 mg/l (Cmin)

Table 11. Pharmacokinetics parameters and chosen information about drugs determined for TDM purposes

Positive result usually means, that the patient ingested the determined substance. But positive result can be also generated by interfering compounds. The interferences are described in chapter about immunoassay tests specificity. When the time from substance ingestion and collecting blood sample is too short (shorter than time, when maximum blood concentration is observed), the determination should be performed once again. The second sampling time should be set correct, in order to reflect the tissues concentration. For example after digoxin ingestion the drug is distributed to muscle tissues and the time of setting equilibrium between serum and tissues is 6-8 h. Blood digoxin concentration measured earlier does not correlate the medical symptoms and severity of poisoning.

Negative result usually means, that the patient didn't ingest the determined substance. But negative result are obtained when the sample is collected in wrong time, too early or too late (out of the detection window). Negative result is obtained, when the method is not sensitive enough or cut-off concentration is too high. The next reason of negative result is limited sensitivity of the test for the measured analyte, when the immunoassay is dedicated for the group of substances. For example diazepam and nordiazepam are detected in benzodiazepine immunotests in low concentration. But lorazepam and chlordiazepoxide are detected in benzodiazepine test in high concentration, sometimes three or four times higher than diazepam. The implication of that can be false negative result, despite drug ingestion and observed poisoning symptoms.

So the result report should contain not only the determination result but information about assay method, its sensitivity (limit of detection, cut-off value), specificity (some most important interfering compounds) and recommendation for confirmation of the result.

7. Summary

Immunoassay methods are commonly used in laboratories. Toxicologists use them as useful screening in medical diagnosis of acute poisoning, checking abstinence, forensic purposes and therapeutic drug monitoring. When short time of analysis is important, immunoassay is the best method.

Despite many positive points, the method has some disadvantages. Commonness and low costs encourage performing the assays by unqualified staff. Forensic toxicologists always perform results confirmation. In medical laboratories the confirmation is not obligatory, and usually is not necessary, when interpretation is made in correlation to patient's condition.

Reporting rapid test result is sometimes dicey, there is a risk of false result. That is why the result report must contain information about the immunological methods used to perform determination, it's sensitivity, specificity and possible interferences.

This would keep confidence in laboratory results.

8. References

[1] AGSA Drug of Abuse Testing Guidelines (2006). www.cscq.ch/agsa

[2] Alapat P.M., Zimmerman J.L.: Toxicology in the critical care unit. Chest. 2008, 133, 1006-1013.

[3] Apollonio L.G., Whittall I.R., Pianca D.J., Kyd J.M., Maher W.A.: Matrix effect and cross-reactivity of select amphetamine-type substances, designer analogues, and putrefactive amines using the Bio-Quant direct ELISA presumptive assays for amphetamine and methamphetamine. J Anal Toxicol. 2007, 31, 208-213.
[4] Baselt R.C.: Disposition of Toxic Drugs and Chemicals in Man. Sixth Edition. Biomedical Publications Foster City, California USA, 2002.
[5] Boettcher M., Haenseler E., Hoke C., et. al.: Precision and comparability of Abuscreen OnLine assays for drugs of abuse screening in urine on Hitachi 917 with other immunochemical tests and with GC/MS. Clin. Lab. 2000, 46, 49-52.
[6] Brent J., Wallace K, Burkhart K., Phillips S., Donovan J.: Critical Care Toxicology. Diagnosis and Management of the Critically Poisoned Patient. Elsevier Mosby. 2005, 533-544.
[7] Compton P.: The Role of urine toxicology in chronic opioid analgesic therapy. Pain Manag. Nurs. 2007, 8, 166-172.
[8] Fermann G.J., Suyama J.: Point of care testing in the emergency department. Journal of Emerg. Med. 2002, 22, 393-404.
[9] Flanagan R.J.: Developing an analytical toxicology service: principles and guidance. Toxicol. Rev. 2004, 23, 251-263.
[10] Fraser A.D., Worth D.: Monitoring urinary excretion of cannabinoids by fluorescence-polarization immunoassay: a cannabinoid-to-creatinine ratio study. Ther. Drug Monit. 2002, 24, 746-750.
[11] Garcia-Jimenez S., Heredia-Lezama K., Bilbao-Marcos F., et. al.: Screening for marijuana and cocaine abuse by immunoanalysis and gas chromatography. Ann. NY Acad. Sci. 2008, 1139, 422-425.
[12] George S., Braithwaite R.A.: Use of On-Site Testing for Drugs of Abuse. Clinical Chemistry. 2002, 48, 1639-1646.
[13] Haddad L., Shannon M., Winchester J.: Clinical Management of Poisoning And Drug Overdose. W.B. Saunders Comp. 1998, 609-626.
[14] Harris C.R.: The toxicology Handbook for Clinicians. Philadelphia, Mosby Elsevier Inc. 2006.
[15] Holler J.M., Bosy T.Z., Klette K.L., et. al.: Comparison of the Microgenic CEDIA heroin metabolite (6-AM) and the Roche Abuscreen ONLINE opiate immunoassays for the detection of heroin use in forensic urine samples. Journal of Analytical Toxicol. 2004, 28, 489-493.
[16] Huestis M.A., Cone E.J., Wong C.J., et. al.: Monitoring opiate use in substance abuse treatment patients with sweat and urine drug testing. Journal of Analytical Toxicol. 2000, 24, 509-521.
[17] Janus T.: Diagnostics and interpretation of results in forensic toxicology of amphetamines. Ann Acad Med Stetin. 2006, 52. 47-59.
[18] Korte T., Pukalainen J., Lillsunde P., Seppalla T.: Comparison of RapiTest with Emit d.a.u. and GC-MS for the analysis of drugs in urine. Journal of Analytical Toxicology. 1997, 21, 49-53.
[19] Kraemer T., Paul L.D.: Bioanalytical procedures for determination of drugs of abuse in blood. Anal. Bioanal. Chem. 2007, 388, 1415-1435.

[20] Kroener L., Musshoff F., Madea B.: Evaluation of immunochemical drug screenings of whole blood samples. A retrospective optimization of cutoff levels after confirmation-analysis on GC-MS and HPLC-DAD. Journal of Analytical Toxicology. 2003; 27(4):205-212.
[21] Lachenmeier D.W., Sproll C., Musshoff F.: Poppy seed foods and opiate drug testing - where are we today? Therap. Drug Monit. 2010, 32, 11-18.
[22] Lewandowski K., Flood J., Finn C., Tannous B., et. al.: Implementation of Point-of-Care Urine Testing for Drugs of Abuse in the Emergency Department of an Academic Medical Center. American Journal of Clinical Pathology. 2008, 129, 796-801.
[23] Lu NT, Taylor BG.: Drug screening and confirmation by GC-MS: comparison of EMIT II and Online KIMS against 10 drugs between US and England laboratories. Forensic Science International. 2006; 157(2-3):106-116.
[24] Maravalias C., Stefanidou M., Dona A., et al.: Drug-facilitated sexual assault provoked by the victim's religious beliefs: a case report. American Journal of Forensic Med. Pathol. 2009, 30, 384-385.
[25] Maurer H.H.: Current role of liquid chromatography-mass spectrometry in clinical and forensic toxicology. Anal. Bioanal. Chem. 2007, 388, 1315-1325.
[26] Melanson S.E.: Drug-of-abuse testing at the point of care. Clin. Lab. Med. 2009, 29, 503-509.
[27] Meyler's Side Effect of Drugs. The International Encyclopedia of Adverse Drug Reactions and Interactions Fifteenth Edition. 2006 Elsevier B.V.
[28] Moffat A.C.: Clarke's Analysis of Drugs and Poisons. Third Edition. Pharmaceutical Press, 2004.
[29] Moody D.E., Fang W.B., Andreynak D.M., et. al.: A comparative evaluation of the instant-view 5-panel test card with OnTrak TesTcup Pro 5: comparison with gas chromatography-mass spectrometry. Journal of Anal. Toxicol. 2006, 30, 50-56.
[30] Penders J., Verstraete A.: Laboratory guidelines and standards in clinical and forensic toxicology. Accred. Qual. Assur. 2006, 11, 284-290.
[31] POISINDEX, Micromedex Health Care System v. 2.00. Thomson Micromedex 2011.
[32] Saugy M., Robinson N., Saudan C.: The fight against doping: back on track with blood. Drug Testing and Analysis. 2009, 1, 474-478.
[33] Schwettmann L., Kulpmann W.R., Vidal C.: Drug Screening in urine by cloned enzyme donor immunoassay (CEDIA) and kinetic interaction of microparticles in solution (KIMS): a comparative study. Clin. Chem. Lab. Med. 2006. 44, 479-487.
[34] Tang J.M., Lewandrowski K.B.: Urine drugs of abuse testing at the point-of-care: clinical interpretation and programmatic considerations with specific reference to the Syva Rapid Test (SRT). Clin. Chim. Acta. 2001, 307, 27-32.
[35] Tsai S.C., ElSohly M.A., Dubrovsky T., et. al.: Determination of five abused drugs in nitrate-adulterated urine by immunoassays and gas chromatography-mass spectrometry. Journal of Anal. Toxicol. 1998, 22, 474-480.
[36] Vandevenne M., Vandenbussche H., Verstraete A.: Detection time of drugs of abuse in urine. Acta Clin. Belg. 2000, 55, 323-333.

[37] Wu A.H.B., McKay C., Broussard L.A., et. al.: National Academy of Clinical Biochemistry Laboratory Medicine Practice Guidelines: Recommendations for the Use of Laboratory Tests to Support Poisoned Patients Who Present to the Emergency Department. Clinical Chemistry. 2003, 49, 357-379.
[38] Zimmerman J.L.: Poisonings and overdoses in the intensive care unit: general and specific management issues. Crit. Care Med. 2003, 31, 2794-2801.

7

Development of an Ultra-Sensitive Enzyme Immunoassay for Insulin and Its Application to the Evaluation of Diabetic Risk by Analysis of Morning Urine

Seiichi Hashida[1,2], Yusuke Miyzawa[1], Yoshie Hirajima[1], Asako Umehara[2,3], Mayumi Yamamoto[1] and Satoshi Numata[4]

[1]*Human Life Science, Tokushima Bunri University,*
[2]*Life Style Diseases, Institute for Health Sciences, Tokushima Bunri University,*
[3]*Dietetics and Nutrition, Takamatsu Red Cross Hospital,*
[4]*Health Science, University of Kochi,*
Japan

1. Introduction

1.1 Principle of immunoassay for peptides

Currently available enzyme immunoassay methods for peptides can be divided into two groups, homogeneous and heterogeneous methods. Homogeneous enzyme immunoassay methods, in which signals that are directly obtained from a mixture of test samples and reagents correlate with the amount of peptide in test samples, are simpler and quicker but less sensitive than heterogeneous enzyme immunoassay methods, in which free and bound forms of enzyme-labeled reactants are separated from each other.

Heterogeneous enzyme immunoassay methods can be divided into competitive and noncompetitive methods. In a typical competitive enzyme immunoassay method, a fixed amount of labeled peptide is reacted with the corresponding antibody in the absence and presence of the unlabeled peptide whose level is to be measured. The amount of the peptide to be measured correlates with the amount of labeled peptide that is bound to the antibody, which can only be measured within a certain range of error (approx. 5%). Assay sensitivity increases as the concentration of labeled peptide and antibody are decreased. However, the concentration of labeled peptide and antibody should be high enough so that more than 50% of the labeled peptides and antibody used are in bound form. In other words, the minimum concentration of labeled peptide that can be used is limited by the affinity of the antibody. The sensitivity of a competitive enzyme immunoassay that is modified using a labeled antibody is also limited in a similar manner. In this type of assay, it makes no difference whether radioisotopes or enzymes are used as labels. In most cases the detection limit for peptides using such a modified competitive enzyme immunoassay is at femtomole

($\times 10^{-15}$ moles) or higher levels. [Aikawa, 1979; Fyhrquist, 1976; Glänzer, 1984; Morton, 1975; Mukoyama, 1988; Scharpé, 1987; Tikkanen, 1985; Uno, 1985]

In contrast to competitive assay methods, in noncompetitive immunoassay methods, the excess of enzyme-labeled antibody is efficiently eliminated by simple washing, and the amount of enzyme-labeled antibody nonspecifically bound to an antibody-coated solid phase in the absence of the antigen to be measured (background noise) can be minimized. This reduction in background noise makes it possible to achieve attomole sensitivities, provided that antibodies with sufficiently high affinity are used. Indeed, the reported detection limit for peptides, using noncompetitive enzyme immunoassay methods with appropriate techniques, is at attomole ($\times 10^{-18}$ moles) levels, as described below [Hashida, 1991 & 1993; Ishikawa, 1983a & 1989].

Twenty years ago, a novel method (immune complex transfer method) was developed to lower the nonspecific binding of enzyme-labeled antibody without reducing the size of the solid phase surface or the reaction mixture volume used for immunoreactions [Hashida, 1988]. For this method, the antigen to be measured was reacted simultaneously with a 2,4-dinitrophenylated IgG antibody and a Fab' antibody that was labeled with β-D-galactosidase from Escherichia coli. The resulting immune complex, which was comprised of all three components, was trapped on polystyrene beads that were coated with affinity-purified anti-2,4-dinitrophenyl group IgG. These polystyrene beads were then washed to eliminate the excess Fab'-β-D-galactosidase conjugate. The immune complex was eluted from the polystyrene beads with an excess of *εN*-2,4-dinitrophenyl-L-lysine and was transferred to polystyrene beads coated with anti-IgG Fc portion IgG. This transfer resulted in more complete elimination of the Fab'-β-D-galactosidase conjugate that was nonspecifically bound to the polystyrene beads coated with the affinity-purified (anti-dinitrophenyl group) IgG, thereby markedly reducing the background noise of the two-site enzyme immunoassay. Since there was also a smaller decrease in specific binding than in previous types of assays, these two features of the assay significantly improved assay sensitivity. Using this two-site immune complex transfer enzyme immunoassay, the detection limit of human ferritin was 1 zmol (zeptomole; 1×10^{-21} moles) per assay [Hashida, 1990 & 1995].

1.2 Ultra-sensitive assay for insulin

Insulin levels have typically been measured in serum using ELISA, which is a noncompetitive assay method [Lindström, 2002]. In order to determine insulin secretion ability, an oral glucose tolerance test (OGTT) is performed for which blood samples have to be collected every 30 min for 2 h. However, blood sampling involves risks of pain and infection. In contrast, urine samples can be collected more easily than serum samples. The insulin level in urine, collected at a specific time after serum insulin changes, may reflect these serum insulin levels. Thus urinary insulin levels may provide useful information regarding insulin secretion.

In order to overcome the problem that urinary insulin levels are too low to be measured by conventional ELISA, we developed an ultra-sensitive immune complex enzyme immunoassay (ICT-EIA) to measure urinary insulin.

2. Materials and methods

2.1 Buffers

The following buffers were used. Buffer A: 10 mM sodium phosphate buffer (pH 7.0) containing 0.1 M NaCl, 1.0 g/l bovine serum albumin (BSA), 1.0 mM MgCl2 and 1.0 g/l NaN3; buffer B: 10 mM sodium phosphate buffer (pH 7.0) containing 0.4 M NaCl, 0.1 g/l BSA, 1 mM MgCl2 and 1.0 g/l NaN3. Bovine serum albumin (BSA; fraction V) was obtained from Intergen Co. (Purchase, NY).

2.2 Human insulin, antibodies and ELISA

Recombinant human insulin was purchased from Millipore (St. Charles, MO). Human resistin and human Insulin-like growth factors-I (IGF-I) were purchased from R&D Systems, Inc. (Minneapolis, MN). Human chorionic gonadotropin (hCG) was purchased from Roche Diagnostics K.K. (Tokyo, Japan). Human growth hormone (hGH) was purchased from JCR Pharmaceuticals Co., Ltd (Hyogo, Japan)

Mouse anti-human insulin monoclonal antibodies (Ab-1; 16E9 and Ab-2; 6F7) were purchased from Japan Clinical Laboratories, Inc. (Nagoya, Japan). Guinea Pig anti-human insulin (Ab-3; N2PP05) antibody was purchased from Meridian Life Sci., Inc. (Saco, ME). Mouse anti-human resistin monoclonal antibodies (184305 and 184320) were purchased from R&D Systems. Rabbit (anti-2,4-dinitrophenyl (DNP)-BSA) serum was purchased from Shibayagi Co., Ltd. (Gunma, Japan). Rabbit anti-mouse Fc IgG was purchased from Thermo Sci. (Rockford, IL).

The ELISA for insulin was purchased from Mercodia (Uppsala, Sweden).

2.3 Subjects

A total of 141 Japanese non-diabetic, non-obese (NDNO) and non-diabetic obese (NDO) volunteers and 42 Japanese diabetic patients (DM) from our clinic participated in the study (Table 1). Criteria for obese subjects in this study included: body mass index (BMI) of >25 kg/m^2 or percentage body fat ratio of >25% for men and >30% for women. The study protocol was approved by the ethics committees of Tokushima Bunri University and Tokushima University and all participants gave written informed consent.

Parameters measured	NDNO	NDO	DM
(mean ± SD)			
No. of subjects (male/female)	106 (10/96)	35 (12/23)	42 (27/15)
Age (years)	30.3 ± 18.1	48.4 ± 7.0a	55.2 ± 27.7a,b
BMI (kg/m2)	21.9 ± 2.9	27.0 ± 4.1a	25.1 ± 3.3a
Fasting plasma glucose (mg/dl)	80.0 ± 12.7	84.5 ± 9.4a	119.6 ± 25.5a,b
HbA1c (%)	4.8 ± 0.4	5.1 ± 0.3a	7.2 ± 1.5a,b

aP < 0.01, compared with NDNO; bP < 0.01, compared with NDO.
NDNO, non-diabetic, non-obese volunteers; NDO, non-diabetic obese volunteers; DM, diabetic patients

Table 1. Clinical characteristics of the study groups

2.4 Blood and urine sampling

Blood samples were drawn early in the morning from an antecubital vein of subjects who had fasted overnight. Samples were then transferred into chilled glass tubes and kept on ice for <30 min. Serum was separated from the samples by centrifugation at 1,500 x g for 15 min at 4 °C and kept frozen at -30 °C until analysis.

Urine samples were collected early in the morning from non-diabetic and diabetic subjects who had fasted for 16 h. The urine samples (10 ml) were mixed with 0.1 ml of both BSA (100 g/l) and NaN3 (100 g/l) and were kept frozen at -30 °C until analysis. Urinary albumin and creatinine were also measured using standard methods. Urine samples with micro- and macro-albuminuria were excluded. Urinary insulin levels were expressed as a ratio to the concentration (mg) of urinary creatinine (Cre).

2.5 Antibody preparation

IgG was prepared from serum by fractionation with Na_2SO_4 followed by passage through a column of diethylaminoethyl cellulose. Both polyclonal rabbit and monoclonal mouse IgGs were digested with pepsin to $F(ab')_2$, which was further reduced to obtain Fab′ [Hashida, 1995].

2.6 Preparation of capture antibody and enzyme-labeled antibody

Mouse anti-insulin Fab′ monoclonal antibody (Ab-1), guinea pig anti-insulin Fab′ polyclonal antibody (Ab-3) and mouse anti-human resistin monoclonal antibodies (184305) were each conjugated with 6-maleimidohexanoyl-DNP-biotinyl-BSA and used as a capture antibody [Hashida, 1995; Ishikawa, 1983b]. Mouse anti-insulin Fab′ monoclonal antibody (Ab-2) and mouse anti-human resistin monoclonal antibodies (184320) were conjugated with β-D-galactosidase from Escherichia coli using o-phenylenedimaleimide, or with horseradish peroxidase or alkaline phosphatase from calf intestine, using *N*-succinimidyl-6-maleimidehexanoate and was used as an enzyme-labeled antibody [Hashida, 1995; Ishikawa, 1983b].

Thiol groups were introduced into mouse anti-insulin IgG monoclonal antibody (Ab-4) using S-acetylmercaptosuccinic anhydride (Nacalai Tesque, Inc., Kyoto, Japan) and the antibody was then conjugated with 6-maleimidohexanoyl-DNP and 6-maleimidohexanoyl-biocytin and used as a capture antibody [Hashida, 1995; Ishikawa, 1983b].

2.7 Preparation of protein-coated polystyrene beads

Polystyrene beads (3.2-mm diameter; Immuno Chemical, Inc., Okayama, Japan) were coated with affinity-purified anti-DNP-BSA IgG (0.01 g/l), anti-mouse Fc IgG or biotinyl-BSA (0.01 g/l) by physical adsorption [Hashida, 1995; Ishikawa, 1983b]. Biotinyl-BSA-coated polystyrene beads were then reacted with streptavidin (0.01 g/l) [Hashida, 1995; Ishikawa, 1983b].

2.8 Immunoenzymometric assay (IEMA) for insulin

The protocol of the IEMA for insulin was as follows (Fig. 1): An aliquot (100 µl) of standard human insulin, or urine sample, was incubated overnight at 4 °C with 100 µl buffer B containing 100 fmol Ab-1 Fab′ conjugated with DNP-biotinyl-BSA and 30 fmol Ab-2 Fab′-β-

D-galactosidase conjugate (Complex formation). Thereafter, one streptavidin-coated polystyrene bead was added and incubated for 30 min. The bead was then washed, and the bound β-D-galactosidase activity was assayed fluorometrically with 4-methylumbelliferyl-β-D-galactoside (0.2 mM) as the substrate for 1 h at 30 °C [Ishikawa, 1983b].

2.9 Two-site immune complex transfer enzyme immunoassay (ICT-EIA) for insulin

The protocol of the ICT-EIA for insulin was as follows (Fig. 1): An aliquot (100 μl) of standard human insulin diluted in buffer B, or urine sample, was incubated overnight at 4 °C with 100 μl buffer B containing 100 fmol of capture antibody conjugate; Ab-1 or Ab-3 Fab′ conjugated

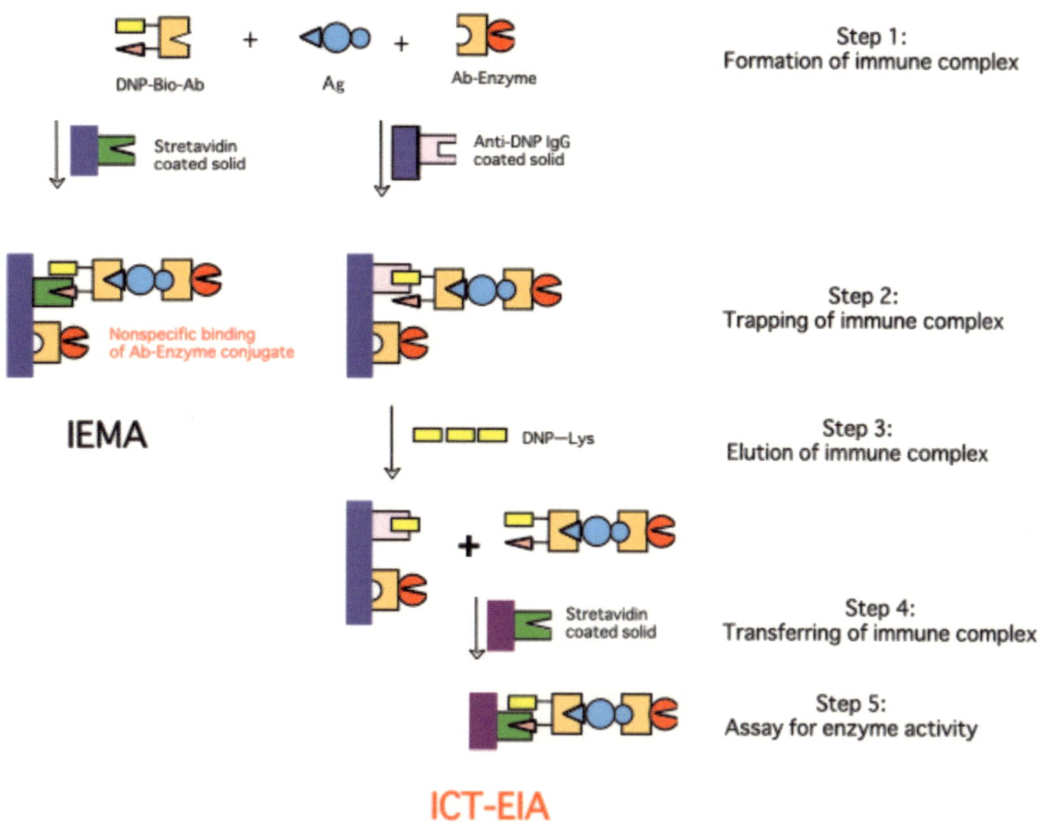

The ICT-EIA assay entails five steps: 1. Complex formation, during which the three assay components of capture antibody, antigen, and enzyme-conjugated antibody form a complex; 2. Entrapment, during which the formed complex is trapped on an anti-DNP solid phase; 3. Elution, during which the bound immune complex is eluted with DNP-Lysine solution; 4. Transfer, during which the eluted immune complex is transferred onto a streptavidin solid phase; 5. Enzyme assay, during which the activity of the enzyme bound to the immune complex is assayed fluorescently. The IEMA assay is outlined at the left for comparison.
Ab, antibody; Ag, antigen; Lys, lysine.
Color key: Blue

Fig. 1. Schematic outline of the IEMA and ICT-EIA for insulin with DNP-biotinyl-BSA or a DNP-biotinyl-Ab-1 IgG conjugate, and 30 fmol Ab-2 Fab'-β-D-galactosidase conjugate (Complex formation). Thereafter, one polystyrene bead coated with affinity-purified IgG (anti-DNP-BSA) was added to the mixture and incubated for 30 min (Entrapment). After removal of the incubation mixture, the polystyrene bead was washed twice with buffer A and then incubated in 150 μl buffer A containing 2 mM *eN*-2,4-DNP-L-lysine for 30 min (Elution). After removal of the polystyrene bead, one streptavidin-coated polystyrene bead was added to the eluate and incubated for 30 min (Transfer). The bead was then washed, and the bound β-D-galactosidase activity was assayed fluorometrically with 4-methylumbelliferyl-β-D-galactoside (0.2 mM) as a substrate for 20 h at 30 °C [Hashida, 1995; Ishikawa, 1983b]. All incubations with polystyrene beads were performed with shaking at 210 strokes/min at room temperature [Hashida, 1995; Ishikawa, 1983b].

To compare the assay of urinary insulin with assay of other urinary hormones derived from serum, ICT-EIAs for resistin were performed using a similar method as that described above for the ICT-EIA for insulin, including similar volumes of standard and samples, concentration of antibody conjugates, buffer, temperature and incubation times, except that, in the ICT-EIA for resistin, both DNP-biotinyl-BSA anti-resistin Fab' (184305) and anti-resistin Fab'(184320)-β-D-galactosidase antibody conjugates were used.

2.10 Measurement of urinary albumin and creatinine levels

Albumin and creatinine levels were measured in first morning urine samples. Albumin levels were assessed with an ICT-EIA as described above but using a specific anti-albumin monoclonal antibody as described in previous report [Umehara, 2009] and creatinine levels were assessed by reaction with picric acid using a commercial kit (Creatinine-test Wako, Wako Pure Chemical Industries, Ltd., Osaka, Japan).

2.11 Laboratory tests

Plasma lipoproteins, total cholesterol, high-density lipoprotein (HDL), low-density lipoprotein (LDL), triglycerides (TG) and HbA1c levels were analyzed consecutively using standard laboratory techniques by Bio Medical Laboratories, Inc. (Tokyo, Japan).

2.12 OGTT test

Eleven healthy young subjects (3 males and 8 females) ingested 75 g glucose. Blood samples were then obtained at 0, 60 and 120 min and urine samples at 0 and 120 min following ingestion. The levels of blood glucose and insulin, as well as levels of urinary insulin, were measured.

2.13 Statistical analysis

All data are presented as means ± SD. The detection limit of ICT-EIA or ELISA for insulin was expressed as the minimal amount of insulin which gives a significant bound enzyme activity (fluorescence or absorbance signal) after subtraction of the background signal (no insulin). A significant difference from the background was confirmed using Student's t-test ($P < 0.001$, $n = 5$).

Statistical analysis was performed using SPSS version 20.0.0. Correlations were performed using Spearman's correlation coefficient. Differences between two and three groups were compared using the Mann-Whitney U test and the Kruskal-Wallis test, respectively.

3. Results

3.1 IEMA for insulin

To compare the newly developed ICT-EIA with other methods of insulin assay we performed an IEMA for insulin as outlined in Fig. 1. Insulin was simultaneously incubated with a mixture of a monoclonal (Mc) Ab-1 Fab′ conjugated with DNP-biotinyl-BSA (Mc-DNP) and a monoclonal (Mc) Ab-2 Fab′-β-D-galactosidase conjugate (Mc-Gal), resulting in the formation of an immune complex consisting of all three components. This immune complex was then trapped onto a streptavidin-coated solid phase. The solid phase was washed to eliminate unbound conjugates and the bound β-D-galactosidase activity was measured fluorometrically.

Using this assay the detection limit for insulin was 0.01 μU, which was 3-fold lower than that of a conventional ELISA (Fig. 2).

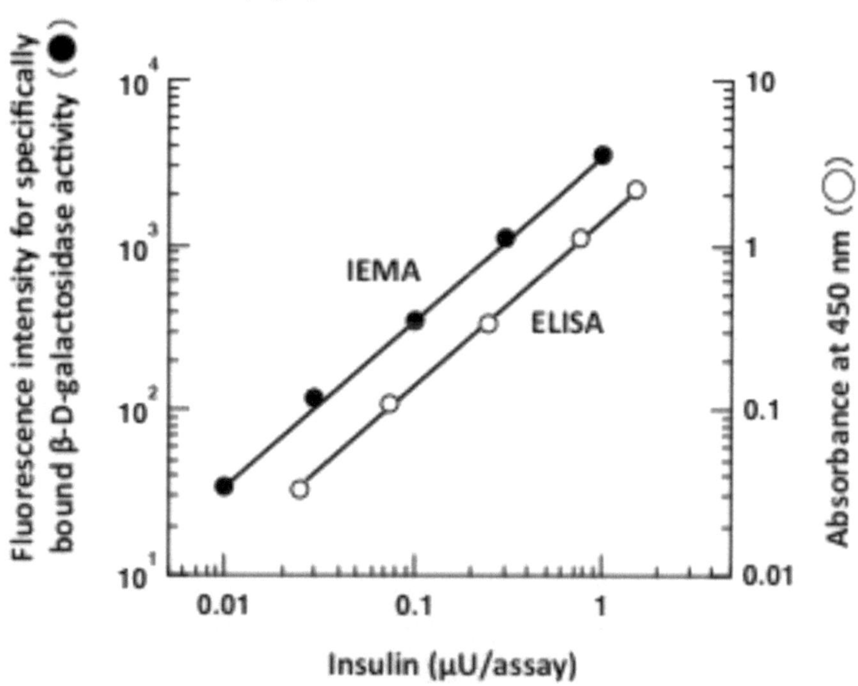

The open symbols indicate the specifically bound peroxidase activity in the conventional ELISA. The closed symbols indicate the specifically bound β-D-galactosidase activity in the IEMA performed using monoclonal capture and enzyme-conjugated antibodies

Fig. 2. Calibration curves for insulin assay using IEMA and ELISA.

3.2 ICT-EIA for insulin

The ICT-EIA for insulin was performed as outlined in Figure 1. Insulin was simultaneously incubated with a mixture of Mc-DNP and Mc-Gal, to form an immune complex as described for the IEMA method. This immune complex was first trapped onto a solid phase coated with anti-DNP IgG. Subsequently, the solid phase was washed to eliminate unbound conjugates and the immune complex was then specifically eluted from this solid phase using DNP-Lys and transferred onto a second solid phase coated with streptavidin. Finally, the bound β-D-galactosidase activity was measured fluorometrically.

When the same two mouse monoclonal antibodies that were used for IEMA were used for ICT-EIA, the fluorescence signal from the bound β-D-galactosidase activity in the ICT-EIA was strongly decreased compared to that obtained in the IEMA at low insulin concentrations and was not linear with the lowest insulin concentrations. This effect resulted in a detection limit for insulin of 0.03 μU, which was 3-fold higher than that of the IEMA (Fig. 3). Similar results were obtained even if the high molecular weight β-D-galactosidase (540 kDa) enzyme with which the antibody was conjugated was exchanged for a lower molecular weight enzyme such as peroxidase (40 kDa) or alkaline phosphatase (120 kDa) (data not shown).

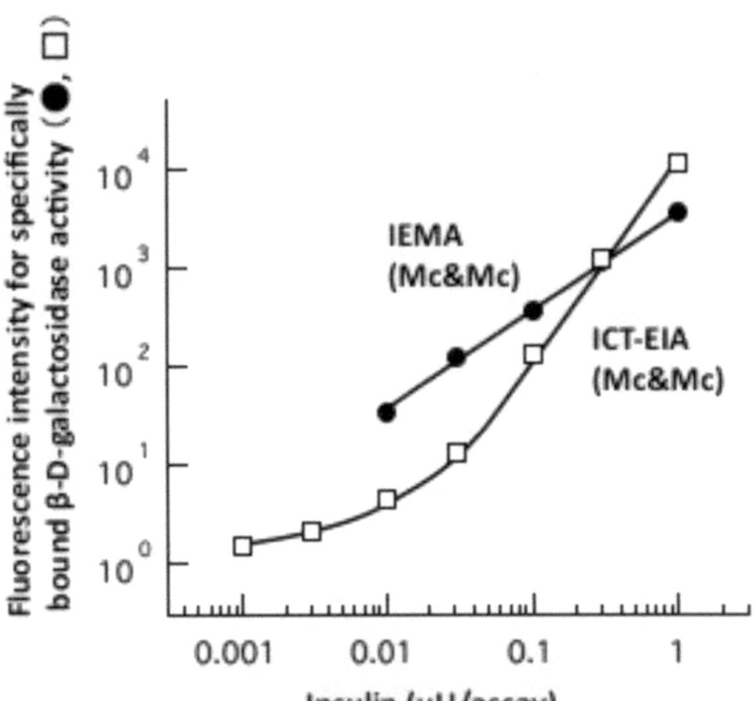

The closed symbols indicate the specifically bound β-D-galactosidase activity in the IEMA as described in Fig. 1 using monoclonal capture (Mc-DNP) and enzyme-conjugated (Mc-Gal) antibodies respectively. The open symbols indicate the specifically bound β-D-galactosidase activity in the ICT-EIA using the same two monoclonal antibodies that were used for IEMA.

Fig. 3. Calibration curves for insulin assay using IEMA and ICT-EIA.

We next tested the effect of using a combination of an enzyme labeled monoclonal mouse antibody (Mc-Gal) and a non-affinity purified polyclonal capture antibody (Pc-DNP) for formation of the immune complex in ICT-EIA (Mc-Gal & Pc-DNP). The resulting fluorescence signal decreased linearly in accordance with insulin dilution. The detection limit for insulin was 0.0003 μU (12 fg; 1.8 amol) (Fig. 4), which was 30-fold lower than that of IEMA. When a polyclonal antibody was used for enzyme labeling and a monoclonal antibody for capture (Pc-Gal & Pc-DNP), or when both antibodies were the same polyclonal antibody, the insulin detection limit increased, but the linearity with insulin dilution was preserved (Fig. 5).

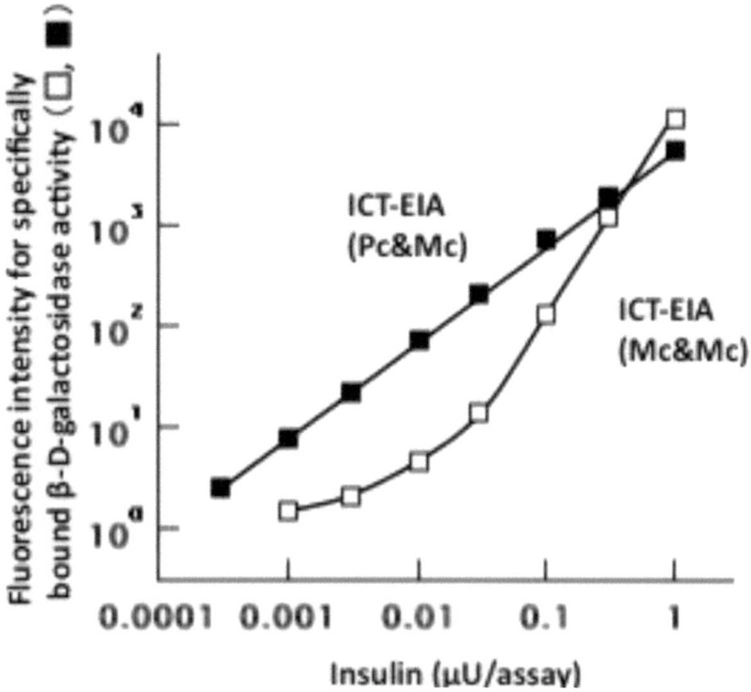

The open symbols indicate the specifically bound β-D-galactosidase activity in the ICT-EIA performed as described in Fig. 3. The closed symbols indicate the specifically bound β-D-galactosidase activity in the ICT-EIA in which a combination of a polyclonal capture antibody (Pc-DNP) and a monoclonal enzyme-labeled antibody (Mc-Gal) was used.

Fig. 4. Calibration curves for insulin assay using two different ICT-EIAs.

3.3 Improved ICT-EIA for insulin and limit of urinary insulin detection

Figure 5 shows typical calibration curves of the ICT-EIAs for insulin using various combinations of polyclonal/monoclonal capture and enzyme-conjugated antibodies. The detection limit and sensitivity for insulin using a polyclonal capture antibody and a monoclonal enzyme labeled antibody (Pc-DNP & Mc-Gal) was 0.0003 μU (0.3 nU) and 0.15 μU/ml of urine, respectively, using 2-μl samples for complete recovery of the added insulin. This detection limit was 100-fold lower than that of a sensitive ELISA and of IEMA using Mc-DNP & Mc-Gal (Fig.2 and 3). The assay range (CV < 10%) for insulin in urine was 0.5-150 μU/ml, using urine samples with a volume of 2 μl. Based on these data the ICT-EIA using a polyclonal capture antibody and a monoclonal enzyme labeled antibody was used for the remainder of the study.

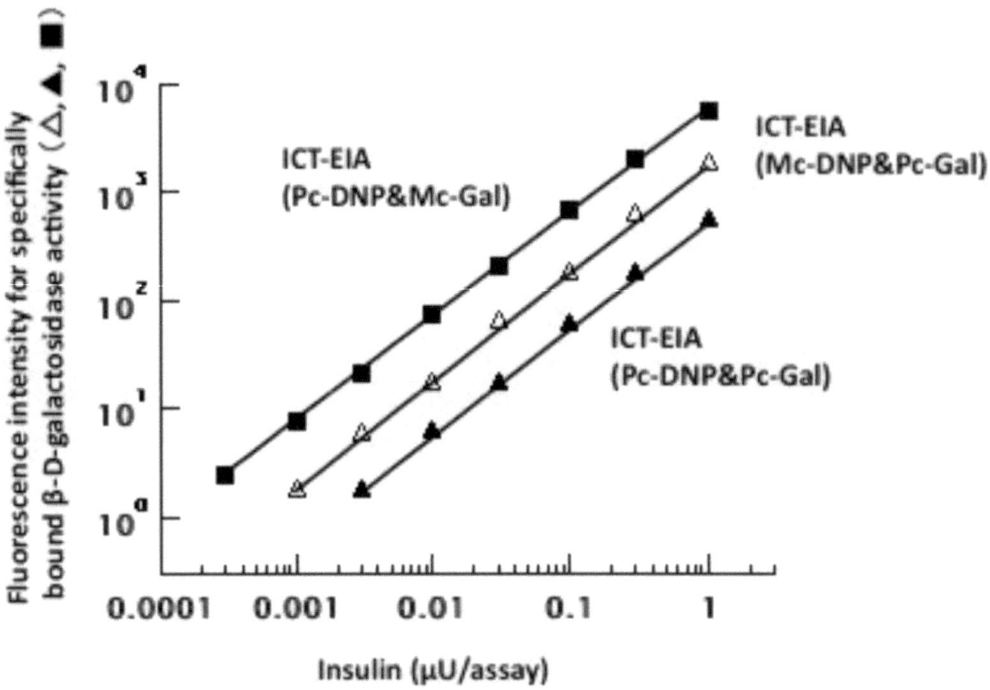

The closed squares indicate the specifically bound β-D-galactosidase activity in the ICT-EIA in which a polyclonal capture antibody (Pc-DNP) and a monoclonal enzyme-labeled antibody (Mc-Gal) were used as described in Fig. 4. The open triangles indicate the specifically bound β-D-galactosidase activity in an ICT-EIA in which the polyclonal (Pc-Gal)/monoclonal antibody (Mc-DNP) combination was reversed. The closed triangles indicate the specifically bound β-D-galactosidase activity in an ICT-EIA in which the same polyclonal antibody was used for the capture and enzyme-labeled antibody (Pc-DNP & Pc-Gal).

Fig. 5. Calibration curves for insulin assay using three different ICT-EIAs.

3.4 Assay precision

The reproducibility of ICT-EIA for analysis of insulin in urine was estimated using two or three samples containing different concentrations of insulin (range, 0.5-22.5 μU/ml). The within-assay and between-assay CVs for insulin were 2.5-6.2% (n = 10) and 3.5-7.5% (n = 10), respectively.

3.5 Recovery and dilution tests

Analytical recovery of exogenously added insulin to 2-μl and 5-μl urine samples (range, 1.2-25.3 μU/ml) was 92.8-106% and 72.5-103%, respectively. Dilution curves for the urine samples paralleled those for standard insulin. Based on these data, 2 μl of urine was used for all experiments described below.

3.6 Specificity of ICT-EIA

The cross-reactivity of ICT-EIA for insulin and other hormones was evaluated. In the ICT-EIA for insulin, cross-reactions on a molar basis with hIGF-I, hCG and hGH were all <0.1%, indicating that ICT-EIA can specifically measure insulin concentrations.

3.7 Comparison with ELISA

Insulin levels measured in 35 serum samples (3.3-23.1 μU/ml) using ICT-EIA correlated well with those determined by ELISA (r = 0.924, P < 0.001) (Fig. 6).

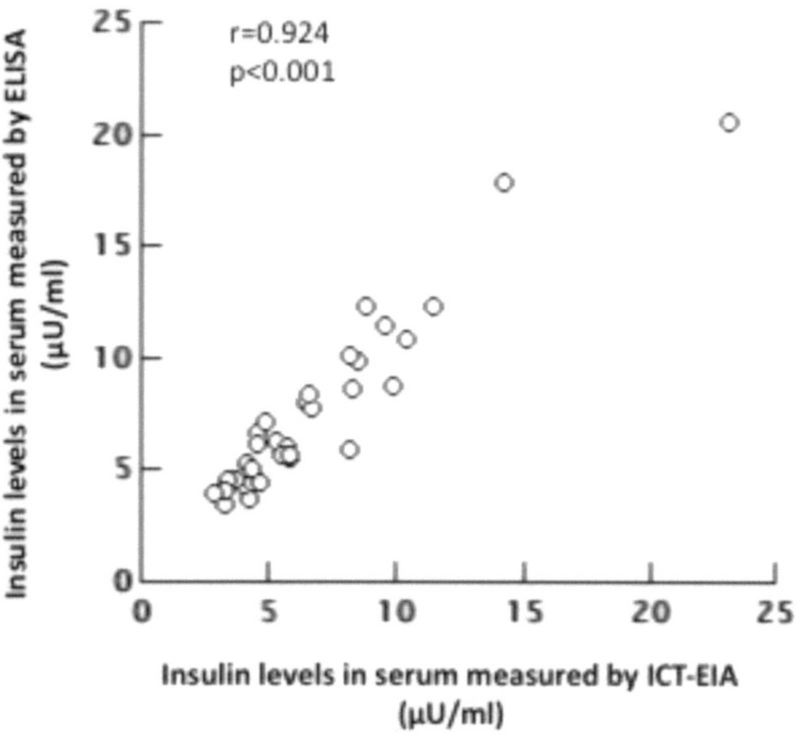

The regression equation and the calculated correlation coefficient (n = 35, r = 0.924, P < 0.001) are shown.

Fig. 6. Correlation between serum insulin levels measured by ELISA and by ICT-EIA.

3.8 Effects of increased blood glucose levels after OGTT on the insulin concentration in serum and urine

In order to determine whether the urinary insulin level reflects the blood insulin level, insulin levels in both serum and urine from non-diabetic healthy subjects were measured after OGTT using the ICT-EIA. Blood was collected at 0, 0.5, 1.0, 1.5 and 2.0 h, and urine was collected at 0 and 2 h after glucose ingestion. Blood glucose, serum insulin and insulin in the urine were measured (Table 2). Increases in the blood glucose level corresponded to significant increases in the blood insulin level, which were followed by increases in the urinary insulin level two hours later. The total quantity of insulin in urine was calculated based on the urine volume. A strong correlation was found between serum insulin levels at 60 min after glucose ingestion and total insulin values in urine during 2 h after ingestion (r = 0.87, P < 0.001), suggesting that measurement of insulin in urine may be useful for assessing the relative insulin levels in serum (Fig. 7).

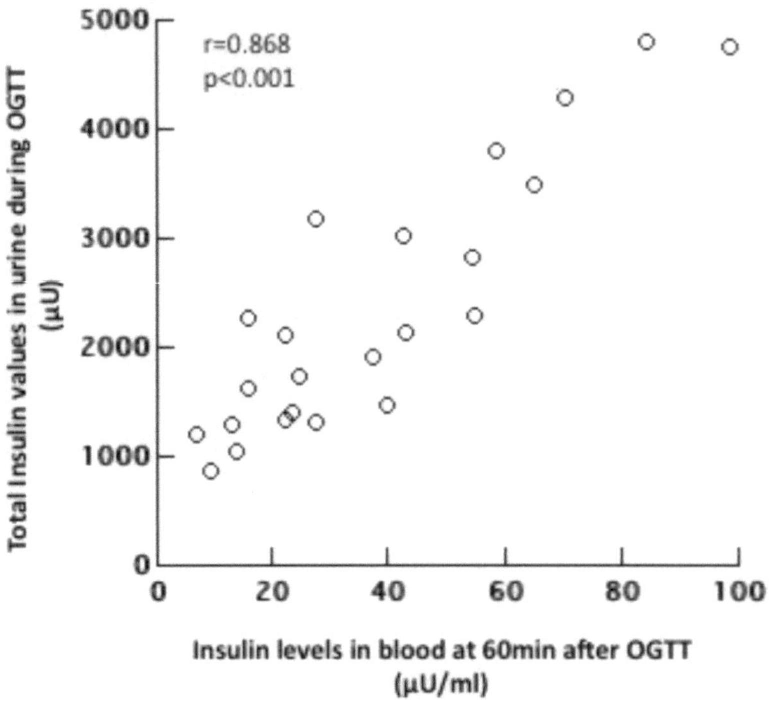

Blood was collected at 1 h, and urine was collected at 0 and 2 h, after glucose ingestion. The regression equation and the calculated correlation coefficient (n = 23, r = 0.868, P < 0.001) are shown.

Fig. 7. Correlation between serum and urinary insulin levels after OGTT.

Serum and urine levels	Time after OGTT (h)		
	0	1	2
Blood glucose (mg/dl)	82 ± 11	135 ± 29*	118 ± 18*
Serum insulin (μU/ml)	3.1 ± 1.7	33.3 ± 25.9*	39.1 ± 45.0*
Urine insulin (μU/mg creatinine)	3.0 ± 1.9	-	15.2 ± 8.1*

*P < 0.01, compared with that at 0 h.
Urine: 0 h, before OGTT; 2 h, during 2 h after the OGTT.

Table 2. Concentration of glucose and insulin in serum, and of insulin in urine, in the oral glucose tolerance test (OGTT).

3.9 Measurement of insulin and resistin concentrations in urine

Urine samples were collected in the early morning from fasting NDNO and NDO subjects, and from fasting DM patients. Urinary insulin was measured by ICT-EIA and expressed in terms of μU/mg creatinine. The insulin concentrations determined in urine from NDNO and NDO subjects and from DM patients were 4.3 ± 2.8, 9.0± 5.5 and 13.9 ± 17.6 μU/mg creatinine, respectively (Fig. 8); the insulin concentration was significantly higher in DM patients than in NDNO subjects (P < 0.001).

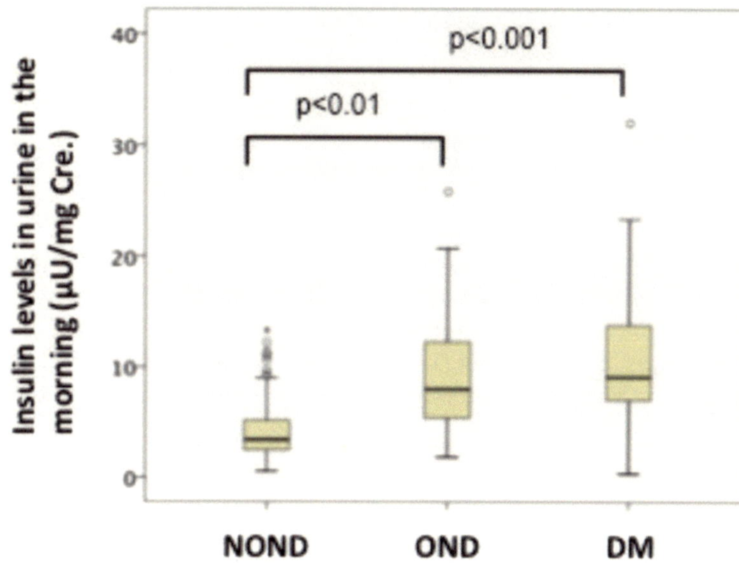

Urinary insulin levels are expressed as a boxplot (box-and-whisker diagram); scale bars indicate sample minimum and maximum, boxes indicate lower quartile, median and upper quartile. DNO (n = 106), NDO (n = 35) and DM (n = 42). Insulin levels are expressed relative to urinary creatinine (Cre).

Fig. 8. Insulin levels in the urine of NDNO subjects, NDO subjects and DM patients.

Resistin concentrations were also measured in urine from NDNO and NDO subjects and from DM patients and were determined to be 18.6 ± 20.9, 15.4 ± 17.2 and 30.0 ± 36.2 ng/mg creatinine, respectively (Fig. 9); the resistin concentration in DM subjects was significantly higher than in NDO and NDNO subjects ($P < 0.05$) (Fig. 9).

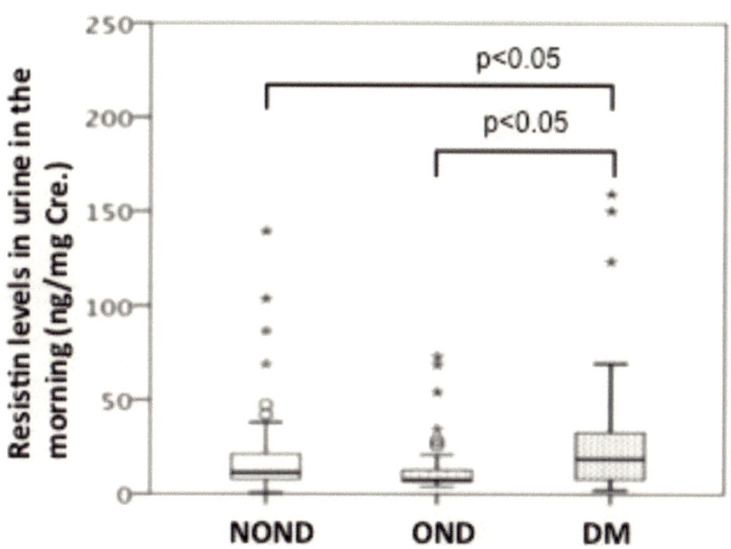

Urinary resistin levels are expressed as a boxplot similar to that described in Fig. 8.

Fig. 9. Resistin levels in the urine of NDNO and NDO subjects and of DM patients.

3.10 Correlation of insulin level to resistin levels in urine

We analyzed the correlation of urinary insulin level to urinary resistin level in 42 DM patients. The urinary insulin level was significantly and positively correlated to urinary levels of resistin ($r = 0.426$, $P < 0.001$) (Fig. 10).

4. Discussion

We developed a new ultra-sensitive technique for the measurement of insulin by employing a non-competitive two-site binding method that utilizes two different types of anti-insulin antibodies and an immune-complex transfer method (ICT-EIA). This new method can measure insulin levels as low as 0.3 nU (12 fg; 1.8 amol), with a sensitivity of 0.15 μU/ml, using 2-μl urine samples. This assay is 100-fold more sensitive than a sensitive ELISA.

Various kinds of peptides can be measured at attomole levels by a non-competitive two-site enzyme immunoassay (ICT-EIA). For this purpose, the peptide molecules to be measured have to have two or more epitopes that are sufficiently separated from each other to allow simultaneous binding of two antibody molecules. A previous study using a single chain peptide provided a hint as to the distance required between epitopes for simultaneous binding of two antibodies. Human α-atrial natriuretic peptide (α-hANP) is a single chain polypeptide consisting of 28 amino acids with a ring structure that is formed by an intramolecular disulfide bound [Hashida, 1988b]. Ten amol of α-hANP were measured by a two-site enzyme immunoassay using a peroxidase-labeled antibody Fab′ against the C-terminus of the peptide and a solid phase coated with IgG against the N-terminal half of the ring structure. The distance between the two epitopes recognized by the two antibody molecules in this single chain peptide appeared to correspond to 12-15 amino acids.

Since most polyclonal antibodies used in assays are now being replaced with monoclonal antibodies, a non-competitive two-site binding assay using two kinds of monoclonal antibody has recently been developed. When two kinds of monoclonal antibody were used in the ICT-EIA method, it was possible to measure most proteins at concentrations of less than attomole levels [Hashida, 1988b, 1990 & 1995].

However, it has not been possible to measure peptides, insulin, CRH, α-ANP, adrenomedullin or PAMP at less than attomole levels with an ultra-sensitive assay (ICT-EIA) using two monoclonal antibodies [Hashida, 2004; Katakami, 2002; Yamaga, 2003]. The major reason for this failure appeared to be due more to a decreased signal rather than because of dilution degree. Two factors have been considered that might contribute to this phenomenon. One factor is insufficient antibody affinity and the other is steric hindrance within an immune complex consisting of two antibodies (each of 50 kDa) and a peptide (6 kDa). Both of these factors would contribute to weak binding of the antibodies to the peptide in the immune complex resulting in dissociation of the peptide from antibody during the transfer from the first to the second solid phase.

We tested a number of combinations of ten different monoclonal anti-insulin antibodies, which varied in affinity and epitope, in the development of the ICT-EIA for insulin, but the results of all of the assays were the same (data not shown). We further examined the study due to the multi-antibody which several kinds of different monoclonal antibodies to insulin were caused by, but the results of these assays were again the same (data not shown). When the same polyclonal antibody, which was not insulin affinity-purified, was used as both the capture and the enzyme labeled antibody for ICT-EIA, a linear standard curve in accordance with insulin dilution was obtained, but the assay was of lower sensitivity than the other ICT-EIA assays (Fig. 5). Subsequently, a combination of one monoclonal and one non-affinity purified polyclonal antibody to insulin was used and, in this assay, the detection limit of insulin was 1.8 amol and a linear standard curve in accordance with insulin dilution was obtained.

When an affinity-purified polyclonal rabbit antibody was used in an ICT-EIA for assay of ferritin (450 kDa), 1 zmol (0.001 amol; 1×10^{-21} moles) of ferritin was detected [Hashida, 1990]. The average number of β-D-galactosidase labeled antibody Fab′ molecules bound per ferritin molecule was calculated to be 1.0-1.4. In addition, the detection limit of the β-D-galactosidase activity was 1 zmol. On the other hand, the average number of bound enzyme-labeled antibody molecules per peptide molecule was calculated to be 0.001-0.01. Therefore, the peptide detection limit of this immunoassay was estimated to be between 0.1-1 attomoles. Thus, it is likely that detection of 0.1 amol (0.02 μU) of a insulin will be possible if an affinity-purified antibody is used.

As described in the " Introduction ", blood samples have to be collected every 30 min for 2 h to assess the secretion of insulin in the OGTT. If the urinary insulin level reflects the serum insulin level, then the secretion of insulin after glucose ingestion may be easily assessed by measurement of urinary insulin levels. In the ICT-EIA of this study, the urinary insulin levels correlated well with the serum insulin levels at 1 h after glucose ingestion (Fig. 7). Thus, the level of insulin in urine appears to reflect the level in serum suggesting that measurement of insulin in urine may be useful for assessing insulin secretion.

A comparison of the insulin levels in urine collected early in the morning from NDNO and NDO subjects and from DM patients showed that the levels were significantly higher in NDO subjects and in DM patients than in NDNO subjects ($P < 0.01$ and $P < 0.001$ respectively) (Fig. 8). These results indicate that an increase in insulin levels may be a clinically important biomarker of obesity and diabetes risk.

We previously developed a highly sensitive ELISA for urinary growth hormone (GH) [Hashida, 1987, Sukegawa, 1988], which showed that assay of GH during nocturia was useful as a supporting diagnostic index of the pituitary dwarf. We have also recently developed an ultra-sensitive ICT-EIA for urinary soluble human insulin receptor ectodomain (sIR) and found that urinary sIR levels correlated well with sIR blood levels [Umehara, 2009]. Furthermore, the levels of urinary sIR in DM patients were significantly higher than those in NDO subjects and DM patients. Therefore, urinary biomarkers can be useful for both physiological and clinical studies.

In this study, urine samples with micro- and macro-albuminuria were excluded. Urinary insulin and resistin levels were expressed as ratios of urinary concentration to milligrams of urinary creatinine. Urinary insulin levels correlated well with urinary resistin levels ($r = 0.426$, $P < 0.01$) (Fig. 10). Further studies with larger numbers of patients will be needed to determine the cut-off value and criteria for insulin as a diabetic risk biomarker.

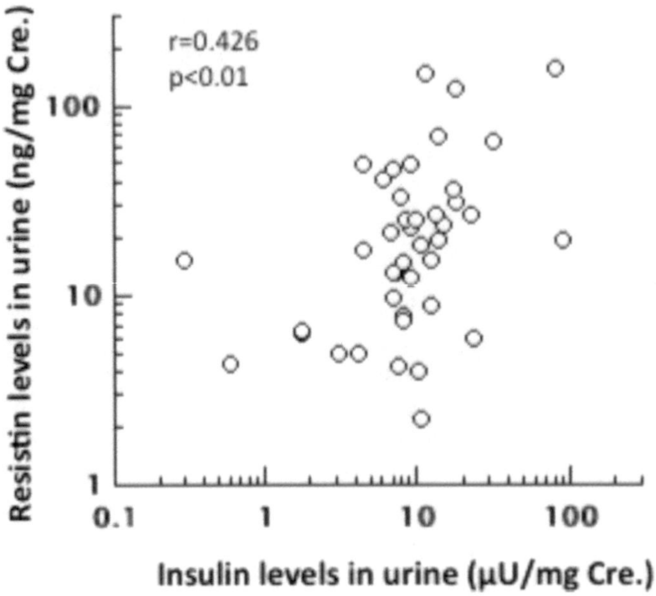

Insulin and resistin levels in the urine of 42 DM patients were measured and are expressed relative to urinary creatinine (Cre). The regression equation and the calculated correlation coefficient (r = 0.426, P < 0.01) are shown.

Fig. 10. Correlation between urinary insulin and resistin levels.

In summary, we have presented a new ultra-sensitive enzyme immunoassay for insulin, the ICT-EIA. This ICT-EIA can specifically measure insulin in urine, without any requirement for sample extraction or concentration. Urinary insulin and resistin levels were increased in patients with diabetes. ICT-EIA may be useful for both physiological and clinical studies of diabetic risk and urinary insulin may be used as a non-invasive maker that is relative to serum insulin. Therefore, measurement of urinary insulin levels will be useful in studies on dietary counseling and exercise guidance for patients with diabetes.

5. Acknowledgments

This study was supported in part by Grant-in-Aids for the Promotion of Science and Technology in Regional Areas (Life Science) from the Ministry of Education, Culture, Sports, Science and Technology, Japan. The authors thank Y. Yamahashi for assistance with experiments.

6. References

Aikawa T, Suzuki S, Murayama M, Hashiba K, Kitagawa T, Ishikawa E. (1979). Enzyme immunoassay of angiotensin I. *Endocrinology*, 105, pp1-6

Fyhrquist F, Soveri P, Puutula L, Stenman U-H. (1976). Radioimmunoassay of plasma renin activity. *Clinical Chemistry*, 22, pp250-256

Glänzer K, Appenheimer M, Krück F, Vetter W, Vetter H. (1984). Measurement of 8-arginine-vasopressin by radioimmunoassay: development and application to urine and plasma samples using one extraction method. *Acta endocrinologica*, 106, pp317-329

Hashida S, Ishikawa E, Kato Y, Imura H, Mohri Z, Murakami Y. (1987). Human growth hormone (hGH) in urine and its correlation to serum hGH examined by a highly sensitive sandwich enzyme immunoassay. *Clinica chimica acta*, 162, pp229-235

Hashida S, Ishikawa E, Mukoyama M, Nakao K, Imura H. (1988a). Direct measurement of a-human atrial natriuretic polypeptide in plasma by sensitive enzyme immunoassay. *Journal of Clinical Laboratory Analysis*, 2, pp161-167

Hashida S, Tanaka K, Kohno T, Ishikawa E. (1988b). Novel and ultrasensitive sandwich enzyme immunoassay (sandwich transfer enzyme immunoassay) for antigens. *Analytical Letters*, 21, pp1141-1154

Hashida S, Ishikawa E. (1990). Detection of one milliattomole of ferritin by novel and ultrasensitive enzyme immunoassay. *Journal of Biochemistry*, 108, pp960-964

Hashida S, Ishikawa E, Mukoyama M, Nakao K, Imura H. (1991). Highly sensitive two-site enzyme immunoassays for human atrial natriuretic polypeptides. in Atrial and Brain Natriuretic Peptides , *Proceedings of the Kyoto Symposium on ANP (1988)*, pp. 97-119, Kodansha Scientific Ltd., Tokyo, Japan

Hashida S, Tanaka K, Yamamoto N, Ishikawa E. (1993). Ultrasensitive enzyme immunoassay for peptide. *Methods in neurotransmitter and neuropeptide research*, pp. 279-304, Elsevier Science Publishers B.V., Amsterdam, Netherlands.

Hashida S, Hashinaka K, Ishikawa E. (1995). Ultrasensitive enzyme immunoassay. *Biotechnology Annual Review Vol.1*, pp. 403-451, Elsevier Science Publishers B.V., Amsterdam, Netherlands.

Hashida S, Kitamura K, Nagatomo Y, Shibata Y, Imamura T, Yamada K, Fujimoto S, Kato J, Morishita K, Eto T. (2004). Development of an ultra-sensitive enzyme immunoassay for human proadrenomedullin N-terminal 20 peptide (PAMP) and direct measurement of two molecular forms of PAMP in plasma from healthy subjects and patients with cardiovascular disease. *Clinical Biochemistry*, 37, pp14-21

Ishikawa E, Imagawa M, Hashida S. (1983a). Ultrasensitive enzyme immunoassay using fluorogenic, luminogenic, radioactive and related substrates and factors to limit the sensitivity. *Developments in Immunology*, 18, pp219-232

Ishikawa E, Imagawa M, Hashida S, Yoshitake S, Hamaguchi Y, Ueno T. (1983b). Enzyme-labeling of antibodies and their fragments for enzyme immunoassay and immunohistochemical staining. *Journal of Immunoassay*, 4, pp209-227

Ishikawa E, Hashida S, Tanaka K, Kohno T. (1989). Ultrasensitive enzyme immunoassay for antigens: technology and applications – a review. *Clinical Chemistry and Enzymology Communications*, 1, pp199-215

Katakami H, Hashida S, Oki Y, Murakami O, Ikenoue T, Ono H, Matsukura S. (2002). Immunoreactive corticotropin-releasing hormone (CRH) in plasma and hypothalamic incubation media as assessed by a novel and highly sensitive immune complex transfer EIA. *Clincal Pediatrics Endocrinology*, 11(Suppl 17), pp93-97

Lindström T, Hedman CA, Arnqvist HJ. (2002). Use of a novel double-antibody technique to describe the pharmacokinetics of rapid-acting insulin analogs. *Diabetes Care*, 25, pp1049-1054

Morton JJ, Padfield PL, Forsling ML. (1975). A radioimmunoassay for plasma arginine-vasopressin in man and dog: application to physiological and pathological states. *Journal Endocrinology*, 65, pp411-424

Mukoyama M, Nakao K, Yamada T, Itoh H, Sugawara A, Saito Y, Arai H, Hosoda K, Shirakami G, Morii N, Shiono S, Imura H. (1988). A monoclonal antibody against N-terminus of a-atrial natriuretic polypeptide (a-ANP): a useful tool for preferential detection of naturally circulating ANP. *Biochemical and Biophysical Research Communications*, 151, pp1277-1284

Scharpé S, Verkerk R, Sasmito E, Theeuws M. (1987). Enzyme immunoassay of angiotensin I and renin. *Clinical Chemistry*, 33, pp1774-1777

Sukegawa I, Hizuka N, Takano K, Asakawa K, Horikawa R, Hashida S, Ishikawa E, Mohri Z, Murakami Y, Shimizu K. (1988). Urinary growth hormone (GH) measurements are useful for evaluating endogenous GH secretion. *The Journal of clinical endocrinology and metabolism*, 66, pp1119-1123

Tikkanen I, Fyhrquist F, Metsärinne K, Leidenius R. (1985). Plasma atrial natriuretic peptide in cardiac disease and during infusion in healthy volunteers. *Lancet*, 2, 66-69

Umehara A, Nishioka M, Obata T, Ebina Y, Shiota H, Hashida S. (2009). A novel ultra-sensitive enzyme immunoassay for soluble human insulin receptor ectodomain and its measurement in urine from healthy subjects and patients with diabetes mellitus. *Clinical Biochemistry*, 42, pp1468-1475

Uno T, Uehara K, Motomatsu K, Ishikawa E, Kato K. (1982). Enzyme immunoassay for arginine vasopressin. *Experientia*, 38, pp786-787

Yamaga J, Hashida S, Kitamura K, Tokashiki M, Aoki T, Inatsu H, Ishikawa N, Kangawa K, Morishita K, Eto T. (2003). Direct measurement of glycine-extended adrenomedullin in plasma and tissue using an ultrasensitive immune complex transfer enzyme immunoassay in rat. *Hypertension research*, 26, pp45-53.

8

Ovarian Biomarkers in Infertility

Ivailo Vangelov, Julieta Dineva, Krassimira Todorova,
Soren Hayrabedyan and Maria D. Ivanova
Institute of Biology and Immunology of Reproduction "Acad. K. Bratanov",
Bulgarian Academy of Sciences,
Bulgaria

1. Introduction

The female infertility is a complex phenomenon that at least in part resides in the manifestation, possible perturbations and interplay of innate and adaptive immunity, with the participation of apoptotic and reactive oxygen species pathways, and some paracrine factors as causative and implementing factors in this process. The spread of the assisted reproduction technologies provided an unseen before opportunity to the intimacy of the ovarian follicle – the oocyte cellular surroundings and the oocyte itself, enabling research and medical community to boost the pursuit of new ovarian function biomarkers in the context of gamete fertilization and embryo development competence. The notion of infertility markers would be presented in a comprehensive viewpoint based on the importance of the folliculogenesis, oocyte-cumulus-granulosa cells interactions and oocyte genesis. This approach is aimed on the provision of non-invasive means for oocyte and embryo competence evaluation and improved reproductive medicine outcome.

2. Autoimmunity and ovarian function impairment

2.1 Anti-ovarian antibodies and infertility

The human ovary can be target of an autoimmune attack in various circumstances, including several organ-specific or systemic autoimmune diseases. One important issue concerning autoimmunity and infertility is the role of autoimmune responses against ovary, adrenal and thyroid glands in the development of premature ovarian failure.

Premature Ovarian Failure (POF) or Primary Ovarian Insufficiency (POI)) is the loss of function of the ovaries before age of 40. It has been estimated that POF affects 1% of the population (Chatterjee et al., 2007). Hormonally, POF is defined by abnormally low levels of estrogen and high levels of follicle stimulating hormone (FSH), which demonstrate that the ovaries are no longer responding to circulating FSH by producing estrogen and developing fertile oocyte.

One of the reasons to suspect an autoimmune etiology of POF is the frequent association of POF with some organ-specific autoimmune diseases but the absence of associated disease cannot exclude an autoimmune mechanism. Among organ - specific autoimmune diseases, the thyroid and adrenal diseases (Addison's disease) are frequently associated with POF. In regard to association with adrenal autoimmunity (Addison's disease) three different situations have to be distinguished: POF associated with adrenal autoimmunity, POF associated with nonadrenal autoimmunity, and isolated or idiopathic POF (Forges et al., 2004). Among POF patients with adrenal autoimmunity 4–5% are positive for autoantibodies directed against steroidogenic cytochrome P450 enzymes, such as 21-hydroxylase autoantibodies, 17α-hydroxylase autoantibodies and cholesterol side-chain cleavage enzyme (side-chain cleavage autoantibodies or steroid cell autoantibodies, SCAs)(Chen et al., 1996). Positivity for these autoantibodies identifies POF due to autoimmunity to steroid-producing cells - SCA-POF (Hoek et al., 1997, Betterle et al., 2002, Bakalov et al., 2005). In these patients the ovarian pathology has been associated with selective mononuclear cell infiltration of large antral follicles (Hoek et al., 1997) and with autoimmune destruction of theca cells (Welt et al 2005). The autoimmune damage of the ovarian theca cells and adrenal cortex are thought to be a T cell-mediated process (Hoek et al., 1997) as POF patients with adrenal autoimmunity have predominantly expressed IgG1 isotype SCA (Brozzetti et al., 2010). The predominant IgG1 isotype of the specific autoantibodies can be interpreted as a sign of Th1 immune response (Hawa et al., 2000). The presence of SCA is a risk factor for development of POF. Relatively higher percentage of women with normal menstrual cycle, who have polyendocrinopathy and SCA become susceptible to ovarian failure development within 8–15 years). The pathophysiological significance of SCA seems to be restricted to patients whose ovarian failure is associated with adrenal autoimmunity. These antibodies are very useful markers of ovarian failure in Addison's disease patients. In 90% of these patients at least one type of SCA can be detected (Falorni et al., 2002) whereas the prevalence of SCA in <10% of cases has been detected in the patients with POF associated with nonadrenal autoimmunity and in the patients with idiopathic POF (Dal Pra et al., 2003).

On the other hand, two-thirds of women with recently diagnosed POF due to SCA-associated autoimmunity have normal serum Anti-Müllerian hormone (AMH) concentrations (La Marca et al., 2010). AMH is expressed by granulose luteinized cells (GLCs) of the ovary during the reproductive years, and controls the formation of primary follicles by inhibiting excessive follicular recruitment by FSH. It therefore, has a role in folliculogenesis and some authors suggest it is a measure of certain aspects of ovarian function (Broer 2011) and useful in assessing conditions such as polycystic ovary syndrome (PCOS) and POF. However, the normal AMH levels in women recently diagnosed for SCA-POF imply that this form of ovarian failure have association with a preserved pool of functioning follicles (La Marca et al., 2010). Indeed, in such patients this is selective autoimmune destruction of theca cells with preservation of GLCs that produce low amounts of estradiol because of lack of substrates. Therefore, the more exact term of this complication, as well as other forms of ovarian failure, would be primary ovarian insufficiency (POI) (Nelson 2009), since the term POI implies more appropriately the continuous nature of the impaired ovarian function.

Among systemic autoimmune diseases, the systemic lupus erithemathosus (SLE) is thought to be most frequently associated with POF (Hoek et al., 1997). Anti- corpus luteum antibodies could represent the first stage of altered ovarian function in SLE patients (Pasoto et al., 1999). An autoantigenic 67 kDa target recognized by autoantibodies from 22% of patients (age<40) with SLE has been described to correlate with elevated serum FSH levels. In general, anti ovarian antibodies (AOA) were found in 84% of the cases of female SLE patients (Moncayo-Naveda et al., 1989).

Follicle dysfunction could be associated with inadequate follicular function, for example, due to mutated FSH- receptor gene (Doherty et al., 2002), but also due to autoimmune ovarian disease damaging the maturing follicles, but at the same time leaving the primordial follicles intact. In the majority of the cases, the cause of POF is unknown, but some of the causes can lead to absence of oocytes, whereas others can lead to disordered follicle maturation. However, several studies have suggested that some cases of POF could be a direct result of autoimmune-mediated damage of the ovaries (Hoek et al., 1997).

Strong support for an autoimmune character of isolated POF would be the presence of antibodies to ovarian structures or AOA in the serum of these patients. Evidence favors the presence of an autoimmune disease of the ovary. In some cases AOA has been considered to be a suitable marker for identification of autoimmune POF (Luborsky et al., 1990, 2000, Fénichel et al 1997, Pires et al., 2006) as well as immunological- related infertility in "*in vitro*" fertilization (IVF) patients (Gobert et al., 1992, Ivanova et al. 1994, 1999, Barbarino-Monnier et al., 2003, Pires et al, 2007). Screen for the presence of AOA before the initiation of the IVF cycle could be recommended, since AOA are thought to be associated with poor results in infertility patients included in the programs for assisted reproduction (Pires et al., 2007).

Other ovarian disturbances as Polycystic Ovarian Syndrome (PCOS), endometriosis, and unexplained infertility are associated with anti-ovarian autoimmunity. Approximately 15% to 30% of couples will be diagnosed with unexplained infertility after their diagnostic workup (Practice Committee of the American Society for Reproductive Medicine, 2006). The presence of AOA has been detected in patients with unexplained infertility (Luborsky et., al 1999, 2000, 2002). It has been demonstrated that AOA could be detected several months or years before the onset of the clinical symptoms without affecting the serum FSH or inhibin B levels (Luborsky et al 2000). Collectively these findings suggest that the AOA are independent markers for the future onset of ovarian failure.

PCOS is of clinical and public health importance as it is very common, affecting up to one in five women of reproductive age. The prevalence of PCOS depends on the choice of diagnostic criteria. One community-based prevalence study using the Rotterdam criteria found that about 18% of women had PCOS, and that 70% of them were previously undiagnosed (Teede et al., 2010). The association of ovarian autoimmunity with PCOS has been previously evaluated (Luborsky et al., 1999). It has been found that the frequency of AOA is similar (25%) among the normally cycling women and PCOS patients. The possible development of humoral autoimmunity and production of AOA consequent to ovarian damage has also been determined in clomiphene citrate-resistant PCOS patients (Alborzi et al., 2009).

Autoimmunity to endometrium and ovary has been studied in patients with endometriosis (Mathur et al., 1982). It has been demonstrated the presence of elevated autoantibody titers to whole ovary, theca cells, granulosa cells and endometrium in the patient sera, and to GLCs in the cervical secretions. Endometriosis and PCOS have been associated with higher values of anti-FSH IgA autoantibodies, and endometriosis also has association with anti-FSH IgG autoantibodies). One of the major epitopes identified was a 78-93 amino acid sequence belonging to part of the human FSH beta-chain (Gobert et al., 2001). This autoantigenic determinant is recognized most frequently by human serum samples from women with AOA. Anti-FSH are thought to be naturally occurring autoantibodies associated with peripheral FSH concentrations, but increased in infertile women with dysregulation of immune reactions and repeatedly performed in vitro fertilization (IVF) (Haller et al., 2005).

Significant progress was made towards the identification of candidate biomarkers involved in human ovarian autoimmunity. The presence of anti-oocyte antibodies has been demonstrated in the sera of POF patients (Damewood et al., 1986) with or without associated autoimmune diseases (Luborsky et al., 1990) and in the sera of infertile patients (Pires et al., 2006, 2007), as well as in mice after neonatal thymectomy (Tong & Nelson 1999). In the mouse model of autoimmune ovarian failure, the autoantigenic oocyte protein has been identified and called Maternal Antigen That Embryos Require (MATER), (Tong & Nelson, 1999). Using specific and sensitive immunoassays (Pires et al., 2007) demonstrated that AOA in infertile women identified an immunodominant antigen- heat shock protein 90-beta, which was localized predominantly in the oocyte cytoplasm. Therefore, anti-HSP90 antibodies could be used as one of the diagnostic markers for ovarian failure and thereby infertility (Pires et al., 2007).

Anti-Zona pellucida autoantibodies bind to the oocyte Zona pellucida (ZP), and therefore, could prevent sperm-zona interaction (Kyurkchiev et al., 1988, Barber & Fayrer Hosken, 2000). Zona pellucida proteins play critical role in oocyte fertilization. Anti-ZP autoantibodies have been linked with human female infertility (Ivanova et al.1994, 1999, Mardesic et al., 2000, Kelkar et al., 2005, Koyama, 2010). Intra cytoplasmic sperm injection (ICSI) is recommended option for IVF therapy of women with anti-ZP autoantibodies (Mardesic et al., 2000). Anti- ZP autoantibodies may induce autoimmune-mediated ovarian damage with follicular depletion and fertility suppression due to impaired ZP formation (Lloyd et al., 2010) and disruption of the gap junctions between the oocyte and granulosa cells, damaging the bidirectional communication necessary for normal folliculogenesis (Calongos et al., 2009).

In addition, novel immunotherapy strategy has been proposed recently for treatment of autoimmune ovarian disease (Li et al., 2008). The continuous presence of physiologically-expressed autoantigen is critical for both tolerance maintenance and autoimmune disease pathogenesis, thus the outcome is determined by the integrity of regulatory T cells, whereas deficiency in the regulatory T-cell function is associated with elevated responsiveness to autoantigen and to environmental stimuli that could potentially promote the autoimmune disease and memory (Tung et al., 2005). Sundblad et al., 2006 showed the presence of circulating autoantibodies directed towards an antigen of approximately 50 kDa, identified subsequently as alpha-enolase. It has been demonstrated that 21 of 110 women with autoimmune POF express this autoantibody, whereas 60 control subjects proved negative. Aldehyde (retinal) dehydrogenase 1A1 (ALDH1A1) and selenium-binding protein 1 (SBP1) are identified as unique autoantigenic targets associated with unexplained infertility (Edassery et al., 2010).

More recently, three immunodominant ovarian autoantigens, α-actinin 4 (αACTN4), heat shock 70 protein 5 (HSPA5) and β-actin (ACTB), have been identified using AOA -positive sera from women with idiopathic POF and women undergoing IVF (Mande et al., 2011). These autoantigens are localized in different structures of the ovary such as the ooplasm of the oocyte, theca, granulosa, corpus luteum and zona pellucida. All the above antigens were found to be expressed in the ooplasm throughout follicular development, and all of them were expressed specifically in the oocyte except αACTN4. Both women with infertility and those with ovarian cancer have autoantibodies to ovarian antigens. Luborsky et al., 2011 showed for the first time that antibodies to mesothelin, a well-characterized ovarian cancer antigen, occur in some of the women with epidemiologic risk for ovarian cancer.

The antibody-mediated autoreactivity directed towards the granulosa cells has been reported in the sera of POF patients (Damewood et al., 1986, Kelkar et al., 2005). AOA in POF patients showed immunoreactivity against the granulosa cells from both the pre-antral and the antral follicles (Damewood et al., 1986). In small percentage of the anti-ZP positive POF sera, a strong autoreactivity directed to granulosa cells has also been detected (Horejsi et al., 2000, Kelkar et al 2005). A 51 kDa protein has been identified as an additional target of SCA (Winqvist et al., 1998). It has been localized in the placenta and in the GLCs by the sera of patients with adrenal insufficiency and associated ovarian failure.

We have developed an ELISA assay to assess the prevalence of anti-granulosa cell antibodies and we have estimated it to be 28.7% in the sera and 44.90 % in the follicular fluids (FFls) of infertile patients undergoing controlled ovarian hyper-stimulations (COHS) for IVF-ET (embryo transfer) compared to 9.1% and 6.67% in the fertile women sera and FFls respectively (Vangelov et al., 2005,2006,2009).For the isolation of granulosa cells, pooled follicular fluids were collected individually for each patient, centrifuged at 200 x g and purified using HISTOPAQUE® -1077 (Sigma Diagnostics, Inc.) gradient centrifugation approach (for details, see Vangelov et al., 2005). The results obtained by this ELISA assay disclosed that antibodies against granulosa cell-antigens occurred more frequently in infertile women undergoing IVF-ET than in fertile normally menstruating women (controls) at the same age, inferring to the conclusion that the detection of anti-granulosa cell antibodies serve as an indicator for their involvement in immunological infertility. Auto-antibodies against GLCs antigens may be considered as a part of the heterogeneous group of AOA (Ghazeeri & Kutteh 2001). The prevalence of anti-granulosa cell autoantibodies in the subgroup with low fertilization rate suggests a negative impact of the anti-granulosa cell autoantibodies on the fertilization outcome. It was suggested that the binding of these antibodies to follicular cells might be a defective signal in the fertilization process (Horejsi et al., 2000). Anti-granulosa cell autoantibodies could play a role as a marker of fertilization failure.

In addition to the mentioned above, the identification of putative granulosa cell antigens recognizable by the antibodies in the infertile women sera, but not by the fertile controls sera is of huge importance. Four undefined GLC autoantigens - 110 kD, 70-80 kD, 47 kD and 37 kD have been identified as autoantigenic targets for the anti-GLCs autoantibodies using immunoblotting assay developed by us (Vangelov et al., 2005). The results from immunoblotting revealed that: 3 patient's sera and none control sera reacted with protein band with MM 37 kD; 14 patient's sera and 3 control sera - at 47 kD; 10 patient's sera and 1 control serum - at 70-80 kD and 8 patient's sera and 3 control sera - at 110 kD. Four patient's sera reacted with all above protein bands. The band with approximate MM of 47 kD was the most frequently occurring antigen in infertile women and the band of 37 kD reacted only with sera from infertile patients studied.

2.2 Cellular immunity, pro-inflammatory cytokines and apoptosis in infertility

The diagnosis of an autoimmune mechanism involvement in infertile patients relies not only on the presence of autoantibodies directed to ovary, but also on the dynamics of immune cell populations and their soluble products. Natural killer cells (NK cells) constitute a major component of the innate immune system. NK cells have a suppressive action on B cells, and therefore, the impaired NK cell activity has a role in some types of autoimmunity. NK cell abnormalities have been reported in women with POF (Hoek et al., 1995) and in women with POI (van Kasteren et al., 2000), as well as in murine post-thymectomy autoimmune oophoritis (Maity et al 1997), all demonstrating a decreased NK cell number and/or activity. Similarly NK cells suppression is observed in neonatal thymectomy induced mice autoimmune oophoritis (Maity et al., 1997), while treatment by the NK cell-stimulating factor (IL-12) before thymectomy preserves the NK cell activity and ameliorates the associated autoimmune oophoritis. NK cells produce the signature Th1 cytokine IFN-γ. The increased periphery NK cell activity and number during pregnancy might explain the apparent Th1 bias (Ntrivalas et al., 2001) that is also associated with multiple observations of recurrent pregnancy losses (Piccinni et al., 1998, Prado-Drayer et al., 2008). These findings suggested an important role for the innate immune system. The immune activation might cause pregnancy failure by inhibiting the reproductive endocrine system. In this way, for example, the inflammatory cytokines are thought to inhibit both the gonadotropin production at hypothalamus and pituitary gland level (Rivest & Rivier 1995), and the progesterone synthesis in corpus luteum of the ovary as well as to promote the luteal regression (Davis & Rueda 2002). Monocytes (Mo) and the monocyte-derived dendritic cells (DCs) play a prominent role in the initial stages of autoimmune reactions against endocrine organs. The accumulation of monocytes/DCs and the clustering of DCs in endocrine organs is one of the first sign of an autoimmune endocrine disorder. Mo start to replace the resident Macrophages (Ma) and DCs under normal state and in response to inflammation signals, they move in the tissue vicinities and proliferate and differentiate into Ma and DCs. The main function of DCs is to act as antigen presenting cells, being messengers between the innate and adaptive immunity. Immature DCs are found in the bloodstream, but once activated, they migrate to the lymph nodes where they interact with T- and B -cells to initiate and shape the adaptive immune response. Dysfunction of Mo and DCs has been found in patients with ovarian failure (Hoek et al., 1993) long enough - the Mo have abnormal polarization and DCs have abnormal interaction with T -cells, refractive to estrogen substitution correction. Alteration of T cell subsets and T cell mediated injury is likely to play an important role in pathogenesis of autoimmune ovarian failure as evidenced by human studies and animal models of autoimmune oophoritis (Hoek et al., 1995, Mignot et al., 1989b, van Kasteren et al., 2000, Chernyshov et al., 2001). The hypoestrogenic hormone status in ovarian failure patients could be responsible for the elevated numbers of activated blood T cells. It has been demonstrated that the estrogen substitution lowered the number of activated peripheral T cells in ovarian failure patients, although not to completely normal levels (Hoek et al 1995). Despite the fact that the data on the numbers of T cells vary between the reported studies, a consistent pattern of an increased number of activated (MHC II+ or IL-2R+) T cells have been demonstrated in the majority of the studies (Hoek et al., 1997). Elevation in the number of peripheral blood B cells has been reported in patients with ovarian failure (Ho et al., 1988), and in ovarian failure patients during initial period of disease (Chernyshov et al., 2001), and in patients with primary ovarian insufficiency (van Kasteren et al., 2000), and in murine autoimmune ovarian failure (Ivanova et al., 1984), and relationship of the raised numbers of B cells to the presence of various autoantibodies has been also demonstrated (Ho et al., 1988). The elevated numbers of peripheral blood B cells is thought to be a sign of activation of the humoral immune system, which is crucial for autoantibody production. This can be very important because estrogen substitution in patients with ovarian failure did not lower the elevated number of peripheral B cells (Hoek et al., 1995). Similar immunological profile has been shown in patients with POI and in patients with POF (van Kasteren et al., 2000), suggesting that POI is a light form of POF. It has been found a decrease in NK cells and in percentage of T-suppressor cells with a rise in T-helper/T-suppressor cell ratio, as well as an increase in B- cells and HLA-DR+ T cells. The question remains whether these changes are the cause or the consequence of the ovarian failure. Autoimmune damage of the ovary could be the primary cause of POF, whereas in natural menopause autoimmunity is a result of hormone dysfunction (Chernyshov et al., 2001).

The variations of cellular immunity function and its relationship with AOA (Huang et al., 1996) and with anti-granulosa cells autoantibodies (Vangelov et al., 2009) have been investigated in patients with ovarian failure. The patients with ovarian failure have increased AOA, CD4+ T-cells and CD4+/CD8+ ratio. It has been shown also, that AOA positive rate in POF patients is associated with higher CD4+/CD8+ ratio (Huang et al., 1996).

In our study, we used our propriate granulosa cell autoantibody ELISA detection assay, and commercially available TNF-α and IFN-γ ELISA kits (eBioscience, USA) to estimate the abundance of granulosa cell autoantibodies, and the concentrations of TNF-α and IFN-γ in FFls, as well as DNA-DAPI staining for the assessment of granulosa cells apoptotic index in ovarian failure patients. The obtained results reveled several findings: 1) significantly higher levels of IFN-γ, TNF-α and apoptotic cells in women with positive autoantibody ELISA test, and 2) significant correlation of anti- granulosa autoantibodies, and apoptotic index, as well as significant correlation of IFN-γ with TNF-α and apoptotic index. Moreover, we have reported (Vangelov et al., 2008, 2009), that cellular immunity (TNF-α, IFN-γ) and humoral immunity (anti-granulosa cell autoantibodies) to granulosa autoantigens can be concurrently produced in patients with ovarian failure, and we suggested that pathogenesis of ovarian failure may be associated with immune factors and apoptosis of granulosa cells. In this scenario the programmed cell dead (apoptosis) of granulosa cells could be very important player. The ovulatory process represents the classical sequence of an acute sterile inflammation under surveillance of innate immune function (Medzhitov, 2010, Rock et al 2010). The cell damage is associated with the release of danger signals-alarmins (Bianchi 2007). In the preovulatory follicle main source of danger signals are damaged granulosa cells (Spanel-Borowski 2011) and the danger signals could be recognized by CK+(cytokeratin-positive) granulosa cells via TLR-4 or other pattern-recognition receptors (PRRs) (Serke et al., 2009, 2010). The ovarian innate immune function will be activated to orchestrate the ovulatory process (Spanel-Borowski, 2011). CK+ cells are assumed to switch off the CK genes in the corpus luteum (CL) stage of secretion and regression to become granulosa-like cells. The granulosa-like cells are thought to be mature DC in the CL (Spanel-Borowski, 2011). However, the low T cell number in the preovulatory follicle wall is signature for a limited interaction with the adaptive immunity. A disturbed conversation between innate and adaptive immunity is reflected by altered T cell profiles in the FFls of patients with idiopathic infertility and in ovaries with POF due to autoimmune damage (Vujovic 2009, Spanel-Borowski 2011). Because DCs process antigens and train naive T cells to become helper and suppressor cells (Banchereau & Steinman, 1998, Turvey & Broide, 2010), DCs are players between innate and adaptive immunity. The pathway of innate immunity is well balanced to achieve the quick recovery of tissue integrity, but an unbalanced action can cause chronic tissue injury and autoimmune diseases. In this aspect, we have reported the relationship between the level of apoptotic granulosa cells and the level of anti- granulosa cell autoantibodies in studied patient group with ovarian failure (Vangelov et al., 2009). Moreover, the biomolecules are susceptible to glycosylation, glycation, phosphorylation and oxidation. Oxidative stress is the major event causing structural modification of proteins with consequent appearance of neo-epitopes (Buttari et al., 2005). The role for oxidative stress in promoting the autoimmune responses have been reviewed (Kannan 2006). Autoimmune responses may be directed against self-structures altered by high-affinity ligand binding or by chemical damage due to environmental events, such as oxidative stress. Several systems that generate reactive oxygen species catalyze a variety of oxidative damage to nucleic acids, lipids, and proteins. In physiological conditions oxidative stress is well compensated, but when there is an overproduction of reactive oxygen species or a deficiency of antioxidant enzyme activity, a biological damage may occur (Puddu et al., 2009). Oxidative stress and inflammation may determine the modification of self-structures also favoring the formation of Advanced glycation end products (AGEs). Chronic oxidative stress causes an accumulation of AGFs products (Ramasamy et al., 2009). The generation of AFGs products and augmentation of proinflammatory mechanisms provide a potent feedback loop for sustained oxidant stress, ongoing the generation of AFGs products. Therefore, self-molecules modified by oxidative events can become targets of autoimmune reactions, thus sustaining the inflammatory responses. In another hand, the disturbed apoptosis execution and clearance can potentially render apoptotic cells as a source of autoantigens normally sequestered in the intracellular environment. Structural changes occurring during cell death may influence the immunogenicity of clustered self-antigens at the surface of apoptotic body (Navratil et al., 2005). In this scenario, high concentrations of self-antigens are packaged during generation of apoptotic cells; the packages also may contain altered fragments of self-antigens that have not been encountered previously by the immune system; under normal circumstances, apoptotic cells are cleared rapidly by macrophages and DCs; therefore, the apoptosis-altered self-antigens are either ignored by the immune system or tolerance to those antigens is maintained. Clearance is achieved through complex mechanisms that enable macrophages and DCs to recognize apoptotic cells as nonthreatening "self" particles, but defects in this process that cause a delay in clearance could change the appearance of apoptotic cells and cause them to be recognized as "foreign invaders," thereby stimulating an inflammatory response that, in turn, activates an immune response to self-antigens (Navratil et al., 2005).

The ovary is an extremely dynamic organ in which excessive or defective follicles are rapidly and effectively eliminated throughout reproductive life. Greater than 99 % of follicles disappear, due to apoptosis of granulosa cells. The balance between signals for cell death and survival determines the destiny of the follicles. The potential use of scores for apoptosis in granulosa cells and characteristics of FFls have been discussed more recently as prognostic markers for predicting the outcome of assisted reproduction (Lefèvre et al., 2011). Follicular fluid and surrounding tissue contains various lymphocytes that synthesize different cytokines. The other sources of cytokines are ovarian somatic cells. We studed the impact of proinflamatory cytokines TNF-α and IFN-γ concentration in FFls, and apoptotic index of granulosa cells on the results of COH/IVF in women with ovarian failure (Vangelov et al., 2009). The obtained results in this study clearly showed that the elevated levels of TNF-α and IFN-γ were directly related with increased incidences of apoptotic granulosa cells and altogether were associated with poor COH/IVF outcome. Moreover, earlier Cianci et al., 1996 reported association of elevated concentration of TNF-α with reduced fertilization rate in women with immunological infertility and concluded, that the elevated TNF-α concentration in the human follicle may negatively influence both ovulation and fertilization related events.

3. Intra ovarian regulators of survival and apoptosis in preovulatory follicle

3.1 Apoptosis of granulosa luteinized cells (GLCs) and cumulus cells (CCs) – predictive marker for results of COH / IVF outcome in infertile women

The oocyte-cumulus-granulosa cells unit comprises an intimate relation between somatic cell syncytium in conjunction with the oocyte involving gap junctions and complex of hormonal and peptide factors. Granulosa cells and cumulus cells play a critical role in oocyte maturation and fertilization by releasing and mediating signals to oocytes. On the other hand the oocyte also influences granulosa cells steroidogenesis, proliferation and Hyaluronic acid synthesis by CCs. Each participant in this unit can disturb signaling and regulation of apoptotic process. Apoptosis is self-destruction under physiological control and is closely involved with most of the reproductive processes, including follicular atresia. Apoptosis can be used to estimate a function of ovarian reserve in women undergoing IVF (Seifer et al., 1996). Many studies have provided evidence that poor oocyte, low IVF outcome and embryo quality can be associated with apoptosis. The incidence of apoptotic bodies has been used as a morphological marker for physiological cell renewal (Tilly et al., 1991) and the presence of apoptosis in human GLCs and CCs in COHS during IVF treatment, has been used as a very sensitive indicator for evaluation of oocyte quality and the IVF outcome (Nakahara et al., 1997; Suh et al., 2002).

The isolated GLCs (Vangelov et al., 2005) were fixed with formaldehyde. The GLCs suspensions were dropped on poly L-Lysine treated slides. CCs were isolated from individual cumulus-oocyte complexes (COCs) of the same patients, and were divided according to the oocyte maturation (immature - G.V. or MI or mature - MII oocytes). The cumulus masses were dispersed with 150 IU Hyaluronidase and after that were fixed and processed as GLCs.

Apoptosis of GLCs and CCs was assayed using DNA-DAPI staining (Dineva et al., 2006) that allows the observation of morphological changes of nuclear chromatin in GLCs and CCs. Morphological characteristics of apoptosis such as chromatin condensation and/or nuclear fragmentation were identified and counted in randomly selected fields among 800–1000 cells and the percentage of apoptotic cells was calculated. The significant negative correlations between the rate of apoptosis in GLCs and both - the number of preovulatory follicles, and the number of retrieved and fertilized oocytes from patients in stimulated cycles was found.

The most convenient evaluation system for oocyte quality is based on oocyte morphology and status of oocytes–cumulus complexes. Cumulus cells surround and intercommunicate with oocytes during follicular development and after ovulation, suggesting that the incidence of apoptosis in cumulus cells could influence oocyte quality (Lee et al., 2001). In our study we found that the rate of apoptosis in GLCs is higher compared to CCs cells from the same patient. The higher rate of apoptosis in CCs from follicles with immature oocytes than from those with mature showed that the level of CCs apoptosis is directly related to the maturation of oocytes and support the data of Host et al., 2000.

The obtained results showed that the incidence of apoptosis in GLCs as well as in CCs could be a predictive marker for IVF outcome.

3.2 Role of Atrial Natriuretic Peptide (ANP) in the ovarian immunoendorine function

3.2.1 GLCs are the main local source of ANP in the preovulatory human follicle

Many endocrine, paracrine and autocrine factors (gonadotrophic and steroid hormones, peptide hormones, cytokines, highly- reactive free radicals) play an important role in the regulation of GLCs proliferation, differentiation and death.

The expression of natriuretic peptides (NPs) and its receptors (NPRs) has been demonstrated in the mammalian ovary (Gutkowska et al., 1993; Russinova et al., 2001).

The presence of ANP was demonstrated in the follicular fluid (Kim et al., 1987); granulosa cells (Ivanova et al., 2003) and luteal cells (Vollmar et al., 1988). ANP plays an important role in the regulation of different aspects of ovarian physiology, such as oocyte meiosis, cumulus cells expansion, spontaneous oocyte maturation, ovarian steroidogenesis and follicular atresia (Samson WK et al., 1988, Tornel et al., 1990; Gutkowska et al., 1999; Zhang et al., 2005).

The indirect immunofluorescence technique (IIF) was used to investigate the localization patterns of ANP on GLCs isolated from women undergoing IVF. The isolated GLCs were fixed on the protocols mentioned above. The GLCs suspensions were dropped on poly L-Lysine treated slides. The cells were permeabilized with Triton X-100 for 5 min and after washing the cells were incubated with cocktail of monoclonal antibodies (Mabs) against recombinant human ANP (Mabs: 6C3, 6F11, 5D3 supernatants), obtained and characterized at the Department of Molecular Immunology (Institute of Biology and Immunology of reproduction, Sofia, Bulgaria), diluted 1:1 in PBS/BSA, overnight, followed by washing with PBS-Tween 20 and then incubated with secondary antibody (Sw/am IgG labeled with FITC, Sevac, Czech Republic), diluted 1:20, for 1h. After washing in PBS-Tween 20, slides were mounted with Mowiol (Sigma®). The expression and localization of ANP were examined using fluorescence microscope (Leiz Labor-Lux, Zeiss). The immunofluorescent expression level of ANP was scored as the intensity of specific immunofluorescence and the number of positive cells from (+) to (+++) as follows: (+++) – intensive immunoreactive ANP expression in prevailing cells population; (++) - intensive immunoreactive ANP expression in most of cells observed; (+) – intensive expression of immunoreactive ANP in a minority of cells observed.

ANP expression was observed as membrane, submembrane and particular granular cytoplasm localized staining. The mature ANP is generated by proteolytic processing in two steps: generation of pro-ANP (stored in the cytoplasmic granules) from immature pre-pro ANP (Bloch et al., 1985), followed by proteolytic maturation of pro-ANP to mature bioactive ANP (Schwartz et al., 1984). The bioactive ANP gets into extracellular space and in this manner ANP acts as autocrine and/or paracrine factor that modulates different aspects of GLCs functions. We consider that the different patterns of ANP expression in GLCs represent localization of ANP during the different stages of posttranslational processing and/or export of ANP from GLCs.

The women included in this study were divided into two groups: women with high level of ANP expression and women with low level of ANP expression in GLCs.

For us the question of great interest was, whether the GLCs are the principal source of ANP in the human preovulatory follicle? For this reason, we measured the ANP concentrations in FFl obtained from the same woman that donated the GLCs specimens followed by an analysis of relationship between the follicular ANP concentration and the expression levels of immunoreactive ANP in GLCs. The concentration of ANP was measured in FFls, obtained from the same woman using a proANP (1-98) kit, with levels of immunoreactive ANP in GLCs found positively correlating to the corresponding FFls ANP concentrations. The concentration of ANP in the FFls of women with high level of immunoreactive ANP expression in GLCs was found to be significantly higher, compared to the women with low level of ANP expression in GLCs.

Our earlier study showed that, in in vitro luteinized porcine granulosa cells (isolated from prepubertal porcine ovaries) supplemented with FSH and luteinizing hormone (LH), the expression of immunoreactive ANP was increased and was highest among the FSH and LH treated GLCs (Dineva et al., 2007).

The established positive relationship between the levels of ANP in FFls and its immunoreactive expression on GLCs together with findings of in vitro experiment show that the GLCs are the main local source of ANP in the preovulatory human follicle.

3.3 ANP is survival factor for GLCs in preovulatory follicle

Diverse effects of NPs are mediated by the activation of membrane bound receptors with a particulate guanylate cyclase (GC) activity to generate Cyclic Guanosine Monophosphate (cGMP). The physiological activities of ANP are mediated by a specific plasma membrane receptor, guanylate cyclase-type receptor GC-A (Chang et al., 1989). Recent studies have shown that components of cGMP signaling pathways are expressed in the ovary and that cGMP can alter granulosa cell function (La Polt et al., 2003). The cGMP/PKG signaling is a target for the prevention of mitochondrial dysfunction-mediated cell death (Chun SY et al. 1996, Takuma et al. 2001).

The survival role of ANP for GLCs, was studied in cultured human GLCs treated with 2Bu-cGMP (analog of cGMP, Sigma) and with human recombinant ANP (hrANP, Sigma). The higher level of ANP production (after 2Bu-cGMP treatment) and the supplementation of cultured GLCs with hrANP were associated with significant suppression of Caspase-3 activity, that is to say, with the inhibition of apoptosis in GLCs, compared to control cells. For Caspase-3 activity assay, the cultured cells were lysed and the soluble fraction of the cell lysate was assayed using specific substrate (Dineva et al., 2007)

3.4 Role of ANP for folliculogenesis and results of COH/IVF

ANP can affect oocyte maturation via cGMP signaling pathways, and suppress spontaneous oocyte maturation (Zhang et al., 2005) and in this manner ANP may be the factor which determines the development of fertilizable oocytes. We analyzed the relationship between the concentrations of ANP in FFls obtained from women undergoing IVF with the number of punctured follicles and the number of retrieved oocytes (results of COH), as well as with the number of fertilized oocytes (results of IVF). The significant positive correlation of follicular ANP with the number of punctured follicles, the number of retrieved oocytes and with the number of fertilized oocytes were documented. Data analysis showed that the level of expression of ANP in the GLCs and its concentration in FFls are potential prognostic markers for COH/IVF outcome.

The higher levels of ANP were associated with "good" folliculogenesis (a high number of punctured follicles and a high number of oocytes retrieved) and with the development of fertilizable oocytes (high number of fertilized oocytes), as a consequence of its direct actions on somatic cells and on oocytes and of its role as a survival factor in the preovulatory human follicle.

3.5 Immunomodulatory role of ANP in preovulatory follicle

In the ovary, many cytokines play an important role in regulation of ovarian steroidogenesis, corpus luteum formation and function, and ovulation (Adashi, 1990). Atrial natriuretic peptide expression from different components of immune system had demonstrated (Kiemer et al., 2000). Macrophages are capable to synthesize ANP and its active state are associated with elevate level of ANP production (Vollmar & Schulz, 1995). Many data showed, that resident ovarian white blood cells are in situ immunomodulator of processes realize in the ovarian follicle, specially ovulation, an inflammatory-like processes, in which immune cells, including macrophages, play very important role (Bukulmez & Arici, 2000, Richards et al., 2002).

The immunomodulatory effect of ANP was studied on in vitro model of peripheral blood cells. Whole human peripheral blood samples, obtained from at least three healthy women, were used for in vitro culture preparation. The cytokine production in all blood samples was stimulated by lipopolysacharide (LPS). The rest cells were treated with human recombinant ANP in different concentration from 10^{-6} to 10^{-8}M. The part of cells was treated with 10^{-12}M ANP, concentration of ANP measured in FFls obtained of women undergoing IVF procedure.

The concentrations of proinflammatory cytokines, TNF-α and IFN-γ in plasma samples, were determined by sandwich-based TNF-α and IFN-γ kits, respectively (E-Bioscience).

The obtained results showed that ANP dose dependently inhibits synthesis of TNF-α and IFN-γ. The inhibitory effect of ANP on the TNF-α and IFN-γ, increases with the decreases of its concentration and is most pronounced at concentrations of ANP (10^{-8}M and 10^{-12}M), established in FFls.

The level of transcription and synthesis of TNF-α is controlled by two factors: Activation protein 1 (AP-1) and Nuclear factor kappa B (NF-κB) (Rhoades et al.,1992), and ANP inhibits their activation by cGMP mediated pathways (Tsukagoshi et al., 2001; Kiemer & Vollmar, 2001). Furthermore, NF-κB and Nuclear Factor of Activated T cells (NFAT) control transcription of the gene for IFN-γ and hence the synthesis IFN-γ (Sica et al., 1997). The ANP inhibits the activation of NF-κB in cells and tissues which is important for the release of many inflammatory molecules and inflammatory response (Zhang et al., 2008). These data and obtained results by us showed that ANP is an important intra ovarian regulator of inflammatory response and is a potential modulator of immune environment within preovulatory follicle.

3.6 Role of antioxidant enzymes in ovarian function

3.6.1 Survival role of Superoxide dismutase (SOD) and Catalase (CAT) for GLCs

Physiological processes in the ovary have a dynamic character and are accompanied with the change in the intensity of cellular metabolism and cellular oxygen consumption, resulting in the generation of reactive oxygen compounds (ROS, reactive oxygen species). The protection from ROS is realized by both: low molecular weight natural antioxidants (antioxidant vitamins and polyphenols) and antioxidant enzyme systems. The enzymatic antioxidant defense include: superoxide dismutase (SOD) catalase (CAT) and glutathione peroxidases (GPRXs). These three enzymes act in a cooperative or synergistic way to ensure a global cell protection. To cope with ROS, cells express an array of antioxidant enzymes, including the superoxide dismutases (SOD) (e.g. cytosolic Cu/Zn- SOD, mitochondrial Mn-SOD and extracellular (Cu/Zn)- EC- SOD) which convert superoxide anions to hydrogen peroxide, that is then transformed to water by catalase (CAT) and by glutathione S-peroxidase. When the balance between physiological ROS production and the antioxidant defences becomes unbalanced, this disequilibrium may drive the cell to cell death (Orrenius et al., 2007).

Biological reactions that reduce the "harmful" levels of free radicals are of prime importance in reproductive systems in maintaining the quality of gametes and support reproduction.

We used a 48h in vitro model of human GLCs, to investigate how the supplementation with various concentrations of Cu, Zn – SOD or the treatment with various concentrations of Cu-chelating agent sodium diethyldithiocarbamate (DDC) influences GLCs total SOD activity and the GLCs viability (Caspase-3 activity) and how these parameters are interrelated.

The isolated GLCs from at least three women were cultured in 96- well plates (Linbro® Flow Labs, Virginia, USA), (50 µl/well). After 24 h culture period the cells were supplemented with 10, 100, 200 U/ml SOD1 (Cu, Zn-SOD, Inst. Microbiology, Bulg.Acad.Sci.) The purified Cu, Zn-SOD enzyme is a water-soluble homodimeric glycoprotein with a molecular mass of approximately 31700 Da and was isolated from Humicola lutea 103 (Krumova et al., 2007). The rest of cells without control were treated with 10, 100 µM DDC (Sigma). The Caspase-3 activity was measured as mentioned above. The total SOD activity in GLCs at the end of the culture period (48 h), was measured according the method of Beaushap & Fridovich (1971).

Based on measured GLCs total SOD activity, anti-oxidative effect of low dose DDC (10µM) and pro oxidative effect of high dose DDC (100µM) were documented: significantly higher GLCs total SOD activity (10 µM DDC) and significantly lower GLCs total SOD activity (100 µM DDC) was measured, respectively, compared to the control cells.

The highest activity of Caspase-3, measured after the treatment with 100 µM DDC was followed by lowest total GLCs SOD activity, showing the direct role of Cu, Zn- SOD in the prevention of human GLCs from apoptosis. A possible cooperation of SOD and cytochrome C in mitochondria-dependent apoptosis has been described by Li et al 2006. The simultaneous release of SOD with cytochrome C has been shown to regulates mitochondria-dependent apoptosis increasing the susceptibility of mitochondria to oxidative stresses (Li et al 2009), whereas the active enzyme has been reported to be implicated in protecting vital mitochondria (Iñarrea et al., 2007). In this study for first time, we demonstrated that the supplementation with Cu, Zn-SOD (200 U/ml) was closely involved in anti-apoptotic mechanisms and maintains the human GLCs viability in vitro, by the suppression of Caspase-3 activity.

3.6.2 Relationship between activity of antioxidant enzymes SOD and CAT in GLCs with COH / IVF outcome

Oocytes and granulosa cells in all follicular stages are endowed with the major antioxidant and detoxifying enzymes (e.g. SOD and CAT) (Suzuki et al., 1999; Mouatassim et al., 1999). SOD activity and CAT activity have been demonstrated in human FFls (Carbone et al., 2003; Pasqualotto et al. 2009; Bausenwein et al., 2010). The expression of SOD and of CAT at mRNA and protein level have been studied in human follicular somatic cells, such as GLCs and CCs in relation to female reproductive aging and successful outcome of assisted reproductive technologies, respectively (Tatone et al., 2006; Matos et al., 2009). The aim of our study was to investigate the relationship among the activity of superoxide dismutase (SOD) and catalase (CAT) in GLCs and apoptosis of these cells with the results of COH/ IVF in infertile women.

For detection of apoptosis in GLCs the method of DAPI-DNA staining was used. The activity of intracellular SOD and CAT of GLCs were measured using the Beaushap & Fridovich; Beers & Sizer methods, respectively (Beers & Sizer, 1952; Beaushap & Fridovich, 1971).

We studied the relationship between the activity of SOD and CAT in GLCs with the level of apoptosis (% apoptotic hGLCs) and with the parameters of COH and IVF. The balance between the ROS production, cellular antioxidant defenses, activation of stress-related signaling pathways, and the production of various gene products, will determine whether a cell exposed to an increase in ROS will be destined for survival or death (Kregel & Zhang, 2007). The SOD and CAT play a central role in the antioxidative defense in the ovary and they act in tandem to neutralize the supra physiologic levels of ROS.

Within the studied patient's groups we found that the "health" status of human GLCs (low level of apoptosis) is associated positively with both, SOD and CAT activity in GLCs obtained from the same woman.

Oxidative stress in granulosa cells was suggested to decrease both fertilization rate and quality of embryos in IVF cycles (Seino et al., 2002). Elevated level and high activity of SOD are associated with better quality of oocyte, and good embryo development, influenced, probably, by the oxidant/antioxidant (du Plessis et al., 2008). Our results demonstrated that the better outcome in the COH/IVF cycles, such as higher numbers of retrieved and fertilized oocytes are related to higher intra cellular SOD activity in GLCs. We consider that the intra cellular SOD activity in GLCs has contribution to the vital oocyte microenvironment, supported also by SOD activity in cumulus-oophorus cells (Matos et al., 2009) as well as by SOD and CAT activity of FFls (Kably Ambe et al., 2005; Pasqualotto et al., 2009), and that intra cellular SOD activity could be a potential biomarker for ART success.

4. Gene expression in cumulus cells as biomarker for oocyte competence

Pregnancy and birth rates in assisted reproductive technology (ART), following in vitro fertilization (IVF) are unique events but unfortunately 2 out of 3 IVF cycles fail to result in pregnancy. Due to the subjective morphological parameters in selection of healthy embryos used in IVF and ICSI programmes, 8 out of 10 transferred embryos fail to implant (Kovalevsky, G. & Patrizio, P., 2005). Consequently, selecting oocytes with normal developmental competence and embryos with the highest implantation potential is of great importance in assisted reproductive technology.

4.1 Cumulus cells as targets of biomarkers

Ovarian follicle development and maturation are complex processes, involving both the oocyte and its surrounding transcriptionally distinct CCs and GLCs (Eppig et al., 2001). Mammalian oocyte growth and development is critically dependent on the functional two-way communication axis that exists between the germ cell and its immediate companions – the ovarian cumulus cells. This communication is in form of direct gap-junction communications and paracrine signaling mediated via soluble oocyte-secreted factors (McNatty et al., 2004). It is well recognized now, that the oocytes also promote cumulus and granulosa cell proliferation, differentiation and apoptosis, suggesting that the health and function of the granulosa and cumulus cells being may be reflective of the health status of the enclosed oocyte (Eppig et al., 2001). Since the CCs and GLCs transcriptomic profiles are influenced of the bidirectional oocyte-somatic cells communication, and thus these profiles could serve as an approximate reflection of the oocyte developmental competence. Perturbations in the oocyte functionality both genetic and functional would result in an altered oocyte-cumulus signaling and thus an altered cumulus transcriptome. In this way, the study of the CCs transcriptomic profile offers the opportunity, by a non-invasive method, to predict oocyte and eventually embryo competence (Assou et al., 2010).

Derived from this paradigm, we believe that after clinical validation a small subset of particular genes would render relatively cheap and non-invasive test for screening of good competence oocytes in all cases when ART procedures are involved, but pre implantation genetic diagnostic (PGD) of succeeding embryo might be not available or should be avoided.

We have recently investigated several gene transcript products as part of larger set of cumulus-derived oocyte competence-predicting genes as a pilot evaluation study and prove of concept, namely: lysyl oxidase (LOX), basigin (BSG), phosphoglycerate kinase 1 (PGK1) and nuclear factor kappa-light-chain-enhancer of activated B cells (NF-κB) (Todorova et al., 2011a, 2011b). We have also studied known protein transcriptional factors that might also impact the oocyte competence in case of altered abundance, perturbing the oocyte development, maturation or fertilization, and thus the oocyte fertility competence.

4.2 The study concept of the transcript biomarkers

Specimens from multiple oocyte-neighboring cumulus cells were isolated from three investigated patients' groups: women with reproductive problems, participating in ICSI procedures with primary sterility; women with reproductive problems, participating in ICSI procedures with secondary sterility; women with so called *"male factor sterility"* (where reproductive failure is result in male infertility) and women who participated in "healthy donors" *in vitro* programs. All three groups of women were subject to hormonal stimulation short or long protocols, involving at least FSH and Progesterone.

A quantitative reverse transcriptase real-time PCR approach was applied to estimate the differential gene expression levels of the LOX and BSG gene transcripts, normalized to the house keeping gene PGK1, in the cumulus cells surrounding acquired oocytes from ICSI-targeted primary and secondary sterility IVF patients and healthy fertile donors.

After separation of the CCs from each acquired oocyte, the specimens were individually collected and they were subject to consecutive lysis, mRNA extraction, reverse transcriptase gene specific cDNA synthesis and PCR amplification. For this approach we utilized the one step Fastlane Cell RT-qPCR Kit (Qiagen, USA). The assays were run on a qPCR Cycler (Agilent Technologies MX3005P, Stratagene, USA) using the exact thermal protocol supplied by the manufacturer. The primers were produced by Biomers, Germany.

The data obtained by the qPCR reaction were subsequently subject to analysis by Stratagene MxPro software and represented as gene transcript fold change, where donor specimens were set as 0 fold change. The subsequent statistical analyses included non-parametric Kruskal-Wallis non-parametric ANOVA on the normalized expression levels of *lox* and *bsg*, expressed as fold change compared to donor expression.

We used *pgk1* as housekeeping normalizing gene since it is a transferase enzyme that in humans is involved in main biochemical pathway – the glycolysis, transferring a phosphate group from 1,3-biphosphoglycerate to ADP, with formation of ATP and 3-Phosphoglycerate (Singer-Sam et al., 1984). It has been also considered as suitable housekeeping gene for the cumulus cells as it is found in all living organisms and its sequence has been highly conserved throughout evolution (Kumar et al., 1999).

4.3 The putative markers

Lysyl oxidase also known as protein-lysine 6-oxidase is a protein that, in humans, is encoded by the LOX gene. Its upregulation by tumor cells may promote metastasis of the existing tumor, causing it to become malignant and cancerous (Hämäläinen et al., 1991). This enzyme oxidized peptidyl lysine to pepttidyl aldehyde residues within collagen and elastin, initiating formation of the covalent cross-linkages that insolubilize these extracellular proteins (Li et al., 1997). This function of LOX made it implicated so far in both ovary extracellular matrix synthesis and to some extent in policistic ovary cystogenesis in rat models as well (Papachroni et al., 2010). LOX was found to be under endocrine, paracrine, and autocrine control, with FSH being major coordinator of its response to these stimuli (Harlow et al., 2003).

Jiang et al., 2010 investigated whole genome gene expression profiling of mural granulosa cells and the authors demonstrated that mural granulosa cells isolated from follicles containing oocytes with normal developmental competence are distinct from those with oocytes exhibiting poor developmental competence. These authors established that there were genes which profiles are different in two investigated groups. They reported *lox* expression to be 2.8-fold higher in mural granulosa cells isolated from follicles containing oocytes which exhibit normal developmental competence when compared with poor ones. These results were validated by real-time PCR (Jiang et al., 2010).

Our data are in controversy with the above findings observing quite the opposite phenomenon - LOX mRNA expression estimated with comparative quantitative real-time PCR ($2^{-\Delta\Delta Ct}$ method) was almost 4.32-fold higher (mean value) in infertile women with primary sterility and reproductive failure, compared to fertile donors. LOX mRNA is up-regulated in women with primary or secondary sterility. The difference observed in women with secondary sterility was also increased in favor of the donors - 3.85. (Todorova et al., 2011a, 2011b). We believe that one possible explanation would be that in the above mentioned study (Jiang et al., 2010) immature rats were subject of an anti-eCG treatment with subsequent induction of apoptosis in the granulosa cells, and folliclar atresia, an effect that they report as antibody dose-dependent. In our study design (Todorova et al., 2011a, 2011b) human subjects were studied and even though they could have varying degree of hormone levels, those are both medication stimulated, and followed as feedback, and no patient participates in ART program unless normal (target range) hormone levels are achieved, and latter normal oocyte morphology is prerequisite for subsequent IVF/ICSI procedure. The observed LOX levels are most likely related to the stimulation protocol that induced follicle maturation (GnRH or FSH) and later on - oocyte maturation (hCG) and ovulation. FSH and hCG (eCG) were found to downregulate LOX gene expression. Therefore it should be expected that in the cumulus cells of fertile women and healthy donors rather decreased lox mRNA transcript levels would be observed. Parallel to that, the lox gene expression is able to suppress oocyte maturation in experimental model systems, suppressing both RAS and Progesterone induction (Di Donato et al., 1997). Thus some subtle differences between donor's and IVF/ICSI failure oocytes exist, that are neither directly reflected by the woman hormonal levels, nor by the oocyte parameters alone. Besides in Jiang et al., 2010 study mural granulosa were analyzed, rather than human cumulus cells.

It has to be noted that there is growing evidence for functional difference in transcriptomes expressed in the oocyte adjacent cumulus cells and the granulosa cells located further on. Although morphologically they may seem the same, the existence of paracrine signaling axis between oocyte and adjacent somatic cells creates a signaling molecules concentration gradient that renders different responses and hence distinct expression profiles in the somatic cells across the oocyte follicle. Whether there are more stable and long lasting differences remains yet to be established.

A more in depth analysis of oocyte physiology reveals that LOX has been shown to participate in very important processes connected with the cell differentiation of granulosa cells (Jiang et al., 2010). TGF-β1 and GDF9 increase lox mRNA expression in rat granulosa cells (Kendall et al., 2003). The GDF9-induced preantral follicular growth in vitro involves increased mural granulosa cell lox mRNA expression (Assou et al., 2010), and similarly the investigations on rat granulosa cells showed that lox transcripts were significantly suppressed 48h after eCG injection compared with untreated controls (Jiang et al., 2010). Harlow et al. demonstrated that while in primary and especially in preantral follicle GDF-9 increases extremely LOX expression, in antral follicle in which the levels of FHS-receptors are induced, FSH dose-dependently decreases the LOX levels, while GDF-9 induction effect is diminished. In this context the lox mRNA and protein expression levels should be expected to be decreased, rather than increased (Harlow et al., 2003). This could serve as legitimate explanation, why in women with infertility the levels of lox mRNA are actually increased, with highest levels in those who are having primary sterility.

Basigin is a member of the immunoglobulin superfamily that is also known as EMMPRIN, short for extracellular matrix metalloproteinase inducer (Miyauchi et al., 1992). BSG has already been shown to be expressed in the ovary and play key roles in fertility. It appears to be critical for both ovulation and implantation. BSG plays fundamental roles in various immunologic phenomena, differentiation, development and intercellular recognition. Knock-out of BSG in mice results in infertility in both sexes. It was demonstrated that *bsg* gene disruption produces failure of female reproductive processes affecting both implantation and fertilization (Kuno et al., 1998). BSG mRNA expression in cumulus cells and basolateral localization of the BSG protein in the endometrial epithelium further support the importance of BSG in these processes (Smedts, A., & Curry, T. (2005). Our data showed an increase of approximately 6.5 fold for *BSG* in primary sterility women compared to the fertile donors (Todorova et al., 2011a, 2011b). The difference observed in women with secondary sterility was also increased in favor of the donors - 2.5 for *BSG*. Correlation statistical analysis applied to the fold-change expression rates of *LOX* vs. *BSG* using the data acquired for every single specimen of cumulus cells suggested although low power, but positive correlation between the *lox* and *bsg* gene expression levels. The Coefficient of determination (r^2) as measure of the significance of the correlation between *LOX* and *BSG* was 0.5.

4.4 The study concept of the transcriptional factor NFκB involvement

Protein lysates from the same oocyte neighboring cumulus cells were subject to SDS-PAGE and subsequent Western blotting for specific antibody-mediated immunological detection of activated NFκB transcription factor. Lysates from cumulus cells were run under reducing conditions in a 12% SDS-PAGE gel. The separated proteins were transferred to a polyvinylidene fluoride membrane (Sigma, St. Louis, MO, USA). The membranes were blocked and then incubated with anti-NFκB antibody (R&D, USA). The membranes were washed and incubated with anti-mouse ALEXA 488 antibody conjugated. The Western blots were visualized by fluorescent scanner - Ethan DIGE (General Electric, USA), using membrane scanning protocol and appropriate for ALEXA 488 exposure times of the Cy2 preset channel in the acquisition software.

NFκB is a protein complex that controls the transcription of DNA. NF-κB is found in almost all animal cell types and is involved in cellular responses to stimuli such as stress, cytokines, free radicals, ultraviolet irradiation, oxidized LDL, and bacterial or viral antigens. NF-κB plays a key role in regulating the immune response to infection (Gilmore et al., 2006). Resent study has shown that LOX has a binding domain for NFκB making it a putative binding partner and interactor (Li, D., & Mehta J. 2000.; Chen et al., 2006).

As a provisionary Western blot suggest, there is distinct protein level expression of NF-κB among the investigated groups of fertile vs infertile women. Immunoblotting with anti-NFκB antibody demonstrated elevated levels of active NFκB in women with reproductive failure, while in donors this stress molecule was not nuclear translocated and detectable. The expression was higher in women with secondary sterility compared to those, (subject to *ICSI*,) with primary sterility (Todorova et al., 2011). It is controversial why NFκB is increased mostly in secondary sterility patients, since it is stress and inflammation related transcriptional factor, but it has to be noted, that a lot of paracrine singling is mediated by interleukins, and other factors released after NFκB nuclear translocation (Paciolla et al., 2011).

The quality of the oocyte is largely dependent on its follicular environment. Developmental competence of the oocytes is a major determinant in the establishment of successful pregnancy in assisted reproduction. The primary criterion for oocyte selection in the human fertility clinic is the morphological characteristics of oocytes that is highly biased and does not accurately predict the quality of the oocyte (Ebner et al., 2003). Many studies reported that cumulus and granulosa cell gene expression is associated with oocyte health and development (Assou et. al., 2010).

Our studies on LOX expression profile in human cumulus cells is the first investigation ever done on human subjects. Our findings suggest that LOX, and to lesser extent BSG may prove first step and prove of concept as future screening panels incorporated markers for oocyte developmental competence. An ongoing research is currently in progress to confirm our suggestion and extend the suggested panel.

5. Conclusion

The study of the ovarian function in the context of both innate to adaptive immunity interaction and the role of such fundamental processes as apoptosis and oxidative stress challenge with their arising complexity and multimodality. We believe that our research will contribute to the discussed in this text long term exploration of the ovarian biology and immunology by the reproductive biology scientific community, providing us with an insight and new clues regarding the non-invasive evaluation of the biological fertility potential and future technological aids in favor of the reproductive medicine. We believe that these infertility biomarkers will prove significant capacity as fertility and oocyte competence predictors.

6. Acknowledgements

Project DOO2-50/2008 "Establishment of center for research on problems of the reproductive health", National Science Fund, Ministry of Education and Science

Project FP7-REGPOT-2009-1 (ReProForce) "Reinforcement of the Research Capacity of the Bulgarian Institute "Biology and Immunology of Reproduction"

7. References

Adashi, E. (1990). The potential relevance of cytokines to ovarian physiology; the emerging role of resident ovarian cells of the white blood cell series. *Endocrine Reviews*, Vol. 11, No. 3, pp. 454–64, ISSN 1945-7189

Alborzi, S., Tavazoo, F., Dehaghani, A., Ghaderi, A., Alborzi, S. & Alborzi, M. (2009). Determination of antiovarian antibodies after laparoscopic ovarian electrocauterization in patients with polycystic ovary syndrome. *Fertility and Sterility*. Vol. 91, No.4, pp. 1159-1163, ISSN 1556-5653

Assou, S., Haouzi, D., Vos J. & Hamamah, S. (2010). Human cumulus cells as biomarkers for embryo and pregnancy outcomes. *Molecular Human Reproduction*.Vol. 16, No 8, pp. 531-538 ISSN: 13609947

Bakalov, V., Anasti, J., Calis, K., Vanderhoof, V., Premkumar, A., Chen, S., Furmaniak, J., Smith, B., Merino, M. & Nelson, L. (2005) Autoimmune oophoritis as a mechanism of follicular dysfunction in women with 46,XX spontaneous premature ovarian failure. *Fertility and Sterility*. Vol. 84, No. 4, pp. 958-65, ISSN 1556-5653

Banchereau, J. & Steinman,R. (1998). Dendritic cells and the control of immunity. *Nature*. Vol. 392, No. 6673, pp. 245-252, ISSN 1476-4687

Barbarino-Monnier, P., Jouan, C., Dubois, M., Gobert, B., Faure, G.& Béné, M.(2003) Antiovarian antibodies and in vitro fertilization: cause or consequence? *Gynécologie Obstétrique & Fertilite*. Vol. 31, No. 9, pp. 770–773, ISSN 1297-9589

Barber, M. & Fayrer-Hosken, R. (2000). Possible mechanisms of mammalian immunocontraception. *Journal of Reproductive Immunology*. Vol. 46, No. 2, pp. 103-24, ISSN 0165-0378

Batova, I., Ivanova, M., Mollova, M. & Kyurkchiev, S. (1998) Human sperm surface glycoprotein involved in sperm-"zona pellucida" interaction. *International Journal of Andrology*. Vol. 21, No. 3, pp. 141-153, ISSN 1365-2605

Bausenwein, J., Serke, H., Eberle K., Hirrlinger, J., Jogschies, P., Hmeidan, F., Blumenauer, V. & Borowski, K. (2010). Elevated levels of oxidized low-density lipoprotein and of catalase activity in follicular fluid of obese women. *Molecular Human Reproduction*, Vol. 16, No. 2, pp. 117–124, ISSN 1460-2407

Beauchamp, C. & Fridovich, I. (1971). Superoxide dismutase: improved assays and an assay applicable to acrylamide gels. *Analytical Biochemistry*. Vol. 44, No. 1, pp. 276-287, ISSN 1096-0309

Beers, R. & Sizer I. (1952) A spectrophotometric method for measuring the breakdown of hydrogen peroxide by catalase. *Journal of Biological Chemistry*. Vol. 195, No. 1, pp.133-140, ISSN 1083-351X

Betterle, C., Dal Pra, C., Mantero. F. & Zanchetta, R. (2002). Autoimmune adrenal insufficiency and autoimmune polyendocrine syndromes: autoantibodies, autoantigens, and their applicability in diagnosis and disease prediction. *Endocrine Reviews*. Vol. 23, No. 3, pp. 327-64. ISSN 1945-7189

Bianchi, M. (2007). DAMPs, PAMPs and alarmins: all we need to know about danger. *Journal of Leukocyte Biology*. Vol. 81, No. 1, pp. 1-5, ISSN 1938-3673

Bloch, K., Scott, J., Zisfein, J., Fallon, J., Margolies, M., Seidman, C., Matsueda, G., Homcy, C., Graham, R. & Seidman, J. (1985) Biosynthesis and secretion of proatrial natriuretic factor by cultured rat cardiocytes. *Science*, Vol. 230, No. 4730, pp. 1168-1171, ISSN 1095-9203

Broer, S., Eijkemans, M., Scheffer, G., van Rooij, I., de Vet, A., Themmen, A., Laven J., de Jong F., Te Velde, E., Fauser, B. & Broekmans, F. (2011). Anti-mullerian hormone predicts menopause: a long-term follow-up study in normoovulatory women. *Journal of Clinical Endocrinology & Metabolism*. Vol. 96, No. 8, pp. 2532-2539, ISSN 1945-7197

Brozzetti, A. , Marzotti, S. , Torre, D.La , Bacosi, M.L. , Morelli, S. , Bini, V. , Ambrosi, B. , Giordano, R. , Perniola, R. ,De Bellis, A. , Betterle, C. , Falorni, A. (2010). Autoantibody responses in autoimmune ovarian insufficiency and in Addison's disease are IgG1 dominated and suggest a predominant, but not exclusive, Th1 type of response. *European Journal of Endocrinology*. Vol. 163, No. 2., pp 309-317, ISSN 08044643

Bukulmez, O. & Arici, A. (2000). Leukocytes in ovarian function. *Human Reproduction Update*. Vol. 6, No. 1, pp. 1-15, ISSN 1460-2369

Buttari,B., Profumo, E., Mattei, V., Siracusano, A., Ortona, E., Margutti, P., Salvati, B., Sorice, M. & Riganò, R. (2005). Oxidized beta2-glycoprotein I induces human dendritic cell maturation and promotes a T helper type 1 response. *Blood*. Vol. 106, No. 12, pp. 3880-3887, ISSN 1528-0020

Calongos, G., Hasegawa, A., Komori, S. & Koyama, K. (2009). Harmful effects of anti-zona pellucida antibodies in folliculogenesis, oogenesis, and fertilization. *Journal of Reproductive Immunology*. Vol. 79, No. 2, pp. 148-155, ISSN 0165-0378.

Carbone, M., Tatone, C., Delle Monache, S., Marci, R., Caserta, D., Colonna, R. & Amicarelli F. (2003). Antioxidant enzymatic defences in human follicular fluid: characterization and age dependent changes. *Molecular Human Reproduction*. Vol. 9, No. 11, pp. 639-643, ISSN 1460-2407

Chang, M., Lowe, D., Lewis, M., Hellmiss, R., Chen, E. & Goeddel DV (1989). Differential activation by atrial and brain natriuretic peptides of two different receptor guanylate cyclases. *Nature*. Vol. 346, pp. 68-72, ISSN 0028-0836

Chatterjee, S., Modi, D., Maitra, A., Kadam, S., Patel, Z., Gokrall, J. & Meherji, P. (2007). Screening for FOXL2 gene mutations in women with premature ovarian failure: an Indian experience. *Reproductive Biomedicine Online*. Vol.15, No. 5, pp. 554-560, ISSN 1472-6491

Chen, J, Liu, Y., Liu, H., Hermonat, & P., Mehta, J. (2006). Molecular dissection of angiotensin II-activated human LOX-1 promoter. *Arteriosclerosis, Thrombosis and Vascular Biology*. Vol. 26, No 5, pp.1163-1168. ISSN: 10795642

Chen, S., Sawicka, J., Betterle, C., Powell, M., Prentice, L., Volpato, M., Rees Smith, B. & Furmaniak, J. (1996). Autoantibodies to steroidogenic enzymes in autoimmune polyglandular syndrome, Addison's disease, and premature ovarian failure. *Journal of Clinical Endocrinology & Metabolism*. Vol. 81, No. 5, pp. 1871-1876, ISSN 1945-7197

Chernyshov,V., Radysh,T., Gura, I., Tatarchuk, T. & Khominskaya, Z.(2001). Immune disorders in women with premature ovarian failure in initial period. *American Journal of Reproductive Immunology*. Vol. 46, No. 3, 220-225, ISSN 1600-0897

Chun, S., Eisenhauer, K. & Minami, S. (1996). Hormonal regulation of apoptosis in early antral follicles: follicle- stimulating hormone as a major survival factor. *Endocrinology*. 1996; Vol. 137, No. 4, pp. 1447-1456. IISSN 1945-7170

Cianci, A., Calogero, AE., Palumbo, M., Burrello, N., Ciotta, L., Palumbo, G. & Bernardini, R. (1996). Relationship between tumour necrosis factor alpha and sex steroid concentrations in the follicular fluid of women with immunological infertility. *Human Reproduction*. Vol. 11, No. 2, pp. 265-268, ISSN 1460-2350

Dal Pra, C., Chen, S., Furmaniak, J., Smith, B., Pedini, B., Moscon, A., Zanchetta, R. & Betterle, C. (2003). Autoantibodies to steroidogenic enzymes in patients with premature ovarian failure with and without Addison's disease. *Europian Journal of Endocrinology*. Vol. 148, No. 5, pp. 565-570, ISSN 1479-683X

Damewood, M., Zacur, H., Hoffman, G. & Rock, J.(1986). Circulating antiovarian antibodies in premature ovarian failure. *Obstetrics and Gynecology*. Vol. 68, No. 6, pp. 850–854, ISSN 0029-7844

Davis, J. & Rueda, B. (2002) The corpus luteum: an ovarian structure with maternal instincts and suicidal tendencies. *Frontiers in Bioscience*. Vol. 7, pp. 1949-1978, ISSN 1093-4715

Di Donato A., Lacal J., Di Duca, M., Giampuzzi, M., Chiggeri, G., & Gusmano, R. (1997). Micro-injection of recombinant lysyl oxidase blocks oncogenic p21-Ha-Ras and progesterone effects on Xenopus laevis oocyte maturation. *FEBS Letters*, Vol. 419, No1, pp. 63-68, ISSN: 00145793

Dineva, J., Vangelov, I., Nikolov, G., Gulenova, D. & Ivanova, M. (2006). Apoptosis of human Granulosa Luteinized (GLCs) and Cumulus Cells (CCs) as a possible indicator for IVF outcome. *Comptes rendus de l'Acad´emie bulgare des Sciences*. Vol. 59, No.7, pp. 781-784. ISSN 1310-1331

Dineva, J., Wójtowicz, A. Augustowska, K., Vangelov, I., Gregoraszczuk, E. & Ivanova, M. (2007). Expression of Atrial Natriuretic Peptide (ANP), Progesterone (P), Apoptosis-Related Proteins (bcl-2, p53) and Caspase-3 Activity in in vitro Luteinized and Leptin-Treated Porcine Granulosa Cells (pGLCs). *Enodocrine Regulations*. Vol. 41, No. 1, 2006, pp.11-18, ISSN 1336-0329

Doherty, E., Pakarinen, P., Tiitinen, A., Kiilavuori, A., Huhtaniemi, I., Forrest, S. & Aittomäki, K. (2002). Novel mutation in the FSH receptor inhibiting signal transduction and causing primary ovarian failure. *Journal of Clinical Endocrinology & Metabolism*. Vol. 87, No. 3, pp. 1151-1155, ISSN 1945-7197

Du Plessis, S., Desai, M. & Agarwal A (2008) The impact of oxidative stress on in vitro fertilization. *Expert Review of Obstetrics and Gynecology*.Vol. 3, No. 4, pp. 359-554, ISSN: 1747-4108

Ebner, T., Moser, M., Sommergruber, M., Tews, G. (2003). Selection based on morphological assessment of oocytes and embryos at different stages of preimplantation development: a review. *Human Reproduction Update*. Vol.9, No 3, pp251-262. ISSN: 13554786

Edassery, S., Shatavi, S., Kunkel, J., Hauer, C., Brucker, C., Penumatsa, K., Yu, Y., Dias, J. & Luborsky, J. (2010). Autoantigens in ovarian autoimmunity associated with unexplained infertility and premature ovarian failure. *Fertility and Sterility*. Vol. 94, No. 7, pp. 2636-2641, ISSN 1556-5653

Eppig, J. (2001). Oocyte control of ovarian follicular development and function in mammals. *Reproduction*. Vol. 122, No6, pp. 829-838, ISSN 14701626

Falorni, A., Laureti, S., Candeloro, P., Perrino, S., Coronella, C., Bizzarro, A., Bellastella, A., Santeusanio, F. & De Bellis, A. (2002). Steroid-cell autoantibodies are preferentially expressed in women with premature ovarian failure who have adrenal autoimmunity. *Fertility and Sterility*. Vol. 78, No. 2, pp. 270-279, ISSN 1556-5653

Fénichel, P., Sosset, C., Barbarino-Monnier, P., Gobert, B., Hiéronimus, S., Béné, M. & Harter, M. (1997). Prevalence, specificity and significance of ovarian antibodies during spontaneous premature ovarian failure. *Human Reproduction*. Vol.12, No. 12, pp. 2623-2628, ISSN 1460-2350

Forges, T., Monnier-Barbarino, P., Faure, G. & Béné, M. (2004). Autoimmunity and antigenic targets in ovarian pathology. *Human Reproduction Update*. Vol. 10, No. 2, pp. 163-75. ISSN 1460-2369

Ghazeeri, G. & Kutteh, W. (2001). Autoimmune factors in reproductive failure. *Current Opinion in Obstetrics and Gynecology*. Vol. 13, pp. 287-291, ISSN 1473-656X.

Gilmore TD. (2006). Introduction to NF-κB: Players, pathways, perspectives. *Oncogene* Vol. 25, No 51, pp. 6680–6684. ISSN: 09509232

Gobert, B., Barbarino-Monnier, P., Guillet-May, F., Béné, M. & Faure G. (1992). Anti-ovary antibodies after attempts at human in-vitro fertilization induced by follicular puncture rather than hormonal stimulation. *Journal of Reproduction and Fertilility*. Vol. 96, No. 1, pp. 213–218, ISSN 0022-4251

Gobert, B., Jolivet-Reynaud, C., Dalbon, P., Barbarino-Monnier, P., Faure, G. Jolivet, M. & Béné, M. (2001). An immunoreactive peptide of the FSH involved in autoimmune infertility. *Biochemical and Biophysical Resarch Communications*. Vol. 289, No.4, pp. 819-824, ISSN 0006-291X

Gutkowska, J., Jankowski, M., Sairam M., Fujio, N., Reis, A., Mukaddam-Daher S. & Tremblay, J. (1999). Hormonal regulation of natriuretic peptide system during induced ovarian follicular development in the rat. *Biology of Reproduction*. Vol. 61, No. 1, 162–170, ISSN 1529-7268

Gutkowska, J., Tremblay, J., Antakly T., Meyer, R., Mukaddam-Daher, S. & Nemer, M. (1993). The atrial natriuretic peptide system in rat ovaries. *Endocrinology*. Vol. 132, No. 2, pp. 693-700, ISSN 1945-7170

Haller, K., Mathieu, C., Rull, K., Matt, K., Béné, M. & Uibo R. (2005). IgG, IgA and IgM antibodies against FSH: serological markers of pathogenic autoimmunity or of normal immunoregulation? *American Journal of Reproductive Immunology*. Vol. 54, No. 5, pp. 262-269, ISSN 1600-0897

Hämäläinen, E. Jones, T., Sheer, D., Taskinen, K., Pihlajaniemi, T., & Kivirikko, K. (1991). Molecular cloning of human lysyl oxidase and assignment of the gene to chromosome 5q23.3-31.2. *Genomics*, Vol. 11, No 3, pp. 508–516. ISSN: 08887543

Harlow, C., Rae, M., Davidson, L., Trackman, P., & Hillier, S. (2003). Lysyl Oxidase Gene Expression and enzyme activity in the rat ovary: regulation by follicle-stimulating hormone, androgen and transforming growth factor beta superfamily members in vitro. *Endocrinology*. Vol. 144, No 1, pp. 154-162. ISSN: 00137227

Hawa, M., Fava, D., Medici, F., Deng, Y., Notkins, A., De Mattia, G. & Leslie, R. (2000). Antibodies to IA-2 and GAD65 in type 1 and type 2 diabetes: isotype restriction and polyclonality. *Diabetes Care*. Vol. 23, No. 2, pp. 228-33, ISSN 1935-5548

Ho, P., Tang, G., Fu, K., Fan, M. & Lawton, J. (1988). Immunologic studies in patients with premature ovarian failure. *Obstetrics and Gynecology*. Vol. 71, No. 4, pp. 622-626, ISSN 0029-7844

Hoek, A., van Kasteren, Y., de Haan-Meulman, M., Hooijkaas, H., Schoemaker, J. & Drexhage, H.(1995). Analysis of peripheral blood lymphocyte subsets, NK cells, and delayed type hypersensitivity skin test in patients with premature ovarian failure. *American Journal of Reproductive Immunology*. Vol. 33, No. 6, pp. 495-502, ISSN 1600-0897

Hoek, A., Schoemaker, J. & Drexhage, H. (1997). Premature ovarian failure and ovarian autoimmunity. *Endocrine Reviews.* Vol. 18, No1, pp. 107-134, ISSN 0163-769X.

Hoek, A., van Kasteren, Y., de Haan-Meulman, M., Schoemaker, J. & Drexhage, H.A. (1993). Dysfunction of monocytes and dendritic cells in patients with premature ovarian failure. *American Journal of Reproductive Immunology.* Vol. 30, No. 4, pp. 207-217, ISSN 1600-0897

Horejsí, J., Martínek, J., Nováková, D., Madar, J. & Brandejska, M. (2000). Autoimmune antiovarian antibodies and their impact on the success of an IVF/ET program. *Annals of the New York Academy of Science.* Vol. 900, pp. 351-356, ISSN 0077-8923.

Host, E., Mikkelsen, A. Lindenberg, S. & Smidt-Jensen S. (2000). Apoptosis in human cumulus cells in relation to maturation stage and cleavage of the corresponding oocyte. *Acta Obstetrica et Gynecology Scandinavica.* Vol. 79, No. 11, pp. 936-940, ISSN 1600-0412

Huang, Q., Liu, Q. & Wu, J. (1996). Determinations of antiovarian antibodies and cellular immunity functions in patients with premature ovarian failure. *Chinese Journal of Obstetrics* and Gynecology.Vol. 31, No. 10, pp. 603-605, ISSN 0529-567

Iñarrea, P., Moini, H., Han, D., Rettori, D., Aguiló, I., Alava, M., Iturralde, M. & Cadenas E. (2007). Mitochondrial respiratory chain and thioredoxin reductase regulate intermembrane Cu,Zn-superoxide dismutase activity: implications for mitochondrial energy metabolism and apoptosis. *Biochemical Journal.* Vol. 405, pp. 173-179. ISSN 1470-8728

Ivanova, M. & Mollova, M. Zona-penetration in vitro test for evaluating boar sperm fertility (1993) *Theriogenology.* Vol. 40, No. 2, pp. 397- 410, ISSN 0093-691X

Ivanova, M., Bourneva, V., Gitsov, L. & Angelova, Z. (1984). Experimental immune oophoritis as a model for studying the thymus-ovary interaction: 1. Morphological studies. *American Journal of Reproductive Immunology.* Vol. 6, No. 3, pp. 99-106, ISSN 1600-0897

Ivanova, M., Gregoraszczuk, E., Augustowska, K., Kolodziejczyk, J., Mollova, M. & Kehayov IR. (2003). Localization of atrial natriuretic peptide in pig granulosa cells isolated from ovarian follicles of various size. *Reproductive Biology.* Vol. 3, No. 2, pp. 173-181, ISSN 1529-7268

Jiang, J., Xiong, H., Cao, M., Xia, X., Sirard, M., & Tsang, B. (2010) Mural granulosa cell gene expression associated with oocyte developmental competence. *Journal of Ovarian Research,* Vol. 3, No 1:6, ISSN: 17572215

Kably Ambe, A., Ruiz Anguas, J., Carballo Mondragón, E. & Karchmer Krivitsky S. (2005) Intrafollicular levels of sexual steroids and their relation with the antioxidant enzymes on the oocyte quality in an in vitro fertilization program. *Ginecology Obstetrics Mexico.* Vol. 73, No. 1, pp. 19-27, ISSN 0014-4142

Kannan, S. (2006). Free radical theory of autoimmunity. *Theoretical Biology and Medical Modeling.* Vol. 3, No.22, ISSN 1742-4682

Kelkar, R., Meherji, P, Kadam, S., Gupta, S. & Nandedkar, T. (2005). Circulating auto-antibodies against the zona pellucida and thyroid microsomal antigen in women with premature ovarian failure. *Journal of Reproductive Immunoogy.* Vol. 66, No.1, pp. 53-67, ISSN 0165-0378.

Kendall N., Marsters, P., Scaramuzzi, R, & Campbell, B. (2003). Expression of lysyl oxidase and effect of copper chloride and ammonium tetrathiomolybdate on bovine ovarian follicle granulosa cells cultured in serum-free media. *Reproduction*, Vol. 125, No 5, pp. 657-665. ISSN: 14701626

Kiemer, A. & Vollmar A. (2001). Elevation of intracellular calcium levels contributes to the inhibition of inducible nitric oxide synthase by atrial natriuretic peptide. *Immunology and Cell Biology*. Vol. 79, pp. 11-17, ISSN 1440-1711

Kiemer, A., Hartung, T. & Vollmar, A. (2000). cGMP-mediated inhibition of TNF-α production by the atrial natriuretic peptide in murine macrophages. *Journal of Immunology*. Vol. 165, No. 1, pp. 175-181, ISSN 1550-6606

Kim, S., Shinjo, M., Usuki S., Tada,M., Miyazaki, H. & Murakami, K. (1987). Binding sites for atrial natriuretic peptide in high concentration in human ovaries. *Biomedical Research*. Vol. 8, pp. 415–420, ISSN 0970938X

Kovalevsky, G. & Patrizio, P. (2005) High rates of embryo wastage with use of assisted reproductive technology: A look at the trends between 1995 and 2001 in the United States *Fertility and Sterility*., Vol. 84 ,No2, pp. 325-330, ISSN 00150282

Koyama, K. (2010). Anti-gonad antibodies, anti-sperm antibodies. *Nihon Rinsho*. Vol. 68, No. 6, pp. 622-624. ISSN 0047-1852.

Kregel, K. & Zhang, H. (2007). An integrated view of oxidative stress in aging: basic mechanisms, functional effects, and pathological considerations. *American Journal of Physiology*. Vol. 292, No.1, pp. 18-36, ISSN 1522-1490

Krumova, E., Dolashka-Angelova, P., Pashova, S., Stefanova, L., Van Beeumen, J., Vassilev, S. & M. Angelova (2007). Improved production by fed-batch cultivation and some properties of Cu/Zn-superoxide dismutase from the fungal strain Humicola lutea 103. *Enzyme and Microbial Technology*. Vol. 40, No. 4, pp. 524-532, ISSN 0141-0229

Kumar, S., Ma, B., Tsai, C., Wolfson, H., & Nussinov, R. (1999). Folding funnels and conformational transitions via hinge-bending motions. *Cellular Biochemistry and Biophysics*. Vol. 31, No2, pp: 141–164. ISSN: 10859195

Kuno, N., Kadomatsu, Fan, K., Hagihara Q., Senda, T., Mizutani, S., & Muramatsu, T. (1998). Female sterility in mice lacking the basigin gene, which encodes a transmembrane glycoprotein belonging to the immunoglobulin superfamily. *FEBS Lett*. Vol. 425, No 2, pp. 191-194. ISSN: 00145793

Kyurkchiev, S., Surneva-Nakova, T., Ivanova, M., Nakov, L. & Dimitrova, E. (1988). Monoclonal antibodies to porcine zona pellucida that block the initial stages of fertilization. *American Journal of Reproductive Immunology and Microbiology*. Vol. 18, No. 1, pp. 11-16, ISSN 8755-8920

La Marca, A., Brozzetti, A., Sighinolfi, G., Marzotti, S., Volpe, A. & Falorni A. (2010). Primary ovarian insufficiency: autoimmune causes. *Current Opinion in Obstetrics and Gynecology*. Vol. 22, No. 4, pp. 277-82. ISSN 1473-656X.

La Polt Ps., Leung, K., Ishimaru, R., Tafoya, M. & Chen J. (2003). Roles of cyclic GMP in modulating ovarian functions. *Reproductive Biomedicine Online*, Vol. 6, No.1, pp.15–23, ISSN 1472-6491

Lee, K., Joo, B., Yong, J., Yoon, M., Choi, O. & Kim, W. (2001). Cumulus Cells Apoptosis as an Indicator to Predict the Quality of Oocytes and the Outcome of IVF–ET. *Journal of Assisted Reproduction and Genetics*. Vol. 18, No. 9, pp. 490-498, ISSN 1573-7330

Lefèvre, B. (2011). Follicular atresia: Its features as predictive markers for the outcome of assisted reproduction. *Gynecologie Obstetrique Fertilite.* Vol. 39, No. 1, pp. 58-62, ISSN 1769-6682

Li, D., & Mehta, J. (2000). Upregulation of endothelial receptor for oxidized LDL (LOX-1) by oxidized LDL and implications in apoptosis of coronary artery endothelial cells: Evidence from use of antisense LOX-1 mRNA and chemical inhibitors. *Arteriosclerosis, Thrombosis, and Vascular Biology.* Vol. 20, No 4, pp. 1116-22, ISSN 1079-5642

Li, J., Jin, H., Zhang, F., Du, X., Zhao, G., Yu, Y. & Wang, B. (2008). Treatment of autoimmune ovarian disease by co-administration with mouse zona pellucida protein 3 and DNA vaccine through induction of adaptive regulatory T cells. *Journal of Gene Medicine.* Vol. 10, 7, pp. 810-20, ISSN 1521-2254

Li, Q., Sato, E., Kira, Y., Nishikawa, M., Utsumi, K. & Inoue M., (2006). A possible cooperation of SOD1 and cytochrome C in mitochondria-dependent apoptosis. *Free Radical Biology and Medicine.* Vol. 40, No. 1, pp.173-181, ISSN 0891-5849

Li, Q., Sato, E., Zhu, X. & Inoue M. (2009) A simultaneous release of SOD1 with cytochrome C regulates mitochondria-dependent apoptosis. *Molecular and Cellular Biochemistry.* Vol. 322, No. 1-2, pp. 151-159, ISSN 1573-4919

Li, W., Nellaiappan, K., Strassmaier, T., Graham, L., Thomas, K., & Kagan, H. (1997). Localization and activity of lysyl oxidase within nuclei of fibrogenic cells. *Proc Natl Acad Sci* USA, Vol. 94, No24, pp.12817-12822, ISSN 00278424

Lloyd, M., Papadimitriou, J., O'Leary, S., Robertson, S. & Shellam, G.R. (2010). Immunoglobulin to zona pellucida 3 mediates ovarian damage and infertility after contraceptive vaccination in mice. *Journal of Autoimmunity.* Vol. 35, No. 1, pp. 77-85, ISSN 0896-8411

Luborsky, J. (2002).Ovarian autoimmune disease and ovarian autoantibodies. *Journal of Womens Health and Gender Based Medicine.* Vol. 11, No. 7, pp. 585-99, ISSN 1931-843X

Luborsky, J., Llanes, B., Davies, S., Binor, Z., Radwanska, E. & Pong, R. (1999). Ovarian autoimmunity: greater frequency of autoantibodies in premature menopause and unexplained infertility than in the general population. *Clinical Immunology.* Vol. 90, No. 3, pp. 368-74, ISSN 1521-6616

Luborsky, J., Llanes, B., Roussev, R.& Coulam C. (2000). Ovarian antibodies, FSH and inhibin B: independent markers associated with unexplained infertility. *Human Reprodoction.* Vol. 15, No. 5, pp. 1046-51, ISSN 1460-2350

Luborsky, J., Visintin, I., Boyers, S., Asari, T., Caldwell, B. & DeCherney, A. (1990). Ovarian antibodies detected by immobilized antigen immunoassay in patients with premature ovarian failure. *Journal of Clinical Endocrinology & Metabolism.* Vol.70, No. 1, pp. 69-75, ISSN 1945-7197

Luborsky, J.L., Yu, Y., Edassery, S., Jaffar, J., Yip, Y., Liu, P., Hellstrom, K.& Hellstrom, I.(2011). Autoantibodies to mesothelin in infertility. *Cancer Epidemiology, Biomarkers and Prevention.* Vol. 20, No. 9, pp. 1970-1978, ISSN 1538-7755

Maity, R., Nair, S., Caspi, R.. & Nelson, L. (1997). Post-thymectomy murine experimental autoimmune oophoritis is associated with reduced natural killer cell activity. *American Journal of Reproductive Immunology.* Vol. 38, No. 5, pp. 360-5, ISSN 1600-0897

Mande, P.V., Parikh, F., Hinduja, I., Zaveri, K., Vaidya, R., Gajbhiye, R. & Khole, V. (2011). Identification and validation of candidate biomarkers involved in human ovarian autoimmunity. *Reproductive Biomedicine Online.* ISSN 1472-6491

Mardesic, T., Ulcova-Gallova, Z., Huttelova, R., Muller, P., Voboril, J., Mikova, M. & Hulvert, J. (2000). The influence of different types of antibodies on in vitro fertilization results. *American Journal of Reproductive Immunology.* Vol. 43, No. 1, pp. 1-5, ISSN 1600-0897

Mathur, S., Peress, M., Williamson, H., Youmans, C., Maney, S., Garvin, A., Rust, P. & Fudenberg, H. (1982). Autoimmunity to endometrium and ovary in endometriosis. *Clinical and Experimental Immunology.* Vol. 50, No. 2, pp. 259-266, ISSN 1365-2249

Matos, L., Stevenson, D., Gomes, F., Silva-Carvalho, J. & Almeida, H. (2009). Superoxide dismutase expression in human cumulus oophorus cells. *Molecular Human Reprodoction.* Vol.15, No. 7, pp. 411-419, ISSN 1460-2407

McNatty, K., Moore, L., Hudson, N., Quirke, L., Lawrence, S., Reader, K., Hanrahan, J., Smith, P., Groome, N., Laitinen, M., Ritvos, O., & Juengel, J. (2004). The oocyte and its role in regulating ovulation rate: a new paradigm in reproductive biology. *Reproduction,* Vol. 128, No 4, pp: 379-386, ISSN: 14701626

Medzhitov, R. (2010). Inflammation 2010: new adventures of an old flame. *Cell.* Vol. 140, No. 6, pp. 771-6, ISSN 0092-8674

Mignot, M., Drexhage, H., Kleingeld, M., Van de Plassche-Boers, E.M., Rao, B. & Schoemaker, J.(1989). Premature ovarian failure. II: Considerations of cellular immunity defects. *Europian Journal of Obstetrics & Gynecology & Reproductive Biology.* Vol. 30, No. 1, pp. 67-72, ISSN 1872-7654

Miyauchi, T., Masuzawa, Y., & Muramatsu, T. (1991). The basigin group of the immunoglobulin superfamily: complete conservation of a segment in and around transmembrane domains of human and mouse basigin and chicken HT7 antigen *Journal of Biochemistry.,* Vol. 110, No 5, pp.770–774. ISSN: 0021924X

Moncayo-Naveda, H., Moncayo, R., Benz, R., Wolf, A. & Lauritzen C. (1989). Organ-specific antibodies against ovary in patients with systemic lupus erythematosus. *American Journal of Obstetrics and Gynecology.* Vol. 160, No. 5, pp. 1227-1229, ISSN 0002-9378

Mouatassim S., Guérin, P. & Ménézo, Y. (1999). Expression of genes encoding antioxidant enzymes in human and mouse oocytes during the final stages of maturation. *Molecular Human Reprodoction.* Vol. 5, No. 8, pp. 720-725, ISSN 1460-2407

Nakahara, K., Saito, H., Saito, T., Ito, M., Ohta, N., Sakai, N., Tezuka, N,. Hiroi, M. & Watanabe, H. (1997). The incidence of apoptotic bodies in membrana granulosa can predict prognosis of ova from patiens participating in in vitro fertilization programs. *Fertility and Sterility.* Vol. 68, No. 2, 312-317, ISSN 1556-5653

Navratil, J., Sabatine, J. & Ahearn, J. (2005). Apoptosis and immune responses to self. *Rheumatic Disease Clinics of North America.* Vol. 30, No. 1, pp. 193-212, ISSN 1558-3163

Nelson, L. (2009). Clinical practice. Primary ovarian insufficiency. *The New England Journal of Medicine.* Vol. 360, No. 6, pp. 606-614, ISSN 1533-4406

Ntrivalas, E., Kwak-Kim, J., Gilman-Sachs, A., Chung-Bang, H., Ng, S., Beaman, K., Mantouvalos, H. & Beer, A. (2001). Status of peripheral blood natural killer cells in women with recurrent spontaneous abortions and infertility of unknown aetiology. *Human Reprodoction*. Vol. 16, No. 5, pp. 855-861, ISSN 1460-2350

Orrenius, S., Gogvadzejavas V. & Zhivotovsky B. (2007). Mitochondrial Oxidative Stress: Implications for Cell Death. *Pharmacology and Toxicolology*. Vol. 47, pp. 143-183, ISSN 1600-0773

Paciolla, M., Boni, R., Fusco, F., Pescatore, A., Poeta, L., Ursini, M., Lioi, M. & Miano, M. (2011). Nuclear factor-kappa-B-inhibitor alpha (NFKBIA) is a developmental marker of NF-κB/p65 activation during in vitro oocyte maturation and early embryogenesis. *Human Reproduction*. Vol. 26, No 5, ISSN: 02681161

Papachroni, K., Piperi, C., Levidou, G., Korkolopoulou, P., Pawelczyk, L., Diamanti-Kandarakis, E., & Papavassiliou, A. (2010). Lysyl oxidase interacts with AGE signalling to modulate collagen synthesis in polycystic ovarian tissue. *Journal of Cellular and Molecular Medicine*., Vol. 14, No 10, pp. 2460-2469 ISSN: 15821838

Pasoto, S., Viana, V., Mendonca, B., Yoshinari, N. & Bonfa, E. (1999). Anti-corpus luteum antibody: a novel serological marker for ovarian dysfunction in systemic lupus erythematosus. *Journal of Rheumatology*. Vol. 26, No. 5, pp. 1087-93, ISSN 1499-2752

Pasqualotto, E., Lara, L., Salvador, M., Sobreiro, B., Borges, E. & Pasqualotto F. (2009). The role of enzymatic antioxidants detected in the follicular fluid and semen of infertile couples undergoing assisted reproduction. *Human Fertilility* (Cambridge). Vol. 12, No. 3, 166-71, ISSN 1464-7273

Petríková, J., Lazúrová, I., Yehuda, S. (2010). Polycystic ovary syndrome and autoimmunity. *European Journal of International Medicine*. Vol. 21, No. 5, pp.369-371, ISSN 0953-6205

Piccinni, M., Beloni, L., Livi, C., Maggi, E., Scarselli, G. & Romagnani, S. (1998). Defective production of both leukemia inhibitory factor and type 2 T-helper cytokines by decidual T cells in unexplained recurrent abortions. *Nature Medicine*. Vol. 4, No. 9, pp.1020-1024, ISSN 1546-170X

Pires, E., Meherji, P., Vaidya, R., Parikh, F., Ghosalkar, M. & Khole V. (2007). Specific and sensitive immunoassays detect multiple anti-ovarian antibodies in women with infertility. *Journal of Histochemistry and Cytochemistry*. Vol. 55, No. 12, pp.1181–1190, ISSN 1551-5044

Pires, E., Parte, P., Meherji, P., Khan, S. & Khole V. (2006). Naturally occurring anti-albumin antibodies are responsible for false positivity in diagnosis of autoimmune premature ovarian failure. *Journal of Histochemistry and Cytochemistry*. Vol. 54, No. 4, pp. 397–405, ISSN 1551-5044

Prado-Drayer, A., Teppa, J., Sánchez, P. & Camejo, M. (2008). Immunophenotype of peripheral T lymphocytes, NK cells and expression of CD69 activation marker in patients with recurrent spontaneous abortions, during the mid-luteal phase. *American Journal of Reproductive Immunology*. Vol. 60, No.1, pp. 66-74, ISSN 1600-0897

Puddu, P., Puddu, G., Cravero, E., De Pascalis, S. & Muscari, A. (2009). The emerging role of cardiovascular risk factor-induced mitochondrial dysfunction in atherogenesis. *Journal of Biomedical Science*. Vol. 6, p. 112, ISSN 1423-0127

Ramasamy, R., Yan, S. & Schmidt, A. (2009). RAGE: therapeutic target and biomarker of the inflammatory response - the evidence mounts. *Journal of Leukocyte Biology*. Vol. 86, No. 3, pp. 505–512, ISSN 1938-3673

Rhoades, K., Golub, S, & Economou J. (1992). The regulation of the human tumor necrosis factor alpha promoter region in macrophage, T cell, and B cell lines. *The Journal of Biological Chemistry*. Vol. 267, No. 31, 22102-22107, ISSN 1083-351X

Richards, J., Russell, D., Ochsner, S. & Espey, L. (2002). Ovulation: new dimensions and new regulators of the inflammatory-like response. *Annual Review of Physiology*. 2002, 64, pp. 69-92, ISSN 00664278

Rivest, S. & Rivier, C. (1995). The role of corticotropin-releasing factor and interleukin-1 in the regulation of neurons controlling reproductive functions. *Endocrine Reviews*. Vol. 16, No. 2, pp. 177-99, ISSN 1945-7189

Rock, K., Latz, E., Ontiveros, F. & Kono, H. (2010). The sterile inflammatory response. *Annual Review of Immunology*. Vol. 28, pp. 321-42, ISSN 0066-4162

Russinova, A., Mourdjeva, M., Kyurkchiev, S. & Kehayov, I. (2001). Immunohistochemical detection of atrial natriuretic factor (ANF) in different ovarian cell types. *Endocrine Regulations*. Vol 35, No. 2, pp. 81-89, ISSN 1336-0329.

Samson, W., Aguila, M. & Bianchi R. (1988). Atrial natriuretic factor inhibits luteinizing hormone secretion in the rat: evidence for a hypothalamic site of action. *Endocrinology*. Vol. 122, No. 4, pp. 1573-82, ISSN 1945-7170

Schwartz, D., Geller, D., Manning, P., Siegel, N., Fok, K., Smith, C. & Needleman P. (1984). Ser-Leu-Arg-Arg-atriopeptin III: the major circulating form of atrial peptide. *Science*. Vol. 229, No. 4711, pp. 397-400, ISSN 1095-9203

Seifer, D., Gradiner, A., Ferreria, K. & Peluso, J. (1996). Apoptosis as a function of ovarian reserve in women undergoing in vitro fertilization. *Fertility and Sterility*. Vol. 66, No. 4, pp. 593–598, ISSN 1556-5653

Seino, T., Saito, H., Kaneko, T., Takahashi, T., Kawachiy, S. & Kurachi, H. (2002). Eight-hydroxy-2'-deoxyguanosine in granulosa cells is correlated with the quality of oocytes and embryos in an in vitro fertilization-embryo transfer program. *Fertility and Sterility*. Vol. 77, No. 6, pp. 1184–1190, ISSN 1556-5653

Serke, H., Bausenwein, J., Hirrlinger, J., Nowicki, M., Vilser, C., Jogschies, P., Hmeidan, F., Blumenauer,V. & Spanel-Borowski, K. (2010). Granulosa cell subtypes vary in response to oxidized low-density lipoprotein as regards specific lipoprotein receptors and antioxidant enzyme activity. *Journal of Clinical Endocrinology & Metabolism*. Vol. 95, No. 7, pp. 3480-90, ISSN 021-972

Serke, H., Vilser, C., Nowicki, M., Hmeidan, F., Blumenauer,V., Hummitzsch, K., Losche, A. & Spanel-Borowski, K. (2009). Granulosa cell subtypes respond by autophagy or cell death to oxLDL-dependent activation of the oxidized lipoprotein receptor 1 and toll-like 4 receptor. *Autophagy*.Vol. 5 , pp. 991–1003, ISSN 1554-8635

Sica, A., Dorman, L., Viggiano, V., Ghosh, P., Rice, N. & Young, H. (1997). Interaction of NF-B and NFAT with the Interferon- Promoter. *The Journal of Biological Chemistry*. Vol. 272, No. 48, pp. 30412-30420, ISSN 1083-351X

Singer-Sam, J., Keith, D. Tani, K., Simmer, R. Shively, L., Lindsay, S. Yoshida, A & Riggs, A. (1984). Sequence of the promoter region of the gene for human X-linked 3-phosphoglycerate kinase. *Gene*, Vol. 32 , No 3, pp.409–417. ISSN: 03781119

Smedts, A., & Curry, T. (2005). Expression of basigin, an inducer of matrix metalloproteinases, in the rat ovary. *Biology of Reproduction*., Vo. 73, No1, pp.80-87. ISSN: 00063363

Spanel-Borowski, K. (2011). Footmarks of innate immunity and cytokeratin-positive cells as potential dendritic cells. *Advances in Anatomy, Embryology and Cell Biology.* Vol 209, Springer Heidelberg. ISBN 978-3-642-16076-9.

Suh, Ch., Jee, B., Choi, Y., Kim, J., Lee, J., Moon, S. & Kim, S. (2002). Prognostic Implication of Apoptosis in Human Luteinized Granulosa Cells During IVF–ET. *Journal of Assisted* Reproduction *and Genetics.* Vol. 19, No. 5, pp. 209-214, ISSN 1058-0468

Sundblad, V., Bussmann, L., Chiauzzi, V., Pancholi, V. & Charreau, E. (2006). α-enolase: a novel autoantigen in patients with premature ovarian failure. *Clinical Endocrinology.* Vol. 65, pp. 745–751, ISSN 1365-2265

Suzuki, T., Sugino, N., Fukaya, T., Sugiyama, S., Uda, T., Takaya, R., Yajima, A. & Sasano, H. (1999). Superoxide dismutase in normal cycling human ovaries: immunohistochemical localization and characterization. *Fertility and Sterility.* Vol. 72, No. 4, pp. 720-726, ISSN 1556-5653

Takuma, K., Phuagphong, P., Lee, E., Mori, K., Baba, A. & Matsuda T. (2001). Anti-apoptotic Effect of cGMP in Cultured Astrocytes: inhibition by cGMP-dependent protein kinase of mitochondrial permeable transition. *The Journal of Biological Chemistry.* Vol. 276, No. 51, pp. 48093-48099, ISSN 1083-351X

Tatone, C., Carbone, M., Falone, S., Aimola, P., Giardinelli, A., Caserta, D., Marci, R., Pandolfi, A., Ragnelli, A. & Amicarelli, F. (2006). Age-dependent changes in the expression of superoxide dismutases and catalase are associated with ultrastructural modifications in human granulosa cells. *Molecular Human Reprodoction.* Vol. 12, No. 11, pp. 655-60, ISSN 1460-2407

Teede, H., Deeks, A.& Moran, L (2010). Polycystic ovary syndrome: a complex condition with psychological, reproductive and metabolic manifestations that impacts on health across the lifespan. *BMC Medicine.* Vol. 30, pp. 8-41. ISSN 1741-7015

Tilly, Y., Kowalski K., Yohanson A. & Hsueh A. (1991) Involvement of apoptosis in ovarian follicular atresia and postovulatory regression. *Endocrinology.* Vol. 129, No. 5, pp. 2799-2801, ISSN 1945-7170

Todorova, K., Vangelov, I., Dineva, J., Penchev, V., Hayrabedyan, S., Nikolov, G., Mollova, M., Ivanova, M. (2011). Lysyl Oxidase as a Potential Biomarker for Predicting Oocyte Quality. *Comptes rendus de l'Acade'mie bulgare des Sciences.* Vol. 64, No9, pp. 1355-1362. ISSN 1310-1331

Todorova, K., Zasheva, D., Hayrabedyan, S, Dineva, J, Vangelov, I, Penchev, V., Nikolov, G., Mollova, M., Ivanova, M. (2011). Gene Panel in Human Cumulus Cells as Biomarker for Successful in vitro Procedures. *Comptes rendus de l'Acade'mie bulgare des Sciences.* Vol. 64, No8, pp. 1143-1150. ISSN 1310-1331

Tong, Z. & Nelson, L. (1999). A mouse gene encoding an oocyte antigen associated with autoimmune premature ovarian failure. *Endocrinology.* Vol. 140, No. pp. 83720–3726

Törnell, J., Carlsson, B. & Billig, H. (1990). Atrial natriuretic peptide inhibits spontaneous rat oocyte maturation. *Endocrinology.* Vol. 126, No. 3, pp. 1504-1508, ISSN 1945-7170

Tsukagoshi, H., Shimizu, Y., Kawata, T., Hisada, T., Shimizu, Y. & Iwamae, S. (2001). Atrial natriuretic peptide inhibits tumor necrosis factor-alpha production by interferon-gamma-activated macrophages via suppression of p38 mitogen-activated protein kinase and nuclear factor-kappa B activation. *Regulatory Peptides.* Vol. 99, No. 1, pp. 21-29, ISSN 0167-0115

Tung, K., Setiady, Y, Samy, E., Lewis, J. & Teuscher, C. (2005). Autoimmune ovarian disease in day 3-thymectomized mice: the neonatal time window, antigen specificity of disease suppression, and genetic control.*Current Topics in Microbiology and Immunology*. Vol. 293, pp. 209-247, ISSN 0070-217X

Turvey, S. & Broide, D. (2010). Innate immunity. *Journal of Allergy and Clinical Immunology*. Vol. 125, pp. 24–32, ISSN 0091-6749

Van Kasteren, Y., von Blomberg, M., Hoek, A., de Koning, C., Lambalk, N., van Montfrans, J., Kuik, J. & Schoemaker, J. (2000). Incipient ovarian failure and premature ovarian failure show the same immunological profile.*American Journal of Reproductive Immunology*. Vol. 43, No. 6, pp. 359-66, ISSN 1600-0897

Vangelov, I., Dineva, J., Nikolov, G., Lolov, S. & Ivanova, M. (2005). Antibodies against granulosa luteinized cells and their targets in women attending IVF program. *American Journal of Reproductive Immunology*. Vol. 53, No. 2, pp. 106-12, ISSN 1600-0897

Vangelov, I., Dineva, J., Nikolov, G., Gulenova, D. & Ivanova, I. (2008). Relationship among Anti-granulosa Luteinized Cells Antibodies, Apoptosis of Granulosa Luteinized Cells, Levels of TNF-a and IFN-g in Follicular Fluids of Infertile Women. *Comptes rendus de l'Acade'mie bulgare des Sciences*. Vol. 61, No. 3, pp. 341-348, ISSN 1310-1331

Vangelov, I., Dineva, J., Nikolov, G., Gulenova, D. & Ivanova, M. (2006). Anti- granulosa cell antibodies in follicular fluids and their impact on the response to controlled ovarian hyperstimulation / fertilization rate. *Comptes rendus de l'Acade'mie bulgare des Sciences*. Vol. 59, No.11, pp. 1191-1196, ISSN 1310-1331

Vangelov, I., Dineva, J., Nikolov, G., Gulenova, D. & Ivanova, M. (2009). Impact of Follicular Cytokines (TNF-α, IFN-γ and Apoptosis of Human Granulosa Luteinized Cells (GLCs) on the Results after Controlled Ovarian Hyperstimulation (COH) and in vitro Fertilization (IVF) in Women with Ovarian Factor of Infertility. *Comptes rendus de l'Acade'mie bulgare des Sciences*. Vol. 62, No. 9, pp. 1169-1176, ISSN 1310-1331

Vollmar, A. & Schulz, R (1995). Expression and differential regulation of natriuretic peptides in mouse macrophages. *Journal of Clinical Investigation*. Vol. 95, No. 6, pp. 2442-2450, ISSN 0021-9738

Vollmar, A., Mytzka, C., & Schulz, R. (1988). Atrial natriuretic peptide in bovine corpus luteum. *Endocrinology*. Vol. 123, No. 2, pp. 762-767, ISSN 1945-7170

Vujovic, S. (2009). Aetiology of premature ovarian failure. *Menopause International*. Vol. 15, pp. 72–75, ISSN 1754-0461

Welt, C., Falorni, A., Taylor, A., Martin, K. & Hall JE. (2005). Selective theca cell dysfunction in autoimmune oophoritis results in multifollicular development, decreased estradiol, and elevated inhibin B levels.*Journal of Clinical Endocrinology & Metabolism*. Vol. 90, No. 5, pp. 3069-76, ISSN 1945-7197

Zhang, M., Tao, Y., Zhou, B., Xie, H., Wang, F., Lei, L., Huo, L., Sun, Q. & Xia, G. (2005). Atrial natriuretic peptide inhibits the actions of FSH and forskolin in meiotic maturation of pig oocytes via different signalling pathways. *Journal of Molecular Endocrinology*. Vol. 34, No. 2, pp. 459-472, ISSN 1479-6813

Zhang, X., Xu, H., Jiang, Y., Yu, S., Cai, Y., Lu, B., Xie, Q. & Ju, T. (2008). Influence of dexamethasone on mesenteric lymph node of rats with severe acute pancreatitis. *World Journal of Gastroenterology*. Vol. 14, No. 22, pp. 3511–3517, ISSN 1007-9327

9

Ferret TNF-α and IFN-γ Immunoassays

Alyson Ann Kelvin[1], David Banner[2], Ali Danesh[2],
Charit Seneviratne[2], Atsuo Ochi[2] and David Joseph Kelvin[1,2,3,4]
[1]*Immune Diagnostics & Research, Toronto, Ontario,*
[2]*Division of Experimental Therapeutics, Toronto General Hospital Research Institute, University Health Network, Toronto, Ontario,*
[3]*International Institute of Infection and Immunity, Shantou University Medical College, Shantou, Guangdong,*
[4]*Sezione di Microbiologia Sperimentale e Clinica, Dipartimento di Scienze Biomediche, Universita' degli Studi di Sassari, Sassari,*
[1,2]*Canada*
[3]*China*
[4]*Italy*

1. Introduction

Despite the prominent use of ferrets in medical research, the immune system of ferrets remains poorly characterized (Svitek & von, V, 2007). Here we describe ferret TNF-α and IFN-γ immunoassays.

Specifically, this covers the following topics:

- Background: The use of ferrets in medical research
- TNF-α and IFN-γ cloning and sequencing
- Expression and purification of recombinant ferret TNF-α and IFN-γ proteins
- Cytokine real-time PCR based assays
- Development of IFN-γ and TNF-α hybridoma clones
- ELISA and ELISPOT assays for the ferret cytokine IFN-γ

2. Background

This Background describes the current use of ferrets in medical research but also includes a description of past uses. The importance of ferrets is highlighted in human disease modeling and in prophylactic and vaccine development. The various uses of ferrets in medical research demonstrate the need for immune profiling reagents and assays.

2.1 Biology of the ferret

The ferret, *Mustela putorius furo,* is a relatively small and inexpensive animal in terms of its potential for research use, although mice remain the traditional influenza model for virus pathogenesis.

Essentially, mice are low cost animals that have a broad availability of corresponding reagents for immunological investigation. Mice are easily mutated and there exists a plethora of currently available transgenic mice with immune targeted gene deletions or gene knock-ins (Belser, Szretter, Katz, & Tumpey, 2009). Two factors against the use of mice in influenza immune studies are 1) most human influenza strains must be mouse adapted prior to initiation of infection studies due to the inability of human influenza viruses to replicate in the mouse and 2) mice do not exhibit human-like clinical signs of influenza such as sneezing and temperature fluxes.

In contrast to mice, ferrets do develop respiratory illnesses that are similar to human disease. Although the ferret is not considered a large laboratory animal, it is able to provide many biological samples for pathological testing during an infection study. For instance, frequent and sizable blood sampling is feasible in the ferret that is not practical in smaller rodents such as in mice and rats.

Furthermore, clinical features of disease are easily observed. Such as clinical fever manifested as an elevation in body temperatures can be detected as early as 1 day following infection with many viruses. Our own as well as previously published studies have shown that high fevers can persist for many days following infection of viruses such as H1N1pdm influenza (Rowe et al., 2010b; Sweet et al., 1979; Zitzow et al., 2002). As well as fever, nasal discharge, sneezing and activity level can also be observed in ferrets infected with influenza viruses (Rowe et al., 2010b). Taken together, these clinical features along with the feasibility for blood and pathological sampling suggest the ferret to be an optimal animal for the study of human infectious diseases, including influenza viruses. For example, our group has recently used the ferret model successfully to characterize and compare immunopathology caused by several strains of currently circulating influenza A and B viruses (Huang et al., 2011).

2.2 Respiratory viral infections

Viral respiratory infectious diseases are a major worldwide concern which causes significant morbidity and mortality (Kolling et al., 2001). Respiratory viral diseases such as the severe acute respiratory syndrome coronavirus (SARS-CoV), avian influenza H5N1 and pandemic influenza H1N1 virus are potential epidemic and/or pandemic threats (Dushoff, Plotkin, Viboud, Earn, & Simonsen, 2006; Weiss & McMichael, 2004; Dawood, Dalton, Durrheim, & Hope, 2009; Dawood et al., 2009). Specifically, influenza is a significant contributor to morbidity and mortality worldwide and is the focus of our laboratory and the focus disease of this chapter.

The World Health Organization estimates the burden of season influenza to be approximately one billion cases annually, including 3-5 million severe cases and 300,000-500,000 deaths (Girard, Cherian, Pervikov, & Kieny, 2005). Influenza illness in humans is caused by an influenza RNA virus of the *Orthomyxoviridae* family. The influenza virus can be categorized as one of three types: A, B, or C (Steinhauer & Skehel, 2002). Importantly, the influenza viral genome is susceptible to two primary types of genetic mutations that cause variation in the immunogenic proteins and subsequently in disease presentation and clinical features (Kasowski, Garten, & Bridges, 2011; Steinhauer & Skehel, 2002). Firstly, antigenic drift is defined by minor changes to the viral genome introduced during virus RNA replication (Steinhauer & Skehel, 2002). Second, antigenic shift is when a host is infected by various influenza strains at the same time allowing entire genome segments to be reassorted during co-infection. This results in novel influenza strains markedly distinct from their progenitors (Steinhauer & Skehel, 2002; Kasowski et al., 2011). From these reassortments, novel influenza strains may arise with new clinical symptoms and disease features that have the potential to be highly pathogenic, easily transmissibility with pandemic potential.

The most significant recent reassortant to emerge was the 2009 pandemic H1N1 influenza A (H1N1pdm) strain (Perez-Padilla et al., 2009). H1N1pdm is closely related to the reassortant swine influenza A viruses previously isolated in North America, Europe, and Asia (Trifonov, Khiabanian, & Rabadan, 2009). Infection with H1N1pdm resulted in diverse clinical outcomes. The majority of reported cases were mild and self-limiting (Gilsdorf, Poggensee, & Working Group, 2009; Nicoll & Coulombier, 2009; Writing Committee of the WHO Consultation on Clinical Aspects of Pandemic, 2010) and typical symptoms include fever, sore throat, malaise, and headache (Health Protection Agency, Health, National Public Health Service for Wales, & HPA Northern Ireland Swine influenza investigation team, 2009). A small proportion of pandemic influenza cases required hospitalization and patient ventilator support (Centers for Disease Control and Prevention (CDC), 2009; Kumar et al., 2009; Perez-Padilla et al., 2009; Writing Committee of the WHO Consultation on Clinical Aspects of Pandemic, 2010). Common complications in there severe cases were severe hypoxemia, shock, pneumonia, and acute respiratory distress syndrome (ARDS)(Perez-Padilla et al., 2009; Kumar et al., 2009; Centers for Disease Control and Prevention (CDC), 2009). Nonpulmonary acute organ dysfunction has also been reported (Uyeki, Sharma, & Branda, 2009; Kumar et al., 2009). Since ferrets show signs of illness and are easily infected with human strains of H1N1pdm, we are currently investigating and have published on the immunopathogenic mechanisms and possible therapeutics for H1N1pdm illness in ferrets (Rowe et al., 2010a; Huang S.S.H. et al., 2011; Cameron et al., 2008).

2.3 Host immune responses

Host immunity can be broken down into an innate and adaptive immune response. The innate immune response is a nonspecific attack on the invading agent while the adaptive immune response is an attack tailored to the individual pathogen (Ryan & Majno, 1977). What determines the type of triggered immune response is the invading agent itself. The agent is recognized first by the innate immune arm and together the innate and adaptive immune responses lead to a unique immune signature that for each pathogen. Furthermore, the clinical outcome is the biological consequence of the immune response that has developed toward the pathogen (Belz, Bedoui, Kupresanin, Carbone, & Heath, 2007; Zheng et al., 2007).

In order to evaluate the immune response during the course of viral infection, it is important to be able to determine the activity of the immune cells. Cell identity and their activation status are distinguished by the molecules expressed at the cell surface. Furthermore, cells of the immune system can be described as innate or adaptive immune cells. Innate immune cells include neutrophils, esosinophils, basophils, macrophages and NK cells. Adaptive immune cells include T lymphocytes, B lymphocytes and Dendritic cells (Hauge, Madhun, Cox, Brokstad, & Haaheim, 2007). Many of these cells have yet to be characterized in the ferret.

As well as understanding the cell activation and cellular populations during an immune response, it is also important to elucidate the intracellular activation and intercellular events which occur following infection. Cells are often activated by cytokines, soluble extracellular proteins that mediate signals from one cell to another. Once the cell has been in contact with a cytokine, intracellular signalling cascades are activated. The activation of these signalling cascades leads to cell effector function.

One of the most prominent branches of cytokine-cell signalling events is of the inflammatory interferon (IFN) cytokines which connect the innate immune response with the activation of the adaptive immunity. The IFN family of cytokines can be categorized as either Type I IFN or Type II. IFN-α and IFN-β are of the Type I IFN cytokines and have a prominent role during viral infection. IFN-γ is of the Type II IFN family. IFN-γ also plays a role in viral infections but also functions during bacterial infections.

The release of IFN-γ leads to cellular activation through signalling pathways. Ligation of the interferon receptors 1 and 2 (IFNAR1 and IFNAR2 for IFN-α and IFN-β; IFNGR1 and IFNGR2 for IFN-γ) with an IFN cytokine induces IFN signaling pathways and promotes IFN gene induction. Both the Type I and Type II cytokines signal through JAK-STAT pathways to activate IFN genes and promote immune responses (Marijanovic, Ragimbeau, van der Heyden, Uze, & Pellegrini, 2007). IFN induced JAK-STAT signalling often involves interferon regulatory factor 9 (IRF9) (Takaoka & Yanai, 2006). The interferon stimulatory factor 3 complex (ISGF3) binds to interferon-stimulated response element (ISRE) and activates transcription of IFN-α inducible genes, including 2'–5' oligoadenylate synthase 1 (OAS1), myxovirus resistance 1 (MX1), interferon stimulated gene 15 (ISG15) and many other IFN-response genes (IRGs) (Uddin & Platanias, 2004). The expression of IFN-γ-induced protein IP10, or CXCL10, following IFN stimulation, is often considered a hallmark of virus infection in host organisms. IFN-α stimulation ultimately promotes a cellular antiviral state which is hallmarked by the upregulation of IRGs (Chevaliez & Pawlotsky, 2009). Although IFN signalling gene upregulation during viral infection has been the subject of previous reports, there is little information regarding the host immune responses directly induced by viruses versus those that are upregulated due to secondary IFN stimulation (Chelbi-Alix & Wietzerbin, 2007; Haagmans et al., 2004; Loutfy et al., 2003; Cameron et al., 2007). Therefore there is a need for the study of IFN signalling and IFN stimulated events during viral infection which can be investigated using the ferret model.

TNF (Tumor Necrosis Factor) -α is a cytokine produced mainly by activated macrophages and T-lymphocytes, and exerts a multitude of biological activities including cytotoxic effects upon certain tumours and virus- infected cells, immunomodulation, and regulation of cellular proliferation (Vilcek & Lee, 1991). TNF-α is a potent inhibitor of influenza replication in vitro (Seo & Webster, 2002), and the induction of TNF-α expression has been associated with ARDS-like symptoms in H5N1 infected mice (Xu et al., 2006). Depletion of TNF-α in influenza or respiratory syncytial virus-infected animals significantly reduced pulmonary inflammation and cytokine production without compromising viral clearance, and almost completely abolished any associated weight loss and observable illness (Hussell, Pennycook, & Openshaw, 2001). There is evidence to suggest that hyper-production of TNF-α contributes to the high degree of virulence exhibited by H5N1 strains in humans. Using primary cultures of human monocyte-derived macrophages, Cheung et al. demonstrated a significant increase in TNF-α gene transcription and protein expression in H5N1-infected cells compared to that of H1N1- or H3N2- infected cells (Cheung et al., 2002). Dysregulation of cytokines, including TNF-α, is thought to contribute to the immunopathogenesis of influenza and SARS CoV virus infections, however, the *in vivo* mechanism is unknown.

2.4 Examining the ferret host immune response in respiratory diseases

When infected with respiratory viruses ferrets display many of the symptoms and pathological features seen in infected humans (Darnell et al., 2007; Martina et al., 2003; Peltola, Boyd, McAuley, Rehg, & McCullers, 2006). The ferret model has been used in influenza research since the influenza virus was first isolated (Bouvier & Lowen, 2010; Lambkin et al., 2004; Small, Jr., Waldman, Bruno, & Gifford, 1976). Importantly, ferrets and humans have similar lung physiology allowing influenza to infect both species through a comparable mechanism, sialic receptors the host receptor for influenza (Maher & DeStefano, 2004; van et al., 2007). Furthermore, as ferrets are highly susceptible to influenza virus, they can also transmit the influenza virus from infected to healthy ferrets (Smith et al., 1933).

As well as influenza, ferrets have shown promise as a model for other respiratory viruses such as Severe Acute Respiratory Syndrome Corona virus (SARS Covirus), the BSL-4 Nipah virus and morbilliviruses and other pathogens such as gastro-intestinal bacteria and prions (Bouvier, Lowen, & Palese, 2008; van den Brand et al., 2008; Bossart et al., 2009; Svitek & von, V, 2007; ter et al., 2006; Martina et al., 2003).

2.5 The use of ferrets for the investigation of influenza therapeutics

Not only are ferrets useful for infectious disease modeling but they are also a good platform for testing and developing viral therapeutics. Currently ferrets are used for influenza drug testing; for example, neuraminidase inhibitors are effective during ferret influenza infection (Mendel et al., 1998; Govorkova et al., 2007; Yun et al., 2008). As well, ferrets display immunological memory and are thus useful for testing the safety and efficacy of vaccines (Bouvier & Lowen, 2010; Maher & DeStefano, 2004; Gupta, Earl, & Deem, 2006). Ferrets have been used to investigate SARS and influenza vaccines (Bouvier & Lowen, 2010; Maher & DeStefano, 2004; Gupta et al., 2006).

Previously, we sought to elucidate the ferret immune response during viral infection and identify potential therapeutic drug targets (Danesh et al., 2011). We investigated the genetic programs and cell signaling pathways that were regulated by SARSCoV infection compared to IFN-α2b stimulation in the ferret model (Danesh et al., 2011). The phosphorylation status of signaling molecules in IFN-α2b-stimulated peripheral blood mononuclear cells (PBMCs) was examined with the end of identifying kinase inhibitors that may be useful in SARS pathogenesis. We found IFN-α2b caused STAT1 phosphorylation in *in vitro* experiments (Danesh et al., 2011). Importantly, gene expression profiles of PBMCs as well as lung necropsies of SARS-CoV-infected ferrets identified 7 upregulated IRGs that were similarly upregulated in response to IFN-α2b injection (Danesh et al., 2011). In summary, IFN-α2b injection and SARS-CoV infection led to both similar as well as unique gene expression signatures (Danesh et al., 2011). Taken together, increased knowledge of these gene expression signatures and signalling pathways will improve the understanding of the ferret immune system and lead to possible therapeutic drug targets.

2.6 Recent advances in ferret reagent development

Although researchers are able to use direct infection of human influenza strains and monitor biological clinical signs with the ferret model, there is a paucity of reagents for influenza investigative studies in the ferret. As well, there is a lack of information on the ferret immune system that has slowed the progress of this system. Specifically, the lack of ferret specific antibodies capable of detecting surface molecules of immune cells and reagents for ferret inflammatory mediators such as cytokines has hindered the immune profiling in ferret infectious disease models.

Recently, we reported the characterization of the ferret chemokines, CXCL9, CXCL10 and CXCL11, which are important in migration of mononuclear cells to sites of infection (Danesh et al., 2008). We have previously characterized ferret cytokine and chemokine genes as well as have developed immunological assays for evaluating the ferret immune system following SARS and influenza infection (Cameron et al., 2008; Danesh et al., 2008; Ochi et al., 2008). As both IFN-γ and TNF-α are significant hallmarks of adaptive immunity, these cytokines are useful markers when studying the viral immune response.

3. Ferret immunoassays

3.1 TNF-α and IFN-γ cloning and sequencing

The methods used for cloning ferret TNF-α and IFN-γ genes are covered in this section. ClustalW alignments of ferret genes with orthologues from other mammalian species such as canine are also shown.

3.1.1 Methods

Animals

Six-month-old male ferrets (*Mustela putorius furo*) were obtained from Triple F Farms Inc. (Sayre, Pa. USA). Animals were housed at Toronto General Research Institute animal facility and the animal use protocol was approved by the animal care committee of the University Health Network, Toronto, Ontario. Animals were quarantined and monitored for one week before tissue, blood collection and project initiation. Animal diets are based on a low fat, high protein regimen, recommended by Triple F Farms for small carnivores.

Total RNA purification of ferret IFN-γ and TNF-α

Ferret whole blood was diluted at a ratio of 1:1 with RPMI (Invitrogen, Mississauga, Canada) and blood was stimulated with mitogens, LPS (1ug/ml, Sigma Chemicals, St. Louise, MO, USA), PMA (50 ng/ml, Sigma), ionomycin (0.1 mM, Sigma) or poly I:C (25 µg/ml, Sigma) by incubating at 37°C in 5% CO2 for 2, 4, 8, and 12 hrs. Following cell stimulation, RNA was isolated using the Paxgene RNA isolation method (Qiagen, Missisauga, Canada) according to manufacturer's protocols. cDNA was synthesized from purified total RNA by reverse transcriptase II (Invitrogen) according to supplier's instructions.

Cloning, sequencing and expression of ferret TNF-α and IFN-γ

Gene specific primers were used to amplify ferret TNF-α and IFN-γ by PCR. Primers were designed based on highly conserved regions of the nucleotide gene sequences. These regions were identified through ClustalW-based multiple sequence alignments of the TNF-α and IFN-γ genes from several species (ClustalW 1.83, European Bioinformatics Institute (http://www.ebi.ac.uk/clustalw/) and are shown in Table 1. Accession numbers used for ClustalW alignments of INF-γ are as follows: Eurasian badger; Y11647, rabbit; P30123, cat; P46402, dog; P42161, mouse; P01580, and human; P01579. The Gene peptide accession numbers for IFN-γ are: badger, CAA72346; dog, AAD314233; panda, ABE02189; cat, BAA06309; rhinoceros, ABC18310; donkey, AAC42595; pig, ABG56234; dolphin, BAA82042; sheep, ABD64367; buffalo, BAE75855; cow, NP_776511; armadillo, AAZ57195; woodchuck, AAC31963; rabbit, BAA24439; human, P01579; monkey, AAM21477; mouse, P01580; rat, NP_620235; chicken, CAA69227; zebrafish, BAD06253.

Primers	5'-3' sequence
Consensus cloning primers*	
Forward	**ATG**AGCACTGAAAGCATGATCC
Reverse	GTCTACTTTGGGATCATTGCCCTG**TGA**
5' RACE Primers	
Adapter outer primer	GCTGATGGCGATGAATGAACACTG
Adapter inner primer	GCGGATCCGAACACTGCGTTTGCTGGCTT TGATG
Gene specific primers	
Inner primer	CGACGAGGAGGAAGGAGAAGA
Outer primer	CAGAGGTTTGATTAGTTGGAGGCC
3' RACE Primers	
Adapter outer primer	GCGAGCACAGAATTAATACGACT
Adapter inner primer	CGCGGATCCGAATTAATACGACTCACTAT AGG
Gene specific primers	
Inner primer	ATCAACCTGCCTGCCTATCTCG
Outer primer	TCAACCTCCTGTCTGCCATCAAG
Expression-construct cloning primers	
Forward primer	AACGCCATGAGTACTGAAAGCATGATCC
Reverse prime	CAGGGCAATGATCCCAAAGTAGA

*In consensus primers, translation initiation and termination codons depicted in bold.

Table 1. Primers used to clone and express full length cDNA for ferret TNF-α

To ensure correct sequencing of 3' and 5' cDNA ends or the genes, we used RNA ligase-mediated rapid amplification of cDNA ends (RLM-RACE) as per manufacturer's instructions (FirstChoice RLM-RACE Kit, Ambion, Ausin, Texas, USA). Briefly, 1-2µg of total RNA from mitogen-stimulated ferret blood cells (described above) was used as starting material. The RNA was treated with calf intestinal alkaline phosphatase (CIP) and subsequently with tobacco acid pyrophosphate (TAP). RNA adapter was ligated and the RNA was reverse transcribed to cDNA followed by PCR amplification with nested primers (outer and inner) to adapter and gene (for TNF-α see Table 1.). 3' RACE was also performed as per manufacturer's protocol with gene-specific nested primers (Table 1.).

The primers were tested in silico using Primer Express (Applied Biosystems). Standard PCR was performed using these consensus primers and template cDNA. Bands at the appropriate size were excised, gel purified and sub-cloned into pCR2.1-TOPO vector (Invitrogen). DNA sequences of positive clones were confirmed by sequencing with ABI 3730XL DNA analyzers (Center for Applied Genomics, Toronto, ON, Canada). Gene identification was confirmed using Basic Local Alignment Search Tool (BLAST) analyses against the National Centre for Biotechnology Information databases.

3.1.2 Results

Cloning and sequencing of the ferret TNF-α and IFN-γ genes

To determine the consensus regions for both ferret TNF-α and IFN-γ ClustalW analysis was performed for human, cat and dog TNF-α and IFN-γ nucleotide sequences. The coding region for all three species was predicted to encode a 702 bp transcript and a 501 bp transcript, respectively for TNF-α and IFN-γ.

Using the consensus sequence for TNF-α and IFN-γ genes, forward and reverse primers (Table 1. for TNF-α) were designed and used to amplify full-length ferret TNF-α and IFN-γ from a ferret cDNA library derived from mitogen-stimulated ferret PBMCs. When necessary, RACE was used to identify the endogenous ferret sequences at the 5′ and 3′ ends of the transcript. The nucleotide sequence of ferret TNF-α and IFN-γ (previously published (Ochi et al., 2008)) are shown in Figure 1. and Figure 2., respectively. In addition to the 702 bp coding region, we have determined the sequence of the 65 bp 5′ and 175 bp 3′ untranslated regions, respectively.

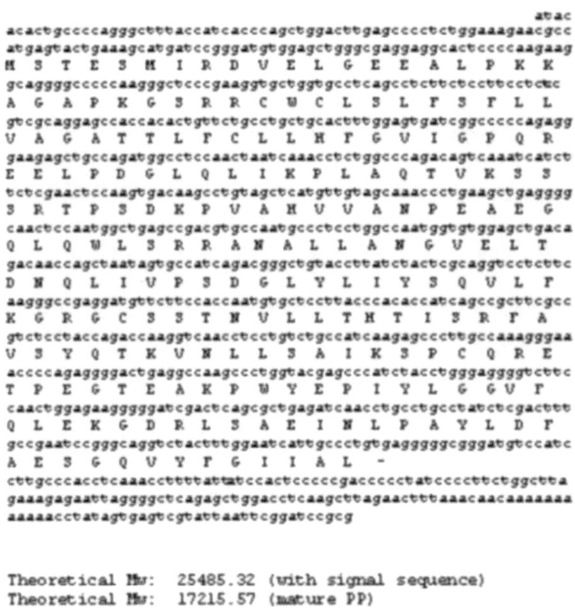

The ferret cDNA was 942 bp, and the predicted protein 314 aa. Numbers on the right indicate cDNA bp. The 5′-UTR was 65 base pairs, the complete coding region of 702 base pairs, and 175 bp of the 3′UTR. Calculated molecular weight (MW) of the predicted protein is indicated at the bottom.

Fig. 1. Full-length ferret TNF-α cDNA nucleotide sequence and predicted amino acid sequence.

Multiple amino acid sequence alignment revealed that the predicted ferret TNF-α protein shares a high level of homology with cat (91% similarity) and dog (95% similarity) sequences (Figure 3). The sequence similarity to ferret TNF-α was lower when compared to human (78%) and mouse (88%) TNF-α sequences. The TNF ligand family consists of 19 proteins characterized by a conserved C-terminal domain called the TNF-α homology domain (THD) (Bodmer et al., 2002). The ferret TNF-α THD domain was found to be significantly conserved with dog and cat TNF-α sequences (Figure 3).

```
agatcagctcagtctttcagacctgatcaacttaaactgggagctactgatttcagctac   60

ttcagcctaactacgaaacaatgaattatacaaactatatcttagcttttcagctttgcg  120
                      M  N  Y  T  N  Y  I  L  A  F  Q  L  C  V

tgattttctgttcttctggctattactgtcaggccatgtttttaaagaaatagaagacc  240
 I  F  C  S  S  G  Y  Y  C  Q  A  M  F  F  K  E  I  E  D  L
taaaggaatattttaatgcaagtaatccagatgtagcagatggtgggcctcttttcttag  300
 K  E  Y  F  N  A  S  N  P  D  V  A  D  G  G  P  L  F  L  D
atattttgaagaactggagagaggagagtgacaaaaaaatcattcaaagccaaattgtct  360
 I  L  K  N  W  R  E  E  S  D  K  K  I  I  Q  S  Q  I  V  S
ccttctacttgaaactgtttgaaaacttcaaagataaccagatcattcaaaggagcatgg  420
 F  Y  L  K  L  F  E  N  F  K  D  N  Q  I  I  Q  R  S  M  D
ataccatcaaggaagacatgcttgtcaggttcttcaataacagcagcagtaagctggagg  480
 T  I  K  E  D  M  L  V  R  F  F  N  N  S  S  S  K  L  E  D
acttccttaagctgattcgaattcctgtgaatgatctgcaggtccagcgcaaagcgataa  540
 F  L  K  L  I  R  I  P  V  N  D  L  Q  V  Q  R  K  A  I  N
atgaactcatcaaagtgatgaatgatctctcaccaagatctaacctaaggaagcggaaaa  600
 E  L  I  K  V  M  N  D  L  S  P  R  S  N  L  R  K  R  K  R
ggagtcacagtgtgtttcccggccgcagagcatcgaaataattgtcatcctgtctgcaat  660
 S  H  S  V  F  P  G  R  R  A  S  K  -
atttgaattttaaatctaaatctatttatttatatttaatattttacattatttatatg  720

aagaatatattttagactcataagtcatagtatttataatagcaacttttatgtaatga  780
aaatgactattaatatatgtattatttataattcctttatcctgtgactatttcactcaa  840
cctcctcccttctttttcctgaccaactaggcaagactgtgattttaagacataatctca  900
ggaaccaactaggcagctgacttaagtaagaccctgtgggttatgcatttatttcacttg  960
ataccatgagcacttataaatgaaacgatgccgtccagtcgctgcctacctgggaacatg 1020
tctgtattatgagccactgctctaa                                    1045
```

Full length ferret IFN-γ cDNA sequence including 80 base pairs in the 5′ untranslated region (UTR), 501 base pairs of coding sequence with predicted amino acid sequence, and 404 base pairs in the 3′UTR.

Fig. 2. Ferret IFN-γ cDNA (Ochi et al., 2008).

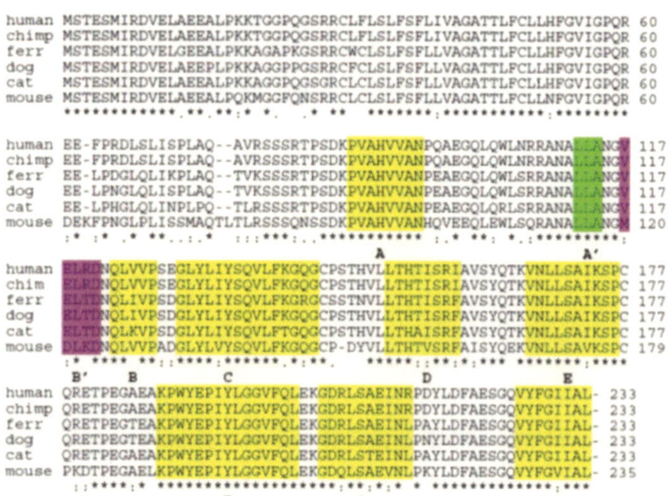

Name	Length(aa)	(%)
human	233	88
chimpanzee	233	88
mouse	235	78
dog	233	95
cat	233	91

Conserved regions of the TNF-α homology domains (THD) are indicated by the highlighted regions. The table below indicates the overall aa homology (including conservative substitution) with ferret TNF-α.

Fig. 3. Multiple protein sequence alignment analysis of TNF-α from various species.

A clustal alignment of the amino acid sequences of ferret, Eurasian badger, rabbit, cat, dog, mouse, and human IFN-γ was performed using the ClustalW program. In contrast to ferret TNF-α, INF-γ amino acid clustal alignment showed the predicted ferret IFN-γ most similar to the Eurasian badger (*Meles meles*) (97%), followed by the canine (86%) and feline (83%) sequences (Figure 4) (Ochi et al., 2008). The homology of ferret IFN-γ to human and mouse IFN-γ was 63% and 48%, respectively. Phylogenetic tree, previously published by our group (Ochi et al., 2008) depicting the relationship of IFN-γ to its orthologues, shows the proximity of ferret IFN-γ to badger (Figure 5) .

```
human    MKYTSYILAFQLCIVLGSLGCYCQDPYVKEAENLKKYFNAGHSDVADNGTLFLGILKNWK 60
rabbit   MSYTSYILAFQLCLILGSYGCYCQDTLTRETEHLKAYLKANTSDVANGGPLFLNILRNWK 60
ferret   MNYTNYILAFQLCVIFCSSGYYCQAMFFKEIEDLKEYFNASNPDVADGGPLFLDILKNWR 60
badger   MNYTNFILAFQLCVIFCSSGYYCQAMFFKEIEDLKEYFNASNPDVADGGPLFLDILKNWR 60
cat      MNYTSFIFAFQLCIILCSSGYYCQAMFFKEIEELKGYFNASNPDVADGGSLFVDILKNWK 60
dog      MNYTSYILAFQLCVILCSSGCNCQAMFFKEIENLKEYFNASNPDVSDGGSLFVDILKKWR 60
mouse    MNATHCILALQLFLMAVS-GCYCHGTVIESLESLNNYFNSSGIDVEEK-SLFLDIWRNWQ 58
         *. *  *:*:** ::  * *  *:     .. * *: *:::.  ** :  .**:.* ::*:

human    EESDRKIMQSQIVSFYFKLFKNFKDD-QSIQKSVETIKEDMNVKFFNSNKKKRDDFEKLT 115
rabbit   EESDNKIIQSQIVSFYFKLFDNLKDH-EVIKKSMESIKEDIFVKFFNSNLTKMDDFQNLT 115
ferret   EESDKKIIQSQIVSFYLKLFENFKDN-QIIQRSMDTIKEDMLVRFFNNSSSKLEDFLKLI 115
badger   EESDKTIIQSQIVSFYLKLFENFKDN-QIIQRSMDTIKEDMLVRFFNSSSSKREDFLKLI 115
cat      EESDKTIIQSQIVSFYLKMFENLKDDDQRIQRSMDTIKEDMLDKLLNTSSSKRDDFLKLI 120
dog      EESDKTIIQSQIVSFYLKLFDNFKDN-QIIQRSMDTIKEDMLGKFLNSSTSKREDFLKLI 115
mouse    KDGDMKILQSQIISFYLRLFEVLKDN-QAISNNISVIESHLITTFFSNSKAKKDAFMSIA 117
         ::.*  .*:****:***:::*. :**. : *...:. *:..:   ::...  * : * .:

human    NYSVTDLNVQRKAIHELIQVMAELSPAAKTGKRKRSQMLFRGRRASQ- 166
rabbit   RISVDDRLVQRKAVSELSNVLNFLSPKSNLKKRKRSQTLFRGRRASKY 167
ferret   RIPVNDLQVQRKAINELIKVMNDLSPRSNLRKRKRSHSVFPGRRASK- 166
badger   RIPVNDLQVQRKAINELIKVMNDLSPRSNLRKRKRSHSVFPGRRASK- 166
cat      QIPVNDLQVQRKAINELFKVMNDLSPRSNLRKRKRSQNLFRGRRASK- 167
dog      QIPVNDLQVQRKAINELIKVMNDLSPRSNLRKRKRSQNLFRGRRASK- 166
mouse    KFEVNNPQVQRQAFNELIRVVHQLLPESSLRKRKRSRC---------- 155
         .  * :  ***:*. ** .*:  * * :.  *****:
```

SeqA	Name	Len(aa)	SeqB	Name	Len(aa)	Score
1	ferret	166	2	badger	166	97
1	ferret	166	3	cat	167	83
1	ferret	166	4	human	166	63
1	ferret	166	5	dog	166	86
1	ferret	166	6	rabbit	167	62
1	ferret	166	7	mouse	155	48

Alignment of the amino acid sequences of ferret, Eurasian badger, rabbit, cat, dog, mouse, and human IFN-γ precursor proteins is shown. Asterisks indicate positions of identical amino acid residues in all sequences. Periods indicate positions with semiconserved substitutions. Amino acid homology score between ferret IFN-γ and orthologues are shown in the lower panel.

Fig. 4. Ferret IFN-γ amino acid clustal alignment (Ochi et al., 2008).

3.2 Development of recombinant TNF-α and IFN-γ proteins

The cloning of ferret TNF-α and IFN-γ are detailed in the following section, including the primers used, PCR program, and vector generation. We present expression of the sub-cloned genes in COS-7 cells by SDS-PAGE and flow cytometry.

3.2.1 Methods

Generation of an expression vector for ferret TNF-α and IFN-γ inflammatory cytokines

PCR was used to engineer a Kozak sequence at the 5′ end of the ferret TNF-α and IFN-γ open reading frames, and the 3′ termination codons were removed by PCR prior to subcloning into the pcDNA3.1/ His6.V5/ TOPO expression vector (Invitrogen). Removal of the termination codon enabled the cloned gene to be expressed as a fusion protein with two C-terminal epitope tags, His6 and V5.

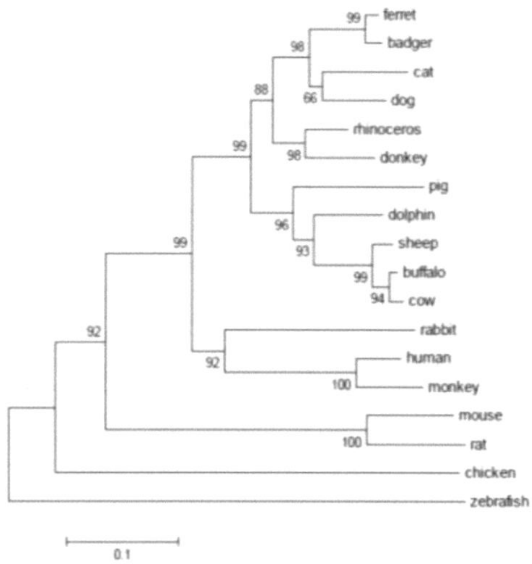

Phylogenetic tree analysis showing the relationship between ferret and other known vertebrate IFN-γ sequences. This tree was constructed using ClustalW and MEGA 3.1 packages and bootstrapped 10,000 times. †Bootstrapping confidence values are between 66 and 100.

Fig. 5. Ferret IFN-γ phologenetic analysis (Ochi et al., 2008).

Transfection and purification of recombinant His-tagged TNF-α

COS-7 cells (ATCC, Manassas, Virginia, USA) were maintained in Dulbecco's modified eagle's medium (DMEM), supplemented with 10% fetal bovine serum (Invitrogen) at 37°C, 5% CO2. COS-7 cells (1x10^7) were transfected with Effectene transfection reagent according to manufacturer's instructions (Qiagen, Mississauga, Ontario, Canada). Twenty-four to forty-eight hours following transfection, the cell culture media from the cells were run through Ni-NTA metal immobilized affinity columns to bind the His-tagged recombinant protein (Novogen, Oakville, ON, Canada). The columns were washed and the protein was eluted according to the manufacturer's protocols. Fractions containing the recombinant proteins were pooled and dialyzed against phosphate buffered saline (PBS) at 4°C and subsequently concentrated by spin column (Nanosep 10k OMEGA, Pall Life Science,East Hills, NY, USA). TNF-α and IFN-γ protein concentrations were determined by protein assay kit (Pierce, Rockford, IL, USA).

Expression and purification of GST-IFN-γ using a bacterial expression system

Ferret IFN-γ cDNA was subcloned into pGEX-6P1 vector (GE Healthcare) and purified as a GST fusion protein from Escherichia coli strain BL21 (DE3) by glutathione affinity chromatography.

Western Blot analysis

SDS-Poylacrylamide gel electrophoresis (10-15% SDS-PAGE) was performed with pre-cast gels (Bio-Rad, Hercules, CA, USA) according to standard protocols. Protein blots were blocked with 5% milk protein in 0.01% Tween-20 in PBS (T-PBS) for 1 hour at room

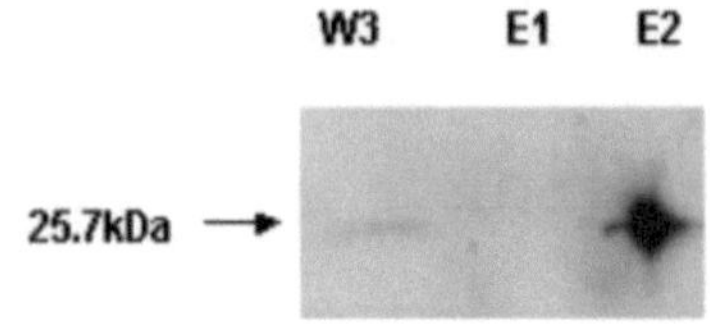

The expression construct encoding full-length ferret TNF-α was transfected into COS-7 cells and purified using with ion (Ni2+) immobilized affinity chromatography. The eluted protein fractions were subjected to SDS-PAGE and western blotting. Arrow depicts the band at predicted molecular weight of ferret TNF-α. W3 denotes wash fraction 2, and E1 and E2 denote elution fractions 1 and 2.

Fig. 6. Purified recombinant ferret TNF-α protein molecular weight determined by western blot analysis.

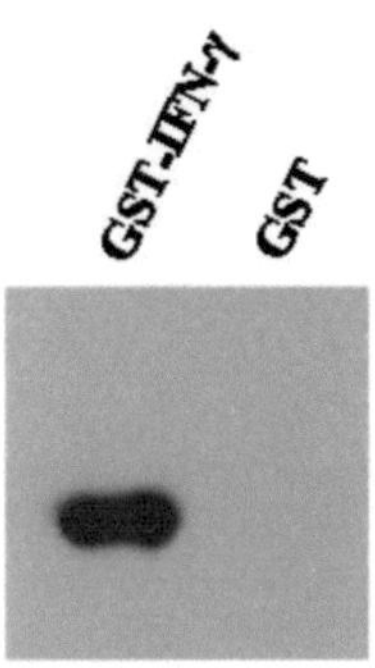

Detection of recombinant ferret IFN-γ by polyclonal antibody-specific immunoblotting.

Fig. 7. Detection of ferret recombinant IFN-γ.

temperature followed by an incubation of 16 hours at 4°C with mouse-anti-His6 primary antibody (Invitrogen) at 508 ng/ml concentration or monoclonal anti-V5 Ab (1:1000) (Invitrogen). The blots were washed and incubated with goat-anti-mouse-HRP secondary antibody (Santa Cruz, Santa Cruz, CA, USA). Bands were visualized using enhanced chemiluminiscent (ECL) reagents according to manufacturer's protocol (GE Healthcare, Peterborough, Ontario, Canada).

3.2.2 Results

Expression and purification of the recombinant ferret TNF-α and IFN-γ

In order to obtain recombinant ferret TNF-α and IFN-γ protein to be used in immunoassays and monoclonal antibody generation, TNF-α and IFN-γ genes were first subcloned. Specifically, TNF-α and IFN-γ cDNA were individually subcloned into expression plasmid to generate expression tag fusion proteins (described previously). Ferret TNF-α was expressed and purified from a mammalian cell line and IFN-γ from a bacterial expression system.

The native human TNF-α polypeptide is cleaved at amino acid 76 to form the mature TNF-α signal peptide at 17215 Da (Wang et al., 1985). We predicted the ferret signal sequence cleavage site to be at the junction of 46 and 47 by SignalP 3.0 analysis. The observed molecular weight of ferret TNF-α according to our results was closer to that of human TNF-α at 25.7 kDa (including the His6 and V5 tags). In agreement, western blot analysis of the eluted fractions of ferret TNF- α protein purified from COS-7 transfected cell media resulted in a single band of approximately 25.7 kDa molecular weight (Figure 6).

For IFN-γ, purified recombinant ferret IFN-γ protein was expressed as a GST fusion protein and purified from chemically competent E. coli cells. Ferret recombinant IFN-γ protein migrated as a 40 kDa band when subjected to SDS-PAGE and western blotting using a polyclonal anti-IFN-γ antibody (Figure 7).

3.3 Cytokine real-time PCR based assay

Cytokines are important inflammatory and immune mediators. Here we present primers designed using ClustalW alignment analysis for studying ferret cytokines by real-time PCR.

3.3.1 Methods

ClustalW analysis for cytokine primer design

Cytokine Primers were designed as previously described (Section: Cloning, sequencing and expression of ferret TNF-α and IFN-γ in 4.2.1). Gene specific primers were designed based on highly conserved regions of orthologue nucleotide gene sequences. Conserved regions were identified through ClustalW-based multiple sequence alignments of the orthologues from several species using the ClustalW 1.83 from the European Bioinformatics Institute (http://www.ebi.ac.uk/clustalw/). The Primers are presented in Tables 2, Table 3 and Table 4.

IL-1alpha F	ACCCACTTCATGAGGACTGC
IL-1alpha R	TGCTACTGATCTGGGCTTCA
IL-1beta F	CGACTGCAAATTCCAGGACATAA
IL-1beta R	TTGGTTCACACTAGTTCCGTTGA
Il2 F3	CTTCGCAAACAGTGCACCTA
Il2 R3	GCCTTCTTGGGCATGTAGAA
IL4 F	TCACCGGCACTTTCATCCA
IL4 R	TTCTCGCTGTGAGGATGTTCA
IL5 F	GGGGAGGCTGTGGATAAACT
IL5 R	CAACTTTCCCGGTGTCCACTC
IL6 F	AGTGGCTGAAACACGTAACAATTC
IL6 R	ATGGCCCTCAGGCTGAACT
IL8 F	AAGCAGGAAAACTGCCAAGAGA
IL8 R	GCCAGAAGAAACCTGACCAAAG
Il10 F	CCTGTCGGAGATGATCCAGT
Il10 R	CAAGCTCACTCATGGCTTTG
IL11 F	CTGAGCCTGTGGCCAGATA
IL11 R	GGGAATCCAGGTTGTGGTC
Il12BF	CACCAGCAGCTTCTTCATCA
Il12BR	AGGTCTTGTCCACGCAGAGT
IL13F	TGGTTGACTGTGGTCATTGC
IL13R	GATGCCTGATTCTGGGTGAT
IL-16 Fnew	GGGGAGCCGGATCTAGAAAAC
IL-16 Rnew	CGAGGAGGAGTTCAGGTCAG
Il17AF	CCTCAGCATGTGAAGGTCAA
Il17AR	AACCAGGATCTCTTGCTGGA
IL18F	GACGATATGCCCGATTCTGA
IL18R	ATCATGGCCTGGAACACTTC

Table 2. Ferret Interleukine Primers

TNF-alpha F	CCAGATGGCCTCCAACTAATCA
TNF-alpha R	GGCTTGTCACTTGGAGTTCGA
IFN-gamma F	TCAAAGTGATGAATGATCTCTCACC
IFN-gamma R	GCCGGGAAACACACTGTGAC

Table 3. Ferret Inflammatory Cytokine Primers

Real-time PCR

Real-time PCR analysis was performed as previously described (Bosinger et al., 2004). Briefly, experiments were carried out using the SYBR Green qPCR kit (Applied Biosystems, Foster City, California, USA) on an an ABI 7900 System (Applied Biosystems). The PCR mixture contained 25 pmol primers and 250 nmol of cDNA. Amplification was performed with the following program: pre-heating for 15 minutes at 95°C followed by 40 cycles of 95°C for 15 seconds, 60°C for 1 minute, and 72°C for 1 minute. Subsequent to the completion of PCR amplification, the temperature was raised from annealing temperature to 95°C for melting curve analysis.

CCL2 (MCP-1) F	GCTCCCTATTCACTTGCTGTTTC
CCL2 (MCP-1) R	GATTCGATAGCCCTCCAGCTT
CCL 4 F	TGTGACCGTCCTTTCTCTCC
CCL 4 R	GAATCTTCCGCAGGGTGTAA
CCL5 F	GCTGCTTTGCCTACATTTCC
CCL5 R	CCCATTTCTTCTGTGGGTTG
CCL 7 F	TATCTCAACCACCTGCTGCT
CCL 7 R	GCTTGGGTTTTCTTGTCCAG
CCL8 F	CATCCCAATTACCTGCTGCT
CCL8 R	ACTGGCTGTTGGTGATCCTC
CCL 11 F	AGGTCTCCGCAGCACTTCT
CCL 11 R	TATCCTTGGCCAGTTTGGTC
CCL 17 F	CGGGAGTGCTGCCTAGAGTA
CCL 17 R	CTTCACCCTCTTGTCCTTGG
CCL21 F	TCAGGCAGAGCTATGTGCAG
CCL21 R	TCAGTCCTCTTGCAGCCTTT
CCL22 F	ACTGCACTCCTGGTTGTCCT
CCL22 R	ATCTTCACCCAGGGCACTCT
CCL 23 F	ACGAATTCGATGTGCAAACA
CCL 23 R	AGCTGGCCCCTACTACCATT
CXCL5 F	GAGCTGCGTTGTGTGTGTTT
CXCL5 R	ACTTCCACCTTGGAGCACTG
CXCL9 (MIG) F	GGTGGTGTTCCTCTTTTGTTGAGT
CXCL9 (MIG) R	GGAACAGCGTCTATTCCTCATTG
CXCL10 (IP10) F	CTTTGAACCAAAGTGCTGTTCTTATC
CXCL10 (IP10) R	AGCGTGTAGTTCTAGAGAGAGGTACTC
CXCL 11 F	AGAGGACGCTGTCTTTGCAT
CXCL 11 R	TGGGATTTAGGCATCGTTGT
CXCL12 F	ACAGATGTCCTTGCCGATTC
CXCL12 R	CCACTTCAATTTCGGGTCAA
CXCL 13 F	TCCAAGGTGTTCTGGAGGTC
CXCL 13 R	GGGAATCTTTCTCTTAAACACTGG
CXCL 14 F	CCCTCCGGTCAGCATGAG
CXCL 14 R	CCAGGCGTTGTACCACTTG

Table 4. Ferret CC and CXC Chemokine Primers

3.3.2 Results

Ferret cytokine and chemokine specific real-time PCR primers

Primers specific toward ferret cytokine and chemokine genes were designed by ClustalW analysis. Primers for ferret interleukins (Table 2), ferret inflammatory cytokines (Table 3) and ferret CC and CXC chemokines (Table 4) are described.

Induction of TNF-α target genes by treatment of ferret blood cells with recombinant ferret TNF-α

Once confirming that the recombinant TNF-α protein was of proper molecular weight, we then went on to assess the biological potential of the recombinant protein *in vitro*. Ferret whole peripheral blood was stimulated with recombinant ferret TNF-α and the RNA was extracted. Following extraction, the expression level of a panel of known TNF-α target cytokine/chemokine genes were measured by real-time PCR. CXCL8 (120-fold), IFN-γ (12-fold), IL-1R (6-fold), IL-6 (3-fold) and IL-1β (2-fold) were increased following stimulation (Figure 8). These results indicated that the recombinant ferret TNF-α protein had biological activity.

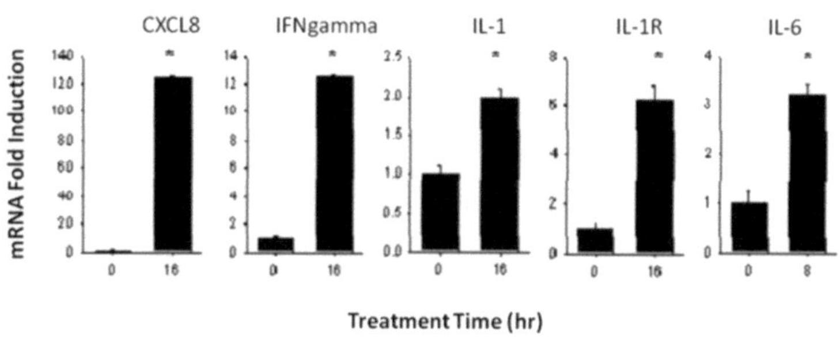

Fig. 8. Real-Time PCR analysis of ferret cytokines transcript stimulated by TNF-α

3.4 Development of IFN-γ and TNF-α hybridoma clones

The generation of monoclonal antibodies specific to ferret IFN-γ and TNF-α are vital to the development of ELISAs and ELISPOTs. In this section we outline the development of these monoclonal antibodies using recombinant IFN-γ and TNF-α conjugated to a carrier protein, KLH (keyhole limpet hemocyanin) using glutaraldehyde. Furthermore, the KLH-IFN-γ/TNF-α complexes injected and cell fusion to establish IFN-γ/TNF-α reactive B cell hybridomas is described along with downstream hybridoma clones slection.

3.4.1 Methods

Monoclonal anti-ferret TNF-α antibody production

Monoclonal antibodies to recombinant ferret TNF-α were manufactured by Open Biosystems (Birmingham, AL, USA).

Mouse B cell hybridoma preparation for anti-ferret-IFN-γ

Recombinant ferret IFN-γ (50 μg) along with 2 mg of keyhole limpet hemocyaine (KLH) (Calbiochem, San Diego, CA, USA) were diluted in 0.5 ml PBS. Five μl of glutaraldehyde were added and the mixture was incubated for 1 hr at room temperature. The whole mixture was washed on a spin column (Nanosep 10k OMEGA, Pall Life Science) and then concentrated to 0.1 ml volume. PBS (0.5 ml) was then added and the mixture was centrifuged. After two PBS washes, the mixture was filled to 0.5 ml with PBS. This mixture was used as the priming antigen. Mice were immunized with 25 µl antigen suspension in emulsified Complete Freund's Adjuvant and further injected at bi-weekly intervals with 5 µg of recombinant ferret IFN-γ. Three days following the third injection, spleen cells were removed and isolated for fusion with Sp2/0-Ag14 using polyethylene glycol (Roche, Mannheim, Germany). HAT (hypoxanthine aminopterin thymidine) resistant hybridomas were selected. Hybridoma cells were screened for the reactivity against IFN-γ by ELISA using Nunc MaxiSorp 96 well plates coated with ferret IFN-γ (100 µl, 0.1 µg/ml).

3.4.2 Results

Monoclonal ferret TNF-α antibody recognizes endogenous TNF-α isolated secreted from mitogen-stimulated ferret blood cells

A monoclonal anti-ferret TNF-α antibody was commercially manufactured by immunizing mice with recombinant ferret TNF-α. Isolated ferret peripheral blood cells were then stimulated with the mitogens: SEB (Staphylococcal enterotoxin B), IFN-γ, ionomycin and PMA plus ionomycin. Following stimuation, cell supernantants were run on SDS-PAGE and analyzed by western blotting using the manufactured monoclonal ferret TNF-α antibody. Endogenous ferret TNF-α protein was recognized in samples that had been stimulated with SEB, IFN-γ and PMA plus ionomycin. In contrast, TNF-α was not present in the supernatant from cells treated with ionomycin alone or unstimulated cells (Figure 9). These results suggested that the manufactured ferret monoclonal TNF-α antibody was able to recognize endogenous secreted ferret TNF-α.

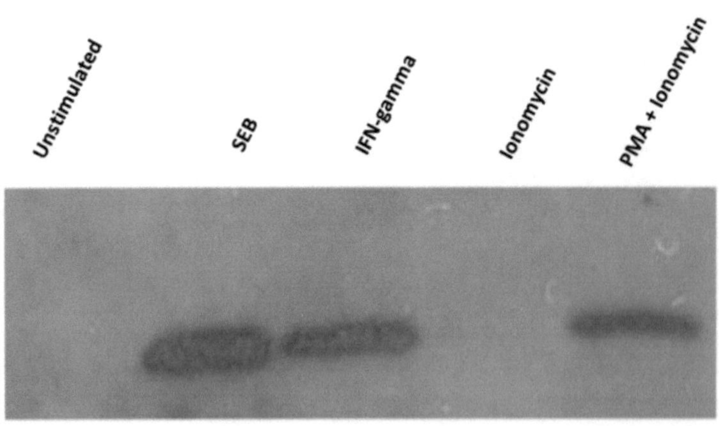

PBMCs were isolated and stimulated with SEB (100 µg/ml), IFN-γ (2000IU/ml), ionomycin alone (1 ug/ml) or PMA (50 ng/ml) with ionomycin (1 µg/ml), for 24 hrs at 37°C. Cell supernatant was run on SDS-PAGE and subjected to western blotting with a monoclonal antibody (2µg/ml) against recombinant ferret TNF-α.

Fig. 9. Ferret monoclonal TNF-α antibody recognizes secreted endogenous TNF-α.

Generation of monoclonal Abs specific for ferret IFN-γ

Prior to the generation of ferret IFN-γ monoclonal antibodies, we attempted to monitor IFN-γ levels from ferret cell cultures using human and mouse commercially available cytometric bead arrays. Neither human nor mouse-specific arrays resulted in the positive detection of ferret IFN-γ. The failure in detection was most likely due to the inablility of the human and mouse IFN-γ antibody to recognize the ferret IFN-γ protein. These results prompted us to generate our own monoclonal antibodies specific to ferret IFN-γ. To produce ferret IFN-γ specific antibodies, recombinant IFN-γ was conjugated to a carrier protein, KLH (keyhole limpet hemocyanin) using glutaraldehyde (as described in the methods). The resulting KLH-IFN-γ complex was injected intraperitoneal into Balb/c mice. Following fusion of splenocytes with hybridoma parent cells, IFN-γ-reactive B cell hybridomas were established and clones were selected by ELISA reactivity. Clone 1H1H12 and 4A4B7 recognized recombinant ferret IFN-γ evident by a 40 kDa band (Figure 10).

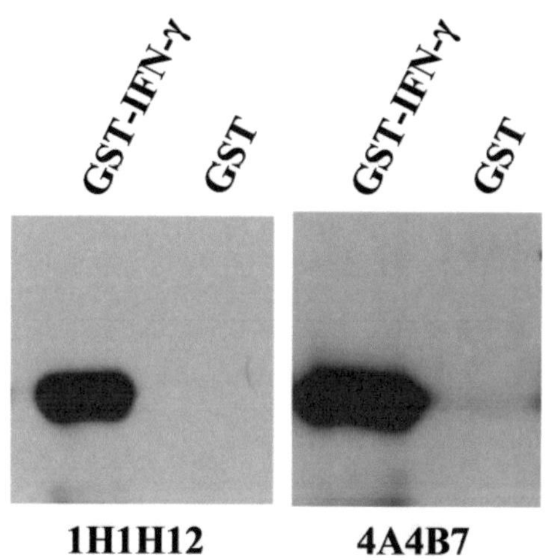

Fig. 10. Ferret IFN-γ monoclonal antibody detects recombinant and endogenous ferret IFN-γ protein.

Lysates from COS-7 cells transfected with recombinant ferret IFN-γ samples were analyzed by western blot using a monoclonal antibody established from mouse immunized by recombinant ferret IFN-γ (left panel). Supernatants derived from ferret PBMC cultures stimulated with PMA plus ionomycin, were also analyzed by western blot using anti-ferret IFN-γ monoclonal antibody (right panel). Arrows at the right of each panel indicate the dimers for lower molecular weight protein bands and putative tetramer as higher molecular weight species.

3.5 ELISA and ELISPOT assays for the ferret cytokine IFN-γ

An important application for monoclonal anti-ferret IFN-γ antibodies is the detection and quantitation of IFN-γ protein in biological samples. In this section the protocols for both IFN-γ ELISA and ELISPOT are described. This includes the selection and testing of the monoclonal antibodies and ELISAs to measure IFN-γ levels in sera obtained from influenza A-infected ferrets. Furthermore, a ferret-specific IFN-γ ELISPOT assay is outlined using the same set of monoclonal ferret IFN-γ antibodies used in the ELISA.

3.5.1 Methods

Ferret IFN-γ-specific ELISA

ELISA plates (96-well) (MaxiSorb, Nunc) were coated with 100 μl/well with monoclonal anti-IFN-γ (2 μg/ml) overnight at 4°C. Wells were blocked with 150 μl 1% BSA in PBS for 1 hour at 37°C. Supernatants from mitogen-stimulated PBMC cultures or serum from influenza A virus infected ferrets were loaded into the wells at appropriate dilutions and incubated for 1 hour at 37°C. Wells were washed with PBS/0.5% Tween-20 and then incubated for 1 hour at room temperature with biotin conjugated anti-IFN-γ antibody (1 μg/ml in 0.5% Tween-20/1%BSA). Following secondary antibody incubation, the wells were washed three times with PBS/0.5% Tween-20 before incubation with HRP-Avidin for 30 minutes. The substrate, (o-phenylenediamine, Sigma) was applied for 15 minutes at room temperature. Colorimetric changes were quantitated using an automated ELISA reader (μQuant, BIO-TEK Instruments, Winooski, VT, USA).

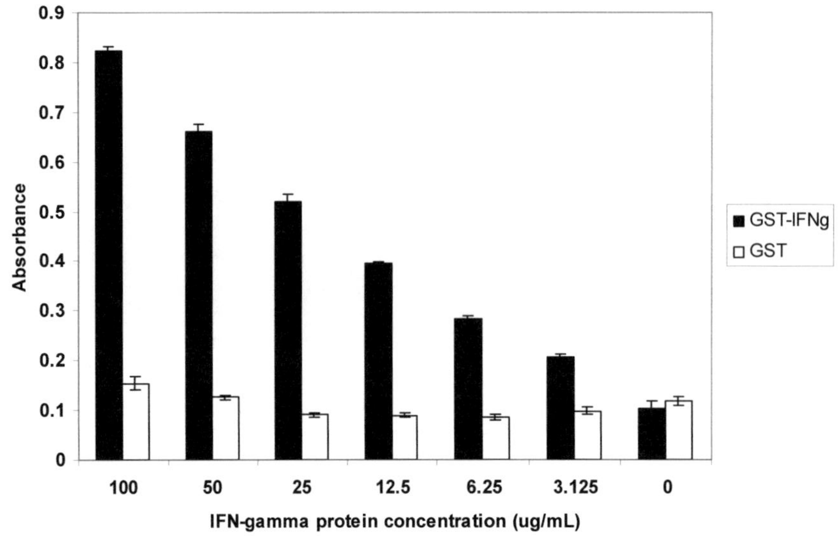

ELISA plate wells were coated with a monoclonal anti-ferret antibody. Recombinant ferret IFN-γ was sequentially diluted and added to the wells. Ferret IFN-γ was detected by a second monoclonal anti-ferret IFN-γ biotin conjugated antibody. Logarithmic dilution was used to derive a standard curve for downstream applications of the ELISA.

Fig. 11. Recombinant IFN-γ protein quantification by ELISA.

Ferret IFN-γ-specific ELISPOT assay

PVDF plates (Millipore, MAIPS4510) or MaxiSorp plates (Nunc) were coated with a monoclonal anti-ferret IFN-γ antibody, and subsequently blocked with 1% BSA in PBS. Isolated ferret PBMCs from peripheral blood were stimulated for 18 hours. The wells were then washed with water to remove cells and captured IFN-γ was detected by a biotin-conjugated detection antibody coupled to HRP-avidin (Sigma). The ELISPOT was developed using DAB (Vector Laboratories, Burlingame, CA, USA).

3.5.2 Results

Detection of ferret IFN-γ by ELISA and ELISPOT immunoassays

An important application for monoclonal antibodies is the detection and quantitation of protein in biological samples. Here we tested our monoclonal antibodies for use in a ferret IFN-γ-specific ELISA by first determining the antibody pair for IFN-γ recognition. Clone 4A4B7 was conjugated to biotin and used as the detection antibody against ferret IFN-γ. Clone 1H1H12 was used to coat the assay wells and be used as a capture antibody.

This clone pair showed an increased optical density that correlated directly with the concentration of purified recombinant IFN-γ (Figure 11).

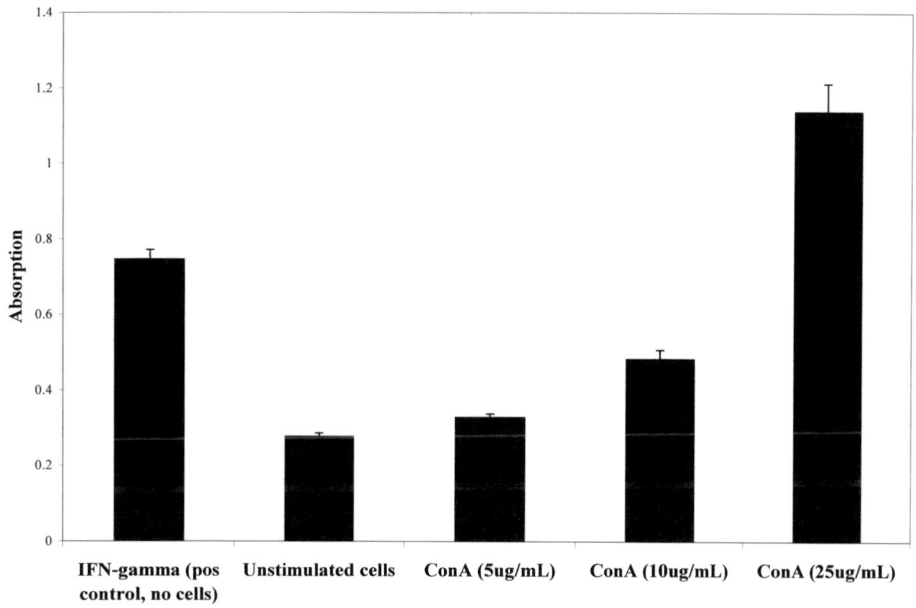

IFN-γ ELISA was performed on supernantant from isolated ferret PMBCs treated with ConA. Results represent the mean values of triplicate samples.

Fig. 12. ELISA detection of IFN-γ from mitogen-stimulated PBMCs.

We then used the ELISA assay to detect endogenous IFN-γ from ConA-stimulated ferret PBMCs. Our assay showed that IFN-γ was only present in samples that were treated with ConA and no detection in the negative control unstimulated samples (Figure 12). These results indicated that the monoclonal antibodies selected are applicable for ferret IFN-γ-specific ELISA and that the pair was a reliable detection system.

ELISPOT assays are also key tools in the determining the activation of cellular immune responses. Specifically, ELISPOT assays directly quantitate the number of cytokine secreting cells as opposed to the ELISA which quantitates the amount of cytokine produced. To develop a ferret-specific IFN-γ ELISPOT assay we employed the same set of monoclonal ferret IFN-γ antibodies, clone 4A4B7 and 1H1H12. Isolated ferret PBMCs were subjected to an ELISPOT assay (as described in the methods) with stimulation of ConA. As expected, increasing numbers of IFN-γ secreting cells were detected in direct proportion to the number of stimulated cells plated. Furthermore, the number of IFN-γ positive cells did not increase above background when increasing numbers of unstimulated cells were plated (Figure 13). These results suggested that 4A4B7 and 1H1H12 anti-ferret IFN-γ monoclonal antibodies will be useful for not only quantitating ferret IFN-γ levels but also for quantitating IFN-γ producing ferret cells in an ELISPOT assay.

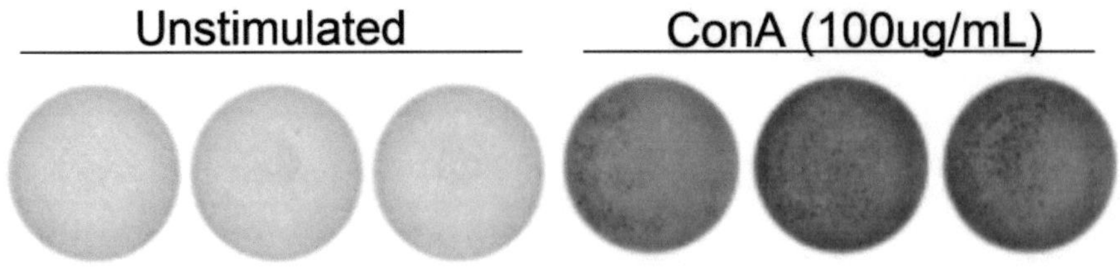

ELISPOT assay was performed in the same manner outlined for Figure 12 for capture and detection. PBMCs were plated and stimulated with ConA 18 hours and IFN-γ secreting cells were captured and detected by biotinylated IFN-g antibody.

Fig. 13. ELISPOT assay for the IFN-γ producing cells in mitogen-stimulated ferret PBMCs.

4. Conclusion

The development of ferret specific immune reagents will significantly improve knowledge gained by ferret infectious disease studies. The importance of the ferret as an animal model in the study of respiratory diseases is increasing. Currently, the use of the ferret model to investigate the immune response as well as immunotherapeutics in respiratory infections by viruses such as SARS CoV and influenza has been slowed by the lack of immunological reagents and immune response assessment tools. In this chapter we highlighted immune reagents and immunoassays that are successful at monitoring the ferret immune response, specifically focusing on cytokines.

Currently, there is much interest to determine the immunological role of TNF-α during influenza infection, as TNF-α is thought to play a pathogenic role in other respiratory infections (Headley, Tolley, & Meduri, 1997). Here we have described the cloning and sequence of the ferret TNF-α gene with the purpose of generating reagents and assays for the investigation of ferret immune responses. With the generated ferret TNF-α expression vector we were able to express and purify recombinant protein for downstream uses. Importantly, the recombinant ferret TNF-α protein was able to stimulate ferret peripheral blood cells and induce the expression of TNF-α target genes such as: CXCL-8, IFN-γ, IL-1β, IL-6 and IL-1R (Vassalli, 1992; Baumann & Gauldie, 1994; Dinarello, 1996; Gabay & Kushner, 1999). Furthermore, we have successfully generated monoclonal antibodies that specifically recognized ferret TNF-α as well as primers that measured TNF-α transcripts in cells stimulated with LPS, a known stimulant of TNF-α (Curnis & Corti, 2004; Mestan et al., 1986; Wang et al., 1985). In summary, we have cloned, sequenced and expressed recombinant ferret TNF-α and demonstrated its biological activity. Our ferret TNF-α protein has enabled us to generate several useful reagents that will be important tools for immune modeling in respiratory diseases.

IFN-γ is an essential regulator in the viral host immune response. Here the cloning of a full length ferret IFN-γ and expression of the recombinant IFN-γ protein was described. Furthermore, we described the generation of two monoclonal antibodies specific for ferret IFN-γ and the subsequent development of immunoassays for the detection of native IFN-γ. We anticipate that the IFN-γ immunoassays established in this study will be useful in gaining insight into ferret antiviral responses and in other immune processes in general.

Previous studies on IFN-γ have shown that there is a strict species-specific activity of IFN-γ. IFN-γ genes isolated from diverse species such as guinea pig, turkey, rhino, and catfish have been previously described in the literature (Jeevan et al., 2006; Loa, Hsieh, Wu, & Lin, 2001; Milev-Milovanovic et al., 2006; Morar et al., 2007; Svitek & von, V, 2007). Our monoclonal antibodies detected recombinant IFN-γ in Western blotting. These two clones were paired successfully during the development of ferret IFN-γ-specific ELISA and ELISPOT bioassays. Previously, we infected ferrets with H3N2 influenza A strain (A/Panama/2007/99) and sampled serum from the animals 6 days post infection (Ochi et al., 2008). The ELISA showed a marked increase in the levels of circulating IFN-γ on day 6 post-infection compared to the uninfected control. Specifically, the level of IFN-γ in serum from the non-infected control ferret was below the detection limit. These results suggested that our developed ELISA assay for quantitation of ferret IFN-γ will be invaluable in monitoring systemic IFN-γ responses during a host response against virus infection.

There is an overwhelming need for experimental models that enable the evaluation of therapeutic treatments and vaccines for use in infectious diseases such as emerging influenza viruses. Ferrets have been used as an animal model of infection with influenza A viruses to test the severity of the disease and also to evaluate efficacy of potential vaccines (Suguitan, Jr. et al., 2006; Cameron et al., 2008; Danesh et al., 2011; Rowe et al., 2010b). Specifically, TNF-α and IFN-γ have been identified as major inducers of pathogenesis in respiratory illnesses which includes SARS (Cheung et al., 2005), (Roberts & Subbarao, 2006) and influenza virus (Maher & DeStefano, 2004; Cheung et al., 2002; de Jong et al., 2006). From these findings comes the hypothesis that these inflammatory cytokines may be the key to potential future therapies.

TNF-α antibodies have been shown to have therapeutic potential in disease either as therapeutic targets or as biomarkers. In a mouse model of influenza-induced pneumonia, a neutralizing antibody to TNF-α significantly reduced the lung pathology and prolonged survival of infected animals thereby suggesting TNF-α as a therapeutic target (Peper & Van, 1995). With the antibodies generated, it is now possible to investigate the therapeutic potential of targeting TNF-α to modulate the immunopathology during influenza infection. Alternatively, IFN-γ has been shown to be a useful biomarker. ELISPOT and ELISA assays are excellent techniques that can be employed in studies monitoring vaccine and therapeutic efficacy by measuring the levels of biomarkers such as IFN-γ. Taken together, these reagents will be helpful in the assessment of vaccine efficacy against influenza A and other emerging infectious viruses.

In conclusion, this work has expanded the potential of the ferret model for respiratory disease investigation as well as other diseases that involved the immune response.

5. References

Anglen, C. S., Truckenmiller, M. E., Schell, T. D., & Bonneau, R. H. (2003). The dual role of CD8+ T lymphocytes in the development of stress-induced herpes simplex encephalitis. J.Neuroimmunol., 140, 13-27.

Baumann, H. & Gauldie, J. (1994). The acute phase response. Immunol.Today, 15, 74-80.

Belser, J. A., Szretter, K. J., Katz, J. M., & Tumpey, T. M. (2009). Use of animal models to understand the pandemic potential of highly pathogenic avian influenza viruses. Adv.Virus Res., 73, 55-97.

Belz, G. T., Bedoui, S., Kupresanin, F., Carbone, F. R., & Heath, W. R. (2007). Minimal activation of memory CD8(+) T cell by tissue-derived dendritic cells favors the stimulation of naive CD8(+) T cells. Nat.Immunol., 8, 1060-1066.

Boon, A. C., de Mutsert, G., Fouchier, R. A., Osterhaus, A. D., & Rimmelzwaan, G. F. (2005). Functional profile of human influenza virus-specific cytotoxic T lymphocyte activity is influenced by interleukin-2 concentration and epitope specificity. Clin.Exp.Immunol., 142, 45-52.

Bossart, K. N., Zhu, Z., Middleton, D., Klippel, J., Crameri, G., Bingham, J. et al. (2009). A neutralizing human monoclonal antibody protects against lethal disease in a new ferret model of acute nipah virus infection. PLoS.Pathog., 5, e1000642.

Bouvier, N. M. & Lowen, A. C. (2010). Animal Models for Influenza Virus Pathogenesis and Transmission. Viruses., 2, 1530-1563.

Bouvier, N. M., Lowen, A. C., & Palese, P. (2008). Oseltamivir-resistant influenza A viruses are transmitted efficiently among guinea pigs by direct contact but not by aerosol. J.Virol., 82, 10052-10058.

Brown, T. J., Crawford, S. E., Cornwall, M. L., Garcia, F., Shulman, S. T., & Rowley, A. H. (2001). CD8 T lymphocytes and macrophages infiltrate coronary artery aneurysms in acute Kawasaki disease. J.Infect.Dis., 184, 940-943.

Cameron, C. M., Cameron, M. J., Bermejo-Martin, J. F., Ran, L., Xu, L., Turner, P. V. et al. (2008). Gene expression analysis of host innate immune responses during Lethal H5N1 infection in ferrets. J.Virol., 82, 11308-11317.

Cameron, M. J., Ran, L., Xu, L., Danesh, A., Bermejo-Martin, J. F., Cameron, C. M. et al. (2007). Interferon-mediated immunopathological events are associated with atypical innate and adaptive immune responses in patients with severe acute respiratory syndrome. J.Virol., 81, 8692-8706.

Centers for Disease Control and Prevention (CDC) (2009). Intensive-care patients with severe novel influenza A (H1N1) virus infection - Michigan, June 2009. MMWR - Morbidity & Mortality Weekly Report.58(27):749-52.

Chelbi-Alix, M. K. & Wietzerbin, J. (2007). Interferon, a growing cytokine family: 50 years of interferon research. Biochimie, 89, 713-718.

Chen, H. C., Lai, S. Y., Sung, J. M., Lee, S. H., Lin, Y. C., Wang, W. K. et al. (2004). Lymphocyte activation and hepatic cellular infiltration in immunocompetent mice infected by dengue virus. J.Med.Virol., 73, 419-431.

Cheung, C. Y., Poon, L. L., Lau, A. S., Luk, W., Lau, Y. L., Shortridge, K. F. et al. (2002). Induction of proinflammatory cytokines in human macrophages by influenza A

(H5N1) viruses: a mechanism for the unusual severity of human disease? Lancet, 360, 1831-1837.

Cheung, C. Y., Poon, L. L., Ng, I. H., Luk, W., Sia, S. F., Wu, M. H. et al. (2005). Cytokine responses in severe acute respiratory syndrome coronavirus-infected macrophages in vitro: possible relevance to pathogenesis. J.Virol., 79, 7819-7826.

Chevaliez, S. & Pawlotsky, J. M. (2009). Interferons and their use in persistent viral infections. Handb.Exp.Pharmacol., 203-241.

Curnis, F. & Corti, A. (2004). Production and characterization of recombinant human and murine TNF. Methods Mol.Med., 98, 9-22.

Danesh, A., Cameron, C. M., Leon, A. J., Ran, L., Xu, L., Fang, Y. et al. (2011). Early gene expression events in ferrets in response to SARS coronavirus infection versus direct interferon-alpha2b stimulation. Virology, 409, 102-112.

Danesh, A., Seneviratne, C., Cameron, C. M., Banner, D., DeVries, M. E., Kelvin, A. A. et al. (2008). Cloning, expression and characterization of ferret CXCL10. Mol.Immunol., 45, 1288-1297.

Darnell, M. E., Plant, E. P., Watanabe, H., Byrum, R., St Claire, M., Ward, J. M. et al. (2007). Severe acute respiratory syndrome coronavirus infection in vaccinated ferrets. J.Infect.Dis., 196, 1329-1338.

Dawood, F. S., Dalton, C. B., Durrheim, D. N., & Hope, K. G. (2009). Rates of hospitalisation for acute respiratory illness and the emergence of pandemic (H1N1) 2009 virus in the Hunter New England Area Health Service. Med.J.Aust., 191, 573-574.

Dawood, F. S., Jain, S., Finelli, L., Shaw, M. W., Lindstrom, S., Garten, R. J. et al. (2009). Emergence of a novel swine-origin influenza A (H1N1) virus in humans. N.Engl.J.Med., 360, 2605-2615.

de Jong, M. D., Simmons, C. P., Thanh, T. T., Hien, V. M., Smith, G. J., Chau, T. N. et al. (2006). Fatal outcome of human influenza A (H5N1) is associated with high viral load and hypercytokinemia. Nat.Med., 12, 1203-1207.

Dinarello, C. A. (1996). Biologic basis for interleukin-1 in disease. Blood, 87, 2095-2147.

Dushoff, J., Plotkin, J. B., Viboud, C., Earn, D. J., & Simonsen, L. (2006). Mortality due to influenza in the United States--an annualized regression approach using multiple-cause mortality data. Am.J.Epidemiol., 163, 181-187.

Foxwell, A. R., Kyd, J. M., Karupiah, G., & Cripps, A. W. (2001). CD8+ T cells have an essential role in pulmonary clearance of nontypeable Haemophilus influenzae following mucosal immunization. Infect.Immun., 69, 2636-2642.

Gabay, C. & Kushner, I. (1999). Acute-phase proteins and other systemic responses to inflammation. N.Engl.J.Med., 340, 448-454.

Gilsdorf, A., Poggensee, G., & Working Group (2009). Influenza A(H1N1)v in Germany: the first 10,000 cases. Euro Surveillance: Bulletin Europeen sur les Maladies Transmissibles = European Communicable Disease Bulletin.14(34).

Girard, M. P., Cherian, T., Pervikov, Y., & Kieny, M. P. (2005). A review of vaccine research and development: human acute respiratory infections. [Review] [107 refs]. Vaccine.23(50):5708-24.

Govorkova, E. A., Ilyushina, N. A., Boltz, D. A., Douglas, A., Yilmaz, N., & Webster, R. G. (2007). Efficacy of oseltamivir therapy in ferrets inoculated with different clades of H5N1 influenza virus. Antimicrob.Agents Chemother., 51, 1414-1424.

Gupta, V., Earl, D. J., & Deem, M. W. (2006). Quantifying influenza vaccine efficacy and antigenic distance. Vaccine, 24, 3881-3888.

Haagmans, B. L., Kuiken, T., Martina, B. E., Fouchier, R. A., Rimmelzwaan, G. F., van, A. G. et al. (2004). Pegylated interferon-alpha protects type 1 pneumocytes against SARS coronavirus infection in macaques. Nat.Med., 10, 290-293.

Hauge, S., Madhun, A. S., Cox, R. J., Brokstad, K. A., & Haaheim, L. R. (2007). A comparison of the humoral and cellular immune responses at different immunological sites after split influenza virus vaccination of mice. Scand.J.Immunol., 65, 14-21.

Headley, A. S., Tolley, E., & Meduri, G. U. (1997). Infections and the inflammatory response in acute respiratory distress syndrome. Chest, 111, 1306-1321.

Health Protection Agency, Health, P. S., National Public Health Service for Wales, & HPA Northern Ireland Swine influenza investigation team (2009). Epidemiology of new influenza A (H1N1) virus infection, United Kingdom, April-June 2009. Euro Surveillance: Bulletin Europeen sur les Maladies Transmissibles = European Communicable Disease Bulletin.14(22).

Hoji, A. & Rinaldo, C. R., Jr. (2005). Human CD8+ T cells specific for influenza A virus M1 display broad expression of maturation-associated phenotypic markers and chemokine receptors. Immunology, 115, 239-245.

Huang S.S.H., Banner, D., Fang, Y., Ng, D. C., Kanagasabai T., Kelvin, D. J. et al. Comparative Analyses of Pandemic H1N1 and Seasonal H1N1, H3N2, and Influenza B Infections Depict Distinct Clinical Pictures In Ferrets. PLoS One, (in press).

HULL, R. B. & LOOSLI, C. G. (1951). Adrenocorticotrophic hormone (ACTH) in the treatment of experimental air-borne influenza virus type A infection in the ferret. J.Lab Clin.Med., 37, 603-614.

Hussell, T., Pennycook, A., & Openshaw, P. J. (2001). Inhibition of tumor necrosis factor reduces the severity of virus-specific lung immunopathology. Eur.J.Immunol., 31, 2566-2573.

Jeevan, A., McFarland, C. T., Yoshimura, T., Skwor, T., Cho, H., Lasco, T. et al. (2006). Production and characterization of guinea pig recombinant gamma interferon and its effect on macrophage activation. Infect.Immun., 74, 213-224.

Kasowski, E. J., Garten, R. J., & Bridges, C. B. (2011). Influenza pandemic epidemiologic and virologic diversity: reminding ourselves of the possibilities. [Review]. Clinical Infectious Diseases.52 Suppl 1:S44-9.

Kolling, U. K., Hansen, F., Braun, J., Rink, L., Katus, H. A., & Dalhoff, K. (2001). Leucocyte response and anti-inflammatory cytokines in community acquired pneumonia. Thorax, 56, 121-125.

Kumar, A. M., Zarychanski, R. M., Pinto, R. P., Cook, D. J. M., Marshall, J. M., Lacroix, J. M. et al. (2009). Critically Ill Patients With 2009 Influenza A(H1N1) Infection in Canada. [Miscellaneous Article]. JAMA, 302, 1872-1879.

Lambkin, R., Oxford, J. S., Bossuyt, S., Mann, A., Metcalfe, I. C., Herzog, C. et al. (2004). Strong local and systemic protective immunity induced in the ferret model by an intranasal virosome-formulated influenza subunit vaccine. Vaccine, 22, 4390-4396.

Loa, C. C., Hsieh, M. K., Wu, C. C., & Lin, T. L. (2001). Molecular identification and characterization of turkey IFN-gamma gene. Comp Biochem.Physiol B Biochem.Mol.Biol., 130, 579-584.

Loutfy, M. R., Blatt, L. M., Siminovitch, K. A., Ward, S., Wolff, B., Lho, H. et al. (2003). Interferon alfacon-1 plus corticosteroids in severe acute respiratory syndrome: a preliminary study. JAMA, 290, 3222-3228.

Maher, J. A. & DeStefano, J. (2004). The ferret: an animal model to study influenza virus. Lab Anim (NY), 33, 50-53.

Marijanovic, Z., Ragimbeau, J., van der Heyden, J., Uze, G., & Pellegrini, S. (2007). Comparable potency of IFNalpha2 and IFNbeta on immediate JAK/STAT activation but differential down-regulation of IFNAR2. Biochem.J., 407, 141-151.

Martina, B. E., Haagmans, B. L., Kuiken, T., Fouchier, R. A., Rimmelzwaan, G. F., Van Amerongen, G. et al. (2003). Virology: SARS virus infection of cats and ferrets. Nature, 425, 915.

Mendel, D. B., Tai, C. Y., Escarpe, P. A., Li, W., Sidwell, R. W., Huffman, J. H. et al. (1998). Oral administration of a prodrug of the influenza virus neuraminidase inhibitor GS 4071 protects mice and ferrets against influenza infection. Antimicrob.Agents Chemother., 42, 640-646.

Mestan, J., Digel, W., Mittnacht, S., Hillen, H., Blohm, D., Moller, A. et al. (1986). Antiviral effects of recombinant tumour necrosis factor in vitro. Nature, 323, 816-819.

Milev-Milovanovic, I., Long, S., Wilson, M., Bengten, E., Miller, N. W., & Chinchar, V. G. (2006). Identification and expression analysis of interferon gamma genes in channel catfish. Immunogenetics, 58, 70-80.

Morar, D., Tijhaar, E., Negrea, A., Hendriks, J., van, H. D., Godfroid, J. et al. (2007). Cloning, sequencing and expression of white rhinoceros (Ceratotherium simum) interferon-gamma (IFN-gamma) and the production of rhinoceros IFN-gamma specific antibodies. Vet.Immunol.Immunopathol., 115, 146-154.

Nicoll, A. & Coulombier, D. (2009). Europe's initial experience with pandemic (H1N1) 2009 - mitigation and delaying policies and practices. Euro Surveillance: Bulletin Europeen sur les Maladies Transmissibles = European Communicable Disease Bulletin.14(29).

Ochi, A., Danesh, A., Seneviratne, C., Banner, D., Devries, M. E., Rowe, T. et al. (2008). Cloning, expression and immunoassay detection of ferret IFN-gamma. Dev.Comp Immunol., 32, 890-897.

Peltola, V. T., Boyd, K. L., McAuley, J. L., Rehg, J. E., & McCullers, J. A. (2006). Bacterial sinusitis and otitis media following influenza virus infection in ferrets. Infect.Immun., 74, 2562-2567.

Peper, R. L. & Van, C. H. (1995). Tumor necrosis factor as a mediator of inflammation in influenza A viral pneumonia. Microb.Pathog., 19, 175-183.

Perez-Padilla, R., Rosa-Zamboni, D., Ponce, d. L., Hernandez, M., Quinones-Falconi, F., Bautista, E. et al. (2009). Pneumonia and respiratory failure from swine-origin influenza A (H1N1) in Mexico. New England Journal of Medicine.361(7):680-9.

Pinto, R. D., Nascimento, D. S., Vale, A., & Santos, N. M. (2006). Molecular cloning and characterization of sea bass (Dicentrarchus labrax L.) CD8alpha. Vet.Immunol.Immunopathol., 110, 169-177.

Roberts, A. & Subbarao, K. (2006). Animal models for SARS. Adv.Exp.Med.Biol., 581, 463-471.

Rowe, T., Banner, D., Farooqui, A., Ng, D. C., Kelvin, A. A., Rubino, S. et al. (2010a). In vivo ribavirin activity against severe pandemic H1N1 Influenza A/Mexico/4108/2009. J.Gen.Virol., 91, 2898-2906.

Rowe, T., Leon, A. J., Crevar, C. J., Carter, D. M., Xu, L., Ran, L. et al. (2010b). Modeling host responses in ferrets during A/California/07/2009 influenza infection. Virology, 401, 257-265.

Ryan, G. B. & Majno, G. (1977). Acute inflammation. A review. The American journal of pathology, 86, 183.

Seo, S. H. & Webster, R. G. (2002). Tumor necrosis factor alpha exerts powerful anti-influenza virus effects in lung epithelial cells. J.Virol., 76, 1071-1076.

Small, P. A., Jr., Waldman, R. H., Bruno, J. C., & Gifford, G. E. (1976). Influenza infection in ferrets: role of serum antibody in protection and recovery. Infect.Immun., 13, 417-424.

Somamoto, T., Yoshiura, Y., Nakanishi, T., & Ototake, M. (2005). Molecular cloning and characterization of two types of CD8alpha from ginbuna crucian carp, Carassius auratus langsdorfii. Dev.Comp Immunol., 29, 693-702.

Steinhauer, D. A. & Skehel, J. J. (2002). Genetics of influenza viruses. [Review] [175 refs]. Annual Review of Genetics.36:305-32.

Suguitan, A. L., Jr., McAuliffe, J., Mills, K. L., Jin, H., Duke, G., Lu, B. et al. (2006). Live, attenuated influenza A H5N1 candidate vaccines provide broad cross-protection in mice and ferrets. PLoS Med., 3, e360.

Svitek, N. & von, M., V (2007). Early cytokine mRNA expression profiles predict Morbillivirus disease outcome in ferrets. Virology, 362, 404-410.

Sweet, C., Bird, R. A., Cavanagh, D., Toms, G. L., Collie, M. H., & Smith, H. (1979). The local origin of the febrile response induced in ferrets during respiratory infection with a virulent influenza virus. Br.J.Exp.Pathol., 60, 300-308.

Takaoka, A. & Yanai, H. (2006). Interferon signalling network in innate defence. Cell Microbiol., 8, 907-922.

ter, M. J., van den Brink, E. N., Poon, L. L., Marissen, W. E., Leung, C. S., Cox, F. et al. (2006). Human monoclonal antibody combination against SARS coronavirus: synergy and coverage of escape mutants. PLoS.Med., 3, e237.

Trifonov, V., Khiabanian, H., & Rabadan, R. (2009). Geographic dependence, surveillance, and origins of the 2009 influenza A (H1N1) virus. New England Journal of Medicine.361(2):115-9.

Uddin, S. & Platanias, L. C. (2004). Mechanisms of type-I interferon signal transduction. J.Biochem.Mol.Biol., 37, 635-641.

Uyeki, T. M. M., Sharma, A. M. D., & Branda, J. A. M. (2009). Case 40-2009: A 29-Year-Old Man with Fever and Respiratory Failure. [Miscellaneous Article]. New England Journal of Medicine, 361, 2558-2569.

van den Brand, J. M., Haagmans, B. L., Leijten, L., van, R. D., Martina, B. E., Osterhaus, A. D. et al. (2008). Pathology of experimental SARS coronavirus infection in cats and ferrets. Vet.Pathol., 45, 551-562.

van, R. D., Munster, V. J., de, W. E., Rimmelzwaan, G. F., Fouchier, R. A., Osterhaus, A. D. et al. (2007). Human and avian influenza viruses target different cells in the lower respiratory tract of humans and other mammals. Am.J.Pathol., 171, 1215-1223.

Vassalli, P. (1992). The pathophysiology of tumor necrosis factors. Annu.Rev.Immunol., 10, 411-452.

Vikman, S., Giandomenico, V., Sommaggio, R., Oberg, K., Essand, M., & Totterman, T. H. (2007). CD8(+) T cells against multiple tumor-associated antigens in peripheral blood of midgut carcinoid patients. Cancer Immunol.Immunother..

Vilcek, J. & Lee, T. H. (1991). Tumor necrosis factor. New insights into the molecular mechanisms of its multiple actions. J.Biol.Chem., 266, 7313-7316.

Wang, A. M., Creasey, A. A., Ladner, M. B., Lin, L. S., Strickler, J., Van Arsdell, J. N. et al. (1985). Molecular cloning of the complementary DNA for human tumor necrosis factor. Science, 228, 149-154.

Wang, Y., Lobigs, M., Lee, E., & Mullbacher, A. (2003). CD8+ T cells mediate recovery and immunopathology in West Nile virus encephalitis. J.Virol., 77, 13323-13334.

Weiss, R. A. & McMichael, A. J. (2004). Social and environmental risk factors in the emergence of infectious diseases. Nat.Med., 10, S70-S76.

Willemsen, R. A., Sebestyen, Z., Ronteltap, C., Berrevoets, C., Drexhage, J., & Debets, R. (2006). CD8 alpha coreceptor to improve TCR gene transfer to treat melanoma: down-regulation of tumor-specific production of IL-4, IL-5, and IL-10. J.Immunol., 177, 991-998.

Writing Committee of the WHO Consultation on Clinical Aspects of Pandemic ((2010). Clinical Aspects of Pandemic 2009 Influenza A (H1N1) Virus Infection. [Review]. New England Journal of Medicine, 362, 1708-1719.

Xu, T., Qiao, J., Zhao, L., Wang, G., He, G., Li, K. et al. (2006). Acute respiratory distress syndrome induced by avian influenza A (H5N1) virus in mice. Am.J.Respir.Crit Care Med., 174, 1011-1017.

Yun, N. E., Linde, N. S., Zacks, M. A., Barr, I. G., Hurt, A. C., Smith, J. N. et al. (2008). Injectable peramivir mitigates disease and promotes survival in ferrets and mice infected with the highly virulent influenza virus, A/Vietnam/1203/04 (H5N1). Virology, 374, 198-209.

Zheng, B., Zhang, Y., He, H., Marinova, E., Switzer, K., Wansley, D. et al. (2007). Rectification of age-associated deficiency in cytotoxic T cell response to influenza a virus by immunization with immune complexes. J.Immunol., 179, 6153-6159.

Zitzow, L. A., Rowe, T., Morken, T., Shieh, W. J., Zaki, S., & Katz, J. M. (2002). Pathogenesis of avian influenza A (H5N1) viruses in ferrets. J.Virol., 76, 4420-4429.

10

A Modified Enzyme Immunoassay Method for Determination of cAMP in Plant Cells

Lidia A. Lomovatskaya, Anatoly S. Romanenko, Nadya V. Filinova and Olga V. Rykun
Siberian Institute of Plant Physiology and Biochemistry, Siberian Branch of the Russian Academy of Sciences, Irkutsk, Russia

1. Introduction

A substantial experimental material shown that an adenylate cyclase signaling system is active in plants (Yavorskaya and Kalinin, 1984; Cooke et al. 1994; Newton et al., 1999; Moutinho et al., 2001; Richards et al., 2002). Convincing data have been obtained, which are related to the main components of the scrutinized system: cAMP, adenylate cyclase, phosphodiesterase, cAMP-binding proteins (Brown et al., 1980; Polya and Bowman, 1981; Phedenko et al., 1983; Yavorskaya and Kalinin, 1984; Tarchevsky, 2001), nucleotide-gated channels (Martinez-Atienza et al., 2007). The concentration of the endogenous cAMP is an indicator of the functional activity for this signaling. Several methods are known to be used to the aim of its determination, of which Gilman's method was the most popular (Gilman, 1970). This method is based on the competitive replacement of the unlabelled nucleotide, which is present in the complex containing the cAMP-binding protein in the test sample, with 8-^{3}H-cAMP. The method of radioimmune dilution (Rosenberg et al., 1982) represents another approach to the analysis. It is based on the primary binding together the standard antigen, which is present in excess and is generally labeled with a radioactive iodine isotope, with antibodies, which are deficient. On the next stage, the unlabeled antigen is added to the generated complex, which competitively supplants the radioactive label. On the basis of a decrease in the radioactivity observed, is make conclusion about the amount of the bound antigen. More rarely the following complex and labour-consuming methods are applied: mass spectrometry and high-performance gas-liquid chromatography (Newton et al., 1980), and also the bioluminescent method allowing to monitor the dynamics of cAMP in the living cell (Nicolaev and Lohse, 2006). Application of the all mentioned methods, in general, requires multi-step purification with the use of different ion-exchange resins, high voltage electrophoresis that can result in partial loss of the cyclic nucleotide. Therefore some authors, having detected cAMP with the use of enumerated methods, note that the results achieved are obviously underestimated (Yavorskaya and Kalinin, 1984). In case of application of Gilman's method and the method of radioimmune dilution there appears the hazard of radioactive pollution of the environmental. Furthermore, and this quite important, it is necessary have to possess expensive equipment in order to detect of the levels radioactivity. Mass-spectrometry and gas-liquid chromatography belong to the set of precise methods, but their application presumes i) employment of specially trained operators as well as ii) the process of long-term and multi-step preparing of the sample.

On account of above considerations, the objective of the present research presumed modification of the immunoenzyme method (EIA), which is widely applied in analysis of other substances, in order to determine the level of cAMP in plants.

One of the critical stages in the analysis conducted with the employment of EIA is proper preparing of the plant sample. The main requirement to the sample presumes efficient removal of the admixtures under the condition of maximal retaining of the antigen to be determined in the sample. This is conditioned by the fact that any contamination can cause the process of nonspecific binding the antibodies and hence distortion of the result. Therefore, previously to verify purity of the sample prepared, we applied two independent methods: NMR and capillary electrophoresis. The concentration of cAMP in plant samples (plants of potato *in vitro*) was determined by capillary electrophoresis. We also used this method to compare the value of concentration to the value obtained by EIA (Lomovatskaya et al., 2011).

It has been determined in the comparative experiments conducted earlier (Lomovatskaya et al., 2011) that the sensitivity of modified method is about 5 pM, which is eight to ten times more precise than that obtained using the acetylated version of EIA from Sigma–Aldrich and two times better than that from GE Healthcare. Furthermore, the EIAs from Sigma–Aldrich and GE Healthcare require the use of compounds, which possess lachrymator and corrosive effects; the prices of the reagents used for our modified method are some three times cheaper than those using the method from Sigma–Aldrich. Therefore, modified EIA, compared with that from commercial suppliers, is more sensitive, safer and more economical. The results considered suggest that the application of modified EIA may be useful for further investigations of the cAMP content, and accordingly, properties and functios.

Our modification of the method EIA has given us the possibility to determine the level of cAMP in various plant objects under the influence of stressors of abiotic and biotic natures. The following model systems have been employed: the suspension culture of arabidopsis cells + soft and rough heat shock, the potato plants *in vitro* + exopolysaccharides of bacterial initiators of ring rot pathogen *Clavibacter michiganensis* subsp. *sepedonicus*, and also red beet root-crops (*Betula vulgaris)* + fungus *Botritis cinerea.*

2. Experimental procedures

2.1 The plant material

The cell culture of Arabidopsis thaliana (ecotype Columbia) was growing in 250-mL flasks containing the medium comprised by mineral salts prepared according to Murashige and Skoog (1962), 3% sucrose, 0.5 mg/l thiamin-HCl and 0.1 mg/l 2,4-D. The flasks were placed on a shaker (80 r.p.m.) and incubated in darkness at 26° C. In our experiments, 8-day-old cultures in a logarithmic phase of growth were used. In order to create stress conditions, the suspension (10 ml) was held in conic flasks, under permanent wobbling and in bath-marie at 37°C or 50°C for 2 min. During this time period, an assigned temperature level in the medium of suspension growth was. After that, the samples were additionally incubated during 1, 3, 5 or 15 minutes. The suspension, which did not undergo the effect of thermal shock, was the check sample. After the exposition, the suspension was quickly filtered through fine-meshed fosta nylon and immobilized with the use of liquid nitrogen.

2-week-old potato plants were used. *In vitro* the plants were grown in test-tubes in a growth chamber (16 h light, 6 klux, 20°C/8 h darkness, 15°C) on a liquid salt Murashige and Skoog medium (Murashige and Skoog, 1962). The following chemicals were added: 20 g/L sucrose (Reakhim, Russia), 1.0 mg/L thiamine, 0.5 mg/L pyridoxine, 0.1 mg/L indole-3-butyric acid and 0.02 mg/L ferulic acid (Sigma, USA). To create stress conditions, solution of exopolysaccharides extracted from *Clavibacter michiganensis* subsp. *sepedonicus* bacterium causing potato tubers ring rot was added to potato plants growing medium in final concentration 0.1% and left for 1 min, then the plants were frozen in liquid nitrogen. Vacuoles from red beet root *Betula vulgaris* parenchyma cells were obtained through preparation method (Salyaev et al., 1981). This method allows to obtain fractions of "heavy" and "light" vacuoles, the names being due to the difference in floating density. Red beet root infecting by fungus *Botritis cinerea* was used as a stress factor. Root tissue, which was not infected by fungus, was used for the investigation.

2.2 Preparing samples for analysis of cAMP

Homogenization of plant tissues (stems and roots of potato plants *in vitro,* 10 grams) and suspension cells was conducted with the application of a homogenizer in some isolation medium of the following composition (Fluka, Sweden): 3 ml of 50 mM tris-HCl, pH 7.2, 0.1 mM theophylline (inhibitor of phosphodiesterase), 1 mM dithyothreitol (protector of SH-groups), 0.5 mg/mL polyvinylpyrrolidon (sorbing phenols). To the end of additional binding of phenols (Karimova et al., 1993) we used ione-exchange resin Dowex-50 ("Sigma", USA), which had the weight ratio (i.e. the *resin* to *plant* weight ratio) of 1:5. Crude homogenate was filtered through fine-meshed fosta nylon, this process being followed by centrifugation of the filtrate during 40 minutes at 20 000 g. The level of cAMP was determined in the supernatant.

There were also used vacuole fractions placed in isolation medium (1:1 by volume), where these organelles were destroyed under hypotonic shock. The level of cAMP was determined in the acquired vacuolar sap.

2.3 Supernatant cleaning from admixtures of other nucleotides

1 ml of sample was put into the column with neutral aluminum oxide, the thickness of its layer being 1 sm^3, which was balanced with the buffer. Elution was conducted with the use of the same buffer, and analysis of the substance's spectrum was carried out with the aid of a chromatograph ("Uvicord", Sweden) at the wavelength of 276 nm. The set of standard test specimens included adenosine, 5'-AMP, cAMP, cGMP, cTMP, cCMP ("Sigma", USA) in concentration of 100 pM. In this case, cAMP eluded earlier than other compounds and was discovered already in the second ml, what coordinates with the information, which can be found in the literature (White and Zenser, 1971).

Next, the eluate (of total volume 8 ml) was evaporated on a rotary evaporator under vacuum. Its dry residue was washed in 1 ml 100% dimethylsulfoxide («Reachim», Russia) to remove salts, and then it was centrifuged during 5 min at 20000g. Dimethylsulfoxide was removed and the residue was washed with the use of acetone («ECOS-1», Russia). The specimen was air-dried at room temperature and analyzed to determine the concentration of cAMP by EIA.

2.4 Analysis by EIA to determine the concentration of cAMP in the samples

To the end of antigen immobilization we prepared a mixture, which contained 1 mL of the tested sample dissolved in 1 ml of PBS (i.e. 20 mM of phosphate buffer plus 0.1 M NaCl, pH 7.0), 0.5 mg of the dry plant sample plus 0.08 mL 25% glutaraldehyde plus 1 mg/mL BSA (Sigma), 0.1 mL of which was added into each well of the polystyrene multiwell plate. The plate was incubated during 15 hours at 37°C, and the wells were rinsed three times with the solution of PTBS (20 mM of phosphate buffer plus 0.1 M NaCl plus 0.3% Tween 100, pH 7.0). To avoid non-specific binding of the antibodies with the solid carrier 0.1 mL of horse serum (Allergen, Russia), diluted 1:10 PBS was added to each well, and the plate was left for 1 h at 37° C and next was rinsed three times with PTBS. After that, a solution prepared of primary rabbit antibodies was added to cAMP («Sigma», USA) (60 mkg per ml in PBS plus 0.1% BSA) and incubated during 2 h at 37° C. Next, the samples were flushed in PTBS again and treated with horse serum. After that, secondary goat's antibodies anti rabbit labeled with the use of peroxidase («Sigma», USA) on 0.1 M carbonate-bicarbonate buffer, pH 8.3, were added in each well and incubated during 1 h at room temperature, whereupon these were rinsed three times with PTBS.

In order to remove the detergent from the wells, we conducted its repeated washing with the use of 0.1 M phosphate-citrate buffer, pH 5.3. In case of peroxidase reaction, 0.1 mL 0.15% orthophenylendiamine (Sigma, USA) diluted in the 0.1 M phosphate-citrate buffer, pH 5.3, and 3 µL 3% H_2O_2 was added into each well. Color developed during 20 min. The reaction was stopped by adding 0.1 mL/well 4 N H_2SO_4. The measurements of the intensity of light absorption by the solution were made with the use of spectrophotometer C-101-46 (BioRad, Germany) at the wavelength of 490 nm. The negative control was represented by the buffer of isolation without plant samples. The concentration of cAMP in the sample was determined with the help of the calibration plot built for cAMP ("Sigma", USA), (Fig.1). This calibration plot was represented as positive control.

For the purpose of additional verification of the specificity of binding the antibodies with cAMP, adenosine (0.1 µM concentration), 5'-AMP, and other cyclical nucleotides, such as cGMP, cUMP, cTMP, cCMP, were tested as the anti-genes.

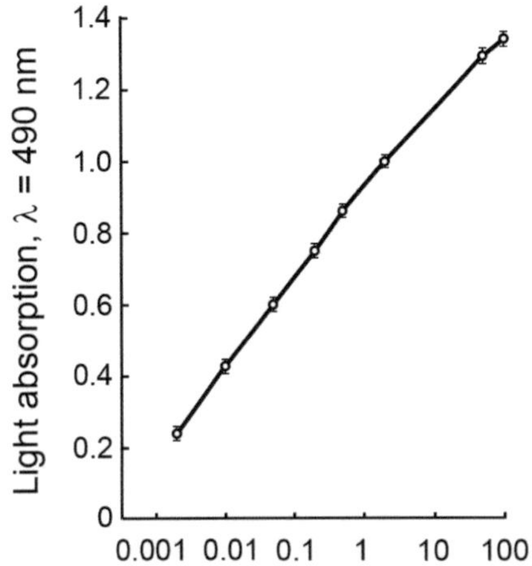

Fig. 1. The calibration plot built for cAMP. Concentrations of cAMP are represented in the logarithmic form.

2.5 Analysis of the data

Eight (EIA) replicates were carried out in experiments, which were repeated two times. Results are expressed as means ± standard errors.

2.6 Results and discussion

2.6.1 Analysis by EIA

Verification of specificity of the process of binding the antibodies, which were harvested against cAMP, has given evidence that such junctions as adenosine, 5'-AMP and other cyclic nucleotides (cGMP, cUMP, cTMP, cCMP) did not react with antibodies. The results turned out to be at the level characteristic of the control sample without any plant material. When employing the radio-immune method with the application of polyclonal antibodies against cAMP, Roef et al. (1996) have obtained similar data related to the specificity of binding cAMP.

Therefore, despite the fact of obvious simplicity of preparing samples and trivial scheme of analysis, the proposed method possesses rather high rates of sensitivity and specificy.

In this connection, it was of interest for us to apply this modification of EIA for revealing variations of cAMP concentrations, if these variations occur in plant cells in response to the abiotic stress, particularly, in case of thermal influences on the cells of arabidopsis.

2.6.2 Results obtained with the use of a modified version of EIA

Our investigations have given evidence that all the kinds of stress had a substantial effect upon the variation of cAMP concentrations in the scrutinized plant objects (Tables 1, 2, 3), what reflects the variations of activities of adenylate cyclase and, obviously, phosphodiesterase as the main components of the adenylate cyclase signaling system.

Temperature and incubation time	cAMP concentration			
	Suspension cells	% to control	Growth medium	% to control
26°C	1,87±0,11	100	3,6±0,25	100
37°C 1 min	32,8±2,40	1754	8,9±0,7	247
37°C 3 min	17,2±1,30	916	8,3±0,8	230
37°C 5 min	17,4±1,30	914	3,6±0,2	100
37°C 15 min	2,7±0,19	144	0,7±0,06	20
50°C 1 min	53,7±4,80	2871	11,5±0,9	321
50°C 3 min	5,5±0,44	294	7,1±0,4	198
50°C 5 min	2,2±0,18	118	5,4±0,3	151
50°C 15 min	13,1±0,90	700	0,7±0,05	20

Table 1. Changes of cAMP concentration, nMol/g raw weight, in Arabidopsis suspension cell culture (*Arabidopsis taliana*) (temperature) stressor and in the environment of their growth under the influence of the short-term abiotic.

The results presented in Table 1 allow to conclude that in Arabidopsis suspension cells both mild and severe heat stresses induce the highest cAMP level already 1 minute after the impact. At 37° C this provokes activation of heat shock protection system, in particular, induction of HSP synthesis (Rikhvanov et al., 2007). Nevertheless, sharp increase of cAMP level at 50° C already 1 minute after, and then its sharp drop, indicated of signal alarm response, due to which there apparently takes place qualitative change-over of intracellular metabolic paths. In Arabidopsis suspension cells this leads, as previously shown, to the development of programmable cell death (apoptosis).

So, both abiotic and biotic stresses cause early activation of adenylate cyclase signal system in different plant species. According to literary data, differences in the induction of early signal pathways are of importance for further adaptive processes. Due to this intensity of the acting stress factor may produce a differentiating effect on the activity of various components of this or that signal system. As Tables 2 and 3 show, biotic stresses also significantly affect activity of adenylate cyclase signal system, despite the fact that in case of *in vitro* potato plants exometabolites of potato ring rot bacterial pathogen act as a stressor, whereas in case of red beet root the stressor is a cultivar of fungus gray rot pathogen.

cAMP concentration			
Resistant cultivar		Susceptible cultivar	
Control	+EPS*, 1 min	Control	+EPS*, 1 min
17,4±0,7	111±4,3	12,8±0,5	0,47±0,02

* EPS – exopolysaccharides of the potato ring rot pathogen *Clavibacter michiganensis* subsp. *sepedonicus*.

Table 2. Changes of cAMP concentration, nMol/g raw weight, in stems of potato plants *in vitro (Solanum tuberosum)* under the influence of the biotic stressor (exopolysaccharides of the potato ring rot pathogen).

cAMP concentration			
Vacuole fractions			
"light"		"heavy"	
control	+*Botritis cinerea*	control	+*Botritis cinerea*
12±0,5	160±7,0	63±3,0	800±37,0

Table 3. Changes of cAMP concentration, nMol/mg protein, in vacuoles isolated from red beet root-crops (*Betula vulgaris)* under the influence of the biotic stressor (infecting with the root-crops by fungus *Botritis cinerea*).

3. Conclusion

The data obtained allow us to assume that variation of the level of intracellular cAMP determines the adaptive and restorative capabilities of plant cells in many respects. We are sure that the proposed modification of EIA may be successfully applied in investigations these or other physiological-biochemical processes in plants. It should be noted that the advantage of this method as compared to analogous method of Sigma-Aldrich and GE Healthcare companies is its hogher sensitivity and relatively lower cost of reagents.

So, for the purpose of determination of cAMP from plant samples we can propose the following scheme (Fig. 2).

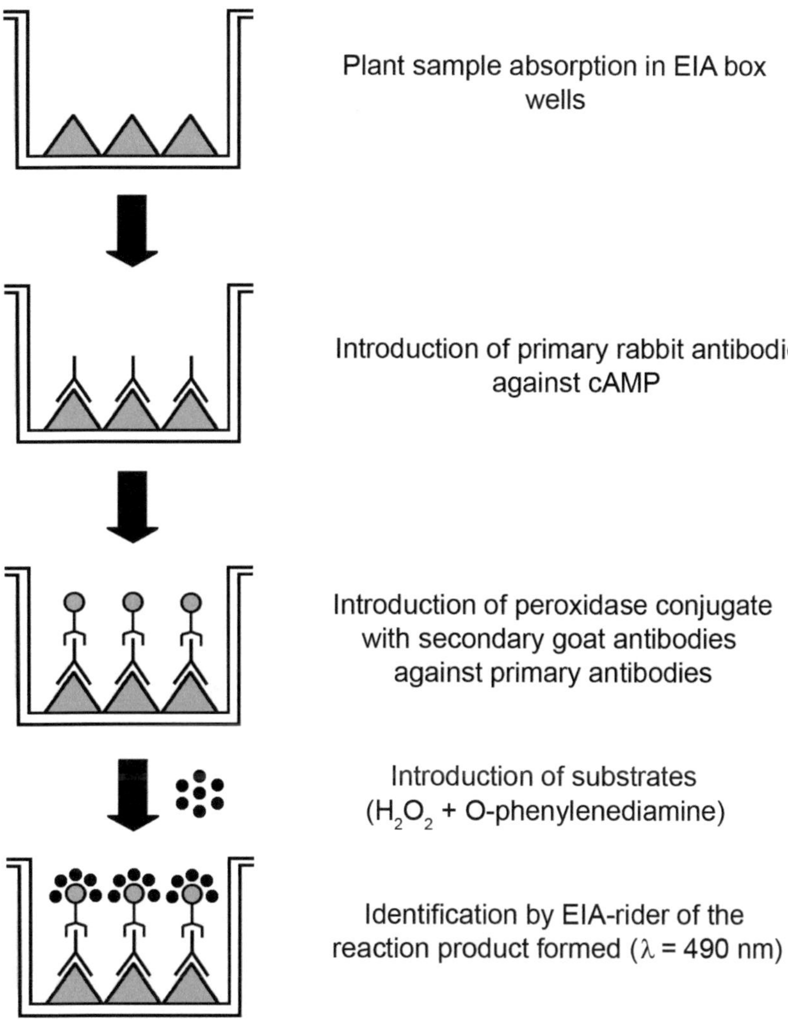

Fig. 2. Major stages of EIA method to determine cAMP concentration in plant sample.

4. References

Brown EG; Newton, R. & Smith, C. (1980) A cyclic AMP binding-protein from barley seedlings. *Phytochemistry,* Vol.19, pp. 2263–2267. doi:10.1002/ps.805

Cooke C,; Smith, C., Walton, J. & Newton RP (1994). Evidence that cyclic AMP is involved in the hypersensitive response of Medicago sativa to a fungal elicitor. *Phytochemistry,* Vol. 35, pp. 889–894. doi: 10.1002/ps.805

Gilman, A. (1970). A protein binding assay for adenosine 3′,5′-cyclic monophosphate. *Proc Natl Acad Sci,* Vol. 67, pp. 305– 312. doi: 10.1073/pnas.0700609104

Karimova, F.; Leonova, S., Gordon, S., Fil'chenkova, V.I. 1993. cAMP secretion by plant cells. *Physiologia Biochemistry Cultivar Plant.* V.25. N.4. P.362-367.

Lomovatskaya, L.; Romanenko, A., Filinova, N. & Dudareva, L. (2011). Determination of cAMP in plant cells by a modified enzyme immunoassay method. *Plant Cell Rep.* Vol. 30, pp. 125–132. DOI 10.1007/s00299-010-0950-5

Martinez-Atienza, J.; Van Ingelgem, C., Roef, L. & Maathuis F. Plant cyclic nucleotide signaling. (2007). Plant *Signaling & Behavior*, Vol. 2, pp. 540–543. doi: 10.4161/psb

Moutinho, A.; Hussey, P., Trevawas, A. & Malho, R (2001). Cyclic AMP act as a second messenger in pollen tube growth and reorientation. *Proc Natl Acad Sci*, Vol. 98, pp. 10481-10486. doi: 10.1073/pnas.0700609104

Murashige, T.; Skoog, F. (1962.) A revised medium for rapid growth and bioassaya with tobacco tissue cultures. *Physiol Plant*, Vol. 15, pp. 473 – 497. doi:10.1104/pp.109.900312

Newton, R.; Gibbs, N., Moyse, C., Wiebers, J. & Brown E. (1980). Mass spectrometric identification of adenosine 3':5'-cyclic monophosphate isolated from a higher plant tissue. *Phytochemistry*, Vpl. 19. pp. 1909–1911. doi: 10.1002/ps.805

Newton, R.; Roef, L., Witters, E. & VanOnckenen, H. (1999). Cyclic nucleotides in higher plants: the enduring paradox. *New Phytol*, Vol. 143, pp. 427–455. doi: 10.1111/j.1469-8137.2007.02063.x.

Nicolaev, V.; Lohse, M. (2006). Monitoring of cAMP synthesis and degradation in living cells. *Physiology*, Vol. 21. pp. 86– 92 doi:10.1152/physiol.00057.2005

Phedenko, E.; Kasumov, K. & Lapko, V. (1995). cAMP system as mediator of phytochrome under light effect. *Russian Physiologia Biochemistry Cultivar Plant*, Vol. 27, pp.3–11

Polya, G.; Bowman J. (1981). Resolution and properties of two high affinity cyclic adenosine 3',5'-monophosphate-binding proteins from wheat germ. *Plant Physiology*, Vol. 68, pp. 577–584.doi:10.1104/pp.108.118935

Richards, H.; Das, S., Smith, C. et al (2002). Cycic nucleotidate content of tobacco BY-2 cells. *Phytochemistry*, Vol. 61. pp.531–537 doi: 10.1002/ps.805

Rikhvanov, E.; Gamburg, K., Varakina N. (2007) Nuclear-mitochondrial crosstalkduring heat shock in Arabidopsis cell culture. *Plant Journal*, Vol. 52, pp. 763.

Roef, l; Witters, E., Gadeyne. J., Marcssen, K., Newton, R. & VanOncenen, H. (1996). Analysis of 3':5'-cAMP and adenylyl cyclase activity in higher plants using polyclonal chicken egg yolk antibodies adenylate cyclase. *Analitlcal biochemistry*, Vol. 233. pp. 188–196 doi: 10.1016/j.ab.2008.08.016

Rosenberg, N.; Pines, M., Sela, J. (1982). Adenosin 3, 5 – cyclic monophosphate – its release in higher by an exogeneous stimulus as detected by radioimmunoassay. *FEBS Letters*, Vol.137, pp. 105–107 doi: 10.1016/j.febslet.2009.12.058

Salyaev, R.; Kuzevanov, V., Khaptagayev, S. & Kopytchuk, V. (1981). Isolation and purification of vacuoles and vacuolar membranes from plant cells. *Russian Plant physiology*. Vol.28, pp. 1295-1305.

Tarchevsky, I. (2001). Plant metabolism at stress. Fan. ISBN 5-7544-0164-7, Kazan, Tatarstan.

White, A.; Zenser, T. (1971). Separation of cyclic 3:5-nucleoside monophosphates from other nucleotides on aluminium oxide columns. Application to the assay of adenyl cyclase and guanyl cyclase. *Analitical Biochemistry*, Vol. 41, pp.372–396 doi: 10.1016/j.ab.2008.08.016

Yavorskaya, V.; Kalinin, F. (1984) About function cAMP-regulation system in plants. *Russian Physiologia Biochemistry Cultivar Plant*, Vol.16, pp. 217–229

11

Toxoplasmosis: IgG Avidity and Its Implication in Serodiagnosis

Veeranoot Nissapatorn[1] and Nongyao Sawangjareon[2]
[1]*University of Malaya,*
[2]*Prince of Songkla University*
[1]*Malaysia,*
[2]*Thailand*

1. Introduction

Toxoplasma gondii (*T. gondii*) is a ubiquitous, coccidian intracellular protozoan parasite that causes toxoplasmosis, a cosmopolitan zoonosis. *Toxoplasma* infections are reported in approximately one-third of the world's population but most are asymptomatic. The infections are mainly acquired through consumption of raw or uncooked meat containing viable tissue cysts or by contamination with highly resistant oocysts in foods, soil and water. In the symptomatic condition, toxoplasmosis occurs congenitally through transplacental transmission from a primarily infected mother during pregnancy that leads to intrauterine death, spontaneous abortion or severe congenital defects such as retinochoroiditis, hydrocephalus or mental retardation (Wong & Remington, 1994; Tenter et al, 2000; Sukthana, 2006). Toxoplasmosis is also a serious and life-threatening disease found in immunocompromised patients such as in organ transplant recipients (Aubert et al, 1996), patients with cancer (Herold et al, 2009) or AIDS (Nissapatorn et al, 2004).

The laboratory diagnosis of toxoplasmosis can be done in many ways including serology, the isolation of *T. gondii* after inoculation into experimental animals, histological examination, and molecular analysis (Fleck & Kwantes, 1980; Meganathan et al, 2010). Of these, serological tests to determine specific antibodies such as IgG, IgM, IgE or IgA are currently the first-line methods of diagnosis to differentiate recent or chronic infections with *T. gondii* (Sensini, 2006). Diagnosis of symptomatic toxoplasmosis is not straight forward due primarily to the clinical manifestations being varied and it can mimic other diseases (Santoni & Santoni-Willians, 1993; Hurt & Tammaro, 2007). Traditionally, the diagnosis of recently acquired toxoplasmosis has been detected either by demonstrating a specific immunoglobulin (Ig) M antibodies, a significant increase in specific IgG antibodies, or both. Due to the high IgG antibodies titres to *T. gondii* infections among the majority of immunocompetents (Remington & Desmonts, 1990) and the persistence of specific IgM antibodies in some individuals this has led to complications in the interpretation of serodiagnostic results even when toxoplasmosis was clinically suspected (Brooks et al, 1987; Bobic et al, 1991; Bertozzi et al, 1999). Moreover, a primary acquired *Toxoplasma* infection during pregnancy and the risk of congenital toxoplasmosis is a medical (clinical and diagnostic) challenge for the clinicians dealing with this tropical and infectious parasitic disease. Therefore, a sensitive and specific method is mandatory for the management of patients with a high probability of being infected by *T. gondii* (Kotresha & Noordin, 2010). In recent years, a number of new methods including new serodiagnostic tools have been developed towards improving the ability to diagnose recently acquired *Toxoplasma* infections during pregnancy in order to limit congenital infections (CI) in the fetus and newborn (Remington et al, 2004). From this point of view, this chapter is aiming to highlight the significant contributions of recently developed serological methods such as the IgG avidity test and serodiagnosis using various recombinant proteins and its implications for the management, including diagnosis and treatment, of toxoplasmosis, particularly in pregnant women or HIV-infected patients among the so called "high risk" population.

2. Recombinant proteins in serodiagnosis of toxoplasmosis

Currently, antigens used for commercial serological assays for the detection of specific anti-*Toxoplasma* antibodies are mainly based on whole tachyzoite lysates. However, the major disadvantage of this kind of antigen is its inconsistant quality due to contamination by extraparasitic components during the processing of preparations that result in interassay variability (Aubert et al, 2000). The use of recombinant antigens cloned in suitable expression vectors has been proven to improve consistency of the tests and to reduce the costs of production (Hiszczyjska-Sawicka et al, 2003). However, because of its complex life cycle, a number of proteins produced at different stages of the parasite life cycle can play different roles in stimulating host immune responses during the infectious process. Furthermore, a precise distinction between acute and latent invasion may be difficult since IgM antibodies, a specific marker for early infection, could be present in sera for many years (Meek et al, 2001). Therefore, certain antigens that are specific to the acute or chronic stages of the infection that produce specific IgG antibodies could serve as a mean to distinguish the recent from a chronic infection.

Tachyzoites, the rapidly multiplying stage of the parasite, is considered to be responsible for active toxoplasmosis. In contrast, bradyzoites, a dormant stage that persists within cysts and is thought to evade the immune response by their absence of expression of immunodominant antigens throughout a prolonged infection (Smith et al, 1996). Several studies have shown that the main targets for antibody production during the acute and chronic phase of *Toxoplasma* infection are the surface antigens (SAG) present in the tachyzoite membrane (Mineo et al, 1980) and their usefulness as antigens has been shown. Secretory proteins: micronemes (MIC), rhoptries (ROP) and dense granules (GRA) released from three distinct tachyzoite parasite organelles during invasion are other potential diagnostic antigens of interest as markers of acute infection. ROP and MIC released during the cell invasion, and GRA that is discharged from parasitophorous vacuoles after invasion, and continues during the intracellular residence of the organism (Carruthers & Sibley, 1997).

The usefulness of several recombinant antigens of *T. gondii* that have been produced and extensively evaluated for their potential use as diagnostic antigens in ELISA to detect specific IgG antibodies during the early phase of infection, allows for differentiation of an acute from a chronic infection. Furthermore, if only a single serum sample is available, an IgG avidity test using recombinant antigens is seen to be more appropriate for detecting a recently acquired infection. The sensitivity and specificity for these antigens have been reported to be in the range of 80% to 100%. These antigens have included:

2.1 Rhoptries antigens (ROP)

Rhoptries are unique secretory organelles shared by all Apicomplexan invasive stages. More than 30 ROPs of *T. gondii* have been identified (Bradley et al, 2005). They are exocytosed upon host cell invasion and their contents are involved in many functions fundamental for the parasite to enter into host cells, and for the establishment and maintenance of the parasitophorous vacuole membrane and acquisition of nutrients (Dubremetz, 2007). The use of recombinant ROP antigens (rROP) has been largely described as the antigenic substrate to use in ELISA tests to detect infection with *T. gondii* (vanGelder et al, 1993; Aubert et al, 2000; Chang et al, 2011). rROP1 has shown its diagnostic value in IgG ELISA avidity tets for identification of acute infections (Holec-Gąsior et al, 2009, 2010a). There is data regarding the potential use of rROP2 for the diagnosis of acute toxoplasmosis that have focused on IgG reactivities (Martin et al, 1998; Chang et al, 2011). In a mouse model, IgM antibody against rROP4 was significantly higher than IgG antibodies with a peak of detection coming on the turn of the acute to a latent infection (Gatkowska et al, 2010).

2.2 Microneme proteins (MIC)

MICs are proteins involved in recognition and/or binding to the host cell (Soldati et al, 2001). At least 12 MICs have been identified from *T. gondii* (Carruthers & Tomley, 2008). However, little is known whether rMIC can be used as an antigen. rMIC1 has thus far been the only protein shown to be highly reactive against sera of patients with acute toxoplasmosis (Holec et al, 2008).

2.3 Dense granule antigens (GRA)

Among identified GRA antigens, at least 12 out of 14 GRA antigens have been detected from *T. gondii* tachyzoites as excretory/secretory antigens (Nam, 2009). They are believed to be involved in parasite survival and virulence (Michelin et al, 2009; Rome et al, 2008). GRA1 is the major secretory antigen recognized in humans chronically infected with *Toxoplasma*. GRA2 has been shown to induce strong antibody and T-cell responses in both humans and experimental mice (Sharma et al, 1984; Brinkmann et al, 1993; Murray et al, 1993; Prigione et al, 2000). While, GRA6 and GRA7 are also shown strong antibody responses in the acute phase of *Toxoplasma* infection (Gatkowska et al, 2006). GRA7 was found in the parasitophorous vacuole and cytoplasm of the host cell infected with the tachyzoite stage (Jacobs et al, 1998). As a consequence, GRA7 is only released after the rupture of infected cells in the acute stage of infection and it is only then that it is exposed to the hosts' immune system. Therefore, detection of GRA7 antibodies would be expected to be a good candidate to use for serodiagnosis. Several rGRA antigens such as rGRA2 (Golkar et al, 2007; Holec-Gąsior et al, 2009), rGRA6 (Aubert et al, 2000; Golkar et al, 2008), rGRA7 (Aubert et al, 2000; Pietkiewicz et al, 2004; Pfrepper et al, 2005; Pietkiewicz et al, 2007), and rGRA8 (Pfrepper et al, 2005; Gatkowska et al, 2006; Babaie et al, 2009) have been proposed as markers to indicate acute infections. rGRA4 and rGRA7, but not rROP2, have been shown to be valuable in differentiating acute and chronically infected individuals for both adult and congenital toxoplasmosis (Nigro et al, 2003; Altcheh et al, 2006). In contrast, rGRA1 was reported to be a marker for chronic infections (Ferrandiz et al, 2004; Pietkiewicz et al, 2004).

2.4 Surface antigens (SAG)

Five major SAG antigens specific to the tachyzoite stage have been identified (Couvreur et al, 1988). Of these, the SAG1, SAG2, and SAG3 antigens are the main proteins expressed on the surface of tachyzoites. They are involved in the process of host cell invasion after infection (Mineo & Kasper, 1994; Grimwood & Smith, 1996), and are highly immunogenic for IgG responses. SAG1 and SAG3 are stage-specific antigens of the tachyzoites and are highly conserved in most isolates (Gross et al, 1996; Wu et al, 2009). In contrast, SAG2 has been identified from both bradyzoites and tachyzoites (Lekutis et al, 2000). SAG4 is another surface protein that is specifically expressed by bradyzoites (Knoll & Boothroyd, 1998). rSAG1 successfully detected IgG antibodies in the acute phase of infection (Pietkiewicz et al, 2004), but the highest response to rSAG1 was found during latent infections (Gatkowska et al, 2010). Some studies did show that rSAG2 was effective in specifically detecting IgG antibody to *T. gondii* in patients with acute toxoplasmosis (Parmley et al, 1992). However, more recent studies showed that rSAG2 was produced in acute and chronic infections (Lau & Fong, 2008), whereas rSAG2A was present only during the acute phase of toxoplasmosis (Béla et al, 2008).

2.5 Combinations of recombinant antigens

A cocktail of recombinant antigens help to improve the serological diagnosis of clinical toxoplasmosis. A combination of rGRA1 and rGRA6 has shown promising results when being preliminary tested (Lecordier, 2000). While, the triple combination of SAG1, ROP1 and GRA7 have also been successfully tested in a preliminary format (Aubert, 2000). Different combinations of recombinant antigens that have been evaluated and successfully increase the sensitivity of serodiagnosis from chronic toxoplasmosis are summarized in Table 1.

References	Combinations of recombinant antigens
Aubert et al, 2000	rSAG1, rROP1, and rGRA7 rGRA7, rGRA8, and rSAG1
Li et al, 2000	rGRA7, rGRA8, rSAG2, and rH4
Nigro et al, 2003	rROP2 and rGRA7
Pietkiewicz et al, 2004	rSAG1, rGRA1, and rGRA7
Holec et al, 2008	rGRA1, rGRA7, and rSAG1 rGRA8, rSAG2, and rGRA6 rMic1ex2, rMAG1, and rMIC3
Cóceres et al, 2010	rHSP20, rSAG1, and rGRA7 rHSP20 and rSAG1 rHSP20 and rGRA7 rSAG1 and rGRA7
Holec-Gąsior & Kur, 2010	rMAG1, rSAG1, and rGRA5 rGRA2, rSAG1, and rGRA5 rROP1, rSAG1, and rGRA5
Holec-Gąsior et al, 2010b	rMAG1 + rSAG1 + rGRA7

Table 1. Selected combination of recombinant antigens that increase the sensitivity of serodiagnosis of chronic toxoplasmosis.

Furthermore, the multiple combinations of recombinant antigens P22, P25, P29, and P35 has confirmed that a cocktail of antigens might be helpful to differentiate between acute and chronic infections when tested against specific IgG antibodies in human samples (Li, 2000). Based on these results, it clearly shows that the combination of recombinant antigens is mandatory in the attempt to distinguish between acute and chronic *Toxoplasma* infections. Nonetheless, the combination of GRA1 and GRA6 for distinguishing between acute and chronic infections was unsuccessful found in pregnant women (Ferrandiz et al., 2004). The combinations of recombinant antigens that could be used to distinguish between acute and chronic infections are summarized in Table 2.

References	Combinations of recombinant antigens
Li et al, 2000	rGRA8, rSAG2, rGRA2, and rGRA7
Beghetto et al, 2003	rGRA3, rGRA7, rMIC3, and rSAG1
Pietkiewicz et al, 2007	rGRA1, rGRA7 and rSAG1

Table 2. Selected combination of recombinant antigens that use to distinguish between acute and chronic infections.

3. IgG-avidity: A real-time serodiagnosis for*Toxoplasma* infection

It seems that a conventional single serum assay does not provide an accurate diagnosis in differentiating between a recently acquired primary infection and a chronic infection (Lappalainen & Hedman, 2004). The IgG-avidity test is an assay that measures the antigen-binding avidity/affinity of IgG antibodies against *T. gondii* infection and was first introduced to try to eliminate this problem (Hedman et al, 1989). This avidity test has significantly lessened the possibility of misdiagnosis, by assisting in determining a difference between a recently acquired (primary/acute) and a chronic (latent/past/remote) infection. This has greatly decreased the requirement for a confirmatory (a single or the first sample) or follow-up serological tests, to remove any doubts or anxiety for further testings (Cozon et al, 1998; Liesenfeld et al, 2001; Montoya et al, 2002; Remington et al, 2004; Press et al, 2005; Reis et al, 2006; Candolfi et al, 2007; Nissapatorn et al, 2011). Hence, the measurement of IgG-avidity has proved to be a highly sensitive method, used to assess the early time of antigenic challenge and it is especially recommended for use in combination with other existing conventional serological assays (Lappalainen & Hedman, 2004; Nissapatorn et al, 2011). The IgG avidity test has so far been the best serological approach that can offer a rapid diagnosis of a recently acquired *Toxoplasma* infection in a single serum sample. Until now the IgG-avidity test has been tested and used in several different clinical scenarios: a recently acquired *Toxoplasma* infection, primary acquired infection during pregnancy, congenital toxoplasmosis, ocular toxoplasmosis (OT), and in immunocompromised individuals such as cancer patients, solid organ transplant recipients or persons living with HIV/AIDS.

3.1 Acute (recently) acquired *Toxoplasma* infection

Approximately, one-third of the world's populations are infected with *T. gondii*. However, the majority of these are either mild with non-specific clinical symptoms or asymptomatic. Lymphadenopathy is significantly present in only 3-7% of clinical cases but is the most common form in immunocompetent individuals (Gard & Magnusson, 1951; McCabe et al, 1987). The clinical features show localized, nontender and nonsuppurative lymphadenopathy as a result of *Toxoplasma* infection. Of note, lymphadenopathy may persist for months and may mimic clinically or histologically with neoplastic diseases such as lymphoma or carcinoma of the head, neck and breast (Lappalainen & Hedman, 2004). The diagnosis of toxoplasmic lymphadenopathy is based on serology and lymphnode biopsy.

Serological techniques have traditionally been used but shown some limitations in evaluating the timing of *Toxoplasma* infections. The IgG avidity test has since been introduced for differentiation between recently acquired and past infections in the course of toxoplasmic lymphadenopathy. The duration of low avidity values in patients with lymphadenopathy is not well defined. Lecolier and Pucheu observed patients whose sera had a low IgG avidity for as long as 20 weeks after the acquisition of infection (Lecolier & Pucheu, 1993). A low IgG avidity occurs during < 3 months of lymphadenopathy (Holliman et al, 1994). In the present study, low IgG avidity values were still observed 5 months after the first serological examination in 6 of 19 patients (31.6%) with lymphadenopathy (Paul, 1999). Whereas, a high IgG avidity test resulted from an individual who had a recent onset of lymphadenopathy of at least 4 months (Montoya et al, 2004). Therefore, a high IgG avidity value strongly excludes a recent infection, that is, one that was acquired during the previous 5 months, but a low avidity is not a safe marker for an early stage of infection (Paul, 1999).

3.2 Primary acquired *Toxoplasma* infection during pregnancy

Based on epidemiological data, the prevalent rate of *Toxoplasma* infection in pregnant women is generally high in many geographical locations and plausible risk factors play an important role in *Toxoplasma* acquisition found among these women. However, the rate of acute (recent) acquired *Toxoplasma* infection is unexpectedly low in pregnant women. The gestational stages of pregnancy are determined by the impacts of vertical transmission from the infected mother to the fetus; primary *Toxoplasma* infection in early trimester of pregnancy may result in severe clinical disease, in contrast, congenital toxoplasmosis as a result of maternal infection during third trimester of pregnancy is usually subclinical at birth (Desmonts, 1979). The clinical symptoms of acute toxoplasmosis during pregnancy are usually subclinical or associated with non-specific symptoms. Therefore, the diagnosis is mainly based on serological responses of pregnant women. Serological results are however difficult to interpret and that has contributed to the most challenging situation during pregnancy

In clinical practice, simultaneous testing for specific IgG and IgM antibodies against *T. gondii* in serial serum samples collected at an interval of 3 weeks is the early step in routine screening for *Toxoplasma* infection. Of note, the presence of specific IgG and/or IgM antibodies against *T. gondii* in a single serum sample drawn during pregnancy cannot be used to determine if the infection was chronic or recently acquired. Therefore, successive tests and the definitive diagnosis are required as a result of this initial screening. Factors such as the trimester of infection and maternal-neonatal therapeutic treatments are the main contributing factors to the variation of immunological responses of both mother and neonate (Sensini, 2006). Early and accurate diagnosis is crucial during pregnancy, as the women then require immediate therapeutic options. In addition, IgG and IgM antibodies against *T. gondii* are the first-line serological diagnosis for the detection of recent or chronic infections. A seropositive woman for only IgG antibodies, is unlikely to have recently acquired toxoplasmosis due to the level of specific *Toxoplasma*-IgG antibodies which is an unreliable indicator for acute infection (Robert et al, 2001). Following an acute *Toxoplasma* infection in the mother, the evidence for a rapidly transmitted infection to the fetus has been observed. Hence, early diagnosis of an acute infection during pregnancy is crucial to determine whether treatment of the infected mother can prevent vertical transmission to the fetus.

The measurement of IgG avidity has been developed to avoid using confirmatory tests from a second serum sample for the possibility of a recently acquired infection obtained from the initial serodiagnostic test. A specific positive IgG test with a low avidity has been used to confirm a recent primary acquired *Toxoplasma* infection by using a single serum indicator (Joynson et al, 1990; Lappalainen et al, 1993; Holliman et al, 1994; Jenum et al, 1997; Liesenfeld et al, 2001; Roberts et al, 2001; Abdel Hameed & Helmy, 2004; Press et al, 2005; Reis et al, 2006; Nissapatorn et al, 2011). Due to it being a safe and useful tool for screening for high sensitivity, an IgG-avidity test is able to verify that the majority of pregnant women who presented with *Toxoplasma* IgM antibodies did not have a recently acquired infection (Lappalainen et al, 1993; Nissapatorn et al, 2011). IgG-avidity is therefore recommended to serve as the primary tool for an IgG assay and a sensitive IgM test (Lappalainen & Hedman, 2004; Olariu et al, 2006). Moreover, the IgG-avidity test can be used as a subsequent measurement to confirm the IgM diagnosis, as shown in suspected cases of acute recent toxoplasmosis in immunocompetent patients (Table 3).

Clinical scenarios	Diagnostic tests
Immunocompetents	
Acute infection (primary acquired infection)	*Toxoplasma*-IgG and *Toxoplasma*-IgM antibodies, followed by the measurement of IgG-avidity test (if *Toxoplasma*-IgM positive)
Immunity (latent/chronic/past infection)	*Toxoplasma*-IgG antibodies
Ocular toxoplasmosis (acute retinochoroiditis)	*Toxoplasma*-IgG and *Toxoplasma*-IgM antibodies for the detection of past exposure; seldom useful to show acute infection.
Congenital toxoplasmosis (maternal-fetal infection)	Serology for *Toxoplasma*-IgG, -IgM and -IgA antibodies of the newborn and the mother. *Toxoplasma*-PCR (and culture, if available) from clinical specimens such as blood, urine and cerebrospinal fluid (CSF).
Immunosuppressed patients (cancer patients, organs transplant or HIV-infected patients)	*Toxoplasma*-IgG and *Toxoplasma*-IgM antibodies for the detection of past exposure; a second sample is needed to show reactivation. *Toxoplasma*-PCR (and culture, if available) to detect ongoing active infection using blood and CSF specimens.

Table 3. Laboratory diagnosis in different clinical scenarios of toxoplasmosis.

When a primary acquired infection in a pregnant mother is diagnosed either by seroconversion for IgG or being seropositive for IgM antibodies followed by a low IgG-avidity, the infected mother should be referred immediately for medical assessment to an obstetrician who should include further tests including molecular analysis using an amniotic fluid sample to determine any fetal infection (Hohlfeld et al, 1994; Jenum et al,

References	Sero-pattern	Interpretation	Comments
Montoya & Liesenfeld, 2004 National committee for clinical laboratory standard, 2004 Remington et al, 2004 Nissapatorn et al, 2011	IgG+IgM+ Mother	(a) Past or recently acquired infection	• Risk for congenital infection (CI) • Take gestation period into account. Serological tests for specific *Toxoplasma*-IgA and -IgE antibodies and IgG-avidity
		(b) False-positive	• No risk for CI • Serological tests for specific *Toxoplasma*-IgA and -IgE antibodies and IgG-avidity
Sharma et al, 1983 Partanen et al, 1984 Villena et al, 1999 Gross et al, 2000 Pinon et al, 2001 Remington et al, 2001 Montoya, 2002 Flori et al, 2004 Nielsen et al, 2005	IgG+IgM+ Newborn	(a) Maternal antibies	• No risk for CI • Collect 2nd serum sample 10 days after birth to confirm contaminating maternal specific *Toxoplasma*-IgM antibodies. Test in parallel maternal and neonatal specific *Toxoplasma*-IgG antibodies by Western blotting (WB) or ELISA. Serological follow-up for 1 year to confirm seronegativity for specific *Toxoplasma*-IgG antibodies. • Check for stable IgG-avidity index.
		(b) Maternal and neonatal antibodies	• CI after maternal infection in the third trimester (IgA+) or in the last month (IgA-) of pregnancy • Collect 2nd serum sample 10 days after birth in parallel maternal and neonatal specific IgG antibodies by WB or ELISA. Serological follow-up for 1 year to demonstrate the persistence of specific *Toxoplasma*-IgG antibodies. • Check for increased IgG-avidity index

Table 4. The measurement of IgG avidity test for toxoplasmosis in pregnant woman and newborn.

1998). The combination of a sensitive test for *Toxoplasma*-specific IgM antibodies and the measurement of IgG avidity had shown the highest predictive value in association with the possible time of infection (Petersen et al, 2005; Press et al, 2005). When a high IgG-avidity result was found in women within their first trimester of pregnancies, it provided a strong indicator against primary infection. As there is a low risk of congenital toxoplasmosis there is no intervention necessarily required. In general, IgG-avidity has been used to confirm past or recently acquired infection or false-positive results in pregnant women who showed seropositive for IgG and IgM antibodies (Table 4) and this has been recommended by several authors (Montoya & Liesenfeld, 2004; National committee for clinical laboratory standard, 2004; Remington et al, 2004).

3.3 Congenital toxoplasmosis

Toxoplasmosis has historically been recognized as one of the most important pathogens causing congenital infection (CI) and it has also been comprised in "TORCHs" infections. Transplacental (vertical, congenital, materno-fetal) transmission of *T. gobdii* can be a serious complication as a result of primary acquired infection during pregnancy. Of note, most infected children are asymptomatic at birth but they can manifest problems during later decades of life associated with ocular (acute retinochoroiditis) and neurological involvements (hydrocephalus).

Postnatal diagnosis is a complex process due to the presence of passive maternal IgG antibodies or the variability of perinatal IgM antibody findings (Desmonts et al, 1985; Daffos et al, 1988). Moreover, the level of specific IgA and IgM antibodies may not be able to be detected in all children with CI. Hence, a combination of specific IgA and IgM antibodies is the recommended approach for serological measurements in affected children (Naessens et al, 1999). In addition, determination of IgG-avidity and/or serological detection of specific IgG could serve as an alternative option for the diagnosis of congenital toxoplasmosis (Said et al, 2011). Combined with serological tests, the role of PCR in detecting *T. gondii* organism in amniotic fluid sample has been found to be more promising in terms of sensitivity and specificity during antenatal testing compared to postnatal diagnosis (Hohlfeld et al, 1994; Jenum et al, 1998; Yamada et al, 2011).

IgG avidity is generally not tested in the neonate due primarily to its having a similar pattern to the infected mother. However, a previous study has demonstrated that a significant maturation of IgG avidity was shown in congenitally infected children during postnatal follow-up (Lappalainen et al, 1995). In contrast, long-term therapy with pyrimethamine-sulphonamide, as opposed to treatment with spiramycin alone, was found to slow the progression of the avidity index (Flori et al, 2004). An IgG-avidity result in the first month of the postnatal period usually represents a combination of both mother and the newborn's own IgG antibodies and that depends on several contributing factors such as the sampling time, the IgG-titre and avidity of the mother as well as the newborn (Lappalainen & Hedman, 2004). In the absence of maternofetal transmission, the avidity index remains stable until the disappearance of passively transmitted specific antibodies from the infected mothers (Sensini, 2006). It is of interest that there is a delay of maturation of IgG-avidity in congenital toxoplasmosis that can be demonstrated by performing the test on antibodies eluted from dried blood spots (Guthrie cards) to detect, at birth, a maternal primary infection acquired during the second or third trimester of pregnancy and to evaluate retrospectively the risk for high suspicion of CI during late infancy (Buffolano et al, 2004). In general, it has been recommended that IgG-avidity should be used to confirm CI in the neonates (Table 4) being seropositive for both IgG and IgM antibodies either from maternal antibodies or both maternal and neonatal antibodies (Sharma et al, 1983; Weiss et al, 1988; Chumpitazi et al, 1995; Flori et al, 2004; Nielsen et al, 2005).

3.4 Ocular toxoplasmosis

Ocular toxoplasmosis (OT) occurs mainly in the uveal tract and it is the most common cause of posterior uveitis in immunocompetent persons. Retinochoroiditris is the most common lesion found among non-specific clinical manifestations of OT. In most cases, OT is the result of reactivated or congenital rather than from acquired *Toxoplasma* infections (Perkins, 1973; Ronday et al, 1995; Montoya & Remington, 1996). Clinical diagnosis of OT is based on the manifestations of characteristic biomicroscopic features (Rothova et al, 1986; de Jong, 1989; Tabbara, 1994).

Over more than three decades, many different serological tests have been introduced to detect specific IgG antibodies against *T. gondii* that can indicate chronic infections (Holliman et al, 1991). The detection of specific IgM antibodies indicates a recently acquired infection, however, it is found to have a high rate of false-positive results due to persisting IgM antibodies (Leisenfeld et al, 1997). Moreover, the absence or low levels of specific IgM antibodies in reactivated OT, cannot therefore serve as a reliable serological marker for this disease (Lappin et al, 1995; Ronday et al, 1995; Garweg et al, 1998; Klaren et al, 1998). Serological diagnosis of OT is insensitive (Rothova et al, 1986; Kijlstra et al, 1989; Holliman et al, 1991) and is of limited value (Lappalainen & Hedman, 2004). Also, the role of an IgG avidity measurement is to confirm the stage of chronic infection and to raise the suspicion of an ongoing reactivated OT (Paul, 1999; Garweg et al, 2000).

3.5 Cerebral toxoplasmosis

In contrast to the majority of immunocompetents persons, toxoplasmosis can cause serious clinical outcomes in immunocompromised individuals such as patients with AIDS or organ transplant recipients. In patients with an advanced HIV infection, toxoplasmosis is one of the most common central nervous system diseases associated with opportunistic infections that cause high rates of morbidity and mortality. Cerebral toxoplasmosis (CT) is the most common clinical disease entity and it causes focal intracerebral lesion(s) in patients with AIDS. Among AIDS patients, >95% of CT is due to the reactivation of latent (chronic) *Toxoplasma* infections as a result of the progressive loss of cellular immunity (Luft & Remington, 1988). In clinical practice, the incidence of CT patients is related both to *Toxoplasma* IgG seropositivity and to the CD4 cell count. The risk of developing CT among seropositive patients with AIDS was 27 times that of seronegative ones (Oksenhendler et al, 1994). The clinical presentations of CT depend on the number of lesions and locations. Headache, hemiparesis and seizure (Porter & Sande, 1992; Nissapatorn et al, 2004; Vidal et al, 2005) are among the most common neurological presentations found in CT patients. Other clinical manifestations include disarthria, movement disorders, memory and cognitive impairments and neuropsychiatric abnormalities. These neurological deficits remain in surviving patients even after a good clinical response to therapy (Hoffmann et al, 2007). More than 50% of CT patients may have focal neurological findings. The empirical diagnosis is based on a low CD4 count of less than 200 cells/cumm, computer tomography scans will show ring enhancing lesions, seroevidence of specific IgG, IgM or both antibodies to *T. gondii*, and a good response to anti-*Toxoplasma* therapy. Specific anti-*Toxoplasma* therapy is initiated in a highly suspicious or confirmed toxoplasmosis. CT is a life-threatening but treatable condition provided there is early diagnosis and treatment.

In HIV-infected patients, serological titres are often low and that makes for disease phase definition and therapeutic decisions difficult (Spausta et al, 2003). The determination of IgG avidity is another serological marker and it has been shown to be of some help in serodiagnosis of *Toxoplasma* infection among immunocompromised individuals. So far, very few studies have used the IgG avidity test for the differentiation of primary and reactivated chronic infections in HIV-infected patients. However, there was no significant difference between the avidity values in HIV-infected patients with CT and those without clinical signs of reactivation (Holliman et al, 1994; Spausta et al, 2003; Adurthi et al, 2010). A liver transplant recipient with reactivated toxoplasmosis was first reported by performing an IgG avidity test (Lappalainen et al, 1998). This patient was seropositive for *T. gondii* with high avidity indicating a chronic infection before the first transplantation. Subsequencely, serological diagnosis showed a rise in specific IgG antibodies, negative for IgM antibodies and with a constantly high IgG avidity, indicating a reactivation before the second transplantation. Serodiagnosis for *T. gondii* was negative for both donors. The presence of *T. gondii* DNA was shown by PCR in blood samples and liver biopsy prior to the death of this patient. Based on the results obtained, an avidity test for the serological status of *T. gondii* is therefore recommended if there are non-specific clinical symptoms of toxoplasmosis and it could be used for the diagnosis in differentiating recently acquired, chronic or secondary reactivation of latent toxoplasmosis in immunocompromised patients.

4. Conclusion

Estimation of the IgG avidity index is a classical serological method. Antibodies with low avidity are detectable at a very early stage of infection whereas high avidity antibodies indicate past infections. The measurement of IgG avidity has demonstrated its superior diagnostic values in serological interpretations of *Toxoplasma* infections in different clinical scenarios, particularly when timing between chronic and recently acquired infections or primary and secondary (reactivated) infections are required. The IgG avidity test represents an important addition to other first-line serological methods such as IgG, IgM and IgA specific antibodies against *T. gondii*. Above all, serological diagnosis should be performed in combination with culture based and molecular techniques to obtain the best and most accurate results.

5. Acknowledgement

The authors sincerely thank Dr. Brian Hodgson for his valuable comments and the University of Malaya Research Grant (UMRG 094/09HTM and UMRG 374/11HTM) for financial support.

6. References

Abdel Hameed, D.M. & Helmy, H. (2004). Avidity IgG: diagnosis of primary *Toxoplasma gondii* infection by indirect immunofluorescent test. *Journal of the Egyptian Society of Parasitology*, Vol. 34, No. 3, pp. 893-902, ISSN 0253-5890

Adurthi, S., Mahadevan, A., Bantwal, R., Satishchandra, P., Ramprasad, S., Sridhar, H., Shankar, S.K., Nath, A. & Jayshree, R.S. (2010). Utility of molecular and serodiagnostic tools in cerebral toxoplasmosis with and without tuberculous meningitis in AIDS patients: A study from South India. *Annals of Indian Academy of Neurology,* Vol. 13, No. 4, pp. 263-270, ISSN 1998-3549

Altcheh, J., Diaz, N.S., Pepe, C.M., Martin, V., Nigro, M., Freilij, H. & Angel, S.O. (2006). Kinetic analysis of the humoral immune response against three *Toxoplasma gondii*-recombinant proteins in infants with suspected congenital toxoplasmosis. *Diagnostic Microbiology and Infectious Disease,* Vol. 56, No. 2, pp. 161-165, ISSN 0732-8893

Aubert, D., Foudrinier, F., Villena, I., Pinon, J.M., Biava, M.F. & Renoult, E. (1996). PCR for diagnosis and follow-up of two cases of disseminated toxoplasmosis after kidney grafting. *Journal of Clinical Microbiology,* Vol. 34, No. 5, pp. 1347, ISSN 0095-1137

Aubert, D., Maine, G.T., Villena, I., Hunt, J.C., Howard, L., Sheu, M., Brojanac, S., Chovan, L.E., Nowlan, S.F. & Pinon, J.M. (2000). Recombinant antigens to detect *Toxoplasma gondii*-specific immunoglobulin G and immunoglobulin M in human sera by enzyme immunoassay. *Journal of Clinical Microbiology,* Vol. 38, No. 3, pp. 1144-1150, ISSN 0095-1137

Babaie, J., Zare, M., Sadeghiani, G., Lorgard-Dezfuli, M., Aghighi, Z. & Golkar, M. (2009). Bacterial production of dense granule antigen GRA8 of *Toxoplasma gondii. Iranian Biomedical Journal,* Vol. 13, No. 3, pp. 145-151, ISSN 1028-852X

Beghetto, E., Buffolano, W., Spadoni, A., Del Pezzo, M., Di Cristina, M., Minenkova, O., Petersen, E., Felici, F. & Gargano, N. (2003). Use of an immunoglobulin G avidity assay based on recombinant antigens for diagnosis of primary *Toxoplasma gondii* infection during pregnancy. *Journal of Clinical Microbiology,* Vol. 41, No. 12, pp. 5414-5418, ISSN 0095-1137

Béla, S.R., Oliveira Silva, D.A., Cunha-Junior, J.P., Pirovani, C.P., Chaves-Borges, F.A., Reis de Carvalho, F., Carrijo de Oliveira, T. & Mineo, J.R. (2008). Use of SAG2A recombinant *Toxoplasma gondii* surface antigen as a diagnostic marker for human acute toxoplasmosis: analysis of titers and avidity of IgG and IgG1 antibodies. *Diagnostic Microbiology and Infectious Disease,* Vol. 62, No. 3, pp. 245-254, ISSN 0732-8893

Bertozzi, L.C., Suzuki, L.A. & Rossi, C.L. (1999). Serological diagnosis of toxoplasmosis: usefulness of IgA detection and IgG avidity determination in a patient with a persistent IgM antibody response to *Toxoplasma gondii. Revista do Instituto de Medicina Tropical de São Paulo,* Vol. 41, No. 3, pp. 175-177, ISSN 1678-9946

Bobic, B., Sibalic, D. & Djurkovic-Djakovic, O. (1991). High levels of IgM antibodies specific for *Toxoplasma gondii* in pregnancy 12 years after primary toxoplasma infection. Case report. *Gynecologic and Obstetric Investigation,* Vol. 31, No. 3, pp. 182-184, ISSN 0378-7346

Bradley, P.J., Ward, C., Cheng, S.J., Alexander, D.L., Coller, S., Coombs, G.H., Dunn, J.D., Ferguson, D.J., Sanderson, S.J., Wastling, J.M. & Boothroyd, J.C. (2005). Proteomic analysis of rhoptry organelles reveals many novel constituents for host-parasite interactions in *Toxoplasma gondii. The Journal of Biological Chemistry,* Vol. 280, No. 40, pp. 34245-34258, ISSN 0021-9258

Brinkmann, V., Remington, J.S. & Sharma, S.D. (1993). Vaccination of mice with the protective F3G3 antigen of *Toxoplasma gondii* activates CD4+ but not CD8+ T cells and induces *Toxoplasma* specific IgG antibody. *Molecular Immunology,* Vol. 30, No. 4, pp. 353-358, ISSN 0161-5890

Brooks, R.G., McCabe, R.E. & Remington, J.S. (1987). Role of serology in the diagnosis of toxoplasmic lymphadenopathy. *Reviews of Infectious Diseases,* Vol.9, No.5, pp. 1055-1062, ISSN 0162-0886

Buffolano, W., Lappalainen, M., Hedman, L., Ciccimarra, F., Del Pezzo, M., Rescaldani, R., Gargano, N. & Hedman, K. (2004). Delayed maturation of IgG avidity in congenital toxoplasmosis. *European Journal of Clinical Microbiology & Infectious Diseases,* Vol. 23, No. 11, pp. 825-830, ISSN 0934-9723

Candolfi, E., Pastor, R., Huber, R., Filisetti, D. & Villard, O. (2007). IgG avidity assay firms up the diagnosis of acute toxoplasmosis on the first serum sample in immunocompetent pregnant women. *Diagnostic Microbiology and Infectious Disease,* Vol. 58, No. 1, pp. 83-88, ISSN 0732-8893

Carruthers, V.B. & Sibley, L.D. (1997). Sequential protein secretion from three distinct organelles of *Toxoplasma gondii* accompanies invasion of human fibroblasts. *European Journal of Cell Biology,* Vol. 73, No. 2, pp. 114-123, ISSN 0171-9335

Carruthers, V.B. & Tomley, F.M. (2008). Microneme proteins in apicomplexans. *Sub-cellular Biochemistry,* Vol. 47, pp. 33-45, ISSN 0306-0225

Chang, P.Y., Fong, M.Y., Nissapatorn, V. & Lau, Y.L. (2011). Evaluation of *Pichia pastoris*-expressed recombinant rhoptry protein 2 of *Toxoplasma gondii* for its application in diagnosis of toxoplasmosis. *The American Journal of Tropical Medicine and Hygiene,* Vol. 85, No. 3, pp. 485-489, ISSN 1476-1645

Chumpitazi, B.F., Boussaid, A., Pelloux, H., Racinet, C., Bost, M. & Goullier-Fleuret, A. (1995). Diagnosis of congenital toxoplasmosis by immunoblotting and relationship with other methods. *Journal of Clinical Microbiology,* Vol. 33, No. 6, pp. 1479-1485, ISSN 0095-1137

Cóceres, V.M., Becher, M.L., De Napoli, M.G., Corvi, M.M., Clemente, M. & Angel, S.O. (2010). Evaluation of the antigenic value of recombinant *Toxoplasma gondii* HSP20 to detect specific immunoglobulin G antibodies in *Toxoplasma* infected humans. *Experimental Parasitology,* Vol. 126, No. 2, pp. 263-266, ISSN 1090-2449

Couvreur, G., Sadak, A., Fortier, B. & Dubremetz, J.F. (1988). Surface antigens of *Toxoplasma gondii*. *Parasitology,* Vol. 97 (Pt 1), pp. 1-10, ISSN 0031-1820

Cozon, G.J., Ferrandiz, J., Nebhi, H., Wallon, M. & Peyron, F. (1998). Estimation of the avidity of immunoglobulin G for routine diagnosis of chronic *Toxoplasma gondii* infection in pregnant women. *European Journal of Clinical Microbiology & Infectious Diseases,* Vol. 17, No. 1, pp. 32-36, ISSN 0934-9723

Daffos, F., Forestier, F., Capella-Pavlovsky, M., Thulliez, P., Aufrant, C., Valenti, D. & Cox, W.L. (1988). Prenatal management of 746 pregnancies at risk for congenital toxoplasmosis. *The New England Journal of Medicine,* Vol. 318, No. 5, pp. 271-275, ISSN 0028-4793

de Jong, P.T. (1989). Ocular toxoplasmosis; common and rare symptoms and signs. *International Ophthalmology,* Vol. 13, No. 6, pp. 391-397, ISSN 0165-5701

Desmonts, G. (1979). [*Toxoplasma,* mother and child (author's transl)]. *Revista Médica de Chile,* Vol. 107, No. 1, pp. 42-50, ISSN 0034-9887

Desmonts, G., Daffos, F., Forestier, F., Capella-Pavlovsky, M., Thulliez, P. & Chartier, M. (1985). Prenatal diagnosis of congenital toxoplasmosis. *Lancet,* Vol. 1, No. 8427, pp. 500-504, ISSN 0140-6736

Dubremetz, J.F. (2007). Rhoptries are major players in *Toxoplasma gondii* invasion and host cell interaction. *Cellular Microbiology,* Vol. 9, No. 4, pp. 841-848, ISSN 1462-5814

Ferrandiz, J., Mercier, C., Wallon, M., Picot, S., Cesbron-Delauw, M.F. & Peyron, F. (2004). Limited value of assays using detection of immunoglobulin G antibodies to the two recombinant dense granule antigens, GRA1 and GRA6 Nt of *Toxoplasma gondii,* for distinguishing between acute and chronic infections in pregnant women. *Clinical and Diagnostic Laboratory Immunology,* Vol. 11, No. 6, pp. 1016-1021, ISSN 1071-412X

Fleck, D.G. & Kwantes, W. (1980). *The laboratory diagnosis of toxoplasmosis. Public Health Laboratory Service Monograph Series 13,* H.M.S.O., ISBN 0118871048, London

Flori, P., Tardy, L., Patural, H., Bellete, B., Varlet, M.N., Hafid, J., Raberin, H. & Sung, R.T. (2004). Reliability of immunoglobulin G antitoxoplasma avidity test and effects of treatment on avidity indexes of infants and pregnant women. *Clinical and Diagnostic Laboratory Immunology,* Vol. 11, No. 4, pp. 669-674, ISSN 1071-412X

Gard, S. & Magnusson, J.H. (1951). A glandular form of toxoplasmosis in connection with pregnancy. *Acta Medica Scandinavica,* Vol. 141, No. 1, pp. 59-64, ISSN 0001-6101

Garweg, J.G., Jacquier, P. & Fluckiger, F. (1998). [Current limits in diagnosis of ocular toxoplasmosis]. *Klinische Monatsblätter für Augenheilkunde,* Vol. 212, No. 5, pp. 330-333, ISSN 0023-2165

Garweg, J.G., Jacquier, P. & Boehnke, M. (2000). Early aqueous humor analysis in patients with human ocular toxoplasmosis. *Journal of Clinical Microbiology,* Vol. 38, No. 3, pp. 996-1001, ISSN 0095-1137

Gatkowska, J., Hiszczynska-Sawicka, E., Kur, J., Holec, L. & Dlugonska, H. (2006). *Toxoplasma gondii*: an evaluation of diagnostic value of recombinant antigens in a murine model. *Experimental Parasitology,* Vol. 114, No. 3, pp. 220-227, ISSN 0014-4894

Gatkowska, J., Dziadek, B., Brzostek, A., Dziadek, J., Dzitko, K. & Długońska, H. (2010). Determination of diagnostic value of *Toxoplasma gondii* recombinant ROP2 and ROP4 antigens in mouse experimental model. *Polish Journal of Microbiology,* Vol. 59, No. 2, pp. 137-141, ISSN 1733-1331

Golkar, M., Rafati, S., Abdel-Latif, M.S., Brenier-Pinchart, M.P., Fricker-Hidalgo, H., Sima, B.K., Babaie, J., Pelloux, H., Cesbron-Delauw, M.F. & Mercier, C. (2007). The dense granule protein GRA2, a new marker for the serodiagnosis of acute *Toxoplasma* infection: comparison of sera collected in both France and Iran from pregnant women. *Diagnostic Microbiology and Infectious Disease,* Vol. 58, No. 4, pp. 419-426, ISSN 0732-8893

Golkar, M., Azadmanesh, K., Khalili, G., Khoshkholgh-Sima, B., Babaie, J., Mercier, C., Brenier-Pinchart, M.P., Fricker-Hidalgo, H., Pelloux, H. & Cesbron-Delauw, M.F. (2008). Serodiagnosis of recently acquired *Toxoplasma gondii* infection in pregnant women using enzyme-linked immunosorbent assays with a recombinant dense granule GRA6 protein. *Diagnostic Microbiology and Infectious Disease,* Vol. 61, No. 1, pp. 31-39, ISSN 0732-8893

Grimwood, J. & Smith, J.E. (1996). *Toxoplasma gondii*: the role of parasite surface and secreted proteins in host cell invasion. *International Journal for Parasitology*, Vol. 26, No. 2, pp. 169-173, ISSN 0020-7519

Gross, U., Bohne, W., Soete, M. & Dubremetz, J.F. (1996). Developmental differentiation between tachyzoites and bradyzoites of *Toxoplasma gondii*. *Parasitology Today*, Vol. 12, No. 1, pp. 30-33, ISSN 0169-4758

Gross, U., Lüder, C.G., Hendgen, V., Heeg, C., Sauer, I., Weidner, A., Krczal, D. & Enders, G. (2000). Comparative immunoglobulin G antibody profiles between mother and child (CGMC test) for early diagnosis of congenital toxoplasmosis. *Journal of Clinical Microbiology*, Vol. 38, No. 10, pp. 3619-3622, ISSN 0095-1137

Hedman, K., Lappalainen, M., Seppäiä, I. & Mäkelä, O. (1989). Recent primary toxoplasma infection indicated by a low avidity of specific IgG. *The Journal of Infectious Diseases*, Vol. 159, No. 4, pp. 736-740, ISSN 0022-1899

Herold, M.A., Kuhne, R., Vosberg, M., Ostheeren-Michaelis, S., Vogt, P. & Karrer, U. (2009). Disseminated toxoplasmosis in a patient with non-Hodgkin lymphoma. *Infection*, Vol. 37, No. 6, pp. 551-554, ISSN 1439-0973

Hiszczynska-Sawicka, E., Brillowska-Dabrowska, A., Dabrowski, S., Pietkiewicz, H., Myjak, P. & Kur, J. (2003). High yield expression and single-step purification of *Toxoplasma gondii* SAG1, GRA1, and GRA7 antigens in *Escherichia coli*. *Protein Expression and Purification*, Vol. 27, No. 1, pp. 150-157, ISSN 1046-5928

Hoffmann, C., Ernst, M., Meyer, P., Wolf, E., Rosenkranz, T., Plettenberg, A., Stoehr, A., Horst, H.A., Marienfeld, K. & Lange, C. (2007). Evolving characteristics of toxoplasmosis in patients infected with human immunodeficiency virus-1: clinical course and *Toxoplasma gondii*-specific immune responses. *Clinical Microbiology and Infection*, Vol. 13, No. 5, pp. 510-515, ISSN 1198-743X

Hohlfeld, P., Daffos, F., Costa, J.M., Thulliez, P., Forestier, F. & Vidaud, M. (1994). Prenatal diagnosis of congenital toxoplasmosis with a polymerase-chain-reaction test on amniotic fluid. *The New England Journal of Medicine*, Vol. 331, No. 11, pp. 695-699, ISSN 0028-4793

Holec, L., Gasior, A., Brillowska-Dabrowska, A. & Kur, J. (2008). *Toxoplasma gondii*: enzyme-linked immunosorbent assay using different fragments of recombinant microneme protein 1 (MIC1) for detection of immunoglobulin G antibodies. *Experimental Parasitology*, Vol. 119, No. 1, pp. 1-6, ISSN 0014-4894

Holec-Gąsior, L., Kur, J. & Hiszczynska-Sawicka, E. (2009). GRA2 and ROP1 recombinant antigens as potential markers for detection of *Toxoplasma gondii*-specific immunoglobulin G in humans with acute toxoplasmosis. *Clinical and Vaccine Immunology*, Vol. 16, No. 4, pp. 510-514, ISSN 1556-679X

Holec-Gąsior, L. & Kur, J. (2010). *Toxoplasma gondii*: Recombinant GRA5 antigen for detection of immunoglobulin G antibodies using enzyme-linked immunosorbent assay. *Experimental Parasitology*, Vol. 124, No. 3, pp. 272-278, ISSN 1090-2449

Holec-Gąsior, L., Drapala, D., Lautenbach, D. &Kuri, J. (2010a). *Toxoplasma gondii*: usefulness of ROP1 recombinant antigen in an immunoglobulin G avidity assay for diagnosis of acute toxoplasmosis in humans. *Polish Journal of Microbiology*, Vol. 59, No. 4, pp. 307-310, ISSN 1733-1331

Holec-Gąsior, L., Kur, J., Hiszczyńska-Sawicka, E., Drapała, D., Dominiak-Górski, B. & Pejsak, Z. (2010b). Application of recombinant antigens in serodiagnosis of swine toxoplasmosis and prevalence of *Toxoplasma gondii* infection among pigs in Poland. *Polish Journal of Veterinary Sciences*, Vol. 13, No. 3, pp. 457-464, ISSN 1505-1773

Holliman, R.E., Stevens, P.J., Duffy, K.T. & Johnson, J.D. (1991). Serological investigation of ocular toxoplasmosis. *The British Journal of Ophthalmology,* Vol. 75, No. 6, pp. 353-355, ISSN 0007-1161

Holliman, R.E., Raymond, R., Renton, N. & Johnson, J.D. (1994). The diagnosis of toxoplasmosis using IgG avidity. *Epidemiology and Infection,* Vol. 112, No. 2, pp. 399-408, ISSN 0950-2688

Hurt, C. & Tammaro, D. (2007). Diagnostic evaluation of mononucleosis-like illnesses. *American Journal of Medicine,* Vol. 120, No. 10, pp. e911-e918, ISSN 1555-7162

Jacobs, D., Dubremetz, J.F., Loyens, A., Bosman, F. & Saman, E. (1998). Identification and heterologous expression of a new dense granule protein (GRA7) from *Toxoplasma gondii*. *Molecular and Biochemical Parasitology,* Vol. 91, No. 2, pp. 237-249, ISSN 0166-6851

Jenum, P.A., Stray-Pedersen, B. & Gundersen, A.G. (1997). Improved diagnosis of primary *Toxoplasma gondii* infection in early pregnancy by determination of antitoxoplasma immunoglobulin G avidity. *Journal of Clinical Microbiology,* Vol. 35, No. 8, pp. 1972-1977, ISSN 0095-1137

Jenum, P.A., Holberg-Petersen, M., Melby, K.K. & Stray-Pedersen, B. (1998). Diagnosis of congenital *Toxoplasma gondii* infection by polymerase chain reaction (PCR) on amniotic fluid samples. The Norwegian experience. *Acta Pathologica, Microbiologica, et Immunologica Scandinavica,* Vol. 106, No. 7, pp. 680-686, ISSN 0903-4641

Joynson, D.H., Payne, R.A. & Rawal, B.K. (1990). Potential role of IgG avidity for diagnosing toxoplasmosis. *Journal of Clinical Pathology,* Vol. 43, No. 12, pp. 1032-1033, ISSN 0021-9746

Kijlstra, A., Luyendijk, L., Baarsma, G.S., Rothova, A., Schweitzer, C.M., Timmerman, Z., de Vries, J. & Breebaart, A.C. (1989). Aqueous humor analysis as a diagnostic tool in toxoplasma uveitis. *International Ophthalmology,* Vol. 13, No. 6, pp. 383-386, ISSN 0165-5701

Klaren, V.N., van Doornik, C.E., Ongkosuwito, J.V., Feron, E.J. & Kijlstra, A. (1998). Differences between intraocular and serum antibody responses in patients with ocular toxoplasmosis. *American Journal of Ophthalmology,* Vol. 126, No. 5, pp. 698-706, ISSN 0002-9394

Knoll, L.J. & Boothroyd, J.C. (1998). Molecular biology's lessons about *Toxoplasma* development: Stage-specific homologs. *Parasitology Today,* Vol. 14, No. 12, pp. 490-493, ISSN 0169-4758

Kotresha, D. & Noordin, R. (2010). Recombinant proteins in the diagnosis of toxoplasmosis. *Acta Pathologica, Microbiologica, et Immunologica Scandinavica,* Vol. 118, No. 8, pp. 529-542, ISSN 1600-0463

Lappalainen, M., Koskela, P., Koskiniemi, M., Ammala, P., Hiilesmaa, V., Teramo, K., Raivio, K.O., Remington, J.S. & Hedman, K. (1993). Toxoplasmosis acquired during pregnancy: improved serodiagnosis based on avidity of IgG. *The Journal of Infectious Diseases,* Vol. 167, No. 3, pp. 691-697, ISSN 0022-1899

Lappalainen, M., Koskiniemi, M., Hiilesmaa, V., Ammala, P., Teramo, K., Koskela, P., Lebech, M., Raivio, K.O. & Hedman, K. (1995). Outcome of children after maternal primary *Toxoplasma* infection during pregnancy with emphasis on avidity of specific IgG. The Study Group. *The Pediatric Infectious Disease Journal,* Vol. 14, No. 5, pp. 354-361, ISSN 0891-3668

Lappalainen, M., Jokiranta, T.S., Halme, L., Tynninen, O., Lautenschlager, I., Hedman, K., Hockerstedt, K. & Meri, S. (1998). Disseminated toxoplasmosis after liver transplantation: case report and review. *Clinical Infectious Diseases,* Vol. 27, No. 5, pp. 1327-1328, ISSN 1058-4838

Lappalainen, M. & Hedman, K. (2004). Serodiagnosis of toxoplasmosis. The impact of measurement of IgG avidity. *Annali dell'Istituto Superiore di Sanità,* Vol. 40, No. 1, pp. 81-88, ISSN 0021-2571

Lappin, M.R., Burney, D.P., Hill, S.A. & Chavkin, M.J. (1995). Detection of *Toxoplasma gondii*-specific IgA in the aqueous humor of cats. *American Journal of Veterinary Research,* Vol. 56, No. 6, pp. 774-778, ISSN 0002-9645

Lau, Y.L. & Fong, M.Y. (2008). *Toxoplasma gondii*: serological characterization and immunogenicity of recombinant surface antigen 2 (SAG2) expressed in the yeast *Pichia pastoris*. *Experimental Parasitology,* Vol. 119, No. 3, pp. 373-378, ISSN 1090-2449

Lecolier, B. & Pucheu, B. (1993). [Value of the study of IgG avidity for the diagnosis of toxoplasmosis]. *Pathologie-Biologie,* Vol. 41, No. 2, pp. 155-158, ISSN 0369-8114

Lecordier, L., Fourmaux, M.P., Mercier, C., Dehecq, E., Masy, E. & Cesbron-Delauw, M.F. (2000). Enzyme-linked immunosorbent assays using the recombinant dense granule antigens GRA6 and GRA1 of *Toxoplasma gondii* for detection of immunoglobulin G antibodies. *Clinical and Diagnostic Laboratory Immunology,* Vol. 7, No. 4, pp. 607-611, ISSN 1071-412X

Lekutis, C., Ferguson, D.J. & Boothroyd, J.C. (2000). *Toxoplasma gondii*: identification of a developmentally regulated family of genes related to SAG2. *Experimental Parasitology,* Vol. 96, No. 2, pp. 89-96, ISSN 0014-4894

Li, S., Galvan, G., Araujo, F.G., Suzuki, Y., Remington, J.S. & Parmley, S. (2000). Serodiagnosis of recently acquired *Toxoplasma gondii* infection using an enzyme-linked immunosorbent assay with a combination of recombinant antigens. *Clinical and Diagnostic Laboratory Immunology,* Vol. 7, No. 5, pp. 781-787, ISSN 1071-412X

Liesenfeld, O., Press, C., Montoya, J.G., Gill, R., Isaac-Renton, J.L., Hedman, K. & Remington, J.S. (1997). False-positive results in immunoglobulin M (IgM) toxoplasma antibody tests and importance of confirmatory testing: the Platelia Toxo IgM test. *Journal of Clinical Microbiology,* Vol. 35, No. 1, pp. 174-178, ISSN 0095-1137

Liesenfeld, O., Montoya, J.G., Kinney, S., Press, C. & Remington, J.S. (2001). Effect of testing for IgG avidity in the diagnosis of *Toxoplasma gondii* infection in pregnant women: experience in a US reference laboratory. *The Journal of Infectious Diseases,* Vol. 183, No. 8, pp. 1248-1253, ISSN 0022-1899

Luft, B.J. & Remington, J.S. (1988). AIDS commentary. Toxoplasmic encephalitis. *The Journal of Infectious Diseases,* Vol. 157, No. 1, pp. 1-6, ISSN 0022-1899

Martin, V., Arcavi, M., Santillan, G., Amendoeira, M.R., De Souza Neves, E., Griemberg, G., Guarnera, E., Garberi, J.C. & Angel, S.O. (1998). Detection of human *Toxoplasma*-specific immunoglobulins A, M, and G with a recombinant *Toxoplasma gondii* rop2 protein. *Clinical and Diagnostic Laboratory Immunology,* Vol. 5, No. 5, pp. 627-631, ISSN 1071-412X

McCabe, R.E., Brooks, R.G., Dorfman, R.F. & Remington, J.S. (1987). Clinical spectrum in 107 cases of toxoplasmic lymphadenopathy. *Reviews of Infectious Diseases,* Vol. 9, No. 4, pp. 754-774, ISSN 0162-0886

Meek, B., van Gool, T., Gilis, H. & Peek, R. (2001). Dissecting the IgM antibody response during the acute and latent phase of toxoplasmosis. *Diagnostic Microbiology and Infectious Disease,* Vol. 41, No. 3, pp. 131-137, ISSN 0732-8893

Meganathan, P., Singh, S., Ling, L.Y., Singh, J., Subrayan, V. & Nissapatorn, V. (2010). Detection of *Toxoplasma gondii* DNA by PCR following microwave treatment of serum and whole blood. *The Southeast Asian Journal of Tropical Medicine and Public Health,* Vol. 41, No. 2, pp. 265-273, ISSN 0125-1562

Michelin, A., Bittame, A., Bordat, Y., Travier, L., Mercier, C., Dubremetz, J.F. & Lebrun, M. (2009). GRA12, a *Toxoplasma* dense granule protein associated with the intravacuolar membranous nanotubular network. *International Journal for Parasitology,* Vol. 39, No. 3, pp. 299-306, ISSN 1879-0135

Mineo, J.R., Camargo, M.E. & Ferreira, A.W. (1980). Enzyme-linked immunosorbent assay for antibodies to *Toxoplasma gondii* polysaccharides in human toxoplasmosis. *Infection and Immunity,* Vol. 27, No. 2, pp. 283-287, ISSN 0019-9567

Mineo, J.R. & Kasper, L.H. (1994). Attachment of *Toxoplasma gondii* to host cells involves major surface protein, SAG-1 (P30). *Experimental Parasitology,* Vol. 79, No. 1, pp. 11-20, ISSN 0014-4894

Montoya, J.G. & Remington, J.S. (1996). Toxoplasmic chorioretinitis in the setting of acute acquired toxoplasmosis. *Clinical Infectious Diseases,* Vol. 23, No. 2, pp. 277-282, ISSN 1058-4838

Montoya, J.G. (2002). Laboratory diagnosis of *Toxoplasma gondii* infection and toxoplasmosis. *The Journal of Infectious Diseases,* Vol. 185, Suppl 1, pp. S73-S82, ISSN 0022-1899

Montoya, J.G., Liesenfeld, O., Kinney, S., Press, C. & Remington, J.S. (2002). VIDAS test for avidity of *Toxoplasma*-specific immunoglobulin G for confirmatory testing of pregnant women. *Journal of Clinical Microbiology,* Vol. 40, No. 7, pp. 2504-2508, ISSN 0095-1137

Montoya, J.G. & Liesenfeld, O. (2004). Toxoplasmosis. *Lancet,* Vol. 363, No. 9425, pp. 1965-1976, ISSN 1474-547X

Montoya, J.G., Huffman, H.B. & Remington, J.S. (2004). Evaluation of the immunoglobulin G avidity test for diagnosis of toxoplasmic lymphadenopathy. *Journal of Clinical Microbiology,* Vol. 42, No. 10, pp. 4627-4631, ISSN 0095-1137

Murray, A., Mercier, C., Decoster, A., Lecordier, L., Capron, A. & Cesbron-Delauw, M.F. (1993). Multiple B-cell epitopes in a recombinant GRA2 secreted antigen of *Toxoplasma gondii. Applied Parasitology,* Vol. 34, No. 4, pp. 235-244, ISSN 0943-0938

Naessens, A., Jenum, P.A., Pollak, A., Decoster, A., Lappalainen, M., Villena, I., Lebech, M., Stray-Pedersen, B., Hayde, M., Pinon, J.M., Petersen, E. & Foulon, W. (1999). Diagnosis of congenital toxoplasmosis in the neonatal period: A multicenter evaluation. *Journal of Pediatrics,* Vol. 135, No. 6, pp. 714-719, ISSN 0022-3476

Nam, H.W. (2009). GRA proteins of *Toxoplasma gondii*: maintenance of host-parasite interactions across the parasitophorous vacuolar membrane. *The Korean Journal of Parasitology,* Vol. 47 Suppl, pp. S29-37, ISSN 1738-0006

National Committee for Clinical Laboratory Standard. (2004). *Clinical use and interpretation of serologic tests for Toxoplasma gondii.* Approved guideline M36-A, NCCLS, ISBN 1-56238-523-2, Wayne, Pennsylvania

Nielsen, H.V., Schmidt, D.R. & Petersen, E. (2005). Diagnosis of congenital toxoplasmosis by two-dimensional immunoblot differentiation of mother and child immunoglobulin G profiles. *Journal of Clinical Microbiology,* Vol. 43, No. 2, pp. 711-715, ISSN 0095-1137

Nigro, M., Gutierrez, A., Hoffer, A.M., Clemente, M., Kaufer, F., Carral, L., Martin, V., Guarnera, E.A. & Angel, S.O. (2003). Evaluation of *Toxoplasma gondii* recombinant proteins for the diagnosis of recently acquired toxoplasmosis by an immunoglobulin G analysis. *Diagnostic Microbiology and Infectious Disease,* Vol. 47, No. 4, pp. 609-613, ISSN 0732-8893

Nissapatorn, V., Lee, C., Quek, K.F., Leong, C.L., Mahmud, R. & Abdullah, K.A. (2004). Toxoplasmosis in HIV/AIDS patients: a current situation. *Japanese Journal of Infectious Diseases,* Vol. 57, No. 4, pp. 160-165, ISSN 1344-6304

Nissapatorn, V., Suwanrath, C., Sawangjaroen, N., Ling, L.Y. & Chandeying, V. (2011). Toxoplasmosis-serological evidence and associated risk factors among pregnant women in southern Thailand. *The American Journal of Tropical Medicine and Hygiene,* Vol. 85, No. 2, pp. 243-247, ISSN 1476-1645

Oksenhendler, E., Charreau, I., Tournerie, C., Azihary, M., Carbon, C. & Aboulker, J.P. (1994). *Toxoplasma gondii* infection in advanced HIV infection. *AIDS,* Vol. 8, No. 4, pp. 483-487, ISSN 0269-9370

Olariu, T.R., Cretu, O., Koreck, A. & Petrescu, C. (2006). Diagnosis of toxoplasmosis in pregnancy: importance of immunoglobulin G avidity test. *Roumanian Archives of Microbiology and Immunology,* Vol. 65, No. 3-4, pp. 131-134, ISSN 1222-3891

Parmley, S.F., Sgarlato, G.D., Mark, J., Prince, J.B. & Remington, J.S. (1992). Expression, characterization, and serologic reactivity of recombinant surface antigen P22 of *Toxoplasma gondii. Journal of Clinical Microbiology,* Vol. 30, No. 5, pp. 1127-1133, ISSN 0095-1137

Partanen, P., Turunen, H.J., Paasivuo, R.T. & Leinikki, P.O. (1984). Immunoblot analysis of *Toxoplasma gondii* antigens by human immunoglobulins G, M, and A antibodies at different stages of infection. *Journal of Clinical Microbiology,* Vol. 20, No. 1, pp. 133-135, ISSN 0095-1137

Paul, M. (1999). Immunoglobulin G avidity in diagnosis of toxoplasmic lymphadenopathy and ocular toxoplasmosis. *Clinical and Diagnostic Laboratory Immunology,* Vol. 6, No. 4, pp. 514-518, ISSN 1071-412X

Perkins, E.S. (1973). Ocular toxoplasmosis. *The British Journal of Ophthalmology,* Vol. 57, No. 1, pp. 1-17, ISSN 0007-1161

Petersen, E., Borobio, M.V., Guy, E., Liesenfeld, O., Meroni, V., Naessens, A., Spranzi, E. & Thulliez, P. (2005). European multicenter study of the LIAISON automated diagnostic system for determination of *Toxoplasma gondii*-specific immunoglobulin G (IgG) and IgM and the IgG avidity index. *Journal of Clinical Microbiology,* Vol. 43, No. 4, pp. 1570-1574, ISSN 0095-1137

Pfrepper, K.I., Enders, G., Gohl, M., Krczal, D., Hlobil, H., Wassenberg, D. & Soutschek, E. (2005). Seroreactivity to and avidity for recombinant antigens in toxoplasmosis.

Clinical and Diagnostic Laboratory Immunology, Vol.12, No.8, pp. 977-982, ISSN 1071-412X

Pietkiewicz, H., Hiszczynska-Sawicka, E., Kur, J., Petersen, E., Nielsen, H.V., Stankiewicz, M., Andrzejewska, I. & Myjak, P. (2004). Usefulness of *Toxoplasma gondii*-specific recombinant antigens in serodiagnosis of human toxoplasmosis. *Journal of Clinical Microbiology,* Vol.42, No.4, pp. 1779-1781, ISSN 0095-1137

Pietkiewicz, H., Hiszczynska-Sawicka, E., Kur, J., Petersen, E., Nielsen, H.V., Paul, M., Stankiewicz, M. & Myjak, P. (2007). Usefulness of *Toxoplasma gondii* recombinant antigens (GRA1, GRA7 and SAG1) in an immunoglobulin G avidity test for the serodiagnosis of toxoplasmosis. *Parasitology Reseach,* Vol. 100, No. 2, pp. 333-337, ISSN 0932-0113

Pinon, J.M., Dumon, H., Chemla, C., Franck, J., Petersen, E., Lebech, M., Zufferey, J., Bessieres, M.H., Marty, P., Holliman, R., Johnson, J., Luyasu, V., Lecolier, B., Guy, E., Joynson, D.H., Decoster, A., Enders, G., Pelloux, H. & Candolfi, E. (2001). Strategy for diagnosis of congenital toxoplasmosis: evaluation of methods comparing mothers and newborns and standard methods for postnatal detection of immunoglobulin G, M, and A antibodies. *Journal of Clinical Microbiology,* Vol. 39, No. 6, pp. 2267-2271, ISSN 0095-1137

Porter, S.B. & Sande, M.A. (1992). Toxoplasmosis of the central nervous system in the acquired immunodeficiency syndrome. *The New England Journal of Medicine,* Vol. 327, No. 23, pp. 1643-1648, ISSN 0028-4793

Press, C., Montoya, J.G. & Remington, J.S. (2005). Use of a single serum sample for diagnosis of acute toxoplasmosis in pregnant women and other adults. *Journal of Clinical Microbiology,* Vol. 43, No. 7, pp. 3481-3483, ISSN 0095-1137

Prigione, I., Facchetti, P., Lecordier, L., Deslee, D., Chiesa, S., Cesbron-Delauw, M.F. & Pistoia, V. (2000). T cell clones rose from chronically infected healthy humans by stimulation with *Toxoplasma gondii* excretory-secretory antigens cross-react with live tachyzoites: characterization of the fine antigenic specificity of the clones and implications for vaccine development. *Journal of Immunology,* Vol.164, No.7, pp. 3741-3748, ISSN 0022-1767

Reis, M.M., Tessaro, M.M. & D'Azevedo, P.A. (2006). *Toxoplasma*-IgM and IgG-avidity in single samples from areas with a high infection rate can determine the risk of mother-to-child transmission. *Revista do Instituto de Medicina Tropical de São Paulo,* Vol.48, No.2, pp. 93-98, ISSN 0036-4665

Remington, J.S. & Desmonts, G. (1990). Toxoplasmosis. In: Remington, J.S. & Klein, J.O. (eds) *Infectious diseases of the fetus and newborn infant,* WB Saunders Company, Philadelphia, pp. 89-195, ISBN 0721667821

Remington, J.S., McLeod, R., Thulliez, P. & Desmonts, G. (2001). T*oxoplasmosis*. In: Remington, J.S. & Klein, J.O, eds, *Infectious diseases of the fetus and newborn infant*, 5th edn. WB Saunders Company, Philadelphia, pp. 205-346, ISBN 0721667821.

Remington, J.S., Thulliez, P. & Montoya, J.G. (2004). Recent developments for diagnosis of toxoplasmosis. *Journal of Clinical Microbiology,* Vol.42, No.3, pp. 941-945, ISSN 0095-1137

Roberts, A., Hedman, K., Luyasu, V., Zufferey, J., Bessieres, M.H., Blatz, R.M., Candolfi, E., Decoster, A., Enders, G., Gross, U., Guy, E., Hayde, M., Ho-Yen, D., Johnson, J., Lecolier, B., Naessens, A., Pelloux, H., Thulliez, P. & Petersen, E. (2001). Multicenter evaluation of strategies for serodiagnosis of primary infection with *Toxoplasma gondii*. *European Journal of Clinical Microbiology & Infectious Diseases,* Vol. 20, No. 7, pp. 467-474, ISSN 0934-9723

Rome, M.E., Beck, J.R., Turetzky, J.M., Webster, P. & Bradley, P.J. (2008). Intervacuolar transport and unique topology of GRA14, a novel dense granule protein in *Toxoplasma gondii*. *Infection and Immunity,* Vol. 76, No. 11, pp. 4865-4875, ISSN 1098-5522

Ronday, M.J., Luyendijk, L., Baarsma, G.S., Bollemeijer, J.G., Van der Lelij, A. & Rothova, A. (1995). Presumed acquired ocular toxoplasmosis. *Archives of Ophthalmology,* Vol. 113, No. 12, pp. 1524-1529, ISSN 0003-9950

Rothova, A., van Knapen, F., Baarsma, G.S., Kruit, P.J., Loewer-Sieger, D.H. & Kijlstra, A. (1986). Serology in ocular toxoplasmosis. *The British Journal of Ophthalmology,* Vol. 70, No. 8, pp. 615-622, ISSN 0007-1161

Said, R.N., Zaki, M.M. & Abdelrazik, M.B. (2011). Congenital toxoplasmosis: evaluation of molecular and serological methods for achieving economic and early diagnosis among Egyptian preterm infants. *Journal of Tropical Pediatrics,* Vol. 57, No. 5, pp. 333-339, ISSN 1465-3664

Santoni, J.R. & Santoni-Williams, C.J. (1993). Headache and painful lymphadenopathy in extracranial or systemic infection: etiology of new daily persistent headaches. *Internal Medicine,* Vol. 32, No. 7, pp. 530-532, ISSN 0918-2918

Sensini, A. (2006). *Toxoplasma gondii* infection in pregnancy: opportunities and pitfalls of serological diagnosis. *Clinical Microbiology and Infection,* Vol. 12, No. 6, pp. 504-512, ISSN 1198-743X

Sharma, S.D., Mullenax, J., Araujo, F.G., Erlich, H.A. & Remington, J.S. (1983). Western Blot analysis of the antigens of *Toxoplasma gondii* recognized by human IgM and IgG antibodies. *Journal of Immunology,* Vol. 131, No. 2, pp. 977-983, ISSN 0022-1767

Sharma, S.D., Araujo, F.G. & Remington, J.S. (1984). *Toxoplasma* antigen isolated by affinity chromatography with monoclonal antibody protects mice against lethal infection with *Toxoplasma gondii*. *Journal of Immunology,* Vol. 133, No. 6, pp. 2818-2820, ISSN 0022-1767

Smith, J.E., McNeil, G., Zhang, Y.W., Dutton, S., Biswas-Hughes, G. & Appleford, P. (1996). Serological recognition of *Toxoplasma gondii* cyst antigens. *Current Topics in Microbiology and Immunology,* Vol. 219, pp. 67-73, ISSN 0070-217X

Soldati, D., Dubremetz, J.F. & Lebrun, M. (2001). Microneme proteins: structural and functional requirements to promote adhesion and invasion by the apicomplexan parasite *Toxoplasma gondii*. *International Journal for Parasitology,* Vol. 31, No. 12, pp. 1293-1302, ISSN 0020-7519

Spausta, G., Ciarkowska, J., Wiczkowski, A., Adamek, B. & Beniowski, M. (2003). [Anti-*Toxoplasma gondii* IgG antibodies in HIV-infected patients]. *Polski Merkuriusz Lekarski* , Vol. 14, No. 81, pp. 233-235, ISSN 1426-9686

Sukthana, Y. (2006). Toxoplasmosis: beyond animals to humans. *Trends in Parasitology,* Vol. 22, No. 3, pp. 137-142, ISSN 1471-4922

Tabbara, K.F. (1994). A new era of infections. *Annals of Saudi Medicine,* Vol. 14, No. 5, pp. 365, ISSN 0256-4947

Tenter, A.M., Heckeroth, A.R. & Weiss, L.M. (2000). *Toxoplasma gondii*: from animals to humans. *International Journal for Parasitology,* Vol. 30, No. 12-13, pp. 1217-1258, ISSN 0020-7519

vanGelder, P., Bosman, F., de Meuter, F., van Heuverswyn, H. & Herion, P. (1993). Serodiagnosis of toxoplasmosis by using a recombinant form of the 54-kilodalton rhoptry antigen expressed in *Escherichia coli. Journal of Clinical Microbiology,* Vol. 31, No. 1, pp. 9-15, ISSN 0095-1137

Vidal, J.E., Hernandez, A.V., de Oliveira, A.C., Dauar, R.F., Barbosa, S.P.Jr. & Focaccia, R. (2005). Cerebral toxoplasmosis in HIV-positive patients in Brazil: clinical features and predictors of treatment response in the HAART era. *AIDS Patient Care STDS,* Vol. 19, No. 10, pp. 626-634, ISSN 1087-2914

Villena, I., Aubert, D., Brodard, V., Quereux, C., Leroux, B., Dupouy, D., Remy, G., Foudrinier, F., Chemla, C., Gomez-Marin, J.E. & Pinon, J.M. (1999). Detection of specific immunoglobulin E during maternal, fetal, and congenital toxoplasmosis. *Journal of Clinical Microbiology,* Vol. 37, No. 11, pp. 3487-3490, ISSN 0095-1137

Weiss, L.M., Udem, S.A., Tanowitz, H. & Wittner, M. (1988). Western blot analysis of the antibody response of patients with AIDS and toxoplasma encephalitis: antigenic diversity among *Toxoplasma* strains. *The Journal of Infectious Diseases,* Vol. 157, No. 1, pp. 7-13, ISSN 0022-1899

Wong, S.Y. & Remington, J.S. (1994). Toxoplasmosis in pregnancy. *Clinical Infectious Diseases,* Vol. 18, No. 6, pp. 853-861; quiz 862, ISSN 1058-4838

Wu, K., Chen, X.G., Li, H., Yan, H., Yang, P.L., Lun, Z.R. & Zhu, X.Q. (2009). Diagnosis of human toxoplasmosis by using the recombinant truncated surface antigen 1 of *Toxoplasma gondii. Diagnostic Microbiology and Infectious Disease,* Vol. 64, No. 3, pp. 261-266, ISSN 1879-0070

Yamada, H., Nishikawa, A., Yamamoto, T., Mizue, Y., Yamada, T., Morizane, M., Tairaku, S. & Nishihira, J. (2011). Prospective study of congenital toxoplasmosis screening with use of IgG avidity and multiplex nested PCR methods. *Journal of Clinical Microbiology,* Vol. 49, No. 7, pp. 2552-2556, ISSN 1098-660X

12

Immunoassay

Rie Oyama
Iwate Medical University
Japan

1. Introduction

Anti-Müllerian hormone (AMH) is a glycoprotein that belongs to the transforming growth factor-β (TGF-β) superfamily [1]. AMH, also known as a Müllerian inhibiting substance (MIS), has been mainly studied for its regulatory role in male sex differentiation and induces regression of the Müllerian ducts, the anlagen of the female reproductive tract [2]. AMH expression can first be observed in granulosa cells of primary follicles, and its expression is strongest in preantral and small antral follicles (<4mm). AMH expression disappears in follicles as their size increases and is almost completely lost in follicles larger than 8mm, where only very weak expression remains, restricted to the granulosa cells of the cumulus [3]. This expression pattern suggests that, also in women, AMH may play a role in the initial recruitment and in the selection of the dominant follicles. To assess an individual's ovarian reserve, early follicular phase serum levels of FSH, inhibin B and estoradiol (E_2) have been measured. Inhibin B and E_2 are produced rarely by antral follicles in response to FSH, and contribute to the classical feedback loop of the pituitary-gondola axis to suppress FSH secretion. With the decline of the follicle pool, serum levels of inhibin B and E_2 decrease and subsequently serum FSH levels rise [4].The likely explanations are that AMH and FSH are highly correlated [5]. In women undergoing treatment for infertility, ovarian aging is characterized by decreased ovarian responsiveness to exogenous gonadotrophin and poor pregnancy outcome. On the one hand, correct identification of poor responders by assessment of the ovarian reserve before entering an IVF program is important. On the other hand, assessment of the ovarian reserve may also benefit patients that would generally be excluded from an IVF program because of advanced age.

Automatic follicle analysis has the potential to remove any observer bias and to reduce the time needed for measurements, but it must be both valid and reliable [6]. This is particularly true within the field of reproductive medicine, with ultrasound being used on a daily basis to follow the ovarian response to gonadotropins in a process known as follicle tracking [7]. Two-dimensional (2D) measurements are then made and their mean is taken as the true follicular diameter, which is relatively straightforward but follicle tracking becomes more difficult as the number of follicles increases [6]. Therefore, recently, three-dimensional (3D) ultrasound with Sono AVC (Automatic Volume Calculation) has been used to quantify hypoechoic regions within a three-dimensional dataset and provide automatic estimation of their absolute dimensions, mean diameter and volume. Each individual volume is given a specific color and the automated measurements of the mean diameter (relaxed sphere diameter), maximum dimensions (x, y, z diameters) and volume are displayed using these colors in descending order of size. Sono AVC provides measurements of follicular diameter that are more accurate than manual measures and has the potential to improve the clinical workflow because the time taken for the measurements is significantly shorter [8]. The quantification of power Doppler assesses blood flow within the ovary and quantitative 3D-power Doppler angiography has been used to demonstrate the blood flow around the follicles within the ovary. These tools are new methods to analyze the effect of ovary stimulation. The power Doppler data within the 3D dataset can be quantified to generate volumetric measures of blood flow within the dataset as whole or within specific volumes within the dataset. Various software programmes are available to facilitate this, but the one used most frequently is the histogram facility in 4D View (GE Medical System, Zipf, Austria), which generates three indices of vascularity: the vascularization index (VI), the flow index (FI), and the vascularization flow index (VFI). These vascular indices are generated through specific algorithms based on signal intensity and the relative proportion of color voxels (3D pixels) within the defined volume [9]. This study was designed to assess the ability of the combination of AMH and 3D-power Doppler histogram techniques, including the Virtual Organ Computer-aided (VOCAL) software, to generate volume measurements of the ovary. These new combinational ultrasound techniques were used to investigate patient undergoing IVF treatment.

2. Materials and methods

This was a prospective cohort study of 28 patients undergoing controlled ovarian hyperstimulation. All of the patients met the following inclusion criteria: (1) Both ovaries were present with no morphological abnormalities, (2) Regular menstrual cycle lengths ranging between 25 and 34 days, (3) No current or past diseases affecting the ovaries or gonadotrophin or sex steroid section, clearance, or excretion, (4) No clinical signs of hyperandrogenism, (5) Body Mass Indexes ranging from 18 to 25kg/m^2, (6) No current hormone therapy, (7) Adequate visualization of both ovaries in transvaginal ultrasound scans. Informed consent was obtained from all patients and this investigation was approved by our internal Institutional Review Board.

2.1 IVF treatment

Patients were treated with a time-release GnRH agonist from day 2 of menses (Day2). On Day 3, complete pituitary desensitization was confirmed by the detection of low serum levels of E_2 and gonadotrophins. Patients also underwent a conventional ultrasound examination to exclude ovarian cysts and to verify that the endometrium was <5mm. Recombinant FSH therapy (recombinant Follitropin beta) or HMG was then initiated at a dose of 150 IU/day, while daily Gn-RH agonist administration was continued until the day of administration of hCG at 10,000 IU dose.

2.2 AMH

Blood was sampled between days 1 to 16 of menses (Day 1 to 16) from women undergoing IVF treatment. Follicular fluid was obtained from the follicles at Day 14. Blood and follicle fluid were centrifuged at 3,000 bpm/min for 10 minutes, and then stored at -20°C until immunoassay. Serum AMH (S-AMH) levels were assessed using enzyme immunoassay AMH/MIS-EIA (IMMUNOTECH A BECKMAN COULTER COMPANY). Recombinant human AMH was used as a calibration standard to generate a standard curve (conversion factor to pmol/l=ng/ml×7.14).

2.3 3D ultrasound methods.

Ultrasound image sampling was performed on 28 patients undergoing IVF treatment from Day 1 to 16. All assessments were performed using a ultrasound machine and a four-dimensional 9MHz trans-vaginal probe. This provides visualization of the three orthogonal planes so that the central point of the follicle within the right ovary (RO) and the left ovary (LO) were consistent for all three images.

2.4 Sono AVC

The Sono AVC was activated when it had been correctly positioned and magnified. The setting of growth and separation within the software was maintained at a default value of mid for all follicle measurements. The Sono AVC identifies the follicle by giving it a specific color (Figure 1a) and provides automated measurements of the mean diameter (relaxed sphere diameter), maximum dimensions (x y z diameters) and volume (Figure 1b).

2.5 Virtual Organ Computer-aided (VOCAL) and 3D power Doppler volume histogram

3D power Doppler volume histogram was generated based on the VOCAL method. The stimulated ovary was used to measure each index of blood flow in vasculature and vessels per gray scale ratio in the ovary, resulting in the Vacularization Index (VI), Flow Index (FI) and Vascularization Flow Index (VFI). These indexes display on the volume histogram (Figure 2).

2.6 Statistical analysis

Student's *t*-test and Fisher's exact test were conducted using Stat View 5.0 (Abacus Concepts, Inc. Berkeley CA, 1996). Principal component analysis (PCA) and Receiver operating characteristic (ROC) curves were calculated using SPSS 17.0 (SPSS Japan Inc).

3. Results

This study population consisted of 28 patients. The age range was 25 to 44 years (under 35 years: n=6, 35-39 years: n=8, over 40 years: n=14), and the mean age was 36.74±5.88 years. Blood samples were obtained from each patient and 3D ultrasound examination was performed at Day 10.04±5.8 (range: 1 to16). The number of oocytes aspirated was 5.6±3.6 (range; 0 to 16), and the number of embryos generated was 3.3±2.8 (range: 0 to 11).

3.1 AMH

The mean S-AMH level was 0.47±0.125 ng/ml, and the level in the patient under 35 years of age undergoing IVF treatment (0.570±0.216 ng/ml) was significantly higher than that in patient over 40 years of age (0.377±.070 ng/ml; p=0.0003) (Figure 3a), and the mean S-AMH level which was 0.469± 0.181 ng/ml in 35 to 39 years of age. The relationship between the mean S-AMH levels and age of women undergoing IVF treatment was significant (r=0.459, p=0.0004. 95%CI: -0.23 to 0.07) (Figure 3b). These results show that S-AMH levels reduced with the increasing age of women undergoing IVF.

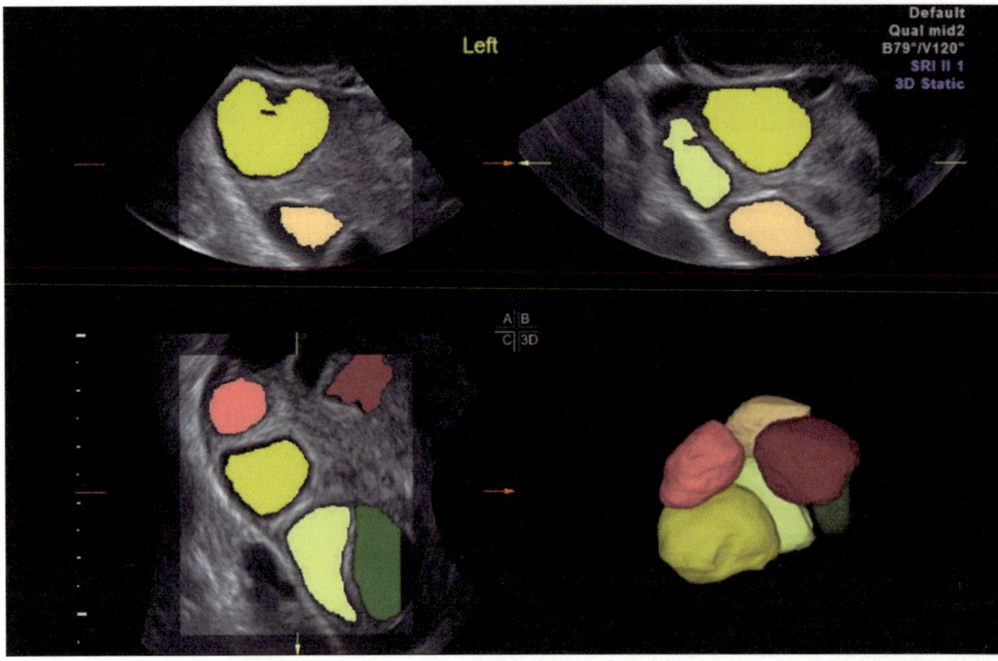

(a)

LMP 2008/10/01 | Day of Cycle 12 | Gravida | AB
Day of stim. | Expected Ovul. | Para | Ectopic

Ovary: Left
Total#: 9

Nr.	d(V) mm	dx mm	dy mm	dz mm	mn. d mm	V cm^3
1	18.9	25.2	20.2	14.6	20.0	3.55
2	18.0	20.3	18.2	16.8	18.4	3.07
3	17.5	30.4	15.9	13.6	20.0	2.82
4	16.0	26.4	16.1	12.1	18.2	2.16
5	15.8	20.9	16.3	12.1	16.4	2.07
6	15.8	22.3	19.5	10.1	17.3	2.07
7	14.7	18.4	15.9	11.6	15.3	1.66
8	12.9	19.0	15.1	9.5	14.5	1.14
9	8.7	13.0	8.3	6.8	9.4	0.35

Ovary: Right
Total#: 9

Nr.	d(V) mm	dx mm	dy mm	dz mm	mn. d mm	V cm^3
1	18.9	25.2	20.2	14.6	20.0	3.55
2	18.0	20.3	18.2	16.8	18.4	3.07
3	17.5	30.4	15.9	13.6	20.0	2.82
4	16.0	26.4	16.1	12.1	18.2	2.16
5	15.8	20.9	16.4	12.1	16.4	2.07
6	15.8	22.3	19.5	10.1	17.3	2.07
7	14.7	18.4	15.9	11.6	15.3	1.66
8	12.9	19.0	15.1	9.5	14.5	1.14
9	8.7	13.0	8.3	6.8	9.4	0.35

Pelvic Floor

funneling yes no
urethral kinking yes no

(b)

1a The Sono AVC identifies the follicle by giving it a specific color
1b many follicles automatically were measured that displayed report on monitor

Fig. 1. Automatic volume calculation (Sono AVC) was used to automatically calculate the volume of the follicle.

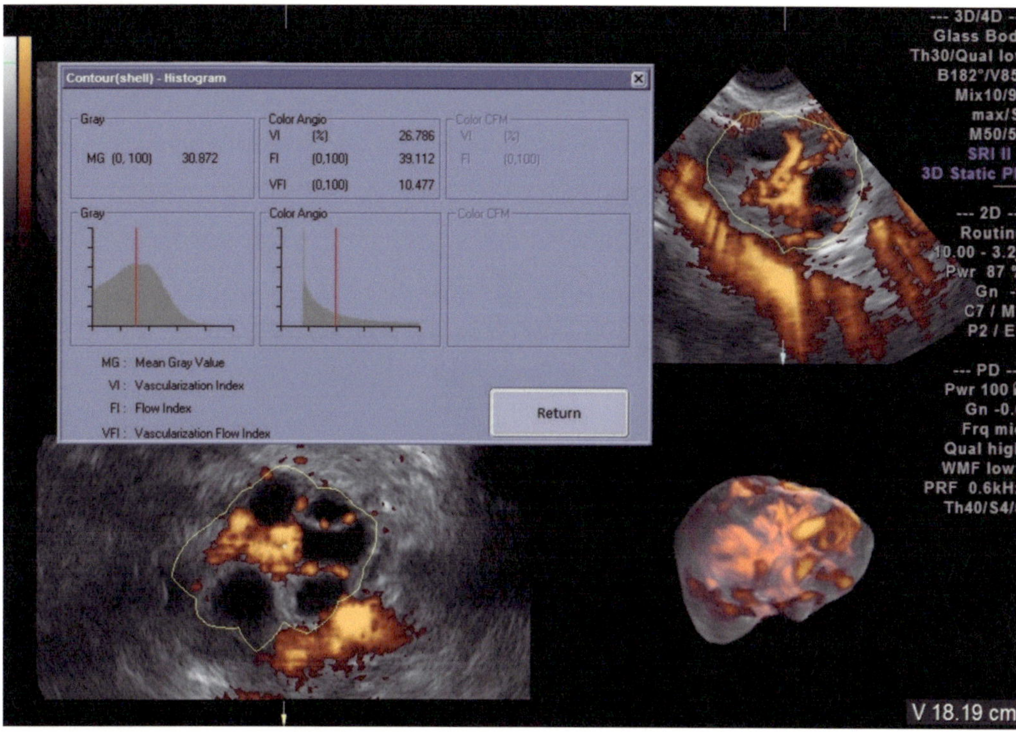

Three-dimensional power Doppler histogram was used to determine the vascular and blood flow, Vascularization indices (VI; vascularization index, FI; flow idex, VFI; vascularization flow index) from computer algorithms.

Fig. 2. Three-dimensional power Doppler image around follicle in ovary.

3.2 3D ultrasound methods

3.2.1 Sono AVC

The mean number of follicles was 5.61±3.28 from the right ovary (range: 0 to 13) vs. 5.46±4.56 from the left ovary (range: 0 to 19). The mean volume of the right follicle was 0.6999±0.613 cm^3 (range: 0.0 to 2.846; cm^3), and the mean volume of left follicle was 0.675±0.845 cm^3 (range: 0.0 to 3.220; cm^3).

3.2.2 3D-power Doppler Volume histogram

The mean FI of the RO and LO were 34.39±9.897 and 29.88±19.66%, respectively. The mean VI of the RO was significant higher LO (RO vs., LO; 7.61±1.121 vs., 3.30±0.679, p=0.013), and the mean VFI of the RO was high compare with LO (RO vs., LO; 2.37±0.337 vs., 0.776±0.844, p=0.024). The mean FI was no difference of index between RO and LO. 0.924) and decreased the S-AMH (oocyte 0.583, embryo 0.647).

3.2.3 The ROC curve

In the embryo, the cut-off value for the S-AMH was 0.2855 ng/ml (AUC; 0.56, sensitivity, 83.3%. specificity, 92.9%; 95% CI, 0.268 to 0.851) (Figure 4a) and the optimum cut-off point

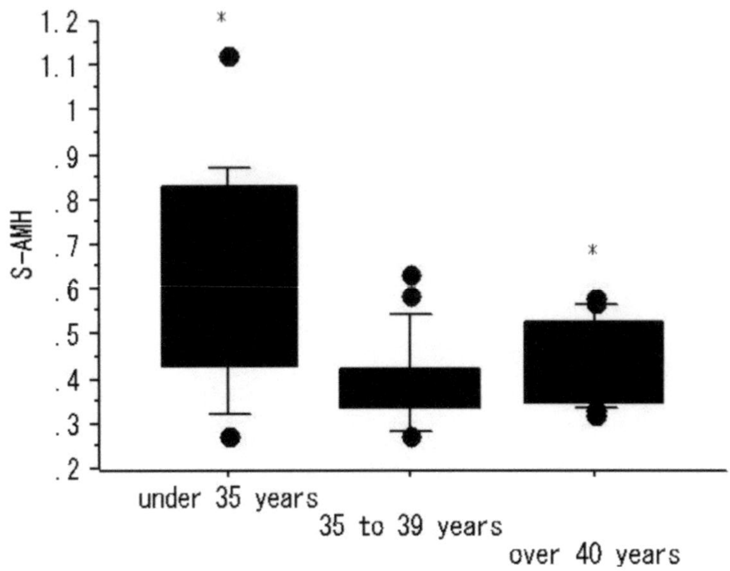

(a)

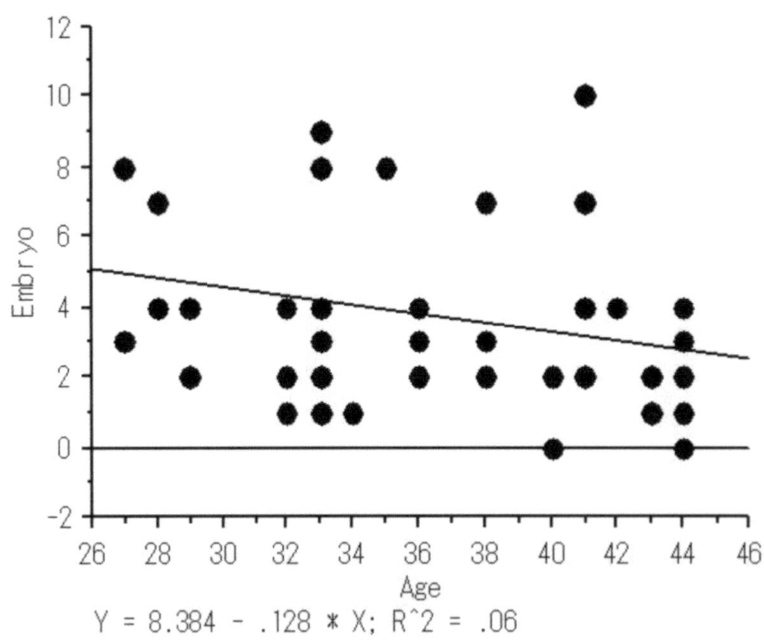

(b)

3a Under 35 years of age of patient (0.47±0.125) was significantly higher than over 40 years of patient (0.377±.070) (p=00003). 35 to39 years of age was 0.570±0.216 ng/ml.
*p<0.05compared to three different group by Fisher's exact test
3b Serum-AMH level corrected for age of patient undergoing *in vitro* fertilization treatment r=0.459, p=0.0004.295%CI: -0.23 to 0.07 by linear regression.

Fig. 3. Serum-AMH level (ng/ml) relation with age of patient undergoing *in vitro* fertilization treatment for the number of embryo was an age of 32.5 years (AUC; Sensitivity; 100%, Specificity; 52.6%, 95% CI 0.542 to 0.892) (Figure 4b).

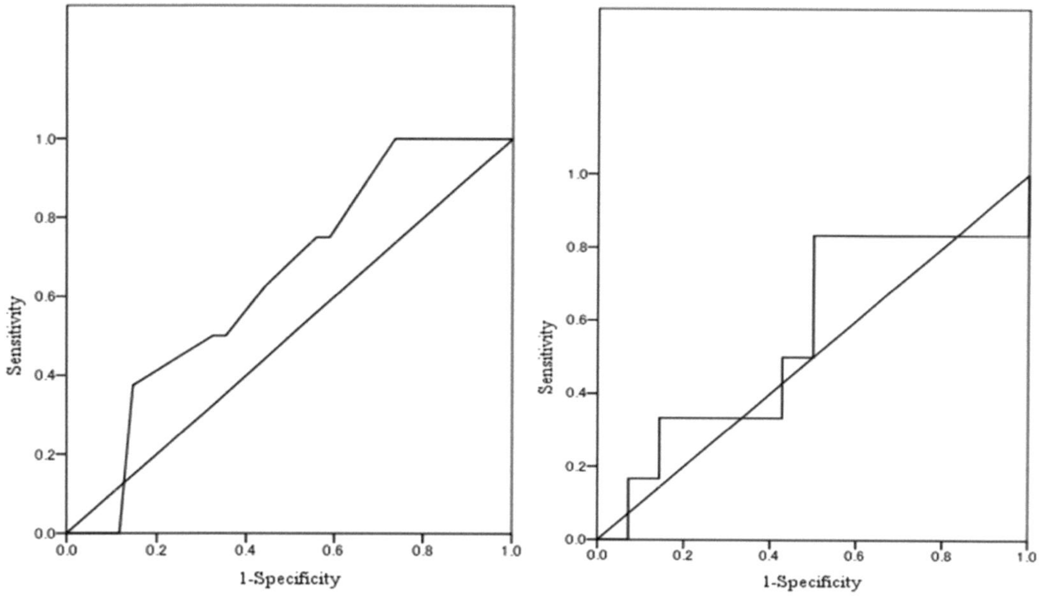

(a) (b)

4a ROC curve that Serum-AMH of cut -off value which took embryo relation with lime of age was 0.2855ng/ml (AUC 0.56. sensitivity, 83.3%. specificity, 92.6 %; 95% CI, 0.268-0.851) (Figure 5c).
4b ROC curve that embryos were taken for the lime of age was 32.5 years (AUC; 0.62, Sensitivity; 100%, Specificity; 52.6%, 95% CI 0.542 to 0.892) (Figure 5d).

Fig. 4. The Receiver-operating characteristic (ROC) curve indicate cut-off value.

4. Discussion

4.1 AMH

In this study, we investigated whether AMH and measurements could be useful markers of successful generation of embryos from patients undergoing IVF treatment, and examined the relationship with the embryo using 3D ultrasonography. We further tested the diagnostic performance of AMH and the age limit of patients undergoing IVF treatment on the number of embryos obtained, by ROC curves. These data led to the conclusion that AMH, Sono AVC and 3D-power Doppler histogram could provide the best available clinical markers of responsiveness to the ovarian stimulation. Our results indicate that AMH is suitable as an effectiveness factor, such as the generation of embryos with IVF treatment, by principal component analysis. We also found that the S-AMH cut-off value was 0.2855 ng/ml (AUC: 0.56. sensitivity, 83.3%. specificity, 92.9%; 95% CI, 0.268 to 0.851) in all cases and the optimum age cut-off was 32.5 years (AUC: 0.643. sensitivity, 100%. Specificity, 52.6%; 95% CI, 0.453 to 0.833). In 2007, Zappacosta et al. reported the Bland-Altman plot analysis (AxSYM Abbott) shows that the immunonephelometric method has a slight positive bias with both HPLC (mean: 1.03μmol/L, 95% confidence interval:0.28-1.79μmol/L) and AxSYM methods (mean: 0.45μmol/L, 95% confidence interval:-0.03-0.94μmol/L) AMH is a significantly correlated with ovarian response in IVF cycles. Indeed, linear regression analysis shows a significant association between AMH and the number of ovocytes collected [11]. AMH levels in women with correct ovarian response range from 0.63 ng/ml [12] to 0.67ng/ml [13]. Scott et al. demonstrated that a single measurement of circulating AMH can be used to individualize treatment strategies for IVF, potentially resulting in reduced clinical risk, along with optimized treatment burden, and clinical pregnancy rates, with the application of the Gn-RH antagonist protocol appearing to be advantageous for patients at the anticipated extremes of ovarian response [14]. In 2009, Singer et al. reported that the use of FSH and AMH in combination might improve the evaluation of ovarian reserve. However, it remains to be determined which of these two ovarian function parameters is superior in assessing ovarian reserve with a single test and which test, or combination of tests is most appropriate [5]. In our study, we did not demonstrate to determine FSH and AMH in combination, and the relationship between S-AMH and successful pregnancy, we think that the reasons which are the first, it is most important determine AMH level compare with FSH level, because FSH levels are effected of FSH stimulate ovarian function undergoing IVF treatment, and the second, likely pregnancy has many factors, including hormones, the immune-cytokine network and the developing syncytium of cells in the endometrium of the uterus. Therefore, the aim of our study was clearly distinct from these studies, as we assessed the combination of AMH and 3D ultrasound methods that automatically measure follicles and blood flow in ovaries during IVF treatment. Particularly, we indicated that the S-AMH relation with the age during IVF treatment from the limit of the S-AMH was 0.2855ng/ml and the number of embryos (≥2) with an optimum cut-off age of 32.5 years. We believe that these cut-off values are predictive of a poor response undergoing IVF treatment. Finally, it is nasally to analyze S-AMH levels and to consider age undergoing IVF treatment. Gnoth et al reported that cut-off that AMH is a predictor of ovarian response and is suitable for screening. A calculated cut-off level≤1.26ng/ml AMH alone detected poor responders (≤4 oocytes) with a sensitivity of 97%, and there was a 98% correct prediction of normal response to IVF treatment if levels were above this threshold. With levels of 0.5ng/ml, a correct prediction of very poor response (≤2 oocytes) was possible in 88% of cases. The Gnoth group report that AMH levels ≥0.5ng/ml did not correlate significantly with clinical pregnancy rates. Measurement of AMH supports clinical decisions, but alone it is not a suitable predictor of IVF success [15]. However, they did not report that a relationship between the cut-off level of serum AMH and the age limit of patient undergoing on the number of embryos obtained. Their level of AMH ≤1.26ng/ml (≤4 oocytes) was higher than our S-AMH level of 0.284ng/ml (oocytes=5; sensitivity, 83.3%. specificity, 92.9%; 95% CI, 0.268 to 0.851). The Gnoth group used a high dose of IVF compared with our dose of IVF treatment, and designated two groups of women; those who were under 35 years and from 35 to 39 years. We suggest that these differences of result occur in between the Gnoth group and our study that it might be due to the doses used during ovarian stimulation and design of group. Other hand, in this study, we showed that the mean FF-AMH level was 0.639±0.290 ng/ml, and there was no relationship between the FF-AMH level and age of women undergoing IVF treatment (r=0.102, p=0.007, 95%CI; -.024 to 0.025). Lee et al. reported that FF-AMH is a marker that reflects ovarian reserve and response to controlled ovarian hyperstimulation. But, FF-AMH levels did not correlate significantly with age, gonadotrophin dose, the number of follicles on the hCG day, and the number of oocytes retrieved [16]. It is interesting that the findings of the FF-AMH in Lee's study were different from our own; for example, the sample sizes were different between these investigations (our study vs. Lee's study; n=28 vs. n=87 patients). Second, the dosing protocols of IVF were different between these studies; Lee's study had two protocols, including the Gn-RH-a long protocol group (n=43,FF-AMH=1.8±0.4ng/ml), in which Gn-RH-a triptorelin (Decapeptyl, 0.1mg/d; Ferring, Malmo, Sweden) was started in the mid-luteal phase of the previous cycle. After pituitary down-regulation, the triptorelin dose was reduced to 0.05mg/dl, and recombinant FSH (Gonal-F; Serono, Genova, Switzerland) was added when two or more follicles reached a diameter of 17 mm, and the other protocol was the GnRH agonist multiple-dose flexible protocol (n=44, FF AMH=1.3±0.3), recombinant FSH (Gonal-F, Serono) was started on the 2nd and 3rd menstrual-cycle day without pretreatment with oral contraceptive [16]. However, our results possibility demonstrated that S-AMH levels exhibits a significant relationship between age of patient undergoing IVF and the successful developed embryos, compared with FF-AMH levels, in the form a protocol that implemented the GnRH agonist- a short protocol in this study.

4.2 3D ultrasound

The vascular indices determined by analysis of the 3D-power Doppler histogram represent the proportion of vascularized tissue (or vascularization index: VI), the amplitude of blood movement in the sampled tissue (or flow index: FI) and the proportion of vascularized and blood movement in the volumetric sample (or vascularization flow index: VFI) [17]. In a recent study, the VI, which was defined as the percentage of the power Doppler signal within a defined volume of interest, was suggested to be representative of the number of vessels in, or the vascularity of, the region of interest [18]. It is that characteristic of FI that is comprised of blood flow and attenuation factors, for example, the signal intensity is a direct consequence of the erythrocyte concentration [19], tissue motion [20], and machine settings [21]. Indeed, Dubiel et al. found in their flow phantom study that a four-fold increase in flow velocity only resulted in a 10% increase in FI. This, together with our data suggests that, despite the often-reported assumption, FI does not represent flow [22]. The 3D-power Doppler vascular indices provide a description of the amount and/or the movement of blood in a volumetric image (tissue). Therefore, vascularization and/or flow in the entire organ may not be represented by an individual tissue sample, or sampled tissues with different volumes will most likely present different vascular indices [20]. Jones et al. found using *in vitro* dual perfusion of human placental lobules, a predictable relationship between flow rates and the vascular indices, VI and VFI, however the FI was a less reliable predictor of flow; thus, it should be interpreted with caution [23]. Our results agree with the report by Jones et al. Furthermore, we explain that the results of FI are related to tissue motion and the specific techniques of each investigator. In the anatomy of the ovary, the ovarian artery, a branch of the aorta, courses along the infundibulopelvic ligament and the mesovarium border of the ovary, where it anastomoses with the ovarian branch of the uterine artery. Approximately 10 arterial branches arise from this arcade and penetrate the ovarian hilus, becoming markedly coiled and branched as they course through the medulla. These helicine arteries have longitudinal ridges of intimal smooth muscle. At the corticomedullary junction, the medullary arteries and arterioles form a plexus, from which smaller, straight cortical arterioles arise and penetrate the cortex in a radial fashion, perpendicular to the ovarian surface. These cortical arterioles branch and anastomose several times, forming sets of interconnected vascular arcades. These arcades give rise to capillaries, which form dense networks within the theca layers of the ovarian follicles [24]. In conclusion, we automatically and quickly detected the number of follicles using Sono AVC, and vascularization around the follicles in the ovary by analysis of the 3D-power Doppler histograms. These results were expected to provide an indicator of ovarian function during IVF treatment. The S-AMH was related to the age of women undergoing COH, further investigations of the level of S-AMH which was necessary to confirm the cut-off level, and the VI might be parameter of vascularized formation around follicle in ovary using 3D-power Doppler histogram.

5. References

[1] Cate RL, Mattalino RJ, Hession C, Tizard R, Farber NM, Cheung A, et al. Isolation of the bovine and human genes for Mullerian inhibiting substance and expression of the human gene in animal cell. Cell. 1986; 45: 685-98.

[2] Josso N, Cate RL, Picard JY, Vigier B, di Clementa N, Wilson C, et al. Anti-Mullerian hormone:the jost factor. Recent Progress in Hormone Reserch. 1993; 48: 1-59

[3] Weenen C, Laven JS, Von Bergh AR, Cranfield M, Groome NP, Visser JA, et al. Anti-Mullerian hormone expression pattern in the human ovary:potential implications for initial and cyclic follicle recruitment. Molecular. Human Reproduction. 2004;10:77-83

[4] Burger HD, Dudley EC, Hopper JL, Groome N, Guthrie JR,Green A, Dennerstein L.Prospectively measured levels of serum follicle-stimulating hormone, estradiol, and the dimeric inhibins during the menopausal transition in a population-based cohort of wowen. Journal of Clinical Endocrinology and Metabolism. 1999;84: 4025-30.

[5] Singer T, Barad DH, Weghofer A, Gleicher N. Correlation of antimüllerian hormone and baseline follicle-stimulating hormone levels. Fertility and Sterility. 2009; 9: 2616-19.

[6] N Raine-Fenning, K. Jayaprakasan, J Clewes. Automated follicle tracking facilitates standardization and may improve work flow. Ultrasound Obstet Gynecol. 2007;30:1015-18.

[7] Wittmaack FM, Kreger DO, Blasco L, Tureck RW, Mastroianni L, Jr,Lessey BA. Effect of follicular size on oocyte retrieval, fertilization,collection. Fertility and Sterility.1994; 62: 1205-10.

[8] Raine-Fenning N, Jayaprakasan K, Chamberlain S, Devlin L, Priddle H, Johnson I. Automated measurements of follicle diameter: a chance to standardize? Fertil Steril. 2009; 91: 1469-72.

[9] Pairleitner H, Steiner H, Hasenoehrl G, Staudach A. Three-dimensional power Doppler sonography: imaging and quantifying blood flow and vascularization. Ultrasound Obstet Gynecol. 1999; 14: 139-43.

[10] S Talbi, A E Hamilton, K C Vo, S Tulac, M T Overgaard, C Doiou, et al. Molecular Phenotyping of Human Endometrium Distinguishes Menstrual Cycle Phase and

Underlying Biological Processes in Normo-Ovulatory Women. 2006; 147: 1097-1121.

[11] Bruno Z, Silvai P, Angelo M, Donata S, Mirca A, Silvoia F, et al. Analytical evaluation of new immunonephelometric method for homcytocyteine measurement. Clinica Chemica Acta. 2006; 375: 165-68.

[12] Nakhuda GS, Chu MC, Wang JG, Sauer MV, Lobo RA. Elevated serum mullerian-inhibiting substance may be a marker for ovarian hyperstimulation syndrome in normal women undergoing in vitro fertilization. Fertil Steril. 2006; 85: 1541-43.

[13] Ficicioglu C, Kutlu T, Baglam E, Bakacak Z.Early follicular antimüllerian hormone as an indicator of ovarian reserve. Fertil Steril. 2006; 85: 592-6.

[14] Scott M Nelson, Robin W Yates, Helen Lyall, Maybeth Jamieson, Isabel Traynor, Marco Gaudoin, et al. Anti-Möllerian hormone-based approach to controlled ovarian stimulation for assisted conception. Human Reproduction. 2009; 24: 867-75.

[15] Gnoth C, Schuring AN, Friol K, Tigges J, Mallmann P, Godehardt E. Relevance of anti-Möllerian hormone measurement in a routine IVF program. Hum Reprod. 2008; 23: 1359-65.

[16] Jung Ryeol Lee, Seok Hyun Kim, Sun Mie Kim, Byung Chul Jee, Seung-Yup Ku, Chang Suk Suh. Follicular Fluid anti-Möllerian hormone and inhibin B concentrations: comparison between gonadotropin-relesing hormone (GnRH) agonist and Groh antagonist cycles. Fertility and Sterility. 2008; 89: 860-67.

[17] C F S de Paula, R Ruano, J A D B Campos, M Zugaib. Quantitative Analysis of Placental Vasculature by Three-Dimensional Power Doppler Ultrasonography in Normal Pregnancies From 12 to 40 weeks of Gestation. Placenta. 2009; 30: 142-48.

[18] Guimaraes Filho H, da Costa L, Araujo Junior E, Nardozza L, Nowak P, Moron A, et al. Plasenta:angiogenesis and vascular assessment through three-dimensional power Doppler ultrasonography. Arch Gynecol Obstet. 2008; 277: 195-00.

[19] Rubin J, Adler R, Fowlkes J, Spratt S, Pallister J, Che J, et al. Fractional moving blood volume: estimation with power Doppler US. Radiology.1995; 197: 183-90.

[20] Preidler K, Szolar D, Uggowitzer M, Stiskal M, Horina J. Technical note:comparison of colour Doppler energy sonography with conventional colour Doppler sonography in detection of flow signal in peripheral renal transplant vessels. Br j Radiol. 1995; 68: 1103-05.

[21] Raine-Fenning N, Nordin N, Ramnarine K, Campbell B, Clewes J, Perkins A, et al.Evaluation of the effect of machine settings on quantitative three-dimensional power Doppler angiography: an in- vitro flow phantom experiment.Ultrasound Obstet Gynecol. 2008; 32: 551-59.

[22] Dubiel M, Hammid A, Breborowicz A, Pietryga M, Sladkevicius P, Olofsson P, et al. Flow index evaluation of 3-D volume flow image:an in vivo and in vitro study. Ulutrasound Med Biol. 2006; 32: 665-71.

[23] N.W.Jones, E.S.Hutchinson, P.Brownbill, I.P.Crocker, D.Eccles, G.J.Bugg, et al. In Vitro Dual Perfusion of Human Placenta Lobules as a Flow Phantom to Investigate the Relationship Between Fetoplasental Flow and Quantitative 3D Power Doppler Angiography. Plasenta. 2009; 30: 130-35.

[24] Philip B, Clement,M.D. Anatomy and Histology of the Ovary. In: Robert J kurman. Blaustein's Pathology of the Female Genital Tract. New York, Springer-Verlag;1994. P. 563-645.

13

Immunological Methods for the Detection of *Campylobacter* spp. – Current Applications and Potential Use in Biosensors

Omar A. Oyarzabal and Cynthia Battie
Alabama State University, Montgomery, Alabama and University of North Florida, Florida, USA

1. Introduction

The genus *Campylobacter* belongs to the epsilon division of the class Proteobacteria. This genus comprises a group of bacteria that occupy diverse habitats and produce a wide range of diseases in different animal hosts (On 2001). Campylobacteriosis is a self-limited gastrointestinal illness that produces diarrhea, fever and abdominal cramps, and antimicrobial therapy is not generally indicated. However, treatment can reduce the duration and severity of illness if caught early, especially in those with the potential for severe illness, including infants, elderly, patients with underlying disease and immunocompromised individuals. In addition to acute enteritis, campylobacteriosis may result in reactive arthritis and Guillain-Barre syndrome (Hannu et al., 2002; Rees et al., 1995). The epidemiology of campylobacteriosis is unique in that most infections are sporadic. Meats, especially undercooked broiler chicken, are the main source of sporadic campylobacteriosis cases, while outbreaks are usually associated with the consumption of raw milk or unchlorinated water (Skirrow 1991). *Campylobacter* spp. are one of the leading agents of bacterial foodborne diseases worldwide (EFSA 2005, 2006). In the USA, there are approximately 12 reported cases per 100,000 persons per year, although the actual number has been estimated at 432 cases per 100,000 (Olson et al., 2008; Samuel et al., 2004). *C. jejuni* is responsible for approximately 95% of the human cases, while *C. coli* is responsible for the rest of the infections. *C. concisus*, *C. fetus*, *C. upsaliensis* and other *Campylobacter* species can cause sporadic cases.

Current methods of identification of campylobacters in stool and food samples rely on their growth on selective agar plates with and without prior broth enrichment. These methods are labor intensive and time consuming, taking four or more days for completion and require robust bacterial growth, which may limit the detection of stressed bacteria that do not grow well but are still infective. More rapid and accurate methods are necessary to identify campylobacters in stool samples in order to treat campylobacteriosis early, and to detect outbreaks as campylobacteriosis is a notifiable disease in the USA. Moreover, rapid detection of campylobacters in environmental samples is important for trace-back investigations to mitigate outbreaks and in food samples to catch contamination during commercial food processing.

During the 1960s and early 1970s, the search for alternative techniques to replace radioactive label reporters to identify biological molecules led to the development of the enzyme-linked immunosorbent assay (ELISA or EIA; Engvall and Perlmann 1971). In the mid-1970s the, the development of the hybridoma technique for monoclonal antibody synthesis (Köhler & Milstein 1975) helped expand the new field of immunodiagnosis and initiate development of immunoassays for the identification of bacterial pathogens. Since then, a variety of immunoassays have been developed for the detection of different foodborne pathogens in food and stool samples, including a few immunoassays for *Campylobacter* spp. detection. The simplest is latex agglutination, in which antibody-coated colored latex beads or colloidal gold particles are used for rapid confirmation of culture results or serotyping of culture isolates. The EIA, the most popular immunoassay used for pathogen detection in foods and stool, is typically designed as a "sandwich" assay, in which an antibody bound to a solid matrix is used to capture the bacterium and a second antibody conjugated to an enzyme then binds to the bacterium. Multi-well microplates are a commonly used solid support but other formats include dipsticks, paddles, membranes, or other solid matrices.

The lateral flow immunochromatographic method is a modified EIA, packaged in a simple device (dipstick or within a plastic casing) and used for rapid pathogen detection. Typically, "sandwich" assays are used for large analytes such as bacteria. Samples migrate from the sample pad through a conjugate pad where the target analyte binds to the antibody conjugated to colored particles. The sample is drawn across the membrane to the capture zone where the target/conjugate complex binds to immobilized antibodies producing a visible line on the membrane. To ensure a working test, the sample migrates further until it reaches the control zone, where excess conjugate is bound to produce a second visible line on the membrane. Two clear lines on the membrane are a positive result. A single line in the control zone is a negative result. Lateral flow immunoassays have many advantages including their simplicity, production of a result within 15 minutes, stability with a long shelf life even in some cases without refrigeration and their low cost, but they may have a higher threshold of detection compared to EIA.

The present chapter reviews commercial and/or published immunological methods, mainly EIA and lateral flow immunoassays used to identify species of *Campylobacter* in food and stool samples. Methods that can be dovetailed with immunoassays to increase bacterial concentration and immunoassay detection, such as sample enrichment, sample filtration and immunomagnetic separation, are described. The strengths and limitations of immunoassays for identification of *Campylobacter* spp. are reviewed, along with suggestions to improve assay performance. The detection of *Campylobacter* spp. by antibody-based biosensors, primarily optical biosensors is also briefly discussed.

2. Identification of *Campylobacter* spp. using immunoassays

The presence of campylobacters in food and stool samples is based on the growth of the bacteria on a selective agar, incubated at 42°C under a reduced oxygen atmosphere (~5% O_2). The limitations of the culture method, especially the need for up to four days to identify campylobacters (Endtz 2000), have dictated the development of culture-independent methods, including immunoassays, for the detection of *Campylobacter* spp. in clinical stool and food samples. Although a variety of immunoassays have been developed for testing clinical and food samples for *Campylobacter* spp., these assays require approval by regulatory bodies, necessitating comparison of immunoassays to culture-based methods, considered the "reference methods." The validation of immunoassays for detection of *Campylobacter* spp. includes testing for **inclusivity**, to assure that different strains of *C. jejuni* and *C. coli* are detected, and **exclusivity**, to assure that closely related, non-target bacteria do not cross-react with the assay (Brunelle 2008). Other performance indicators used to validate assays include:

- Sensitivity: The probability that an assay will yield a positive result when the culture is positive by the reference method.
- Specificity: The probability that an assay will yield a negative result when the sample is negative by the reference method.
- Positive predictive value: The probability that a sample with a positive test contains the bacteria.
- Negative predictive value: The probability that a sample with a negative test does not contain the bacteria.

In the following sections, commercial immunoassays available to detect *Campylobacter* spp. in stool and food samples will be described.

2.1 Clinical stool samples

Several commercial immunological assays are available for identification of *C. jejuni* and *C. coli* in stool samples, including some designed to confirm culture results and others that are culture-independent. Assay formats include latex agglutination, EIAs, and lateral flow formats. Immunoassays based on latex agglutination, developed in the late 1980s, are of limited use because they can only confirm culture results, and may detect closely-related organisms (Haymann 2004). Several EIAs are commercially available for use directly with clinical stool samples, and in some studies have performed as good or better than the standard culture techniques for detecting *C. jejuni* and *C. coli*, and possibly *C. upsaliensis*, and are comparable to nucleic acid tests (Abubakar et al., 2007) but not in all cases. Of the four EIAs commercially available in the USA for direct detection of *Campylobacter* in stool specimens, two are microplate-based and two are incorporated in lateral flow devices (Table 1). These methods are reasonably rapid, from 20 minutes for the lateral flow assays to2-4 h for the microplate assays, and identify specific *Campylobacter* antigens common to *C. jejuni* and *C. coli*.

The ProSpecT™ Campylobacter assay (Remel Inc., Lenexa, KS), a microplate sandwich EIA that uses a polyclonal antibody conjugated to horseradish peroxidase for the detection of common antigen of *C. jejuni* and *C. coli* in fecal specimens and enriched fecal cultures, has received the most scrutiny. The results are read visually or spectrophotometrically, and the analytical sensitivity is approximately 10^{5-6} colony forming units (CFU) per ml^{-1}. The test is accurate for samples stored at 4°C for several days (Dediste et al., 2003; Tolcin et al., 2000). No cross-reactivity with other major fecal bacteria or with other *Campylobacter* spp., including *C. lari* and *C. fetus*, has been identified (Endtz et al., 2000; Hindiyeh et al., 2000). The manufacturer's studies, using three sites in the USA and Canada, demonstrated a pooled sensitivity of 97-100% and specificity of 98-100% using 1,049 stool samples (Table 1). A meta-analysis of the clinical utility of the ProSpecT assay in relationship to standard culture-based methods (Abubakar et al., 2007) included four studies (Dediste et al., 2003;

Endtz et al., 2000; Hindiyeh et al., 2000; Tolcin et al., 2000) that were chosen using QUADAS, an evidence-based tool for the quality assessment of diagnostic studies (Whiting et al., 2003) (Table 1). For the pooled samples (n=2078), the specificity was 98% (95% CI: 89-100%) while the sensitivity was 89% (95% CI: 81-98%). Although the number of false positives was low,

Test Name	Sample Size (% Positive)	Sensitivity (95% CI)	Specificity (95% CI)	Positive Predictive Value	Negative Predictive Value	Source
ProSpecT™ Campylobacter Microplate (Remel, Lenexa, KS)	1049	100 (97-100)	99 (98-100)	-	-	Manufacturer
	164 (30%)	96 (87-99)	99 (95-100)	9	98	Tolcin et al., 2000
	78 (38%)	80 (62-91)	100 (93-100)	100 -	89 -	Endtz et al., 2000
	631 (3%)	89 (67-97)	99 (98-100)	80	99	Hindiyeh et al., 2000
	1205 (8.4%)	89 (82-94)	98 (97-99)	78 -	99 -	Dediste et al., 2003
	182 (34%)	95 (88-98)	94 (84-98)	96 (90, 99)	91 (81,96)	Tribble et al., 2008
	485	99	96	90	99.7	Granato et al., 2010
ImmunoCard STAT!® CAMPY (Meridian Bioscience, Inc., Cincinnati, OH)	420	98 (90-100)	95.9 (93-98)	-	-	Manufacturer
	485	98	94	89.4	99.7	Granato et al., 2010
	242 (9.5%)	90	-	70	-	Bessede et al., 2011
Premier CAMPY EIA (Meridian Bioscience)	2073	97 (89-99)	96 (95-96)	-	-	Manufacturer
	485(6%)	99.2	96	90	99.7	Granato et al., 2010*
	242 (9.5%)	90-95	-	~80	-	Bessede et al., 2011
RIDASCREEN® (R-Biopharm, Darmstadt, Germany)	259	100	99.6	93	100	Manufacturer
	1050 (9.3%)	69	87	36	97	Tissari et al., 2007
	242 (9.5%)	90	-	~89	-	Bessede et al., 2011

Table 1. Performance of selected, commercial kits for direct detection of *C. jejuni* and *C. coli* in stool samples

the positive predictive values ranged from 78-100%, indicating a possible unacceptable number of false negative results especially when screening samples with a low level of contamination. Indeed, a later study showed that when a population has high prevalence of campylobacteriosis, the ProSpecT EIA is sensitive and specific (Tribble et al., 2008). In another study, culture-based methods were less sensitive than PCR and the ProSpecT assay (Granato et al., 2010).

The PREMIER™ CAMPY microplate EIA (Meridian Bioscience, Inc, Cincinnati, OH) uses a monoclonal antibody that binds to an unspecified common antigen of *C. jejuni* and *C. coli*. The limit of detection is 10^{6-7} CFU per ml^{-1}, and according to the manufacturer's literature, this assay had a sensitivity of 97% and specificity of 96% in a study of 2,073 samples (Table 1). High specificity and sensitivity for this EIA were reported by Granato et al. (2010). Another microplate EIA, Ridascreen Campylobacter (R-Biopharm AG, Germany), also uses monoclonal antibodies but does not appear to perform as well as the manufacturer's claims (Bessede et al., 2011; Tissari et al., 2007). The lateral flow assay, ImmunoCard STAT! CAMPY (Meridian Bioscience, Inc.), uses the same monoclonal antibody as the PREMIER CAMPY assay. The capturing of the target bacteria is by an antibody colloidal complex and the assay has similar specificity to the EIA assays, but with a sensitivity of 10^7 CFU per ml^{-1} (Bessede et al., 2011; Granato et al., 2010). The Xpect *Campylobacter* assay (Remel Inc.) is a rapid assay equivalent to the ImmunoCard STAT! CAMPY assay, but preliminary results suggest that it has poor sensitivity (Fitzgerald et al., 2011).

Currently, none of the described assays can be recommended for standalone identification of campylobacters in stool samples, in part because of the limited and conflicting findings regarding the performance of these immunoassays. The performance of these EIAs is variable and suggests a high probability of non-acceptable levels of false negatives in certain situations. The Centers for Disease Control and Prevention (CDC) has recently released preliminary data concluding that EIAs should not be used as standalone tests for direct detection of *Campylobacter* in stool samples. This study investigated 2,767 stool samples with a positive *Campylobacter* prevalence of approximately 3%. Although the specificity and negative predictive values in these tests were excellent, typically >95%, the sensitivities and positive predictive values (PPV) of the four EIAs were not acceptable. For example, the ProSpecT™ Campylobacter assay exhibited a sensitivity of 84% and a PPV of 56%, the PREMIER™ CAMPY assay exhibited a sensitivity of 83% and a PPV of 52%, the ImmunoCard STAT! CAMPY exhibited a sensitivity of 73% and a PPV of 39%, and the Xpect *Campylobacter* assay exhibited a sensitivity of 74% and a PPV of 80%. Therefore, a positive EIA test alone is not sufficient to consider a case "confirmed" and laboratories must confirm positive EIA results by culture methods (Fitzgerald et al., 2011). The basis for discordant results between culture, immunoassay and PCR-based methods needs to be determined.

It is not clear whether the poor performance of these EIAs is inherent in the assays themselves or is due to lack of optimization. The fact that variations appear to be dependent on the test format and manufacturer suggests that these assays could be improved (See Section 4). A limitation for the adoption of EIAs is the prohibitive cost of adopting these rapid tests in combination with routine culture methods (Abubakar et al., 2007).

2.2 Food samples

Current identification methods for *Campylobacter* in foods rely on bacterial growth on one of a variety of selective agar plates which contain antimicrobials to allow for the growth of the target organism, a method adapted from that used for stool samples (Corry et al., 1995). To achieve the required sensitivity of 1 cell per 25 g food, a 25 g food sample is typically enriched in a broth with selective agents to inhibit the growth of competing bacteria while allowing growth of the target organism before plating on selective agar (Oyarzabal 2005; Oyarzabal et al., 2007). Besides increasing bacterial concentration, enrichment is important because campylobacters are randomly distributed and can be present in clumps or aggregates in foods, limiting direct detection. Also, enrichment ensures that stressed or injured bacteria have a chance to recover prior to plating on selective agars. Culture-based methods are the accepted methods outlined in the Food and Drug Administration (FDA)'s Bacteriological Analytical Manual (BAM), the Microbiology Laboratory Guidebook (MLG) of the Food Safety and Inspection Services of the U.S. Department of Agriculture (FSIS USDA) and the International Organization for Standardization (ISO).

These culture-based methods for food screening suffer from the same constraints as those for stool samples: low specificity resulting in false positives, and long lag-time for results (Josefsen et al., 2011). Until recently, the lack of active surveillance and regulatory efforts to control *Campylobacter* spp. in poultry meat, a common vehicle for these pathogens (FSIS USDA 2009a), delayed the development of rapid methods. However, a new performance standard aimed at limiting the prevalence of *Campylobacter*-contaminated poultry meat products in the USA requires the screening of processed carcasses for the presence of this pathogen (FSIS USDA 2009b). Thus, there is a critical need to develop and validate rapid methods for *Campylobacter* identification, including those that are antibody-based.

Although antibody-based methods would speed assay time, only a few latex agglutination assays are included in reference manuals and only for confirmation of positive *Campylobacter* isolates. The FDA's BAM (Hunt et al., 2001), suggests the use of Dryspot *Campylobacter* Test (Oxoid, Basingstoke, Hampshire, England) or Alert for *Campylobacter* (Neogen Corporation, Lansing, MI), but neither are available. The MLG of the FSIS USDA recommends the use of Campy (jcl) (Scimedx Corp., Denville, NJ) or Microgen *Campylobacter* Rapid Test (Microbiology International, Frederick, MD) for confirmation of presumptive isolates (MLG 2011). Commercial EIAs are available for culture-independent identification of campylobacters in food, but these assays have not been extensively validated. Typically applied to enriched cultures, these EIAs reduce assay time and may perform with equal specificity as culture methods, albeit with a sensitivity > 10^4 CFU per ml^{-1}, which is not an improvement over culture methods (Josefsen et al., 2011). Presently, a positive result by a rapid method is only regarded as a presumptive result and must be confirmed by a standard method (Hunt et al., 2001; ISO 2006; MLG 2011). The next paragraphs describe the most common commercial EIAs used with food samples.

The VIDAS/MiniVIDAS CAM (bioMerieux, Hazelwood, MO), an automated EIA for detection of thermotolerant *C. jejuni, C. coli* and C. *lari*, has received the most attention over the last decade. In this assay, food or stool samples are incubated in an enrichment broth for 48 h. After enrichment, samples are boiled for 15 minutes and aliquots are analyzed by an automated enzyme immunoanalyzer. The few published studies indicate that this method performs similarly to culture methods for the identification of naturally occurring

Campylobacter spp. in foods. Hoorfar et al. (1999) found that the MiniVIDAS CAM may provide a faster method for fecal samples from cattle and pigs with the capability of rapid screening of a large number of samples. The reported sensitivity of this assay ranged from 88-94%, which may not be adequate for screening samples with low numbers of *Campylobacter* spp. However, authors used a lower enrichment time (24 h) compared to the manufacturer's recommendation (48 h).

Borck et al. (2002) compared the MiniVIDAS and the EIAFoss, an automated EIA which is no longer available, to culture methods for the identification of *Campylobacter* spp. The reported sensitivity for both EIA assays was higher than the sensitivity of selective agar plates for a variety of turkey meat and turkey fecal samples, but sensitivity varied as a function of sample and enrichment broth. The MiniVIDAS exhibited a sensitivity of approximately 94% for fecal samples with high bacterial loads and 65% for environmental samples with lower bacterial loads, and each methods had a specificity above 93%. Paulsen et el. (2005) has also indicated that the MiniVIDAS is as good as the standard method, with a sensitivity of 97.6% and a reduction in assay time by 24 h for chilled and frozen meat. In this study, Bolton enrichment broth in modified stomacher bags was better than Preston broth for enrichment prior to immunoassay. The MiniVIDAS CAM method has been successful for the detection of *Campylobacter* spp. in tissue samples (tonsils and lymph nodes) and fecal material from pigs during processing (Nesbakken et al., 2003), in a variety of chicken parts with positive results confirmed by culture methods (Reiter et al., 2005), and in artificially-contaminated ground beef and fresh cut vegetables (Chon et al., 2011). Our experiences (OAO) with the MiniVIDAS for screening poultry meat are in accordance with the majority of reports mentioned above. However, the enrichment of the samples for 48 h is indispensable to reduce the high number of false negative samples that otherwise will be encountered (Liu et al., 2009).

Other commercial immunoassays have received less scrutiny than the MiniVIDAS CAM. The TECRA Campylobacter Visual Immunoassay (3M, St. Paul, MN) for *C. jejuni* and *C. coli* employs a 40-h aerobic enrichment in a proprietary broth followed by a 2-h EIA. For 398 broiler carcass rinses from 19 processing plants, TECRA found 317 *Campylobacter* positives, four false positives and 22 false negatives, compared to 48 false negatives with the reference method (Bailey et al., 2008). All these false negatives came from rinses of carcasses collected toward the end of the production process, suggesting that severely injured campylobacters may not recover well in the TECRA enrichment broth. In another study, the TECRA VIA was less sensitive than a PCR method for detection of campylobacters in spiked raw and processed meat and poultry, but performed similarly or better than traditional culture media (Bohaychuk 2005). The low number of false negatives indicates that the TECRA VIA may be a viable screening tool as long as follow-up tests are performed on presumptive positive samples to rule out false positives. Unfortunately, no literature was found describing the antibody target and improvements might be possible with a better choice of antibody because, in the same study, an immunoassay outperformed PCR for detection of *Salmonella*.

Two other commercially available assays for rapid testing of food samples are the Singlepath™ *Campylobacter* microwell sandwich EIA (Merck KGaA, Germany) and the NH Immunochromato *Campylobacter* (Cosmo Bio Co., Tokyo, Japan). The Singlepath was comparable to standard culture methods in a preliminary study with artificially-inoculated meat (Hochel et al., 2004). The NH Immunochromato *Campylobacter* is a two-step enrichment assay using immunochromatographic identification with a reported sensitivity of 55 CFU per 25 g of spiked chicken meat for non-freezer stressed samples. Freezing samples decreased the sensitivity approximately 10-folds (Kawatsu et al., 2010).

Based upon the studies described above, commercial immunoassays show promise as one of the tools to speed food sample screening. However, more studies of these assays with naturally-contaminated samples from a variety of foods is necessary. The effect of bacterial stress that occurs during food processing and storage on assay performance should also be studied. Additionally, the antigen targets of the antibodies used in these assays need to be identified. A concerted effort to improve the performance of these assays should be undertaken now that a new standard for food screening poultry meat for *Campylobacter* spp. has been established in the USA.

3. Increasing concentration of campylobacters prior to immunoassay identification

Because EIA assays have a sensitivity of $\geq 10^4$ CFU per ml^{-1} or g^{-1}, there is a need to increase the number of the target organisms in food samples prior to assay. The enrichment of the sample is the most common method to increase the number of bacterial cells. No enrichment protocol is 100% selective for the organism of concern; therefore other methods are used to separate or concentrate the target bacteria from the rest of the contaminants. This section will review enrichment broths, filtration, and immunomagnetic separation as techniques to increase the number of *Campylobacter* spp. in the food samples prior to identification by EIA.

3.1 Enrichment of the samples

The enrichment of food samples is imperative for the isolation of *Campylobacter* spp. from poultry or raw milk products. The most commonly used enrichment broth is Bolton broth, which has a basal component made up of meat peptone, lactalbumin hydrolysate, yeast extract, alphaketoglutaric acid, ssodium chloride, sodium pyruvate, metabisulphite and carbonate. The use of buffered peptone water performs similarly to Bolton broth for the isolation *Campylobacter* spp., suggesting that the basal medium does not need to be rich in nutrients to support the growth and multiplication of *Campylobacter* spp. (Oyarzabal et al., 2007). An important requirement is the incubation of food samples for at least 48 h in enrichment broth before identification of positive cultures by immunoassay because 24 h incubation results in a high number of false negative samples (Liu et al., 2009).

The antimicrobials added to the basal broth are cefoperazone, trimethoprim and vancomycin, at concentrations of 20 mg per L^{-1} each, and cycloheximide, at a concentration of 50 mg per L^{-1}. Originally, Bolton broth was supplemented with 5% lysed horse blood, but research has shown that the addition of blood is not necessary for isolation of *Campylobacter* spp. from retail broiler meat. Most importantly, blood in the enrichment broth is not necessary if an EIA-based method is employed to detect positive samples (Liu et al., 2009). In the laboratory of one of the authors (OAO), a modification of Bolton broth was made by reducing the antimicrobials added to enrichment and plate media to only cefoperazone, at a concentration of 32 mg per L^{-1}, and amphotericin B at a concentration of 2 to 10 mg per L^{-1} (Liu et al., 2009; Zhou et al., 2011). Although this reduction of antimicrobials may allow for contaminants to grow, we control those contaminants by filtration prior to assay.

3.2 Use of filter membranes to separate contaminating bacteria

Filter membranes were used for the first isolation of *C. jejuni* from human stools (Dekeyser et al., 1972). In this report, the use of 0.65-μm filters was aimed at retaining most of the contaminating bacteria in fecal suspensions while allowing *Campylobacter* organisms to pass through the filter for isolation on agar plates. This differential filtration is different from most of the other filtration protocols in which the target organisms are concentrated by filter retention for subsequent identification. A search for different agar plates with more antimicrobials to control contaminants was initiated in the 1970s and by the early 1990s the filters were not used anymore, except for the isolation of less-known species of *Campylobacter* by Albert Lastovica using the Cape Town protocol (Le Roux & Lastovica 1998; Lastovica & Le Roux 2003). Although filters may not help isolate *Campylobacter* spp. from samples with low number of cells such as water samples (Diergaardt et al., 2003), filters help isolate *Campylobacter* spp. from highly contaminated samples. In enriched samples, the high motility of *Campylobacter* spp. allows for a relatively low number of cells to go through membrane filters and grow as pure colonies on plate media. Thus, filters are highly sensitive for the isolation of naturally occurring *Campylobacter* spp. present on retail broiler meat (Speegle et al., 2009).

A filtration method coupled with a sandwich EIA that uses polymyxin B sulfate (PMB) instead of an antibody to capture *C. jejuni* and *C. coli* was developed by one of the authors (CAB). PMB is used to capture Gram-negative bacteria for EIA detection of *Escherichia coli* and *Salmonella* in a variety of foods (Blais 2005, 2006). PMB binds to lipid A of the lipooligosaccharide (LOS) layer and improves bacterial capture, although treatment of bacteria with zwitterionic detergents is necessary (Blais 2005, 2006; Brooks et al., 1998). In our experiments, various surface waters and tap water were filter sterilized prior to use, and samples of each were spiked with concentrations of 0 to 10^4 CFU ml^{-1} of *Campylobacter* cells. Aliquots (500 ml) were filtered using a conventional EPA filter system with Microfil V 0.2 μm filters and then filters were added to 1 ml phosphate-buffered saline containing CHAPS detergent (3-[(3-cholamidopropyl dimethylammonio]-1-propanesulfonate) with 1-2 minute vortexing. Aliquots of 100 μl were assayed in the PMB-capture ELISA. Sampling (100 μl) of the 500 ml prior to filtration did not yield values above background. Thus, filter concentration coupled with PMB-capture ELISA was able to detect 10^2 CFUml^{-1}, compared to the typical threshold of $10^{4\text{-}5}$ CFU per ml^{-1}, although the net fluorescence intensity was much lower for ocean water (Fig. 1).

3.3 Concentration by immunomagnetic separation

Immunomagnetic separation utilizes magnetic spheres, such as Dynabeads™ (Dynal Biotech), coated with antibodies to capture target bacteria from a variety of matrices. Antibody-bound target cells are separated from the matrix and other bacteria by application of a magnetic field. However, pre-enrichment may still be necessary to obtain a high number of bacteria for detection. Immunocapture followed by plating on selective agar had a threshold of 10^4 CFU per g^{-1} for the detection of *Campylobacter* in ground poultry meat (Yu et al., 2001). The sensitivity did not improve when magnetic beads (Dynabeads™) were coated with a monoclonal antibody to the major 45 KDa porin and coupled with a DNA hybridization assay specific for the 23S rRNA gene of *Campylobacter* spp. (Lamoureux et al., 1997).

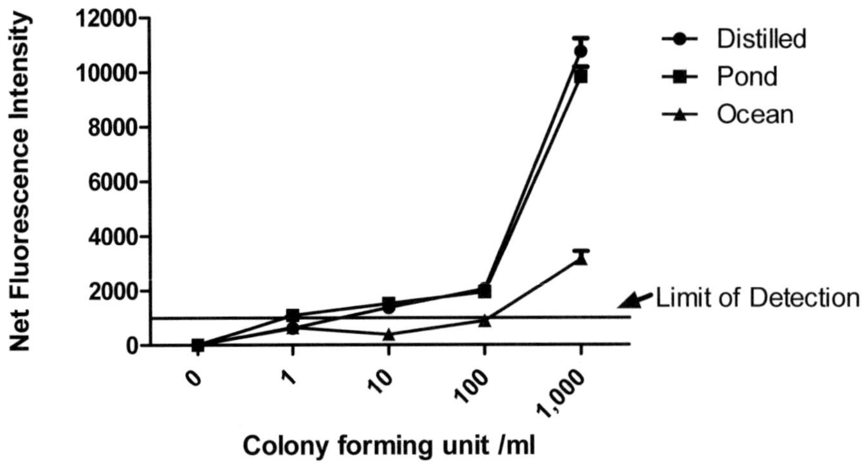

Fig. 1. Capture of *C. jejuni* on Microfil V filters prior to polymyxin B EIA detection. Various water source samples (500 ml) were spiked with different concentrations of *C. jejuni* and then filtered. Net fluorescence intensity was obtained by subtraction of background. Means ± standard error of the means (n= 6 replicates) are plotted as a function of original bacterial concentration.

A modification of immunomagnetic capture uses multiplexed magnetic microspheres, fluorescence-coded microspheres coated with antibodies, to detect bacteria by flow cytometry (MagPlex® Microspheres, Luminex, Austin, TX). Although this technique allows for rapid, multiplexed assays, the desired limit of detection is still a challenge for a variety of food matrices (Kim et al., 2010).

4. Improving antibody-based methods for *Campylobacter* spp. detection

One of the limitations of antibody-based methods for detection of pathogenic bacteria is the high threshold of detection (~10^{4-6} CFUml^{-1}), which results in unacceptable numbers of false negative samples especially for foods (Hochel et al., 2007). The detection limit is not as problematic for rapid detection in stool samples due to the high concentration of campylobacters in fecal samples. As discussed above, bacterial concentrations can be increased to EIA-detectable levels in food, such as retail broiler meats, by broth enrichment of up to 48 h (Liu et al., 2009), although components of enrichment broths may reduce immunoassay sensitivity (Chon et al., 2011). Improvements in EIAs such as reducing background noise or increasing the amplitude of the detection signal can improve performance. Fluorescence-based signaling improves the detection threshold by at least an order of magnitude over colorimetric assays, and the use of biosensors may allow for more efficient signaling to improve sensitivity. If sample matrices reduce EIA performance by increasing background signal, a variety of polymers, such as polyvinylpyrrolidione (Nyquist-Battie 2004) and Biolipiduretm (http://www.biolipidure.com/) can reduce background noise thereby increasing the signal to noise ratio. Another factor that may improve immunoassay performance is the molecular structure of the antibodies. F(ab')$_2$ fragments, or single chain Fv recombinant antibodies because they are smaller resulting in less steric hindrance between antibody molecules, although this premise needs to be investigated.

A possible reason for the high rate of false negatives in EIAs used to detect *Campylobacter* spp. may be the choice of antibody (Hochel et al., 2007; Rice et al., 1996). Some antibodies may not be able to detect all strains of *C. jejuni* and *C. coli*. Antigenic variation is common for externally-exposed molecule, such as outer membrane proteins and LOS, which limits the inclusivity of generic antibodies (Logan & Trust, 1983; Taylor & Chang, 1987, Dubreuil et al., 1990; Hochel et al., 2004). Indeed, surface- exposed immunodominant molecules, such as flagellar proteins (Fernando 2007) and the O-antigen, undergo genetic drift to avoid immunological detection. An alternative target molecule is the core oligosaccharide of the LOS, which has been successfully targeted in EIA assays to detect *C. fetus* (Brooks 2002, 2004; Devenish 2005). High rates of continuous expression of the antigen is another important consideration, especially in *Campylobacter* cells that undergo stress during food production and processing. Detection of stressed bacteria by EIA has been shown to be reduced (Hahm & Bhunia 2006; Nyquist-Battie 2005). In this regard, the structure of the LOS, a target of many antibodies, may vary as a function of the temperature at which *Campylobacter* cells are grown (Semchenko et al., 2010). Thus, identifying stable surface-exposed molecules for detection of *C. jejuni* and *C. coli* could be an avenue to improve antibody-based detection of these pathogens.

Improvements in proteomics over the last decade have made the identification of surface molecules easier (Cordwell et al., 2008; Prokhorova et al., 2006). Once ideal surface molecules are identified, newer methods of antibody production, such as the use of recombinant proteins, peptide fragments or DNA plasmids as immunogens, should be explored. For example, identifying epitopes that are stable but specific for *C. jejuni* in FlaA protein could be undertaken (Fernando 2007), and then peptide fragments with these epitopic sequences could be used to generate antibodies. If an ideal molecular target cannot be identified, it may be necessary to use antibody cocktails to increase the inclusivity of immunoassays (Hochel et al., 2007; Rice et al., 1996).

4.1 Polyclonal versus monoclonal antibodies for *C. jejuni* and *C. coli* detection

Several polyclonal antibodies have been developed for the detection of *C. jejuni* and *C. coli*, but few have been thoroughly tested for the ability to identify most if not all strains. In one study, nine strains were screened using two commercial anti-*Campylobacter* antibodies, B6601R (Biodesign, Saco ME) and 01-92-93 (Kirkegaard and Perry Laboratories; KPL, Gathesburg, MD). Only the former antibody identified all nine *Campylobacter* strains (Wang et al., 2000). Recently, we screened polyclonal antibodies for detection of *C. jejuni* and *C. coli* using a non-sandwich indirect fluorescence ELISA. The KPL antibody 01-92-93, a rabbit anti-*Campylobacter jejuni* C1037-10 (US Biological B10), and C1037-14 (USB14) antibodies recognized all four strains of *C. coli* and all nine strains of *C. jejuni* with a limit of detection of approximately 10^6 CFU per ml^{-1} (unpublished results). The rabbit anti-*Campylobacter* spp. antibody 9-25B-PA (Cygnus Tech.) did not recognize all strains. Given the successful detection of a variety of *C. jejuni* and *C. coli* strains by the USB polyclonal antibodies and the need to determine useful antigenic targets, we performed Western blotting with two *C. jejuni* isolates (ADPH1608 and ADPH 1208, both human isolates). The USB antibodies did not bind to LOS epitopes, as Proteinase K digestion eliminated all bands. Next the surface proteins that are recognized by the USB antibodies were determined by biotinylating surface proteins of the bacteria using a non-membrane penetrant biotinylation agent, EZ-

Link Sulfo-NHS-LC-Biotin, at 5 mg per ml-1 for 1 h at room temperature, a modification of the method of Harding et al. (2007). Membrane proteins were extracted using two membrane protein isolation kits (G Bioscience Focus™ Membrane Protein Extraction kit and BioRad Ready Prep sequential extraction kit). Seven protein bands with the molecular weights of 73, 62, 43, 41, 35, 28, and 24 KDa were both biotinylated and recognized by the USB antibodies using both protein extraction kits. The molecular weight of these bands is similar to many proteins described previously as useful antibody targets for detection of campylobacters. A 62 KDa protein, possibly one of the flagellin proteins, has been mentioned as a useful by previous authors, target for campylobacter detection (Heo et al., 2009; Lu et al., 1997) and is one of the protein targets of the KPL polyclonal antibody (Rice et al., 1996). Lu et al. (1997) demonstrated that a monoclonal antibody to a62 KDa protein was able to detect campylobacters at concentrations of 10^5 CFU per ml^{-1} with great specificity. The 43 Kda protein is another protein that is recognized by *Campylobacter* antibodies such as the KPL antibody (Rice et al., 1996). This 43 KDa protein, bound by a monoclonal antibody developed after injecting mice with whole cell *C. coli,* was determined by MALDI-TOF mass spectrometry to be a major outer membrane protein (Qian et al., 2008a). This antibody was shown to bind to the cell surface using immunogold electron microscopy and detected 10^3 to 10^4 CFU ml^{-1}. A recombinant major outer membrane protein (43 KDa) was used to generate a monoclonal antibody that was specific for *C. jejuni* (Qian et al., 2008b). This antibody recognized an amino acid epitope which is 97% conserved but which is predicted to be exposed to the periplasm not the cell surface. The 28 KDa protein may correspond to PEB1, a surface exposed adhesion protein that is the basis of an ELISA kit (Pei et al., 1991). Antibodies to this protein were able to detect 35 *C. jejuni* and 15 *C. coli* isolates without cross-reactivity (Pei et al., 1991). Taken all together, the 62, 43, 28 KDa proteins may be useful target molecules for *Campylobacter* immunoassays and deserve further scrutiny.

Several monoclonal antibodies have been synthesized for *Campylobacter* detection. Monoclonal antibodies target a single epitope of an antigen, which may limit their use in detection of *Campylobacter* because the epitope may not be conserved across all *Campylobacter* species and strains (Rice et al., 1996), although they exhibit greater specificity than polyclonal antibodies (Velusamy et al., 2010). Indeed, Wang et al. (2000) reported a lack of success with the following monoclonal antibodies: 1744-9029 and 1744-9006 (Biogenesis Ltd, NH), MAB001 (Harlan Sera Lab, GB), and C65701M (Biodesign International, MD). Our experiences with different monoclonal antibodies (AbD Serotec monoclonal antibodies 1745-00, 1744-8508, 1744-9059, and 1744-9109; USB C1037-02A, C1037-04, and C1037-16) support the premise that monoclonal antibodies are not ideal for ELISA detection of *Campylobacter* spp. (data not published). In contrast, the monoclonal antibody to the 62 KDa protein, discussed above, was able to detect whole cells at concentrations of 10^5 CFU pe ml^{-1} with excellent specificity (Lu et al., 1997). Also the monoclonal antibody to the 43 KDa protein was specific for *C. coli,* bound to the cell surface, and detected 10^3 to 10^4 CFU per ml^{-1} (Qian et al., 2008a). However, it is not clear whether these antibodies bind to conserved epitopes expressed under different conditions.

4.2 Capture of *C. jejuni* and *C. coli* in EIAs

The retention of bacteria may be inefficient in EIAs without the use of a capture element such as an antibody as in sandwich EIAs (Hochel et al., 2007) and thus bacteria are typically captured by an antibody in commercial kits. The number of capture antibodies that attach to a microplate may be improved by using biotin-labelled antibodies that can attach to streptavidin coated plates. The use of microplates with bottom filters in conjunction with antibody-capture, such as multi-well filter plates (AcroWell, Pall Corp.), or hydrophobic grid membrane filters may improve capture of antibody-bacterial complexes (Tsai & Slavik 1994; Wang et al., 2000). Another approach is the colony-lift immunoassay. After bacterial colonies are grown on select agar plates, a membrane filter lifts bacteria from the plate for immunoassay. When coupled with an anti-goat polyclonal antibody, the assay was specific and detected all tests strains of *C. jejuni*, *C. coli* and *C. lari* in 18-28 h (Rice et al., 1996). However, field testing of this method has not been published to the best of our knowledge.

Novel capture molecules such as polymyxin B sulfate (PMB), which binds to lipid A of the LOS may improve bacterial capture. The limitation of this method is that treatment of bacteria with zwitterionic detergents is necessary (Blais 2005, 2006; Brooks et al., 1998). Fukuda et al. (2005) demonstrated that PMB capture was superior to antibody capture for detection of *Salmonella* in chicken. Our laboratory demonstrated that PMB-capture enhances ELISA detection of *C. jejuni* as indicated by a 10-fold improvement in the limits of detection with both the USB10 and USB14 antibodies (unpublished results). The PMB-capture ELISA with either of these antibodies detected 19 *C. jejuni* isolates obtained from a variety of sources, including human, pork, turkey and chicken. The minimum cell concentration yielding a positive assay signal was approximately 10^4-10^5 CFU per ml^{-1}, and fluorescence intensity values at 10^6 CFU per ml^{-1} were similar for all isolates with no discernable difference between the two USB antibodies (Fig. 2). The mean signal to noise ratios for the 19 isolates were 16 ± 1 (USB10) and 17±2 (USB14) at 10^6 CFU per ml^{-1}, while the signal to noise ratios for the other Gram-negative bacteria screened at 10^7 CFU per ml^{-1} were below 2.5 except for *H. pylori* (Table 2). Therefore, the assay is specific for *Campylobacter*.

5. Potential use of antibodies in biosensors

Antibodies have the potential to be used in biosensors for the detection of specific bacterial pathogens. Biosensors are defined as analytical devices that combine a bioreceptor, which is a biological or biologically derived element, with a physicochemical transducer (Turner & Newman 2005). The term *immunosensor* describes a sensor that uses antibodies as the sensing element. When antibodies are used in bisosensors, they are the bioreceptors, capturing or sensing elements, and therefore the advantages and limitations in sensitivity and specificity of traditional antibody-based detection methods apply to these biosensors.

The transducers in biosensors are the components in charge of converting the biorecognition event, which happens when antibodies associate to the antigen, into signal that can be quantified. Several different transducers have been developed. In general, transducers can be categorized into four groups: electrochemical, calorimetric, acoustic and optical (Jönsson & Scott 2005). Optical transducers can measure variables such as changes in temperature (thermometric transducers), pressure, flow, etc., and sensors based on optical transducers are called *optical sensors*.

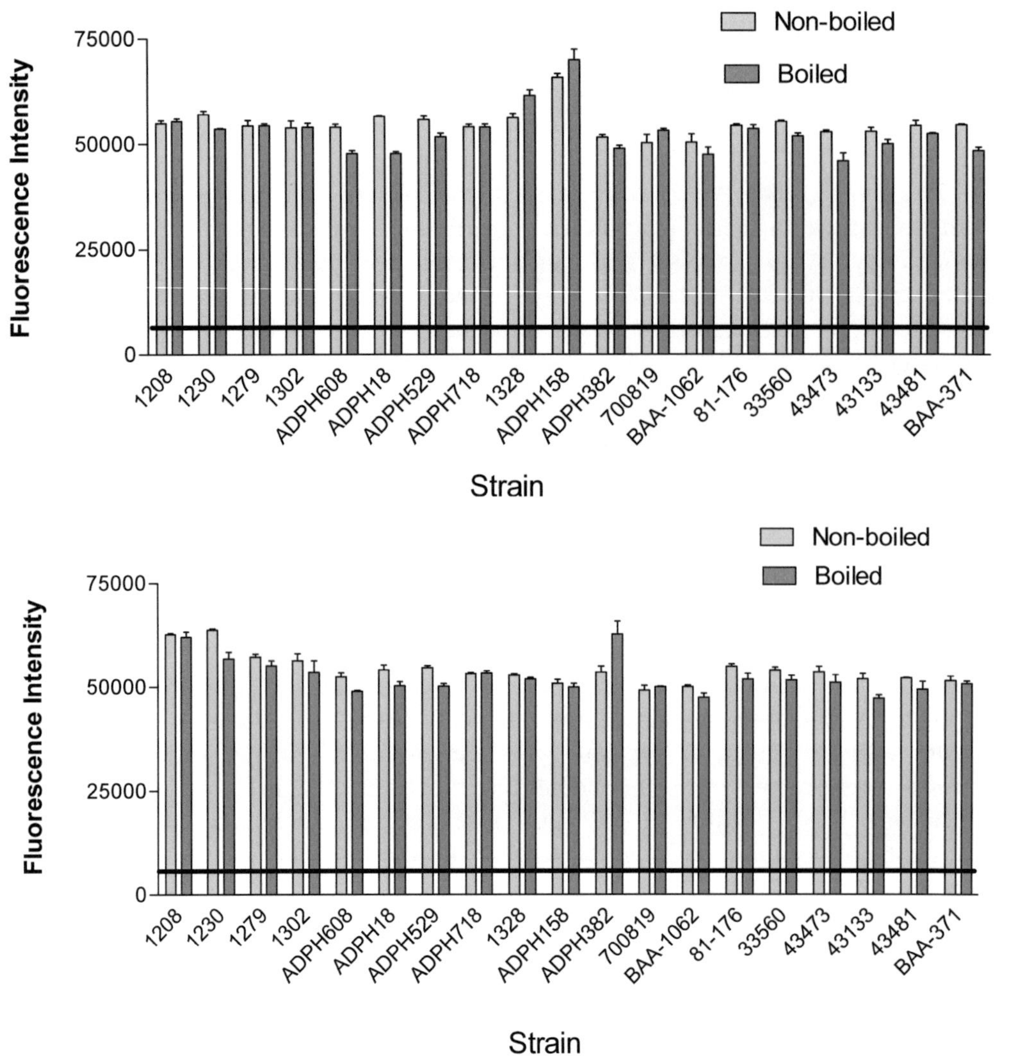

Fig. 2. Detection of 19 *C. jejuni* isolates by a polymyxin B capture ELISA. Representative bacterial colonies were suspended in phosphate buffered saline prior to assay. Fluorescence intensity at 10^6 CFU per ml^{-1} was plotted for both USB10 and USB14 antibodies. Values are means ± SEM for n=5 colonies. The limit of detection was 2.5 greater than background.

5.1 Optical sensors

The optical sensors that use labeled antibodies, e.g. antibodies tagged with fluorescent labels, are similar in design to conventional EIAs. An optical sensor that has been used extensively to detect chemical compounds and bacterial pathogens is surface plasmon resonance (SPR). SPR is an optical phenomenon involving excitation of free oscillating metal electrons and it is based on the phenomenon called *total internal reflection.* When light traveling from a medium more optically dense (refractive index n_1) penetrated into a less optically dense medium (refractive index n_2), the light is bent away from the normal plane to the boundary ($\theta_2 > \theta_1$). The exit angle

Strain	USB10 Antibody	USB14 Antibody
Aeromonas caviae	2.0 ± 0.09	0.8 ± 0.25
A. hydrophila	1.6 ± 0.05	0.74 ± 0.23
Campylobacter coli	19 ± 0.18	18 ± 2.4
C. jejuni	20 ± 0.32	19 ± 2.6
Citrobacter freundii	0.6 ± 0.02	1.4 ± 0.03
Enterobacter cloacae	0.8 ± 0.02	1.8 ± 0.15
E. coli O157:H7	0.98 ± 0.08	1.1 ± 0.01
ECOR 6	1.2 ± 0.02	1.4 ± 0.05
ECOR 15	1.8 ± 0.14	2.2 ± 0.18
EHEC 2-1	0.8 ± 0.05	1.0 ± 0.02
Helicobacter pylori	3.0 ± 0.2	4.0 ± 0.3
Klebsiella oxytoca	0.6 ± 0.01	1.5 ± 0.17
K. pneumoniae	0.5 ± 0.01	1.2 ± 0.14
Morganella morganii	0.7 ± 0.02	1.4 ± 0.09
Pantoea agglomerans	2.8 ± 0.10	1.5 ± 0.40
Plesiomonas shigelloides	0.6 ± 0.02	1.8 ± 0.30
Proteus mirabilis	0.5 ± 0.03	1.3 ± 0.06
Pseudomonas aeruginosa	1.0 ± 0.05	1.0 ± 0.03
Salmonella enterica	1.1 ± 0.07	1.4 ± 0.03
S. enteritidis	1.0 ± 0.08	1.2 ± 0.02
S. typhimurium	1.1 ± 0.08	1.5 ± 0.15
Serratia marcescens	1.7 ± 0.05	0.8 ± 0.23
V. cholerae, classical, Inaba	1.4 ± 0.10	1.5 ± 0.16
O:139	1.7 ± 0.11	2.1 ± 0.10
Vibrio mimicus	2.1 ± 0.06	2.0 ± 0.05
V. parahaemolyticus	1.6 ± 0.08	0.9 ± 0.25

Table 2. Signal to noise ratios for the polymyxin B capture ELISA for various Gram-negative bacteria compared to *C. jejuni* and *C. coli*. Representative bacterial colonies,suspended in PBS at ~ 10^7 CFU per ml^{-1} were assayed using the optimised PMB-capture ELISA. Values are means ± SEM for n=5 experiments. The limit of detection was set at 2.5 or 2.5 greater than background.

(θ_2) approaches 90° when the incident angle (θ_1) increases to a critical angle (θ_c). When the incident angle (θ_1) is equal to or greater than the critical angle (θ_c), the light will be internally reflected (Fig 3 A). The electromagnetic field component of the incident light penetrates a short distance (tens of nanometers) into the less optically dense medium to create an exponentially decaying *evanescent wave* (Fig 3 B). If the incident light is monochromatic and plane-polarized, and a thin film of metal (most frequently gold) is coated at the interface between the two different optically dense media, the photon of the evanescent wave will resonance with free oscillating electrons (plasmons) in the metal film. The evanescent wave can be used to interrogate variations on the surface structure in a distance of up to 300 nm from the surface. The use of SPR as sensor emerged from the realization that SPR signal is sensitive to changes in the refractive index, which is the bending or refraction of a beam of light on entering a denser medium. The refractive index is influenced by the accumulation of mass on the metal surface. The optical excitation of plasmons only "when the energy of the photons of light exactly equals the quantum energy level of the plasmons", a circumstance that is called *attenuated total reflection* (Mol & Fisher 2010).

Some advantages of optical sensors include a wide dynamic range, the possibility of multiplexing to detect several analytes, and a compact, light built that allows for field applications. Another advantage that most commercial SPRs have is that the sensors are based on an open architecture and therefore the sensing element, the antibodies, can be defined by the final user and can be used without any labels to create a label-free biosensor (Ivnitski et al., 1999; Jönsson & Scott 2005). These types of sensors provide a close monitoring of the antibody/antigen reaction in a real-time manner. However, biosensors still have some limitations. For instance, there are constrains on the quantity of antibodies in an active state to capture the target bacteria that can be immobilized on the surface of a sensor. Increasing the density of antibodies is very important to increase sensitivity, but recent studies using three-dimensional aggregation of immunoglobulin G can increase the amount of antibodies by surface area and may provide a way to develop "high performance antibody biosensors" (Feng et al., 2011).

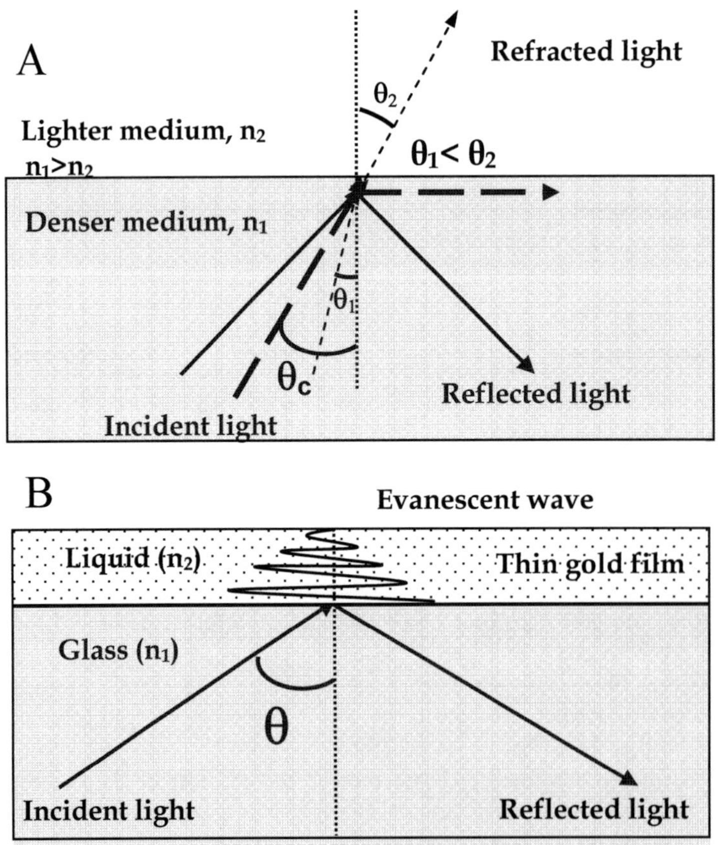

Fig. 3. The optical bases for surface plasmon resonance. Changes in refracted light (A) and the production of evanescent light (B) to interrogate the thin gold surface.

6. Conclusion

Current widely-accepted methods for identifying campylobacters in stool and food samples rely on their growth on selective agar plates with and without prior broth enrichment. These methods are labor-intensive and time-consuming. More rapid and accurate methods, including immunoassays, are necessary to identify campylobacters in stool samples, outbreaks investigations and more recently for screening processed poultry under a new performance standard established in the USA. Yet, the development of antibody-based methods for *Campylobacter* spp. has not received enough attention. At present, none of the commercially-available EIAs are recommended for standalone identification of campylobacters in stool samples, in part because of the limited and conflicting findings regarding their performances. Some of the commercial immunoassays show promise for identification of campylobacters in food although only after broth enrichment for up to 48 hours. More studies of these assays with naturally-contaminated samples from a variety of foods is necessary to validate their performance. Areas of research to improve antibody-based methods should include antibody/antigen characterization, biosensors platforms, and the dovetailing of concentration methods to improve sensitivity.

7. Acknowledgment

The authors wish to acknowledge Deanna Lund for her technical support of this project and Aretha Williams for help with the organization of the manuscript. One of the authors' (CAB) research was supported by Department of Defense grants, DAAD W911SR-05-0020, DAAD W911SR-07-C-0084 and DAAD W911SR-09-C-0005

8. References

Abubakar, I., Irvine, L., Aldus, C., Wyatt, G., Fordham, R., Schelenz, S., Shepstone, L., Howe, A., Peck, M. and Hunter, P. (2007). A systematic review of the clinical, public health and cost-effectiveness of rapid diagnostic tests for the detection and identification of bacterial intestinal pathogens in faeces and food. *Health Technol Assess*, Vol. 11, No. 36, (Sep 2007), pp. (1-216)

Bailey, J. S., Fedorka-cray, P., Richardson, I. J., and Cox, N.A. (2008). Detection of *Campylobacter* from broiler carcass rinse samples utilizing the Tecra visualimmunoassay (VIA). *Journal of Rapid Methods & Automation in Microbiology* Vol. 16, (n.d.), pp. (374–380)

Bessede, E., Delcamp, A., Sifre, E., Buissonniere, A., Megraud, F. (2011). New methods for detection of campylobacters in stool samples in comparison to culture. *J Clin Microbiol*, Vol. 49, (n.d.), pp. (941-944)

Blais, B., Leggate, J., Bosley J., and Martinez-Perez, A. (2005). Detection of *Escherichia coli* O157 in foods by a novel polymyxin-based enzyme-linked immunosorbent assay. *J Food Protect*, Vol. 68, (n.d.), pp. (233-238)

Blais, B., Bosley, J., Martinez-Perez, A., and Popela, M. (2006). Polymyxin-base enzyme-linked immunosorbent assay for the detection *Escherichia coli* O111 and O26. *J Microbiol Methods*, Vol. 65, (n.d.), pp. (468-475)

Bohaychuk, V.M., Gensler, G.E., King, R.K., Wu, J.T., and McMullen, L.M. (2005). Evaluation of detection methods for screening meat and poultry products for the presence of foodborne pathogens. *J Food Prot*, Vol. 68, No. 12, (Dec 2005), pp. (2637-47)

Borck, B., Stryhn, H., Ersbøll, A.K., and Pedersen, K. (2002). Thermophilic *Campylobacter* spp. in turkey samples: evaluation of two automated enzyme immunoassays and conventional microbiological techniques. *J Appl Microbiol*, Vol. 92, No. 3, (n.d.), pp. (574-82)

Brooks, B.W., Mihowich, J.G., Blais, B.W., and Yamazaki, H. (1998). Specificity of monoclonal antibodies to *Campylobacter jejuni* lipopolysaccharide antigens. *Immunol Invest*, Vol. 27, No. 4-5, (Jul - Sep 1998), pp. (257-65)

Brooks, B.W., Robertson, R.H., Lutze-Wallace, C.L., and Pfahler, W. (2002). Monoclonal antibodies specific for *Campylobacter fetus* lipopolysaccharides. *Vet Microbiol*, Vol. 87, No. 1, (Jun 2002), pp. (37-49)

Brooks, B.W., Devenish, J., Lutze-Wallace, C.L., Milnes, D., Robertson, R.H., and Berlie-Surujballi, G. (2004). Evaluation of a monoclonal antibody-based enzyme-linked immunosorbent assay for detection of *Campylobacter fetus* in bovine preputial washing and vaginal mucus samples. *Vet Microbiol*, Vol. 103, No. 1-2, (Oct 2004), pp. (77-84)

Brunelle, S. (2008). Validation of microbiological methods for food. In: *Statistical Aspects of the Microbiological Examination of Foods* 2nd ed. Academic Press, Elsevier, pp. (259-277)

Chon, J.-W., Hyeon, J.-Y., Choi, I.-S., Park, C.-K., Kim, S.-K., Heo, S., Oh, S.-W., Song, K.-Y., & Seo, K.-H. (2011). Comparison of three selective media and Validation of the VIDAS Campylobacter Assay for the detection of *Campylobacter jejuni* in ground beef and fresh-cut vegetables. *J Food Prot*, Vol. 74, No. 3, pp. (456–460)

Cordwell, S.J., Len, A. C. L., Touma, R. G., Scott, N. E., Falconer, L., Jones, D., Connolly, A., Crossett, B., & Djordjevic, S. P. (2008). Identification of membrane-associated proteins from *Campylobacter jejuni* strains using complementary proteomics technologies. *Proteomics*, Vol. 8, (n.d.), pp. (122-139)

Corry, J., Post, D., Colin, P., Laisney, M. (1995). Culture media for isolation of *Campylobacters*. *Int. J. Food Microbiol*, Vol. 26, (n.d.), pp. (43-76)

Dediste, A., Vandenberg, O., Vlaes, L., Ebraert, A., Douat, N., Bahwere, P., and Butzler, J. (2003). Evaluation of the ProSpecT Microplate Assay for detection of *Campylobacter*: a routine laboratory perspective. *Clin Microbiol Infect*, Vol. 9, No. 11, (Nov 2003), pp. (1085-90)

Dekeyser, P., Gossuin-Detrain, M., Butzler, J., and Sternon, J. (1972). Acute enteritis due to a related *Vibrio*: first positive stool cultures. *J Infect Dis*, Vol. 125, (n.d.), pp. (390–392)

Devenish, J., Brooks, B., Perry, K., Milnes, D., Burke, T., McCabe, D., Duff, S., and Lutze-Wallace, C.L. (2005). Validation of a monoclonal antibody-based capture enzyme-linked immunosorbent assay for detection of *Campylobacter fetus*. *Clin Diagn Lab Immunol*, Vol. 12, No. 11, (Nov 2005), pp. (1261-8)

Diergaardt, S., Venter, S., Chalmers, M., Theron, J., and Brözel, V. (2003). Evaluation of the Cape Town protocol for the isolation of *Campylobacter* spp. from environmental waters. *Water SA*, Vol. 29, (n.d.), pp. (225–299)

Dubreuil, J.D., Kostrzynska, M., Logan, S.M., Harris, L.A., Austin, J.W., and Trust, T.J. (1990). Purification, characterization, and localization of a protein antigen shared by thermophilic campylobacters. *J Clin Microbiol*, Vol. 28, pp. (1321-1328)

European Food Safety Authority. (2005). Opinion of the scientific panel on biological hazards on *Campylobacter* in animals and foodstuffs. Vol. 173, (n.d.), pp. (1-10)

European Food Safety Authority. (2006). Trends and Sources of Zoonoses, Zoonotic Agents and Antimicrobial Resistance in the European Union in 2004. (n.d.), pp. (1-275)

Endtz, H., Ang, C., van den Braak, N., Luijendijk, A., Jacobs, B., de Man, P., van Duin, J., van Belkum, A. and Verbrugh, H. (2000). Evaluation of a new commercial immunoassay for rapid detection of *Campylobacter jejuni* in stool samples. *Eur J Clin Microbiol Infect Dis*, Vol. 19, No. 10, (Oct 2000), pp. (794-7)

Engvall, E. and Perlman, P. (1971). Enzyme-linked immunosorbent assay (ELISA). Quantitative Assay of Immunoglobulin G. *Immunochemistry,* Vol. 8, No. 9, (n.d.), pp. (871–4)

Feng, B., Huang, S., Ge, F., Luo, Y., Jia, D., Dai, Y. (2011). 3D antibody immobilization on a planar matrix surface. *Biosensors and Bioelectronics*, Vol. 28, No. 1, (15 October 2011), pp. (91-96)

Fernando, U., Biswas, D., Allan, B., Attah-Poku, S., Willson, P., Valdivieso-Garcia, A., and Potter, A.A. (2008). Serological assessment of synthetic peptides *of Campylobacter jejuni* NCTC11168 FlaA protein using antibodies against multiple serotypes. *Med Microbiol Immunol,* Vol. 197, No. 1, (Mar 2008), pp. (45-53)

Fitzgerald, C., Patrick, M., Jerris, R., Watson, R., Tobin-D'Angelo, M., Gonzalez, A., Polage, C., Wymore, K., Gillim-Ross, L., Sadlowski, J., Monahan, J., Hurd, S., Dahlberg, S., DeMartino, M., Pentella, M., Razeq, J., Leonard, C., Jung, C., Juni, B., Robinson, T., Gittelman, R., Garrigan, C., and I. Nachamkin, (*Campylobacter* diagnostics working group). (2011). Multicenter study to evaluate diagnostic methods for detection and isolation of *Campylobacter* from stool. Annual Meeting of the American Society for Microbiology, New Orleans, LA., (n.d.), 20 Sept 2011, Available from: <http://www.shl.uiowa.edu/educationoutreach/sentclinlabtraining/CampyDx_ASM2011_05182011_FINAL.pdf.>

Food Safety and Inspection Services, U. S. Department of Agriculture. (2009a). The nationwide microbiological baseline data collection program, In: *Young Chicken Survey,* July 2007– June 2008, 20 Sept 2011, Available from: http://www.fsis.usda.gov/PDF/Baseline_Data_Young_Chicken_2007-2008.pdf.>

Food Safety and Inspection Services, U. S. Department of Agriculture. (2009b). Performance standards for *Salmonella* and *Campylobacter,* In: *Young Chicken and Turkey,* 20 Sept 2011, 20 Sept 2011, Available from <http://www.fsis.usda.gov/News_&_Events/Const_Update_123109/index.asp.>

Fukuda, S., Tatsumi, H., Igimi, S. and Yamamoto, S. (2005). Improved bioluminescent enzyme immunoassay for the rapid detection of *Salmonella* in chicken meat samples. *Lett. Appl. Microbiol,* Vol. 41, (n.d.), pp. (379-84)

Granato, P., Chen, L., Holiday I., Rawling, R., Novak-Weekley, S., Quinlan, T. and Musser, K. (2010). Comparison of premier CAMPY enzyme immunoassay (EIA), ProSpecT Campylobacter EIA, and ImmunoCard STAT! CAMPY tests with culture for laboratory diagnosis of Campylobacter enteric infections. *J Clin Microbiol*, Vol. 48, No. 11, (Sept 2010), pp. (4022-7)

Hahm, B.K., and Bhunia, A.K. (2006). Effect of environmental stresses on antibody-based detection of *Escherichia coli* O157:H7, Salmonella enterica serotype Enteritidis and Listeria monocytogenes. *J Appl Microbiol* Vol. 100, pp. (1017-1027)

Hannu, T., Mattila, L., Rautelin, H., Pelkonen, P., Lahdenne, P., Siitonen, A., and Leirisalo-Repo, M. (2002). Campylobacter-triggered reactive arthritis: a population-based study. *Rheumatology* (Oxford), Vol. 41, No. 3, (Mar 2002), pp. (312-318)

Harding S.V., Sarkar-Tyson, M., Smither, S.J., Atkins, T.P., Oyston, P.C., Brown, K.A., Liu, Y., Wait, R., and Titball, R.W. (2007). The identification of surface proteins of Burkholderia pseudomallei. *Vaccine*, Vol. 25, No. 14, Mar 30, pp. (2664-2672)

Heymann, D.L. (Ed.) (2004). *Control of communicable diseases manual, 18th edition,* American Public Health Association, Washington. ISBN: 0-87553-034-6, pp. 700)

Heo, S.A., Nannapaneni, R., Johnson, M.G., Park, J.S., and Seo, K.H. (2009). Production and characterization of a monoclonal antibody to *Campylobacter jejuni. J Food Prot,* Vol. 72, No. 4, (Apr 2009), pp. (870-5)

Hindiyeh, M., Jense, S., Hohmann, S., Benett, H., Edwards, C., Aldeen, W., Croft, A., Daly, J., Mottice, S. and Carroll, K. (2000). Rapid detection of *Campylobacter jejuni* in stool specimens by an enzyme immunoassay and surveillance for *Campylobacter upsaliensis* in the greater Salt Lake City area. *J Clin Microbiol,* Vol. 38, No. 8, (Aug 2000), pp. (3076-9)

Hochel I., Slavíčková, D., Viochna, D., Škvor, J., & Steinhauserová, I. (2007): Detection of *Campylobacter* species in foods by indirect competitive ELISA using hen and rabbit antibodies. *Food Agri Immun,* Vol. 18 (n.d.), pp. (151–167)

Hochel, I., Viochna, D., Skvor, J., and Musil, M. (2004). Development of an indirect competitive ELISA for detection of *Campylobacter jejuni* subsp. *jejuni* O:23 in foods. *Folia Microbiol* (Praha), Vol. 49, No. 5, (n.d.), pp. (579-86)

Hoorfar, J., Nielsen, E.M., Stryhn, H., and Andersen, S. (1999). Evaluation of two automated enzyme-immunoassays for detection of thermophilic campylobacters in faecal samples from cattle and swine. *J Microbiol Methods,* Vol. 38, No. 1-2, (Oct 1999), pp. (101-6)

Hunt, J., Abeyta, C. and Tran, T. (2001). Isolation of *Campylobacter* species from food and water, In: *Food and Drug Administration Bacteriological Analytical Manual,* 20 Sept 2011, Available from: <http://www.fda.gov/Food/ScienceResearch/LaboratoryMethods/BacteriologicalAnalyticalManualBAM/ucm072616.htm>

International Organization for Standardization (ISO). (2006). Microbiology of food and animal feeding stuffs - horizontal method for detection and enumeration of *Campylobacter* spp. Part 1: Detection Methods, 10272-1:2006

Ivnitski, D., Abdel-Hamid, I., Atanasov, P. and Wilkins, E. (1999). Biosensors for detection of pathogenic bacteria. *Biosensor Bioelect,* Vol.14, (n.d.), pp. (599-624)

Jönsson, U. and Scott, A. (2005). Optical affinity biosensors, In: *Biosensors for Food Analysis,* U. Jönsson and A. Scott, pp. (37-45), Woodhead Publishing Ltd., Cambridge, England

Josefsen et al. (2011) In: Hoorfar, Rapid Detection, Identification and Quantification of Foodborne Pathogens, pp. (213, 209-227), ASM Press, Washington D.C.

Kawatsu, K., Taguchi, M., Yonekita, T., Matsumoto, T., Morimatsu, F., and Kumeda, Y. (2010). Simple and rapid detection of *Campylobacter* spp. in naturally contaminated chicken-meat samples by combination of a two-step enrichment method with an immunochromatographic assay. *Int J Food Microbiol,* Vol. 142, No. 1-2, (Aug 2010), pp. (256-9)

Kim, J.S., Taitt, C.R., Ligler, F.S., Anderson, S.P. (2010). Multiplexed magnetic microsphere immunoassay for detection of pathogens in food. *Sens Instrum Food Qual Saf,* Vol. 4, (n.d.), pp. (73-81)

Köhler, G. and Milstein, C. (1975). Continuous cultures of fused cells secreting antibody of predefined specificity. *Nature,* Vol. 256, No. 5517, (n.d.), pp. (495–7)

Lamoureux, M., MacKay, A., Messier, S., Fliss, I., Blais, B.W., Holley, R.A., Simard, R.E. (1997). Detection of *Campylobacter jejuni* in food and poultry viscera using immunomagnetic separation and microtitre hybridization. *J Appl Microbiol,* Vol. 83, No 5, (Nov 1997), pp. (641-651)

Lastovica, A. and Le Roux, E. (2003). Optimal detection of *Campylobacter* spp. in stools. *J Clin Pathol,* Vol. 56, (n.d.), p. (480)

Le Roux, E., and Lastovica, A. (1998). The Cape Town protocol: How to isolate the most campylobacters for your dollar, pound, franc, yen, etc., In: *Campylobacter, Helicobacter & Related Organisms,* A. Lastovica, D. Newell and E. Lastovica (Eds.), pp. (30-33), Institute of Child Health, Cape Town, South Africa

Liu, L., Hussain, S., Miller, R. and Oyarzabal, O. (2009). Efficacy of Mini VIDAS for the detection of *Campylobacter* spp. from retail broiler meat enriched in Bolton broth with or without the supplementation of blood. *Journal of Food Protection,* Vol. 72, (n.d.), pp. (2428-2432)

Logan, S.M., and Trust, T.J. (1983). Molecular identification of surface protein antigens of *Campylobacter jejuni. Infect Immun,* Vol. 42, No. 2 (Nov 1983), pp. (675-682)

Lu, P., Brooks, B.W., Robertson, R.H., Nielsen, K.H., Garcia, M.M. (1997). Characterization of monoclonal antibodies for the rapid detection of foodborne campylobacters. *Int J Food Microbiol,* Vol. 37, (n.d.), pp. (87-9)

Microbiology Laboratory Guidebook, *MLG 41.00.* (2011). Isolation, identification, and enumeration of *Campylobacter jejuni/coli/lari* from poultry rinse and sponge samples, 20 Sept 2011, Available from: <http://www.fsis.usda.gov/PDF/MLG_41_01.pdf>

Mol, N. and Fisher, M. (2010). Surface plasmon resonance: A general introduction, In: *Surface Plasmon Resonance, Methods in Molecular Biology,* N. de Mol and M. Fischer (Eds.), pp. (1-14), Springer , New Yord, NY

Nesbakken, T., Eckner, K., Høidal, H.K., and Røtterud, O.J. (2003). Occurrence of *Yersinia enterocolitica* and *Campylobacter* spp. in slaughter pigs and consequences for meat inspection, slaughtering, and dressing procedures. *Int J Food Microbiol,* Vol. 80, No. 3, (Feb 2003), pp. (231-40)

Nyquist-Battie, C., Frank, L., Lund, D., and Lim, D.V. (2004). Optimization of a fluorescence sandwich enzyme-linked immunosorbent assay for detection of *Escherichia coli* O157:H7 in apple juice. *J. Food Prot,* Vol. 67, (n.d.), pp. (2756-2759)

Nyquist-Battie, C., Mathias, L., Frank, L., Lund, D., and Lim, D.V. (2005). Antibody-based detection of acid-shocked, acid-adapted and apple juice-incubated *Escherichia coli* O157:H7. *J Immunoassay Immunochem,* Vol. 26, (n.d.), pp. (259-271)

Olson, C.K., Ethelberg, S., van Pelt, W. and Tauxe, R.V. (2008). Epidemiology of *Campylobacter jejuni* infections in industrialized nations, In: *Campylobacter 3rd ed,* I.

Nachamkin, C. Szymanski and J. Blaser (Eds.), pp. (163-189), ASM Press, Washington D.C.

On, S. L. W. (2001). Taxonomy of *Campylobacter*, Arcobacter, *Helicobacter* and related bacteria: current status, future prospects and immediate concerns. *J Appl Microbiol*, Vol. 90 (n.d.), pp. 1S-15S.

Oyarzabal, O. A. (2005). Reduction of *Campylobacter* spp. by commercial antimicrobials applied during the processing of broiler chickens: A review from the United States perspective. *Journal of Food Protection*, Vol. 68, (n.d.), pp. (1752–1760)

Oyarzabal, O. A., Backert, S., Nagaraj, M., Miller, R. S., Hussain, S. K. and Oyarzabal, E. A. (2007). Efficacy of supplemented buffered peptone water for the isolation of *Campylobacter jejuni* and *C. coli* from broiler retail products. *Journal of Microbiological Methods*, Vol. 69, (n.d.), pp. (129-136)

Oyarzabal, O., Macklin, K., Barbaree, J. and Miller, R. (2005). Evaluation of agar plates for direct enumeration of *Campylobacter* spp. from poultry carcass rinses. *Applied and Environmental Microbiology*, Vol. 71, (n.d.), pp. (3351-3354)

Paulsen, P., Kanzler, P., Hilbert, F., Mayrhofer, S., Baumgartner, S., Smulders, F.J. (2005). Comparison of three methods for detecting *Campylobacter* spp. in chilled or frozen meat. *Int J Food Microbiol*. Vol. 103, No. 2, (Aug 2005), pp. (229-233)

Pei, Z.H., Ellison, 3rd, R.T., & Blaser, M.J. (1991). Identification, purification, and characterization of major antigenic proteins of *Campylobacter jejuni*. *J Biol Chem*, Vol. 266, (n.d.), p. (16363)

Prokhorova, T.A., Nielsen, P.N., Petersen, J., Kofoed, T., Crawford, J.S., Morsczeck, C., Boysen, A., Schrotz-King, P. (2006). Novel surface polypeptides of *Campylobacter jejuni* as traveller's diarrhoea vaccine candidates discovered by proteomics. *Vaccine*, Vol. 24, (n.d.), p. (6446)

Qian, H., Pang, E., Chang, J., Toh, S.L., Ng, F.K., Tan, A.L., and Kwang, J. (2008a). Monoclonal antibody binding to the major outer membrane protein of *Campylobacter coli*. *J Immunol Methods*, Vol. 339, No. 1, (Nov 2008), pp. (104-13)

Qian, H., Pang, E., Du, Q., Chang, J., Dong, J., Toh, S.L., Ng, F.K., Tan, A.L., and Kwang, J. (2008b). Production of a monoclonal antibody specific for the major outer membrane protein of *Campylobacter jejuni* and characterization of the epitope. *Appl Environ Microbiol*, Vol. 74, No. 3, (Feb 2008), pp. (833-9)

Rees, J.H., Soudain, S.E., Gregson, N.A., and Hughes, R.A.C. (1995). *Campylobacter jejuni* infection and Guillain-Barré syndrome. *N Engl J Med*, Vol. 333, (n.d.), pp. (1374-1379)

Reiter MG, Bueno CM, López C, Jordano R. (2005). Occurrence of *Campylobacter* and *Listeria monocytogenes* in a poultry processing plant. *J Food Prot*. Vol. 2005 Sep;68(9):1903-6

Rice, B.E., Lamichhane, C., Joseph, S.W., and Rollins, D.M. (1996). Development of a rapid and specific colony-lift immunoassay for detection and enumeration of *Campylobacter jejuni*, *C. coli*, and *C. lari*. *Diagn Lab Immunol*, Vol. 3, No. 6, (Nov 1996), pp. (669-77).

Rice, B.E., C. Lamichhane, S.W. Joseph and D.M. Rollins. (1999). Development of a rapid and specific colony-lift immunoassay for detection and enumeration of *Campylobacter jejuni*, *C. coli* and *C. lari*. *Clin. Diagn. Lab. Immunol.*, Vol. 3, pp. (669–677)

Samuel, M., Vugia, D., Shallow, S., Marcus, R., Segler, S., McGivern, T., Kassenborg, H., Reilly, K., Kennedy, M., Angulo, F., and Tauxe, R. (2004). Epidemiology of sporadic

Campylobacter infection in the United States and the declining trend in incidence. *Clin Infect Dis*, Vol. 38, Suppl. 3, (n.d.), pp. (S165-S174)

Sapsford, K.E., Rasooly, A., Taitt, C. and Ligler, F. (2004). Detection of *Campylobacter* and *Shigella* species in food samples using an array biosensor. *Analytica Chimica Acta* Vol. 76, (n.d.), pp. (433–440)

Semchenko, E.A., Day, C.J., Wilson, J.C., Grice, I.D., Moran, A.P., Korolik, V. (2010). Temperature-dependent phenotypic variation of *Campylobacter jejuni* lipooligosaccharides. *BMC Microbiol*, Vol. 10, (n.d.), p. (305)

Skirrow, M. (1991). Epidemiology of *Campylobacter* enteritis. *Int J Food Microbiol*, Vol. 12, (n.d.), pp. (9–16)

Speegle, L., Miller, M., Backert, S. and Oyarzabal ,O. (2009). Use of cellulose filters to isolate *Campylobacter* spp. from naturally contaminated retail broiler meat. *Journal of Food Protection*, Vol. 72, (n.d.), pp. (2592-2596)

Taylor, D.E., Chang, N. (1987). Immunoblot and enzyme-linked immunosorbent assays of *Campylobacter* major outer-membrane protein and application to the differentiation of *Campylobacter* species. *Mol Cell Probes*. Vol. 1, No. 3 (Sep 1987) pp. (261-274)

Tissari, P. and Rautelin, H. (2007). Evaluation of an enzyme immunoassay-based stool antigen test to detect *Campylobacter jejuni* and *Campylobacter coli*. *Diagn Microbiol Infect Dis.*, Vol. 58 No. 2, (Jun 2007), pp. (171-5)

Tolcin, R., LaSalvia, M.M., Kirkley, B.A., Vetter, E.A., Cockerill, F.R., and Procop, G.W. (2000). Evaluation of the Alexon-Trend ProSpecT Campylobacter microplate assay. *J Clin Microbiol*, Vol. 38, (n.d.), pp. (3853-5)

Tribble, D., Baqar, S., Pang, L., Mason, C., Houng, H., Pitarangsi, C., Lebron, C., Armstrong, A., Sethabutr, O. and Sanders, J. (2008). Diagnostic approach to acute diarrheal illness in a military population on training exercises in Thailand, a region of *Campylobacter* hyperendemicity. *J Clin Microbiol*, Vol. 46 No. 4, (Apr 2008), pp. (1418-25)

Tsai, H.C.S. and Slavik, M.F. (1994). Fluoresence concentration immunoassay for rapid detection of *Campylobacter* spp. in chicken rinse water. *J Rapid Meth Aut Microbiol*, Vol. 3, (n.d.), pp. (69–76)

Turner, A. and Newman J. (2005). An introduction to biosensors, In: *Biosensors for Food Analysis*, A. Scott (Ed.), pp. (13-27), Woodhead Publishing Ltd., Cambridge, England

Velusamy, V., Arshak, K., Korostynska, O., Oliwa, K., Adley, C. (2010). An overview of foodborne pathogen detection: In the perspective of biosensors. *Biotech Adv*, Vol. 28, (n.d.), p. (232-254)

Wang, H. (2002). Rapid methods for detection and enumeration of *Campylobacter* spp. in foods. *J AOAC Int*, Vol. 85, No. 4. (Jul-Aug 2002), pp. (996-9)

Wang, H., Boyle, E., and Farber, J. (2000). Rapid and specific enzyme immunoassay on hydrophobic grid membrane filter for detection and enumeration of thermophilic *Campylobacter* spp. from milk and chicken rinses. *J Food Prot*, Vol. 63, No. 4, (Apr 2000), pp. (489-94)

Wei, D., Oyarzabal, O., Huang, T-S., Shankar Ganesh, S., Sista, S. and Simonian, A. (2007). Development of a surface plasmon resonance biosensor for the identification of *Campylobacter jejuni*. *Journal of Microbiological Methods*, Vol. 69, (n.d.), pp. (78-85)

Whiting, P., Rutjes, A.W.S., Reitsma, J.B., Bossuyt, P.M.M., and Kleijnen, J. (2003) The development of QUADAS: a tool for the quality assessment of studies of diagnostic accuracy included in systematic reviews. *BMC Medical Research Methodology*, Vol. 3, (n.d.), p. (25)

Yu, L.S., Uknalis, J., Tu, S.I. (2001). Immunomagnetic separation methods for the isolation of *Campylobacter jejuni* from ground poultry meats. *J Immunol Methods,* Vol. 256, (n.d.), pp. (11-8)

Zhou, P., Hussain, S., Liles, M., Arias, C., Backert, S., Kieninger, J. and Oyarzabal, O. (2011). A simplified and cost-effective enrichment protocol for the isolation of *Campylobacter* spp. from retail broiler meat without microaerobic incubation. *BMC Microbiology,* Vol. 11, No. 175, (n.d.), pp. (1-12)

14

Elisas for Rotavirus Diagnosis, Typing, and Analysis of Antibody Response

Luis Padilla-Noriega
Instituto de Investigaciones Biomédicas, Universidad Nacional Autónoma de México, Mexico

1. Introduction

Enzyme-linked immunosorbent assays (ELISAs) have been widely used to detect antigens and antibodies of a vast number of infectious agents, including viruses. While general approaches to develop and use ELISAs for analysis of antigens and antibodies are the same, different infectious agents differ widely in their complexity, antigenic structure, stability, diversity, and availability of antigens, making it necessary to consider their special characteristics to develop and use these assays. In this review I describe the development and use of ELISAs to detect and analyze rotavirus antigens and antibodies.

Rotaviruses belonging to group/species A (RVA) are the most important cause of severe gastroenteritis in infants throughout the world, and they also cause diarrhea in most mammalian species that have been studied. The main symptoms in infants are vomiting and diarrhea, which are also common to other gastroenteritis agents. Infections can be asymptomatic, mild, or severe leading to dehydration and in some instances death, while in adults asymptomatic infections occur throughout life, with raising levels of circulating anti-rotavirus IgG with increasing age. In the clinical practice diagnosis is facilitated due to the age range of infants with severe symptoms, higher incidence of infections in the cold season, and watery diarrhea. Current vaccines are contributing to relieve the burden of RVA gastroenteritis; however more vaccines are needed due to their high cost and suboptimal efficacy in developing countries (Estes & Kapikian, 2007).

Rotavirus (RV) is a genus of the family *Reoviridae*, classified in 5 species (A-E), formerly known as groups, and 2 tentative species (F and G) (Matthijnssens *et al.*). RV species are identical morphologically, with no cross-reaction antigenically. RVA have a genome consisting of 11 segments of dsRNA that code for 6 structural (VP1-VP4, VP6 and VP7) and 6 non-structural (NSP1-NSP6) proteins. The viral genome in the core of the virion is closely associated with the viral RNA polymerase VP1 and the guanilyl- and methyl-transferase VP3 (RNA-capping enzyme). The virion has icosahedral symmetry and consists of 4 structural proteins in 3 concentric layers: the inner layer formed by 60 dimers of VP2, the intermediate layer formed by 260 trimers of VP6, and the outer layer formed by 260 trimers of VP7 and 60 spikes of VP4 (Jiang *et al.*, 2008). RVA antigens obtained from infected cells contain mature triple-layered particles (TLPs), single-layered particles (SLPs), double-layered particles (DLPs), empty particles of all 3 classes which lack the viral genome, and multimeric complexes of viral proteins that have not been fully characterized (Gallegos &

Patton, 1989). The mature TLPs are unstable in low calcium, in contrast to DLPs which are remarkably stable in environmental settings such as seawater (Loisy *et al.*, 2004). When calcium is chelated the outer layer of the virion disassembles due to the effect of low calcium on the stability of trimeric VP7 capsomers (Dormitzer *et al.*, 2000).

The surface proteins of TLPs consist of a thin layer of the glycoprotein VP7 with a diameter of 90 Å, and VP4 spikes that traverse the VP7 layer, extending outward to a length of 120 Å, and interacting deeply with the intermediate VP6 layer. VP4 needs to be cleaved by trypsin into VP5* and VP8* to enhance viral infectivity, with VP5* subunits occupying the foot, body and stalk regions of the spikes and VP8* the distal heads. Cryo-electron microscopy of TLPs grown in the absence of trypsin show that VP4 is structurally disordered, *i. e.* the spikes cannot be seen, whereas upon trypsination the spikes become conformationally stable and structurally ordered (Jiang *et al.*, 2008). By cryo-electron microscopy the spikes of trypsin-treated TLPs appear to have trimeric foots (Li *et al.*, 2009), with dimeric bodies and two VP8* heads at the tips (Settembre *et al.*). In spite of this apparently dimeric structure, the long bilobed spikes undergo an irreversible conformational change at pH 11 and become trilobed and stunted. The alkali-treated TLPs are non-infectious and bind 3 anti-VP5* Mabs per spike (Pesavento *et al.*, 2005). From these data, it seems that VP4 spikes are trimeric with flexible linked subunits prior to cleavage. Upon treatment with trypsin the spikes rigidify, with one floppy and 2 structured subunits, while treatment with alkali leads to a conformational rearrangement whereby the stalks fold backand rigidify the floppy subunit, thus revealing their trimeric structure (Kim *et al.*).

The outer layer of the TLPs is the machinery for virus attachment and entry into the target cells. In the entry process, VP8* initially interacts with sialic acid (SA)-containing receptors, followed by sequential interactions of VP5* with hsc70 and integrins (Lopez & Arias, 2006). In Madin-Darby canine kidney (MDCK) cells infected with rhesus rotavirus (RRV) entry seems to occur through an endocytosis pathway, since the input RRV proteins colocalize with the early endocytic pathway proteins Rab4 and Rab5. In addition, the entry process is dependent on endocytic calcium concentration, since bafilomycin A1 and elevated extracellular calcium result in accumulation of intact TLPs in the actin network, suggesting a delay in RV decapsidation (Wolf *et al.*). A recombinant VP5* fragment has a trimeric, folded-back structure, that seems to mimic a conformational rearrangement that occurs when the virion uncoats. Such conformational change has been detected with conformational-specific Mabs against the recombinant VP5* fragment. The folding-back of VP5* resembles the conformational changes in enveloped virus fusogenic proteins. It has been proposed that an intermediary in the process of folding back of VP5*, that is able to bind liposomes, leads to membrane disruption of endosomes and virus entry (Trask *et al.*).

RVA replication and early morphogenesis occur in cytoplasmic inclusion bodies known as viroplasms. In MA104 cells the incoming DLPs in the cytoplasm transcribe the viral genome to produce the 11 viral mRNAs. Two of the viral proteins produced contain leader sequences that are targeted to the endoplasmic reticulum (ER), VP7 and NSP4. On the other hand, several viral proteins involved in viral replication and in the initial assembly steps accumulate in viroplasms: NSP2, NSP5, NSP6, VP1 to VP3, and VP6. Initially, viral mRNAs are used as templates to produce the genomic dsRNAs, in a process that occurs simultaneously with assembly of the inner layer of the virion. Further assembly of the intermediate VP6 layer depends on NSP4, and presumably occurs at the interphase between viroplasms and the ER. The DLPs bud into the lumen of the ER, using NSP4 as a receptor. NSP4 presumably also functions as a VP4 receptor, such that budding serves to incorporate both surface proteins of the virion into the transiently enveloped DLPs. Finally, the envelope is lost as the virus matures within the ER to produce TLPs (Patton *et al.*, 2006).

NSP4 primary translation product has 20 kDa that increases to 28 kDa after glycosilation in the ER. The N-terminus contains 3 hydrophobic domains, H1 (aa 7-21) that resides mostly in the ER lumen, H2 (aa 29-47) that traverses the ER lipid bilayer, and H3 (aa 67-85) that is embedded in the surface side of the ER membrane. The protein emerges from the ER approximately at amino acid 44, hence the remaining 131 amino acids reside in the cytoplasm (Bergmann et al., 1989; Chan et al., 1988). The carboxy-terminus of NSP4 has several domains: a heptad repeat (aa 95-137), VP4-bindig (aa 112-148), calcium-binding (aa 114-135), and DLP-binding (aa 161-175) (Estes, 2001). Silencing of NSP4 expression by RNA interference leads to a severe defect in the assembly of both DLP and TLP RVA particles. Upon NSP4 silencing, several viral proteins show altered subcelular distribution, most notably VP6 accumulate as long fibers throughout the cytoplasm instead of being assembled in the viroplasms to form the intermediate layer of the virions. In addition, when NSP4 expression is silenced several proteins that accumulate in the viroplasms show reduced expression levels and viroplasms are small, suggesting that the failure to incorporate VP6 affects the assembly of other proteins that reside in the viroplasms. On the other hand, silencing of VP7 by RNA interference leads to the accumulation of enveloped DLPs in the lumen of the ER and no infectious virions are formed, indicating that VP7 has a role in envelope removal and TLP maturation in the ER (Lopez et al., 2005). Since interference of VP7 expression does not block DLP budding into the ER, the second viral ER-resident protein, NSP4, is most likely responsible of DLP budding into the ER.

The group specificity of RVs depends on VP6, the major antigen of the virion. Within species A, RVs have been classified in 4 subgroups (SG) of VP6, I, II, I/ II, and non-I/II, based on the reactivity with 2 Mabs (Kapikian & Chanock, 1996). In addition, RVAs have been classified in dual serotypes, since both of the surface proteins of the virion induce neutralizing antibodies. By neutralization assays with hyperimmune sera to purified TLPs 15 VP7 serotypes have been identified, known as G serotypes since VP7 is a glycoprotein. The predominance of anti-VP7 neutralizing antibodies in neutralization assays with sera hyperimmune to the whole viral particles preclude typing of VP4 with this assay. In order to determine the serotype-specificity of VP4, hyperimmune sera to recombinant VP4 were developed and used in neutralization assays to identify 14 VP4 serotypes, known as P since VP4 is protease-sensitive. Serotype P1 was further classified as P1A and P1B, based on one-way cross neutralization with hyperimmune sera to the prototype P1A and P1B strains (Hoshino & Kapikian, 1996). RVA G and P serotyping performed by neutralization assays are time consuming, and have been superseded by G and P genotyping based on identities among cognate genes. So far, 25 G genotypes (G[1] to G[25], with square brackets) have been identified with G[1] to G[14] corresponding to the serotypes G1 to G14 (without square brackets). For VP4, 35 P genotypes have been identified, P[1] to P[35], however the numbering of the P genotypes do not coincide with the numbering of P serotypes, since more than one P genotype may correspond to a single P serotype (Matthijnssens *et al.*).

Recently a complete genome classification system was developed for RVA strains based on nucleotide-identity cutoff values for the open reading frames of each of the 11 gene segments. This system assigns a one-letter code to each gene and successive Arabic numbers for the different genotypes, such that the VP7-VP4-VP6-VP1-VP2-VP3-NSP1-NSP2-NSP3-NSP4-NSP5/6 are described using the abbreviations Gx-P[x]-Ix-Rx-Cx-Mx-Ax-Nx-Tx-Ix-Hx. Based on this whole-genome system, human RVA strains were classified in 3 gene constellations that are characteristic of the Wa-like family and porcine RVA strains, the DS-1-like family and bovine RVA strains, and the AU-1-like family that has a mixed canine and feline RVA gene constellation. As an example of the diversity of human and animal RVA strains, 3 genotypes have been identified among human RVA strains based on VP6 (I1, I2, and I3), NSP2 (N1, N2, and N3), or NSP4 (E1, E2, and E3). The diversity considering both human and animal RVA strains is much higher, since 16 I, 9 N, and 14 E genotypes have been identified so far. Among human RVA strains the genotypes I1, N1, and E1 cluster together in the Wa-like family, I2, N2, and E2 in the DS-1-like family; and I3; N3, and E3 in the AU-1-like family (Matthijnssens *et al.*, 2008; Matthijnssens *et al.*).

2. Group/species A rotavirus ELISAs

A commonly used format for ELISAs to diagnose RVAs is based on 2 hyperimmune anti-RVA sera raised in different animal species, one as capture antibody, and the second as detector, followed by an enzyme-conjugate to the second species. Ideally, the capture and conjugate antibodies should be produced in the same species to prevent reactivity of the conjugate to the capture antibody (Yolken & Leister, 1982).

RVA ELISAs depend mostly on VP6, presumably due to the predominance of antibodies to VP6 in the polyclonal sera used for capture and detection, and the predominance of VP6 as an antigen in the assays. The yield of DLPs is usually higher than TLPs in MA104 cells infected with RVAs. In addition, VP6 is the major antigen in TLPs, since it accounts for 51% of its mass (Liu et al., 1988). Using plates coated with rotavirus TLPs or DLPs to screen monoclonal antibodies (Mabs) by solid-phase radioimmunoassay yielded predominantly anti-VP6 Mabs, 70% (Greenberg et al., 1983), as compared to Mabs specific to other viral proteins like VP7, VP4 or VP2. VP6 shows extensive cross-reactivity among RVA strains, such that hyperimmune sera produced to any mammalian RVA can be used in ELISAs to detect a heterotypic response. On the other hand, avian RVA strains are distantly related to mammalian strains (Matthijnssens et al., 2008), hence the performance of hyperimmune sera to mammalian RVA strains may be lower than homologous antisera to detect avian RVA strains by ELISA.

RVA ELISAs have been used in numerous studies to diagnose RVA infections from different animal species. The performance of the assay to detect RVAs from different animal species was similar since 33 human RVAs obtained from stools of naturally infected infants could not be differentiated by an RVA ELISA from strains derived from calves, piglets, foals, monkeys, and mice (Yolken *et al.*, 1978). In one study 1,163 children were analyzed for the presence of RVA particles using two ELISA kits. The kits were evaluated in laboratories of 7 different countries. One of the kits, the DAKO-ELISA, had a sensitivity of 97% and a specificity of 97% as compared to the WHO-ELISA kit. On the other hand, in individual laboratories the range of sensitivity of the DAKO-ELISA was 90-100%, and the range of specificity was 85-100% (Flewett *et al.*, 1989).

3. Subgroup rotavirus ELISAs

RVAs have been classified in four SGs according to the reactivity determined by ELISA of Mabs that specifically reacts with SG I (266/60) or SG II (631/9) (Greenberg *et al.*, 1983).

Other Mabs have been described that also react with SG I or II (Gerna *et al.*, 1989; Liprandi *et al.*, 1990; Taniguchi *et al.*, 1984), however the Mabs developed by Greenberg *et al.* are the most widely used in epidemiological studies.

The antigens used to produce the Mabs 255/60 and 631/30 were the simian genotype I2 strain RRV, and the human genotype I1 strain Wa, respectively. Some murine and avian RVA strains do not react with SG-specific Mabs (Svensson *et al.*, 1990; Theil & McCloskey, 1989), and an equine RV strain reacts with both SG I and II Mabs (Hoshino *et al.*, 1987). No clear correlation has been observed between the subgroup specificity and the VP6 genotyping system, since several of the VP6 genotypes contain strains with different SG specificities (Matthijnssens *et al.*, 2008).

The SG Mabs recognize conformational epitopes that are present in the trimeric but not the monomeric forms of VP6 (Gorziglia *et al.*, 1988). By using *in vitro* translated VP6 from the SG II human Wa strain, single amino acid mutations at position 172 were sufficient for recognition by the SG I Mab 255/60, while retaining the reactivity with the SG II Mab 631/9. On the other hand, the SG I porcine rotavirus YM VP6 with a double mutation at positions 305 and 306 acquires reactivity with the SG II Mab 631/9 and simultaneously loses its capacity to interact with the Mab 255/60 (Lopez *et al.*, 1994). In addition, a single mutation at position 315 was sufficient to change the SG specificity of the murine strain EW from non I/II to II (Tang *et al.*, 1997). All the residues that determine SG specificity are located closely together on the top surface of VP6, which interacts with VP7. Since the SG epitopes also form the VP7 binding structure, the constraints of such interaction have been proposed to be the limiting factor that restricts their antigenic variability (Mathieu *et al.*, 2001).

Epidemiologic studies of the prevalence of SG I and II in infants with gastroenteritis have been done by ELISA. Subgrouping differentiates the SG II Wa-like family from the SGI DS-1-like and AU-1-like families. Among the SG I specimens, the serotype G2 strains are preliminarily assigned to the DS-1-like family. On the other hand, the SG II specimens belonging to the serotypes G1, G3, G4, and G9 are preliminarily assigned to the Wa-like family. Sugroup I strains with serotypes other than G2 are likely to be AU-1-like, animal strains, or genomic reassortants. Apart from the highly prevalent Wa-like and DS-1-like strains, and their characteristic genomic constellations, other SG/serotype combinations are rarely detected (Beards *et al.*, 1989).

4. Serotype-specific rotavirus ELISAs

The development of neutralizing anti-VP7 and anti-VP4 monoclonal antibodies, and their use in epitope-specific ELISAs served to analyze the complexity of RVA serotype-specificity. ELISAs to serotype VP7 have been widely used and are highly sensitive, however the sensitivity has been variable in different studies, prompting for the use of more than one serotype-specific Mab to increase the sensitivity of the method (Ward *et al.*, 1991). On the other hand, ELISAs for VP4 serotyping have been of limited use, presumably due to the antigenic complexity of this protein (Coulson, 1993; Padilla-Noriega *et al.*, 1998). VP4 and VP7 differ in their antigenic structure, exposure on the surface of the virion, conformational flexibility, immunogenicity, role in virus entry to the target cells, and the potency and mechanism of neutralization by antibodies.

Studies of neutralization escape mutants of the G3 simian rotavirus SA11, selected with anti-VP7 Mabs, identified single amino acid substitutions in 3 regions, A, B, and C, localized at amino acids 87-96, 145-150, and 211-223, respectively (Dyall-Smith *et al.*, 1986). Further studies with RVA strains of different G serotypes identified the variable regions designated A and C as major targets recognized by anti-VP7 neutralizing Mabs that are serotype-specific, or cross-reactive (Hoshino et al., 1994; Kobayashi et al., 1991). The breadth of serotype recognition was affected by valency, since the IgM Mab 57-8 has far broader neutralizing range that IgG Mabs (Mackow *et al.*, 1988a). The epitopes recognized by neutralizing Mabs are considered to be operationally related if the escape mutant selected with one Mab acquires resistance to a second Mab. By analysis of the cross-neutralization patterns of several anti-VP7 Mabs with their neutralization escape mutants, the antigenic regions A and C have been shown to be operationally related, and collectively constitute a single large neutralization domain (Morita *et al.*, 1988; Taniguchi *et al.*, 1988a).

Recent analysis of the high resolution structure of VP7 allowed grouping various epitopes identified by Mab escape mutations at intersubunit boundaries designated 7-1a and 7-1b, of the calcium dependent VP7 trimers, corresponding to antigenic regions A and C, respectively. Alternatively, epitopes recognized by neutralizing anti-VP7 Mabs were identified at intrasubunit boundaries designated 7-2, corresponding to antigenic region B. Mabs that bind the 7-1 region are partially dependent on bivalency for neutralization, and Mabs that bind epitopes in the 7-2 region are completely dependent on bivalency for neutralization. In general anti-VP7 Mabs neutralize by cross-linking VP7 trimers (Aoki *et al.*).

The mechanisms of neutralization by Mabs that bind at intersubunit or intrasubunit boundaries of VP7 trimers seem to be different. Mabs that recognize intersubunit boundaries inhibit uncoating of the virion outer layer (Aoki *et al.*; Ruggeri & Greenberg, 1991). Mabs that recognize intrasubunit might interfere with VP4 conformational changes needed for viral entry (Aoki *et al.*).

Anti-VP7 Mabs have been produced that neutralize specific G serotypes by neutralization assays (Coulson *et al.*, 1986; Heath *et al.*, 1986; Shaw *et al.*, 1985; Taniguchi *et al.*, 1987). The structure of the G3-specific neutralizing Mab 4F8 bound to the surface of the G3 strain RRV has been determined (Aoki *et al.*). 4F8 Fabs bind to the intersubunit region 7-1 of VP7 trimers on the surface of the virion. Other serotype-specific Mabs bind the same region on VP7, as determined by the location of mutations that escape neutralization, hence suggesting that binding to the interface of VP7 trimers by divalent Mabs is needed for neutralization by serotype-specific Mabs.

Several sets of serotype-specific anti-VP7 Mabs have been used in ELISAs to detect RVA serotypes G1 to G4 (Coulson *et al.*, 1986; Heath *et al.*, 1986; Shaw *et al.*, 1985; Taniguchi *et al.*, 1988a). The specificity of some of these Mabs has been confirmed by comparison with conventional neutralization tests (Urasawa *et al.*, 1988; Ward *et al.*, 1991). Further development of Mabs that specifically neutralize other RVA serotypes, like G6, G8, G9, and G10, have been useful to increase the coverage of serotyping ELISAs to detect emerging or zoonotic RVA infections (Coulson et al., 1999; Keklar & Ayachit, 2000). Serotype-specific ELISAs have been used in numerous studies to determine the prevalence of different G serotypes in different parts of the world (Beards et al., 1989; Keklar & Ayachit, 2000;

Urasawa et al., 1989). Serotype G1 is the most important serotype in humans throughout the world, accounting for more than 50% of all infections, and other serotypes of the Wa-like family, *i. e.* G3, G4, and G9, are also important, together with the single G2 serotype of the DS1-like family (Santos & Hoshino, 2005). The prevalence of different G serotypes differ by geographic region in the same epidemic season, and it also changes in the same area in consecutive epidemic seasons (Urasawa *et al.*, 1989).

The sensitivity of serotype-specific Mabs to detect all RVA strains in different epidemiologic studies has been variable. Because of epitope variation between RVA strains, the use of several Mabs directed at different epitopes may increase the sensitivity of the method (Ward *et al.*, 1991).

A study of the repertoire of neutralization epitopes on VP4 was done by sequencing the VP4 gene of RVA strain SA11 selected after 39 passages in the presence of hyperimmune anti-SA11 serum. The antiserum selected many mutations in the largest variable region of VP4, localized at amino acids 92-192 in VP8*, and in four positions in VP5*, one in amino acid 393, close to the variable region localized at amino acids 384 to 388, and three in amino acids 453, 588, and 736 (Gorziglia *et al.*, 1990). Studies of neutralization escape mutants selected with neutralizing anti-VP4 Mabs have identified mutations in VP8*, within the variable region of VP8* or very close (Mackow *et al.*, 1988b; Padilla-Noriega *et al.*, 1995; Zhou *et al.*, 1994). Fewer neutralization escape mutants are localized in the second cleavage product of VP4, VP5*, some in the segment 385-392, and also in positions 305, 428, 433, and 494 (Kobayashi *et al.*, 1990; Padilla-Noriega *et al.*, 1995; Taniguchi *et al.*, 1988b). By analyzing the cross-neutralization patterns of several anti-VP4 Mabs with their neutralization escape mutants, 3 independent neutralization domains were identified in human RVA KU, one in VP8* and two in VP5* (Kobayashi *et al.*, 1990). One of the domains in VP5* of KU has been identified only in this strain, using a single Mab, YO-2C2, that selects a neutralization escape mutant in position 305. The same approach was used to study the antigenic structure of the human rotavirus ST3, with a panel of neutralizing Mabs that included 2 anti-KU Mabs that served to define neutralization domains previously established in this strain. By using this approach, 2 neutralization domains were identified in ST3, one in VP8*, and one in VP5* that is operationally related to the large neutralization domain in KU, SA11, and RRV.

From the above studies, VP4 serotypes depend on 3 operationally defined neutralization domains, 2 major domains, one in VP5* and the second in VP8*, and one minor domain on VP5*. The 2 large neutralization domains consist of several operationally related epitopes, and the minor domain consists of a single epitope defined by the Mab YO-2C2.

In one study a VP4 serotyping ELISA was used to characterize the antigenic diversity of VP4 in 569 stool specimens of individuals naturally infected with RVAs. Five neutralizing Mabs were used that had been preliminarily characterized as specific for VP4 serotypes P1A, P1B, and P2. In order to validate the VP4 serotyping ELISA, the genotype of a subset of samples was determined by PCR. Three different patterns of reactivity were found among genotype P[4] strains, corresponding to serotype P1B, and 5 different patterns of reactivity were found among P[8] strains, corresponding to serotype P1A. No genotype P[6] strain was detected in this study, corresponding to serotype P2. The conclusion was that P serotypes can be identified by the patterns of reactivity obtained with multiple Mabs used in serotype specific ELISA (Padilla-Noriega *et al.*, 1998).

5. Anti-rotavirus ELISAs

ELISAs to detect the presence of anti-RVA IgG in individuals or seroprevalence in populations have been successfully developed, using particulate rotavirus antigen. As with ELISAs to detect rotavirus antigen, the dominant antibodies in these assays are anti-VP6. Anti-rotavirus IgM and IgA ELISAs have also been developed, however the sensitivity of these assays is limited (Menchaca *et al.*, 1998; Midthun *et al.*, 1989).

In one study, purified RRV DLPs were used as antigen in ELISA to detect anti-RVA IgG in 125 serum samples from asymptomatic Galapagos sea lion (GSL) pups. Due to the lack of anti-GSL IgG, protein A-peroxidase was used to detect IgG binding to the coat antigen. The sensitivity of the assay was determined by testing 6 serum samples from adult California sea lions (CSL) and one anti-VP6 Mab that had been produced using the human Wa strain as antigen. Adult sera of species susceptible to rotavirus usually contain serum anti-RVA IgG, hence the 6 control sera from adults were expected to contain anti-RVA antibodies. The signal produced in the anti-RVA ELISA by adult sera could be competed to background levels by purified RRV antigen, thus demonstrating the specificity of the assay. Antibodies to rotavirus were detected in 22% of the GSL pups, demonstrating that rotavirus infections are prevalent at an early age in this species (Coria-Galindo *et al.*, 2009).

6. Recombinant rotavirus protein IgG ELISAs

An RVA ELISA to measure the humoral immune response to RRV VP4 and its cleavage products VP5* and VP8* was developed by coating plates with the recombinant baculovirus-expressed proteins, followed by incubation with paired serum samples from infants vaccinated with 2 RVA vaccines, RRV and RRV-derived human RVA reassortant vaccine. In experimental vaccination with live attenuated virus the serotype specificity of the infecting virus is known, thereby allowing the detection of homologous immune responses to the recombinant proteins used in the assay. The presence of anti-VP4, anti-VP5*, and anti-VP8* antibodies was then detected with an anti-IgG conjugate. Of the 44 vaccinated infants studied a high percentage seroresponded to VP4 and VP8*, but fewer infants seroresponded to VP5*, indicating that VP5* is less immunogenic than VP8* (Padilla-Noriega *et al.*, 1992). VP5* induces mostly cross-reactive neutralizing antibodies while VP8* induces mostly strain-specific neutralizing antibodies, hence the low immunogenicity of VP5* might adversely affect the efficacy of rotavirus vaccines. In addition, the failure of natural rotavirus infections to induce a strong cross-reactive neutralizing antibody response might contribute to the short duration of protective immunity, allowing repeated RVA infections throughout life.

An RVA ELISA to measure the humoral immune response to RRV VP7 was developed by coating plates with the recombinant baculovirus-expressed VP7, followed by incubation with paired serum samples from mice immunized with recombinant VP7 (Fiore *et al.*, 1995). The recombinant VP7 was not immunoprecipitated by Mabs that recognize antigenic region 7-1, which are the most potent RVA neutralizing antibodies (Ruggeri & Greenberg, 1991). This finding suggest that unlike TLPs, the recombinant VP7 would not be able to induce neutralizing Mabs to the antigenic region 7-1, due to a conformational difference between the recombinant protein alone or assembled in TLPs.

NSP2 is highly immunogenic in natural RVA infections. In one study, recombinant NSP2 from the N5 strain SA11 was used as antigen in ELISA to detect the IgG and IgA serum antibody responses from 27 children hospitalized for primary RVA gastroenteritis. Heterotypic anti-NSP2 IgG and IgA responses were detected in 100% and 75% of children, respectively. It is of interest that the strong antibody response to NSP2 in natural RVA infections has been useful to detect IgA antibody responses by ELISA to this non-structural protein with high sensitivity (Colomina *et al.*, 1998; Kirkwood *et al.*, 2008).

7. DLP-binding ELISA, a functional assay

A DLP-binding assay was developed that captures purified DLPs from the simian RVA SA11, using recombinant SA11 NSP4 bound to ELISA plates, coupled to detection of the captured DLPs with and anti-VP6 Mab (Jagannath et al., 2006). Upon fusion to the carboxy terminus of glutathione-S-transferase (GST), the C-terminal 20 amino acids of NSP4 were identified as sufficient for DLP-binding, however a C-terminal peptide failed to inhibit the receptor activity of the full-length protein, indicating that DLP binding may somehow depend also on other parts of the protein (Au et al., 1993; O'Brien et al., 2000; Taylor et al., 1993). The N-terminus of NSP4 is relevant for DLP binding, since a deletion mutant lacking the N-terminal 85 amino acids is severely affected in this function. In contrast, ΔN72, a deletion mutant lacking the N-terminal 72 amino acids is fully competent for DLP binding. Site-specific mutations Y166, P168, and M175 in the C-terminus of ΔN72 are totally unable to bind DLPs, supporting the notion that the C-terminus is the primary DLP-binding site, while site-specific mutations in other parts of this protein, F76, Y85, and Y131, exhibit loss of binding which can be regained using higher concentrations of recombinant NSP4 bound to the plates. The dependence of binding upon NSP4 concentration may result from enhanced affinity and cooperativity, suggesting that upon binding of the C-terminus to DLPs, a conformational rearrangement generates a secondary site of interaction in the N-terminus of NSP4, resulting in enhanced affinity (Jagannath et al., 2006).

8. Rotavirus epitope-specific competition ELISAs

RVA epitope-specific competition ELISAs were developed with neutralizing anti-VP4 and anti-VP7 Mabs. These assays were used to analyze the serotype-specificity of the immune response in individuals vaccinated or naturally infected with RVA. Two basic formats have been used for RVA competitive binding ELISA, one to detect binding of Mabs to virus particles bound to the plate and another that allows virus particles to bind Mabs in solution.

To perform competitive biotinilated-Mab ELISA (CBME), the virus has to be purified and bound directly to a plate with a buffer at high pH (*i. e.* bicarbonate buffer, pH 9.6) in the presence of calcium to prevent outer layer disassembly. In order to allow competition to occur, the coated plates are incubated with serial dilutions of the competing antibody and subsequently with a biotinilated Mab. Finally, to detect the amount of biotinilated antibody bound to the viral particles in the solid phase the plates are incubated with avidin-horseradish peroxidase conjugate (Shaw *et al.*, 1987). In a variant of CBME, the epitope-blocking assay (EBA) the virus is bound indirectly to the plate by using a hyperimmune anti-rotavirus serum to the homologous virus strain. At the competition phase, the plates are incubated with serial dilutions of the competing antibody, and subsequently with the Mab of interest. Finally, the amount of Mab bound to the viral particles is determined with anti-mouse IgG conjugated to horseradish peroxidase (Matson *et al.*, 1992).

One format that allows virus particles to bind Mabs in solution, the competitive Mab capture ELISA (CMCE), is performed in plates coated with a Mab. In a separate plate, serial dilutions of the competing antibody are incubated with the viral antigen, and the antigen-antibody complexes are added to the plate containing the capture Mab. Finally, the amount of virus bound to the plates is detected in two steps, by incubation with hyperimmune anti-rotavirus serum and then with horseradish peroxidase-conjugated anti-IgG to the species used to produce the hyperimmune serum (Burns *et al.*, 1988).

The antigenic structure of VP7 from human and simian RVA strains has been analyzed by competition ELISAs. One study compared 3 different sets of neutralizing anti-VP7 Mabs for their ability to bind virus particles in CCME. The antigen used in the competition assays was matched to the antigen used to produce the Mabs that included serotypes G1 to G4. Mabs that recognize epitopes in antigenic regions A and C competed completely, indicating that regions A and C are adjacent to each other on the virus particle (Raj *et al.*, 1992). In contrast, a CBME study with the G3 strain RRV as antigen showed nonreciprocal competition between Mabs that recognize regions A and C of VP7 (Shaw *et al.*, 1987). It is possible that viral particle binding to the plates in CBME rigidifies the outer layer therefore restricting interactions that can occur in solution. From these results, a single large neutralization domain was identified in VP7 with several operationally related epitopes in antigenic regions A, B, and C.

A study of neutralizing and non-neutralizing anti-VP4 Mabs for their ability to bind SA11 particles was performed by CCME. The study included 13 Mabs produced using the P5B P[2] simian strain SA11 as antigen, and two cross-reactive anti-VP4 Mabs made to the P5B P[3] simian strain RRV and the P9 P[7] strain OSU. Of the 6 neutralizing Mabs used in competition assays, 4 selected neutralization escape mutations in VP8* (Zhou *et al.*, 1994), the single Mab 2G4 selected neutralization escape mutants in VP5* and reacted by immunoprecipitation with VP5* (Mackow *et al.*, 1988b; Mackow *et al.*, 1990), and one Mab has not been characterized. As determined by CCME, VP4 has one neutralization domain with 3 antigenic sites, 2 in VP8* and one in VP5*. The different patterns of competition among antigenic sites seem to reflect functional differences between VP5* and VP8* and overall conformational flexibility of VP4, since: i) neutralizing antibodies directed to the antigenic site 1 in VP8* enhanced binding of all non-neutralizing antibodies; ii) the single neutralizing Mab directed to site 2 in VP5* competed with all Mabs, either neutralizing or non-neutralizing; and iii) the single Mab directed to site 3 in VP8* partially competed with all other Mabs, either neutralizing or non-neutralizing. It is of interest that CCME allows conformational alterations of VP4 to occur in solution, thereby revealing that all anti-VP4 neutralizing Mabs seemed to alter the conformational structure of VP4, leading to enhanced binding by other Mabs (Burns *et al.*, 1988). By considering the specificity of the Mabs used in CCME to the cleavage products of VP4, this assay revealed that neutralizing anti-VP8* Mabs are able to allosterically alter the conformation of VP5*.

Studies of the antigenic structure of RRV VP4 by CBME were performed with 11 neutralizing and one non-neutralizing Mab. Of the neutralizing Mabs, 4 selected escape mutations in VP8*, and a single Mab (2G4) on VP5*. As determined by CBME VP4 has one neutralization domain with 2 antigenic sites, one in VP8* and one in VP5*, that is operationally related to the epitope recognized by the single non-neutralizing Mab. The different patterns of competition among antigenic sites determined by CBME seem to reflect more clearly the functional differences between VP5* and VP8* than CCME, since: i) there was no binding enhancement between any pair of Mabs; ii) the single neutralizing Mab directed to the site denominated B in VP5* competed with only one of 10 Mabs directed to the antigenic site A. From these results, CBME, based on the interaction of RVA particles with antibodies in the solid phase, restricts the allosteric changes induced in solution by neutralizing anti-VP8 Mabs on VP5*.

9. Conclusion

The antigenic structure of RVA and the diversity of the antibody response in RVA infections have been studied using a number of ELISAs. Group/species A rotavirus ELISAs and typing ELISAs have been widely used to diagnose RVA infections and to determine the SG and serotype specificities of the field specimens. Anti-rotavirus IgG ELISAs have been used to determine the prevalence of RVA infections in human and animal populations. Recombinant RVA protein IgG ELISAs have been relevant to dissect the antibody response to individual RVA proteins, and to describe the magnitude of the antibody response to the surface proteins of the virion. Epitope-specific ELISAs have been used to analyze the repertoire of neutralizing antibodies induced by natural RVA infections or vaccination, and the antigenicity of cross-reactive and serotype-specific epitopes on the surface proteins of the virion. The knowledge gained on the serotypic diversity and the antigenic structure of RVA particles by using diverse ELISAs are relevant in the design of new vaccines to protect broadly against all relevant RVA serotypes.

10. Acknowledgement

This research was partly supported by grants 51029-Z from Consejo Nacional de Ciencia y Tecnología, Mexico, and IN-224809 from DGAPA-PAPIIT, Universidad Nacional Autónoma de México. I thank Renato León-Rodríguez for technical assistance.

11. References

Aoki, S. T.; Trask, S. D.; Coulson, B. S.; Greenberg, H. B.; Dormitzer, P. R. & Harrison, S. C. Cross-linking of rotavirus outer capsid protein VP7 by antibodies or disulfides inhibits viral entry. *Journal of Virology*, Vol. 85, No. 20, (Oct), pp. 10509-10517

Au, K. S.; Mattion, N. M. & Estes, M. K. (1993). A subviral particle binding domain on the rotavirus nonstructural glycoprotein NS28. *Virology*, Vol. 194, No. 2, (Jun), pp. 665-673

Beards, G. M.; Desselberger, U. & Flewett, T. H. (1989). Temporal and geographical distributions of human rotavirus serotypes, 1983 to 1988. *Journal of Clinical Microbiology*, Vol. 27, No. 12, (Dec), pp. 2827-2833

Bergmann, C. C.; Maass, D.; Poruchynsky, M. S.; Atkinson, P. H. & Bellamy, A. R. (1989). Topology of the non-structural rotavirus receptor glycoprotein NS28 in the rough endoplasmic reticulum. *EMBO Journal*, Vol. 8, No. 6, (Jun), pp. 1695-1703

Burns, J. W.; Greenberg, H. B.; Shaw, R. D. & Estes, M. K. (1988). Functional and topographical analyses of epitopes on the hemagglutinin (VP4) of the simian rotavirus SA11. *Journal of Virology*, Vol. 62, No. 6, (Jun), pp. 2164-2172

Colomina, J.; Gil, M. T.; Codoñer, P. & Buesa, J. (1998). Viral proteins VP2, VP6, and NSP2 are strongly precipitated by serum and fecal antibodies from children with rotavirus infection. *Journal of Medical Virology*, Vol. 56, No. 1, pp. 58-65

Coria-Galindo, E.; Rangel-Huerta, E.; Verdugo-Rodriguez, A.; Brousset, D.; Salazar, S. & Padilla-Noriega, L. (2009). Rotavirus infections in Galapagos sea lions. *Journal of Wildlife Diseases*, Vol. 45, No. 3, (Jul), pp. 722-728

Coulson, B. S. (1993). Typing of human rotavirus VP4 by an enzyme immunoassay using monoclonal antibodies. *Journal of Clinical Microbiology,* Vol. 31, No. 1, (Jan), pp. 1-8

Coulson, B. S.; Gentsch, J. R.; Das, B. K.; Bhan, M. K. & Glass, R. I. (1999). Comparison of enzyme immunoassay and reverse transcriptase PCR for identification of serotype G9 rotaviruses. *Jorunal of Clinical Microbiology,* Vol. 37, No. 10, pp. 3187-3193

Coulson, B. S.; Tursi, J. M.; McAdam, W. J. & Bishop, R. F. (1986). Derivation of neutralizing monoclonal antibodies to human rotaviruses and evidence that an immunodominant neutralization site is shared between serotypes 1 and 3. *Virology,* Vol. 30, No. 2, pp. 302-312

Chan, W. K.; Au, K. S. & Estes, M. K. (1988). Topography of the simian rotavirus nonstructural glycoprotein (NS28) in the endoplasmic reticulum membrane. *Virology,* Vol. 164, No. 2, (Jun), pp. 435-442

Dormitzer, P. R.; Greenberg, H. B. & Harrison, S. C. (2000). Purified recombinant rotavirus VP7 forms soluble, calcium-dependent trimers. *Virology,* Vol. 277, No. 2, (Nov 25), pp. 420-428

Dyall-Smith, M. L.; Lazdins, I.; Tregear, G. W. & Holmes, I. H. (1986). Location of the major antigenic sites involved in rotavirus serotype-specific neutralization. *Proceedings of the National Academy of Sciences U S A,* Vol. 83, No. 10, (May), pp. 3465-3468

Estes, M. K. (2001). Rotaviruses and their replication. In: *Fields Virology,* pp. 1747-1785, Lippincott Williams & Wilkins. Philadelphia

Estes, M. K. & Kapikian, A. Z. (2007). Rotaviruses. In: *Fields Virology,* Fifth (Ed.), pp. 1917-1974, Lippincott Williams & Wilkins, 13:979-0-7817-6060-7. Philadelphia

Fiore, L.; Dunn, S. J.; Ridolfi, B.; Ruggeri, F. M.; Mackow, E. R. & Greenberg, H. B. (1995). Antigenicity, immunogenicity and passive protection induced by immunization of mice with baculovirus-expressed VP7 protein from rhesus rotavirus. *Journal of General Virology,* Vol. 76 (Pt 8), No. (Aug), pp. 1981-1988

Flewett, T. H.; Arias, C. F.; Avendano, L. F.; Ghafoor, A.; Mathan, M. M.; Mendis, L.; Moe, K. & Bishop, R. F. (1989). Comparative evaluation of the WHO and DAKOPATTS enzyme-linked immunoassay kits for rotavirus detection. *Bulletin of the World Health Organization,* Vol. 67, No. 4, pp. 369-374

Gallegos, C. O. & Patton, J. T. (1989). Characterization of rotavirus replication intermediates: a model for the assembly of single-shelled particles. *Virology,* Vol. 172, No. 2, (Oct), pp. 616-627

Gerna, G.; Sarasini, A.; Torsellini, M.; di Matteo, A.; Baldanti, F.; Parea, M. & Battaglia, M. (1989). Characterization of rotavirus subgroup-specific monoclonal antibodies and use in single-sandwich ELISA systems for rapid subgrouping of human strains. *Archives of Virology,* Vol. 107, No. 3-4, pp. 315-322

Gorziglia, M.; Hoshino, Y.; Nishikawa, K.; Maloy, W. L.; Jones, R. W.; Kapikian, A. Z. & Chanock, R. M. (1988). Comparative sequence analysis of the genomic segment 6 of four rotaviruses each with a different subgroup specificity. *Journal of General Virology,* Vol. 69, No. pp. 1659-1669

Gorziglia, M.; Larralde, G. & Ward, R. L. (1990). Neutralization epitopes on rotavirus SA11 4fM outer capsid proteins. *Journal of Virology,* Vol. 64, No. 9, (Sep), pp. 4534-4539

Greenberg, H.; McAuliffe, V.; Valdesuso, J.; Wyatt, R.; Flores, J.; Kalica, A.; Hoshino, Y. & Singh, N. (1983). Serological analysis of the subgroup protein of rotavirus, using monoclonal antibodies. *Infection and Immunity,* Vol. 39, No. 1, (Jan), pp. 91-99

Heath, R.; Birch, C. & Gust, I. (1986). Antigenic analysis of rotavirus isolates using monoclonal antibodies specific for human serotypes 1, 2, 3 and 4, and SA11. *Journal of General Virology,* Vol. 67 (Pt 11), No. (Nov), pp. 2455-2466

Hoshino, Y.; Gorziglia, M.; Valdesuso, J.; Askaa, J.; Glass, R. I. & Kapikian, A. Z. (1987). An equine rotavirus (FI-14 strain) which bears both subgroup I and subgroup II specificities on its VP6. *Virology*, Vol. 157, No. 2, (Apr), pp. 488-496

Hoshino, Y. & Kapikian, A. Z. (1996). Classification of rotavirus VP4 and VP7 serotypes. *Archives of Virology Supplement*, Vol. 12, No. pp. 99-111

Hoshino, Y.; Nishikawa, K.; Benfield, D. A. & Gorziglia, M. (1994). Mapping of antigenic sites involved in serotype-cross-reactive neutralization on group A rotavirus outercapsid glycoprotein VP7. *Virology*, Vol. 199, No. 1, (Feb 15), pp. 233-237

Jagannath, M. R.; Kesavulu, M. M.; Deepa, R.; Sastri, P. N.; Kumar, S. S.; Suguna, K. & Rao, C. D. (2006). N- and C-terminal cooperation in rotavirus enterotoxin: novel mechanism of modulation of the properties of a multifunctional protein by a structurally and functionally overlapping conformational domain. *Journal of Virology*, Vol. 80, No. 1, (Jan), pp. 412-425

Jiang, X.; Crawford, S.; Estes, M. K. & Prasad, B. V. V. (2008). Rotavirus structure. In: *Segmented double-stranded RNA viruses*, pp. 45-60, Caister Academic Press, 978:1-904455-21-9. Norfolk, UK

Kapikian, A. Z. & Chanock, R. M. (1996). Rotaviruses. In: *Fields Virology*, pp. 1657-1708, Lippincott-Raven Publishers. Philadelphia

Keklar, S. D. & Ayachit, V. L. (2000). Circulation of group A rotavirus subgroups and serotypes in India, 1990-1997. *Journal of Health Population and Nutrition*, Vol. 18, No. 3, pp. 163-170

Kim, I. S.; Trask, S. D.; Babyonyshev, M.; Dormitzer, P. R. & Harrison, S. C. Effect of mutations in VP5 hydrophobic loops on rotavirus cell entry. *Journal of Virology*, Vol. 84, No. 12, (Jun), pp. 6200-6207

Kirkwood, C. D.; Boniface, K.; Richardson, S.; Taraporewala, Z. F.; Patton, J. T. & Bishop, R. F. (2008). Non-structural protein NSP2 induces heterotypic antibody responses during primary rotavirus infection and reinfection in children. *Journal of Medical Virology*, Vol. 80, No. 6, (Jun), pp. 1090-1098

Kobayashi, N.; Taniguchi, K. & Urasawa, S. (1990). Identification of operationally overlapping and independent cross-reactive neutralization regions on human rotavirus VP4. *Journal of General Virology*, Vol. 71 (Pt 11), No. (Nov), pp. 2615-2623

Kobayashi, N.; Taniguchi, K. & Urasawa, S. (1991). Analysis of the newly identified neutralization epitopes on VP7 of human rotavirus serotype 1. *Journal of General Virology*, Vol. 72 (Pt 1), No. (Jan), pp. 117-124

Li, Z.; Baker, M. L.; Jiang, W.; Estes, M. K. & Prasad, B. V. (2009). Rotavirus architecture at subnanometer resolution. *Journal of Virology*, Vol. 83, No. 4, (Feb), pp. 1754-1766

Liprandi, F.; Lopez, G.; Rodriguez, I.; Hidalgo, M.; Ludert, J. E. & Mattion, N. (1990). Monoclonal antibodies to the VP6 of porcine subgroup I rotaviruses reactive with subgroup I and non-subgroup I non-subgroup II strains. *Journal of General Virology*, Vol. 71 (Pt 6), No. (Jun), pp. 1395-1398

Liu, M.; Offit, P. A. & Estes, M. K. (1988). Identification of the simian rotavirus SA11 genome segment 3 product. *Virology*, Vol. 163, No. 1, (Mar), pp. 26-32

Loisy, F.; Atmar, R. L.; Cohen, J.; Bosch, A. & Le Guyader, F. S. (2004). Rotavirus VLP2/6: a new tool for tracking rotavirus in the marine environment. *Research in Microbiology*, Vol. 155, No. 7, (Sep), pp. 575-578

Lopez, S. & Arias, C. F. (2006). Early steps in rotavirus cell entry. *Current Topics in Microbiology and Immunology*, Vol. 309, No. pp. 39-66

Lopez, S.; Espinosa, R.; Greenberg, H. B. & Arias, C. F. (1994). Mapping the subgroup epitopes of rotavirus protein VP6. *Virology*, Vol. 204, No. 1, (Oct), pp. 153-162

Lopez, T.; Camacho, M.; Zayas, M.; Najera, R.; Sanchez, R.; Arias, C. F. & Lopez, S. (2005). Silencing the morphogenesis of rotavirus. *Journal of Virology,* Vol. 79, No. 1, (Jan), pp. 184-192

Mackow, E. R.; Shaw, R. D.; Matsui, S. M.; Vo, P. T.; Benfield, D. A. & Greenberg, H. B. (1988a). Characterization of homotypic and heterotypic VP7 neutralization sites of rhesus rotavirus. *Virology,* Vol. 165, No. 2, (Aug), pp. 511-517

Mackow, E. R.; Shaw, R. D.; Matsui, S. M.; Vo, P. T.; Dang, M. N. & Greenberg, H. B. (1988b). The rhesus rotavirus gene encoding protein VP3: location of amino acids involved in homologous and heterologous rotavirus neutralization and identification of a putative fusion region. *Procedings of the National Academy of Sciences U S A,* Vol. 85, No. 3, (Feb), pp. 645-649

Mackow, E. R.; Yamanaka, M. Y.; Dang, M. N. & Greenberg, H. B. (1990). DNA amplification-restricted transcription-translation: rapid analysis of rhesus rotavirus neutralization sites. *Procedings of the National Academy of Sciences U S A,* Vol. 87, No. 2, (Jan), pp. 518-522

Mathieu, M.; Petitpas, I.; Navaza, J.; Lepault, J.; Kohli, E.; Pothier, P.; Prasad, B. V.; Cohen, J. & Rey, F. A. (2001). Atomic structure of the major capsid protein of rotavirus: implications for the architecture of the virion. *EMBO Journal,* Vol. 20, No. 7, (Apr 2), pp. 1485-1497

Matson, D. O.; O'Ryan, M. L.; Pickering, L. K.; Chiba, S.; Nakata, S.; Raj, P. & Estes, M. K. (1992). Characterization of serum antibody responses to natural rotavirus infections in children by VP7-specific epitope-blocking assays. *Journal of Clinical Microbiology,* Vol. 30, No. 5, (May), pp. 1056-1061

Matthijnssens, J.; Ciarlet, M.; Heiman, E.; Arijs, I.; Delbeke, T.; McDonald, S. M.; Palombo, E. A.; Iturriza-Gomara, M.; Maes, P.; Patton, J. T.; Rahman, M. & Van Ranst, M. (2008). Full genome-based classification of rotaviruses reveals a common origin between human Wa-Like and porcine rotavirus strains and human DS-1-like and bovine rotavirus strains. *Journal of Virology,* Vol. 82, No. 7, (Apr), pp. 3204-3219

Matthijnssens, J.; Ciarlet, M.; McDonald, S. M.; Attoui, H.; Banyai, K.; Brister, J. R.; Buesa, J.; Esona, M. D.; Estes, M. K.; Gentsch, J. R.; Iturriza-Gomara, M.; Johne, R.; Kirkwood, C. D.; Martella, V.; Mertens, P. P.; Nakagomi, O.; Parreno, V.; Rahman, M.; Ruggeri, F. M.; Saif, L. J.; Santos, N.; Steyer, A.; Taniguchi, K.; Patton, J. T.; Desselberger, U. & Van Ranst, M. Uniformity of rotavirus strain nomenclature proposed by the Rotavirus Classification Working Group (RCWG). *Archives of Virology,* Vol. 156, No. 8, (Aug), pp. 1397-1413

Menchaca, G.; Padilla-Noriega, L.; Mendez-Toss, M.; Contreras, J. F.; Puerto, F. I.; Guiscafre, H.; Mota, F.; Herrera, I.; Cedillo, R.; Munoz, O.; Ward, R.; Hoshino, Y.; Lopez, S. & Arias, C. F. (1998). Serotype specificity of the neutralizing-antibody response induced by the individual surface proteins of rotavirus in natural infections of young children. *Clinical and Diagnostic Microbiology and Immunology,* Vol. 5, No. 3, (May), pp. 328-334

Midthun, K.; Pang, L. Z.; Flores, J. & Kapikian, A. Z. (1989). Comparison of immunoglobulin A (IgA), IgG, and IgM enzyme-linked immunosorbent assays, plaque reduction neutralization assay, and complement fixation in detecting seroresponses to rotavirus vaccine candidates. *Journal of Clinical Microbiology,* Vol. 27, No. 12, (Dec), pp. 2799-2804

Morita, Y.; Taniguchi, K.; Urasawa, T. & Urasawa, S. (1988). Analysis of serotype-specific neutralization epitopes on VP7 of human rotavirus by the use of neutralizing monoclonal antibodies and antigenic variants. *Journal of General Virology,* Vol. 69 (Pt 2), No. (Feb), pp. 451-458

O'Brien, J. A.; Taylor, J. A. & Bellamy, A. R. (2000). Probing the structure of rotavirus NSP4: a short sequence at the extreme C terminus mediates binding to the inner capsid particle. *J Virol*, Vol. 74, No. 11, (Jun), pp. 5388-5394

Padilla-Noriega, L.; Dunn, S. J.; Lopez, S.; Greenberg, H. B. & Arias, C. F. (1995). Identification of two independent neutralization domains on the VP4 trypsin cleavage products VP5* and VP8* of human rotavirus ST3. *Virology*, Vol. 206, No. 1, (Jan 10), pp. 148-154

Padilla-Noriega, L.; Fiore, L.; Rennels, M. B.; Losonsky, G. A.; Mackow, E. R. & Greenberg, H. B. (1992). Humoral immune responses to VP4 and its cleavage products VP5* and VP8* in infants vaccinated with rhesus rotavirus. *Journal of Clinical Microbiology*, Vol. 30, No. 6, (Jun), pp. 1392-1397

Padilla-Noriega, L.; Mendez-Toss, M.; Menchaca, G.; Contreras, J. F.; Romero-Guido, P.; Puerto, F. I.; Guiscafre, H.; Mota, F.; Herrera, I.; Cedillo, R.; Munoz, O.; Calva, J.; Guerrero, M. L.; Coulson, B. S.; Greenberg, H. B.; Lopez, S. & Arias, C. F. (1998). Antigenic and genomic diversity of human rotavirus VP4 in two consecutive epidemic seasons in Mexico. *Journal of Clinical Microbiology*, Vol. 36, No. 6, (Jun), pp. 1688-1692

Patton, J. T.; Silvestri, L. S.; Tortorici, M. A.; Vasquez-Del Carpio, R. & Taraporewala, Z. F. (2006). Rotavirus genome replication and morphogenesis: role of the viroplasm. *Current Topics in Microbiology and Immunology*, Vol. 309, No. pp. 169-187

Pesavento, J. B.; Crawford, S. E.; Roberts, E.; Estes, M. K. & Prasad, B. V. (2005). pH-induced conformational change of the rotavirus VP4 spike: implications for cell entry and antibody neutralization. *Journal of Virology*, Vol. 79, No. 13, (Jul), pp. 8572-8580

Raj, P.; Matson, D. O.; Coulson, B. S.; Bishop, R. F.; Taniguchi, K.; Urasawa, S.; Greenberg, H. B. & Estes, M. K. (1992). Comparisons of rotavirus VP7-typing monoclonal antibodies by competition binding assay. *Journal of Clinical Microbiology*, Vol. 30, No. 3, (Mar), pp. 704-711

Ruggeri, F. M. & Greenberg, H. B. (1991). Antibodies to the trypsin cleavage peptide VP8 neutralize rotavirus by inhibiting binding of virions to target cells in culture. *Journal of Virology*, Vol. 65, No. 5, (May), pp. 2211-2219

Santos, N. & Hoshino, Y. (2005). Global distribution of rotavirus serotypes/genotypes and its implication for the development and implementation of an effective rotavirus vaccine. *Reviews in Medical Virology*, Vol. 15, No. 1, (Jan-Feb), pp. 29-56

Settembre, E. C.; Chen, J. Z.; Dormitzer, P. R.; Grigorieff, N. & Harrison, S. C. Atomic model of an infectious rotavirus particle. *EMBO Journal*, Vol. 30, No. 2, (Jan 19), pp. 408-416

Shaw, R. D.; Fong, K. J.; Losonsky, G. A.; Levine, M. M.; Maldonado, Y.; Yolken, R.; Flores, J.; Kapikian, A. Z.; Vo, P. T. & Greenberg, H. B. (1987). Epitope-specific immune responses to rotavirus vaccination. *Gastroenterology*, Vol. 93, No. 5, (Nov), pp. 941-950

Shaw, R. D.; Stoner-Ma, D. L.; Estes, M. K. & Greenberg, H. B. (1985). Specific enzyme-linked immunoassay for rotavirus serotypes 1 and 3. *Journal of Clinical Microbiology*, Vol. 22, No. 2, (Aug), pp. 286-291

Svensson, L.; Padilla-Noriega, L.; Taniguchi, K. & Greenberg, H. (1990). Lack of cosegregation of the subgroup II antigens on genes 2 and 6 in porcine rotaviruses. *Journal of Virology*, Vol. 64, No. 1, pp. 411-413

Tang, B.; Gilbert, J. M.; Matsui, S. M. & Greenberg, H. B. (1997). Comparison of the rotavirus gene 6 from different species by sequence analysis and localization of subgroup-specific epitopes using site-directed mutagenesis. *Virology*, Vol. 237, No. 1, (Oct 13), pp. 89-96

Taniguchi, K.; Hoshino, Y.; Nishikawa, K.; Green, K. Y.; Maloy, W. L.; Morita, Y.; Urasawa, S.; Kapikian, A. Z.; Chanock, R. M. & Gorziglia, M. (1988a). Cross-reactive and serotype-specific neutralization epitopes on VP7 of human rotavirus: nucleotide sequence analysis of antigenic mutants selected with monoclonal antibodies. *Journal of Virology,* Vol. 62, No. 6, (Jun), pp. 1870-1874

Taniguchi, K.; Maloy, W. L.; Nishikawa, K.; Green, K. Y.; Hoshino, Y.; Urasawa, S.; Kapikian, A. Z.; Chanock, R. M. & Gorziglia, M. (1988b). Identification of cross-reactive and serotype 2-specific neutralization epitopes on VP3 of human rotavirus. *Journal of Virology,* Vol. 62, No. 7, (Jul), pp. 2421-2426

Taniguchi, K.; Morita, Y.; Urasawa, T. & Urasawa, S. (1987). Cross-reactive neutralization epitopes on VP3 of human rotavirus: analysis with monoclonal antibodies and antigenic variants. *Journal of Virology,* Vol. 61, No. 5, (May), pp. 1726-1730

Taniguchi, K.; Urasawa, T.; Urasawa, S. & Yasuhara, T. (1984). Production of subgroup-specific monoclonal antibodies against human rotaviruses and their application to an enzyme-linked immunosorbent assay for subgroup determination. *Journal of Medical Virology,* Vol. 14, No. 2, pp. 115-125

Taylor, J. A.; O'Brien, J. A.; Lord, V. J.; Meyer, J. C. & Bellamy, A. R. (1993). The RER-localized rotavirus intracellular receptor: a truncated purified soluble form is multivalent and binds virus particles. *Virology,* Vol. 194, No. 2, (Jun), pp. 807-814

Theil, K. W. & McCloskey, C. M. (1989). Nonreactivity of American avian group A rotaviruses with subgroup-specific monoclonal antibodies. *Journal of Clinical Microbiology,* Vol. 27, No. 12, pp. 2846-2848

Trask, S. D.; Kim, I. S.; Harrison, S. C. & Dormitzer, P. R. A rotavirus spike protein conformational intermediate binds lipid bilayers. *Journal of Virology,* Vol. 84, No. 4, (Feb), pp. 1764-1770

Urasawa, S.; Urasawa, T.; Taniguchi, K.; Morita, Y.; Sakurada, N.; Saeki, Y.; Morita, O. & Hasegawa, S. (1988). Validity of an enzyme-linked immunosorbent assay with serotype-specific monoclonal antibodies for serotyping human rotavirus in stool specimens. *Microbiology and Immunology,* Vol. 32, No. 7, pp. 699-708

Urasawa, S.; Urasawa, T.; Taniguchi, K.; Wakasugi, F.; Kobayashi, N.; Chiba, S.; Sakurada, N.; Morita, M.; Morita, O.; Tokieda, M. & et al. (1989). Survey of human rotavirus serotypes in different locales in Japan by enzyme-linked immunosorbent assay with monoclonal antibodies. *Journal of Infectious Diseases,* Vol. 160, No. 1, (Jul), pp. 44-51

Ward, R. L.; McNeaL, M. M.; Clemens, J. D.; Sack, D. A.; Rao, M.; Huda, N.; Green, K. Y.; Kapikian, A. Z.; Coulson, B. S.; Bishop, R. F.; Greenberg, H. B.; Gerna, G. & Schiff, G. M. (1991). Reactivities of serotyping monoclonal antibodies with culture-adapted human rotavirueses. *Journal of Clinical Microbiology,* Vol. 29, No. 3, pp. 449-456

Wolf, M.; Vo, P. T. & Greenberg, H. B. Rhesus rotavirus entry into a polarized epithelium is endocytosis dependent and involves sequential VP4 conformational changes. *Journal of Virology,* Vol. 85, No. 6, (Mar), pp. 2492-2503

Yolken, R. H.; Barbour, B. A.; Wyatt, R. G.; Kalica, A. R.; Kapikian, A. Z. & Chanock, R. M. (1978). Enzyme-linked immunosorbent assay for identification of rotaviruses from different animal species. *Science,* Vol. 201, No. 4352, pp. 259-262

Yolken, R. H. & Leister, F. (1982). Rapid multiple-determinant enzyme immunoassay for the detection of human rotavirus. *Journal of Infectious Diseases,* Vol. 146, No. 1, (Jul), pp. 43-46

Zhou, Y. J.; Burns, J. W.; Morita, Y.; Tanaka, T. & Estes, M. K. (1994). Localization of rotavirus VP4 neutralization epitopes involved in antibody-induced conformational changes of virus structure. *Journal of Virology,* Vol. 68, No. 6, (Jun), pp. 3955-3964

15

Immunochemical Properties of Recombinant Ompf Porin from Outer Membrane of *Yersinia pseudotuberculosis*

Olga Portnyagina, Olga Sidorova, Valentina Khomenko, Olga Novikova, Marina Issaeva and Tamara Solov'eva
Pacific Institute of Bioorganic Chemistry, Far-Eastern Branch, The Russian Academy of Sciences, Russia

1. Introduction

Porins from outer membranes (OM) of Gram-negative bacteria exist in intact membranes as homotrimers forming water-filled pores or channels that provide low-molecular compounds transportation. Surface localization of the porins and their structural peculiarities determine multiplicity of their functions except for the transport one. On the one hand, porins are targets for the host immune system. As the targets they activate factors of the organism fast protection and are involved in the formation of specific immune response. On the other hand, porins serve as the factors of pathogenesis and virulence inhibiting the first stage of the host immune system and providing survival of a pathogen in macroorganism. Porins are species- and genus-specific antigens of Gram-negative bacteria and belong to the highly immunogenic OM components. The antibodies against the porins are found in blood sera both after vaccination and after natural development of infection.

Many researchers have confirmed the existence of two types of porin antigenic determinants. The first type of the determinants is linear (at the level of the primary structure of the protein) and the second one is conformational (or discontinuous) formed at the higher levels of the protein structure. According to some authors, the majority of the conformational determinants (Ranling, et al, 1995) are destroyed during the dissociation of porin trimers under the different denaturing conditions, especially temperature (Lupi et al, 1980). Most the antigenic determinants are believed to be located in the outer loops with unordered structure. In contrast, epitopes located in the transmembrane protein sites are conservative and have a high degree of homology in porins of *Enterobacteriaceae* microorganisms (Singh et al, 1996).

The immune response to OM proteins (including porins) has a number of features, namely, the high level of antibodies (as a result both of artificial immunization and of the natural infection development) and duration of circulation of antibodies (immunological memory). It should be noted that in the organism of experimental animals (mice, rabbits, rats, and monkeys) antibodies to the OM porins are formed independently of a mode of the antigen injected: isolated proteins, whole cells or the cell wall fragments. As shown, antibodies to porin dominated in the monkey infected and pseudotuberculosis patients' sera but not in small laboratory animal sera after experimental infection (Vostrikova et al, 2000).

In the case of antibodies against recombinant porins, both in trimeric and in monomeric forms of the proteins were shown to be highly immunogenic in rabbits, even without adjuvants (Elkins et al, 1994), as well as they stimulated the production of bactericidal and diagnostic IgG antibodies in immune stimulating complex (iscom) or vesicles containing components of the OM (Peeters et al, 1999; Wright et al, 2002). In some cases immunization with recombinant porin was shown to induce not only CD4 + T-cells proliferation but the production of IL-12 as well (Shaw et al, 2002).

Since immunization with pore-forming proteins of bacterial OM leads to the formation of specific antibodies, activates the cellular immune system response and causes no adverse reactions, the porins are considered to be the most promising candidates for vaccines of new generation (Supotnitsky, 1996).

The bacteria of *Yersinia* species belong to the microorganisms that cause intestinal infections in humans and animals. According to the World Health Organization data these diseases are revealed worldwide and more frequently in the economically developed countries where is a wide network of the centralized foodstuffs supply. At the present special interest to the problem of yersiniosis is connected with the immunopathologies, so-called secondary yersiniosis (or second-hearth) forms (arthritis, myocardit, neuralgia, collagenosis) caused in patients by *Yersinia* infection. The etiology of such immunopathologies is not determined in practice because of the absence of specific diagnostic methods (Portnyagina et al, 2010).

Besides, there are no methods of specific protection from the infections caused by pathogenic *Yersinia*. Therefore, the creation of polyvalent vaccine protecting from plague, intestinal yersiniosis, and pseudotuberculosis is the urgent task. The high degree of homology of *Yersinia* porin primary structures (Guzev et al, 2005; Likhatskaya et al, 2005; Issaeva et al, 2003) is a basis for creation of the vaccine preparations that will protect against all infections caused by pathogenic *Yersinia* species (Antonets et al, 2007; Portnyagina et al, 2010).

In this study we have investigated the capacity of the pore-forming recombinant protein from OM of *Y. pseudotuberculosis* to induce immune response in CBA mice. Immunization with the recombinant protein (with and without adjuvants) resulted in IgG antibodies. High-avidity immune serum was obtained as a result of the tree-time immunization. Bactericidal activity of peritoneal macrophages from mice immunized with recombinant protein was significantly higher than that of intact murine macrophages. The use of the recombinant porin instead of native one as the antigen in ELISA for the diagnostics of acute and secondary-hearth forms of pseudotuberculosis does not reduce the efficiency of detection of specific antibodies in the sera of patients. Obtaining of the *Y. pseudotuberculosis* mutant forms of recombinant OmpF porin with outer loops deletions is of particular interest. The study of the relationship between the structure, function, and antigenic properties of mutant proteins will increase the fundamental understanding of the properties of porins and open up new opportunities for the development of highly efficient and specific means for diagnostics and prevention of diseases caused by*Yersinia.*

2. Obtaining of recombinant porin

2.1 Construction of recombinant plasmid with mature *Y. pseudotuberculosis* OmpF porin sequence

The *ompF* gene lacking sequence for the signal peptide was amplified from genomic DNA of the *Y. pseudotuberculosis* 3260 strain using the primer pair of FYm/NdeI (5`-TCGCATATGGCTGAAATCTACAACAAAG- 3`) and RY/BamHI (5`-GGATCCTTAGAACTGATAAACCAAGCC- 3`). GGATCCTTAGAACTGATAAACCAAGCC-3`) was used in the reaction. The primers were designed with Primer Premier 3. The PCR procedure was carried out in a reaction volume of 100 μl containing 1.5 mM $MgCl_2$, dNTP (200 μM of each), direct and reverse primers (0,5 μM of each), 2.5 U *AmpliTaq* DNA polymerase (Applied Biosystems), and DNA template (50 ng). The thermal cycling profile was as follows: (1) preliminary DNA denaturion at 95°C for 5 min; (2) 35 cycles, denaturion at 94°C for 20 sec, annealing at 55°C for 30 sec, and polymerization reaction at 72°C for 1 min 10 sec; and (3) final extension step of 72°C for 5 min. The amplicons were analyzed by electrophoresis in 1% agarose gel. The resulting PCR fragment was purified, digested by restriction endonucleases *Nde*I and *BamH*I (Fermentas), and cloned into expression vector pET41a (Novagen) by the respective restriction sites. The recombinant clones of *E. coli* DH5□ strain were selected in the presence of kanamycin (50 mg/ml), and recombinant plasmids were verified by DNA sequencing on a ABI PRISM 310 Genetic Analyzer (Applied Biosystems) using universal T7 promotor and T7 terminator primers. The recombinant expression plasmid (pET41-m55) was transformed into BL21 (DE3) (Invitrogen), tand selected in the presence of kanamycin (50 mg/ml). The positive clones were used for large-scale culturing experiments.

2.1.1 Isolation and purification of recombinant protein

The resulting pET-m55 plasmid with an intact reading frame was used for transformation of *E. coli* BL21 (DE3) strain. Selection of the recombinant clones was carried out in the presence of kanamycin (50 mg/ml). An empty vector was used as a control. Immunoblot analysis showed that lysate of transformed *E.coli* BL21 (DE3) strain contained a protein with the mobility close to 40 kDa. It interacted with specific antibodies against thermostable porin monomer (OmpF-m) of the pseudotuberculosis microorganisms. At the same time, this protein was not detected in the non-transformed cells lysate (Fig.1a). Based on these data, we concluded that the protein obtained corresponded to the *Y.pseudotuberculosis* porin. The *E. coli* cells transformed were cultured in 1.0 l of the LB medium containing 100 mg/l kanamycin at 37°C for 4–5 h until obtaining suspension with optical density of~0.6 at 600 nm. One mM IPTG was then added to the medium and the cells were cultured again for another 4–5 h. The cells were precipitated by centrifugation at 10000 *g* for 15 min; the precipitate (5 g) was resuspended in 15 ml of 50 mM Tris-HCl, pH 8.0, containing 1 mM EDTA and 100 mM NaCl (TEN buffer). A solution of PMSF (40 μl, 100 mM stock solution in isopropanol) and lysozyme (4 mg) were added to the suspension. The mixture was stirred at room temperature for 30 min, after that DOC (25 mg) was added and the mixture was kept for 20 min on a water bath at 37°C. DNase (30 μl, 1 mg/ml stock solution) was added, the mixture was stirred at room temperature until obtaining of a non-viscous solution. The mixture was then centrifuged at 12000 *g* for 20 min at 4°C. The precipitate of inclusion bodies (IB) was washed twice then urea and PMSF up to final concentrations of 8 M and 0.1 mM, respectively. The mixture was sonicated at 44 MHz for 10 min with intervals of 1 min. The insoluble precipitate was separated by centrifugation at 12000 *g* for 10 min at 4°C. Based on Western-blotting analysis and SDS-PAGE (Fig. 1a) data, we concluded that the transformed *E. coli* cells expressed the porin from pseudotuberculosis pathogen. IB obtained by this method contained a major protein with the mobility correspondent to that of the *Y. pseudotuberculosis* porin in monomeric form (OmpF-m), and a small amount of lower molecular mass proteins. Gel staining with silver ions showed the lack of lipopolysaccharide (LPS) in the IB.

The protein concentration of IB was determined spectrophotometrically. The refolded recombinant porin was obtained using exhaustive dialysis and different types of chromatography in the presence of various detergents. The ionic detergent SDS is widely used for solubilization of membrane proteins but its application for protein refolding is known to prevent the formation of stable porin oligomers (Arockiasamy et al, 2004). Nevertheless, considering the high stability of *Y. pseudotuberculosis* porin to action of SDS (Novikova et al, 1989), we chose the gel chromatography on Sephacryl S-300 (Pharmacia, Sweden) in the presence of SDS for refolding of the recombinant porin. The protein solution was diluted at a ratio of 1 : 2 with TEN buffer containing 4% SDS, sonicated on ice at 44 MHz for 10 min, and loaded onto a Sephacryl S-300 column (2.0 x 70.0 cm) equilibrated with 100 mM Tris-HCl buffer (pH 8.0) containing 10 mM EDTA, 200 mM NaCl, 0.1% SDS, and 0.02% sodium azide. The elution rate was 10 ml/h. According to the SDS-PAGE, protein fractions obtained by chromatography contained only the recombinant porin in monomer form (RP) (Fig. 1*b*).

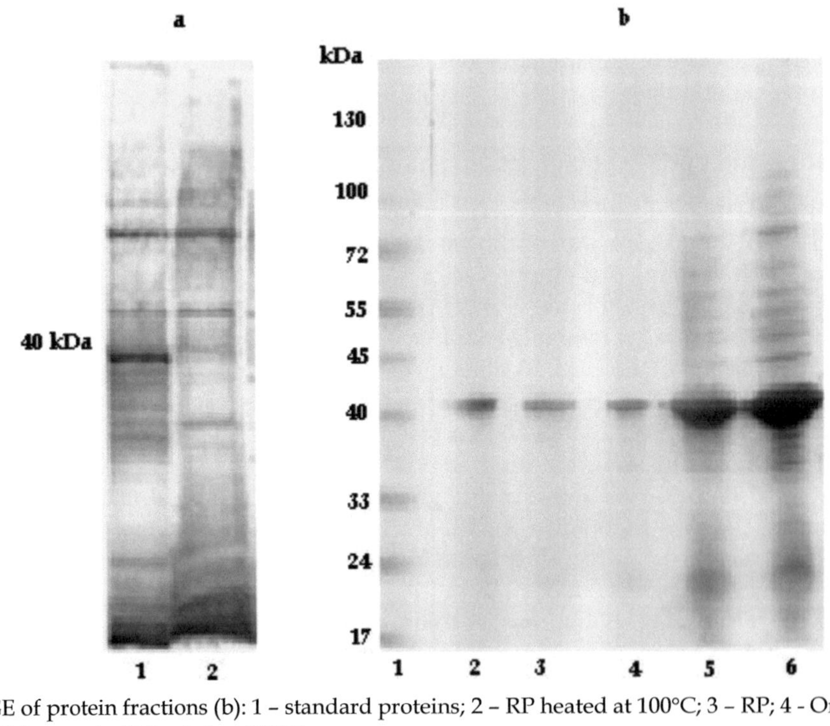

SDS-PAGE of protein fractions (b): 1 – standard proteins; 2 – RP heated at 100°C; 3 – RP; 4 - OmpF-m; 5 – IB in 8 M urea; 6 – IB heated at 100°C.

Fig. 1. Western-blotting of the protein fractions with rabbit antibodies obtained as a result of *Y. pseudotuberculosis* OmpF-m immunization (a): 1 - lysate of transformed *E.coli* cells; 2 - lysate of non-transformed *E.coli* cells.

The results of ELISA showed that the IB isolated from the transformed *E. coli* cells did not contain the *E. coli* OM OmpF porin (Fig. 2).

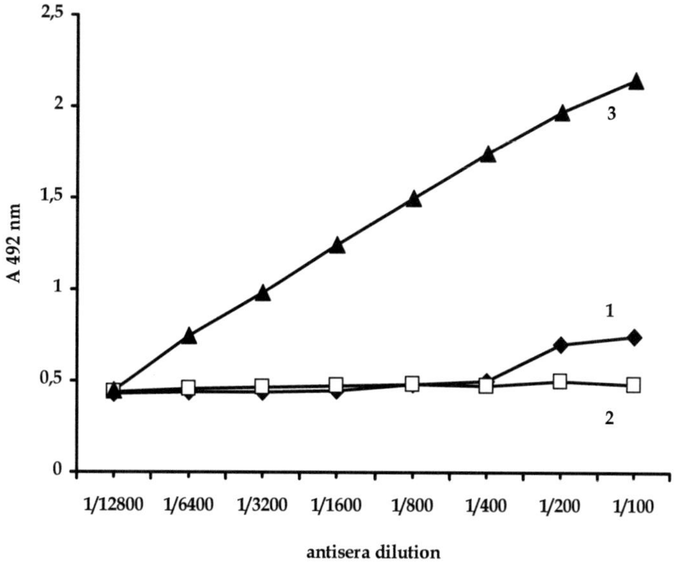

Fig. 2. ELISA of interaction of antiserum obtained after rabbits immunization with OmpF-m from *Y. rseudotuberculosis* OM with: RP (3); IB derived from *E.coli* cells without insertion into the plasmid (2), OmpF porin from *E.coli* OM (1).

2.1.2 Site-directed mutagenesis of the gene OmpF porin

Site-directed mutagenesis of recombinant plasmid pET41a (+)-m55 carrying *ompF* gene was performed to obtain mutant proteins with deletions of loops L1(del 1), L6 (del 6), and L8 (del 8). This plasmid was constructed previously for the expression of the mature OmpF porin. To obtain the original methylated DNA, the plasmid was passed through *E. coli* XL-1 Blue strain. Mutagenic oligonucleotide primers (Table 1) were designed to remove the external loops L1, L6, and L8 (the primers did not contain correspondent sites). Site-directed mutagenesis was performed using polymerase Pfu Ultra II (Stratagene, USA) according to the algorithm proposed in (Wang & Malcolm, 1999).

Name	Sequence (5\`-3\`)	Appointment
T7 prom	TAATACGACTCACTATAGGG	sequencing primer
T7 term	GCTAGTTATTGCTCAGCGG	
Del_L1_for	GTCACTCTTTCTCCGATGGCGACAAGTC	Loop deletion L1
Del_L1_rev	GACTTGTCGCCATCGGAGAAAGAGTGAC	
Del_L6_for	CTCAGAACCTGACTGCGAACAAGACTCG	Loop deletion L6
Del_L6_rev	CGAGTCTTGTTCGCAGTCAGGTTCTGAG	
Del_L8_rev	CAACCTGTTGGACGTTGTTGCTGTTGGC	Loop deletion L8
Del_L8_rev	GCCAACAGCAACAACGTCCAACAGGTTG	

Table 1. Characteristics of primers

The mixture of mutant plasmids resulted after amplification and initial mixture were treated with restriction endonuclease DpnI (Fermentas, Lithuania) for the cleavage of methylated and half-methylated plasmid DNA. This mixture was then used for transforming the cells of *E. coli* Rosetta strain. To select colonies containing "functional" mutant plasmids, the analytical expression of proteins was performed in 30 ml of the LB medium. Results of the expression were assessed by SDS-PAGE (Fig. 3). Colonies 1 and 2 as well as colonies 6 and 8-12 presumably expressing the mutant proteins were selected for the amplification and sequencing of *ompF* gene. PCR amplification was performed using GoTaq polymerase (Promega, USA). PCR fragments were purified using DNA Extraction commercial Kit (Fermentas, Lithuania) and were sequenced using primers T7prom/T7term (Table 1) on an automatized DNA analyzer 3130XL (Applied Biosystems, USA). According to the results of sequencing we selected plasmids containing the deletions of the external loops and maintaining the integrity of the protein encoding sequence of *ompF*. Thus, it was found that the "functional" mutant colonies selected produced a target protein.

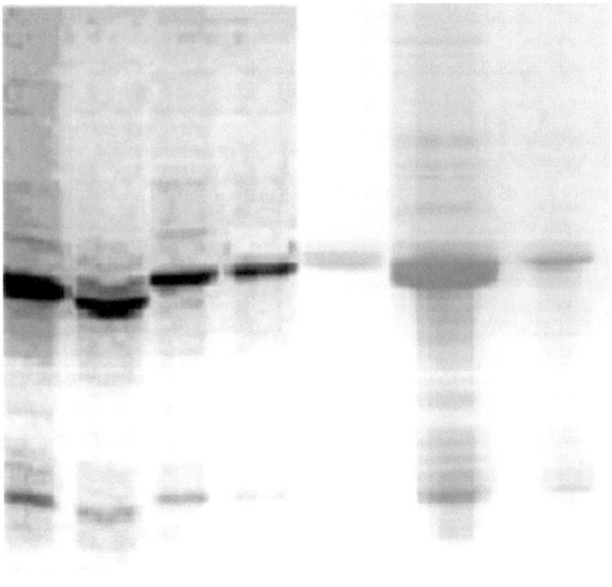

1 2 3 4 5 6 7

Fig. 3. SDS-PAGE of mutant proteins: 1, 2 - del 1 (heated at 100°C and unheated, respectively); 3, 4 - del 6 (unheated and heated at 100°C, respectively), 5 - RP (control, expression in strain BL21 (DE3) *E. coli*); 6, 7 - del 8 (unheated and heated at 100°C, respectively).

2.1.3 Isolation and purification of recombinant mutant forms of the OmpF porin Y. *pseudotuberculosi*

Isolation of proteins with deletions of loops L1, L6, and L8 (samples del 1, del 6, and del 8) was performed according to the procedure developed for RP, except that in the case of mutant proteins we used double amount of lysozyme and DNase. We also isolated full-sized RP as a control. IB containing the mutant porin from urea was purified by exhaustive dialysis (within 4 days). As a result we obtained targeted mutant proteins in monomeric form. According to the SDS-PAGE their electrophoretic mobility coincided with the mobility of RP. The results of refolding of the mutant porin monomers were confirmed by Western-blotting with rabbit antibodies against the native OmpF-m and with murine antibodies against full-sized RP (Fig. 4).

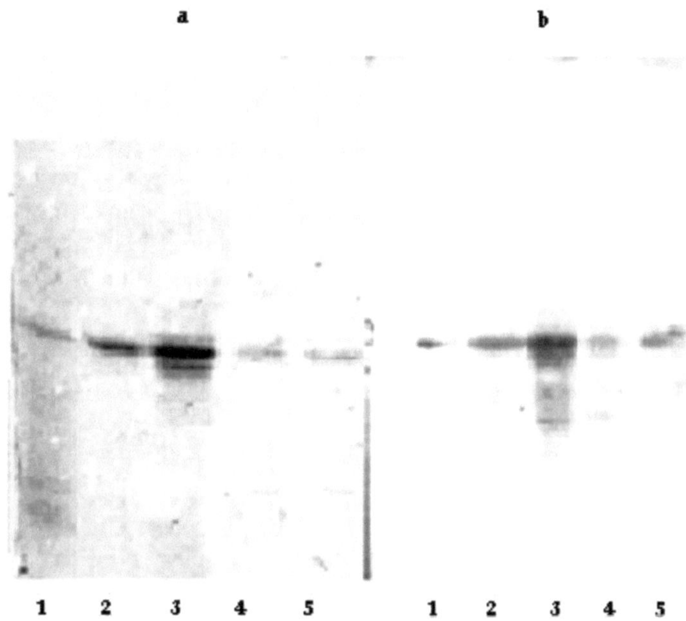

Fig. 4. Western-blotting of protein fractions:
1 - del 1; 2 - del 6; 3 - OmpF-m; 4 - del 8; 5 - RP with rabbit antibodies obtained by immunization of OmpF-m (a);
1 - del 1; 2 - del 6; 3 - RP; 4 - del 8; 5 - native OmpF-m with murine antibodies obtained by immunization of RP (b).

2.2 Antigenic structure of recombinant porins

The antigenic structure of recombinant and mutant proteins was characterized by ELISA. The RP was shown to interact with specific antibodies against OmpF-m. However, complete binding of specific antibodies with the antigen was not observed. The results confirmed that antigen structure of RP only partially corresponded to that of native porin monomer (Fig. 5). Quite possible, the linear antigen determinants (probably formed at the level of primary and/or secondary porin structure) served as common parts of RP and native porin (Portnyagina et al, 1999). At the same time discontinuous (or conformational) antigen determinants (forming by closing in some parts of protein amino acid sequence during assembling 3D protein structure) were absent or were not properly formed.

The mutant porins with the outer loop deletions were found to interact with specific antibodies against the full-sized RP and native OmpF-m (Fig. 6). The results of binding of mutant proteins and RP with antiserum to the latter are similar (Fig. 6a). This suggests that the regions of porin sequence corresponding to the outer loops L8, L1, and L6 do not participate in the formation of the RP antigenic determinants. A similar pattern was observed in the interaction of mutant porins del 1 and del 6 with antibodies to the OmpF-m (Fig. 6b). The exception was the del 8, which reacted with these antibodies 30-40% less efficiently.

It can be assumed that the structure of antigenic determinants of recombinant and native porin monomers has partial coincedence at the region of incomplete forming (in the case of recombinant protein) conformational determinants. This result may also reflect the fact that region of protein sequence corresponding to loop L8 are part of the conformational epitopes of the OmpF-m. Besides, this result was consistent with the antigenic determinants calculated theoretically using various computer programs (ProPred, SYFPEITHI, and RANKPEP) and allowed us to predict the regions of interaction with the T-receptors on the surface of human lymphocytes. According the data obtained by this software it was found that less than 20% of the total number of calculated peptides coincided with the porin external loops areas and the significant part of the latter occured in the loop 8 (Portnyagina et al, 2010).

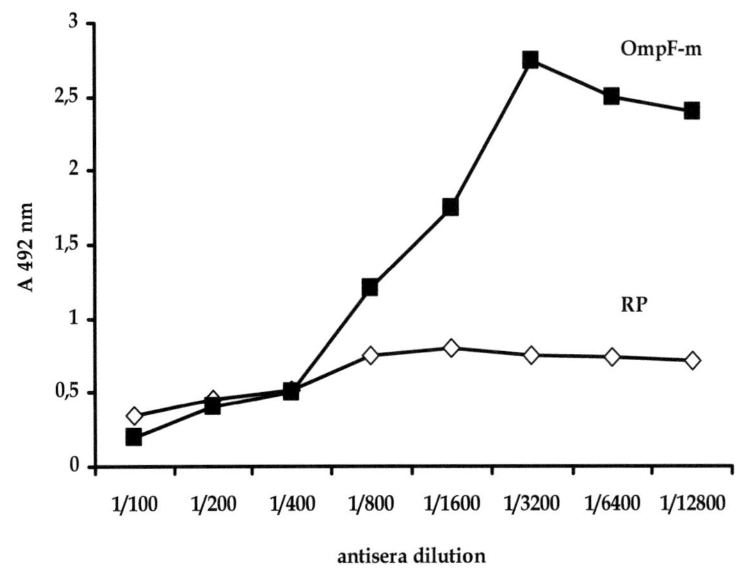

Fig. 5. ELISA of binding of rabbit antisera against OmpF-m with homologous antigen and RP.

2.3 Immunogenic properties of recombinant porins

2.3.1 Obtaining of immune sera

Specific sera to RP were obtained as a result of CBA mice immunization with RP in saline solution mixed with Freund's adjuvant and in detergent solutions. Protein was injected intraperitoneally (100 μg per mouse) three times with intervals of 7 days. The mice of the first group were immunized with purified RP in saline solution. The mice of the second group were immunized by RP mixed with Freund's complete adjuvant (RP/Fr) in ratio 1:1 (v/v), the mice of the third group were immunized by RP in 0.05% octyl-β-D-glucopyranoside (RP/OG) and the mice of the fourth group were immunized by RP in 0.1%

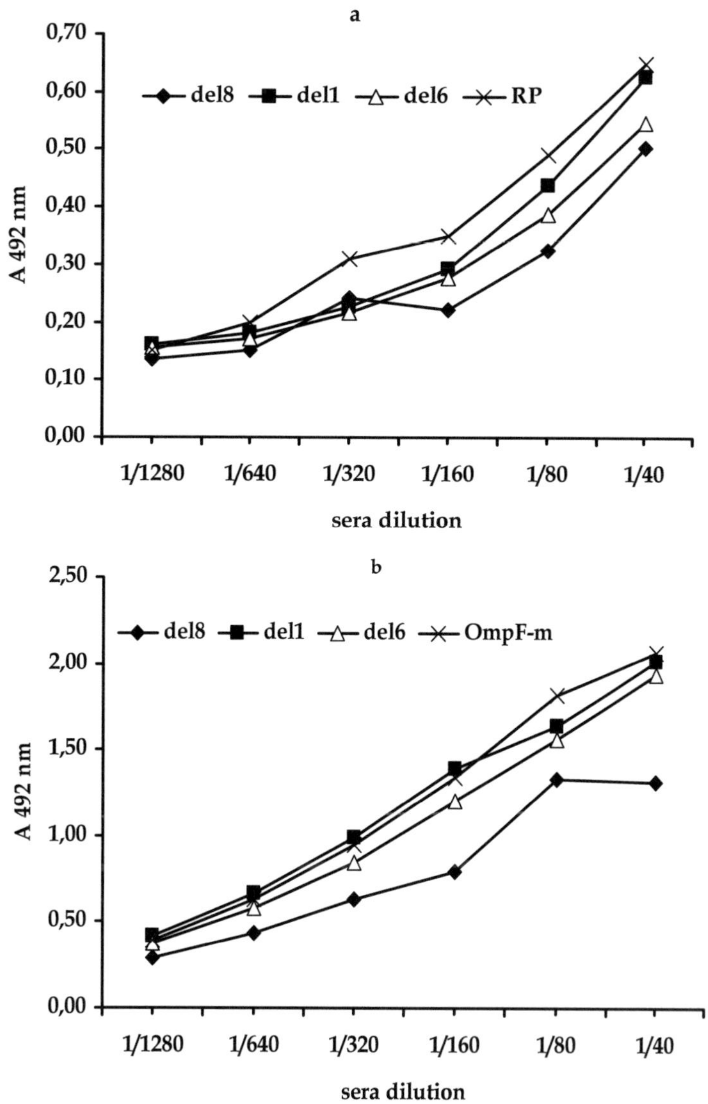

Fig. 6. ELISA of interaction of mutant porins with specific antibodies to: RP (a) and OmpF-m (b).

Zwiterrgent 3 -14 (RP/Zw). To obtain the control serum, we immunized the mice three times with saline solution. Blood sampling was carried out by decapitation of the mice a week after the last immunization. To study the sera obtained, we used indirect ELISA. As second antibodies we used rabbit antibodies against mouse IgG labeled with peroxidase (production of Gamaleya Research Institute of Epidemiology and Microbiology, Moscow). Avidity index (AI) of the sera obtained (which described the ability of a heterogeneous antibodies mixture to bind the antigen and depended on the specificity of the antigen/antibody interaction) was determined by ELISA as described in (Vermot et al, 2002). To remove the low-avidity antibodies, we used 6 M urea solution as a reagent (AppliChem, Germany).

Using ELISA, we determined antibody titers of the immune sera obtained (-lg) (Table 2). It was shown that the serum with the highest titers was obtained by animal immunization with RP/Fr. The titer values of the serum obtained by the immunization with RP/Zw 3-14 and RP were 1-2 dilution lower than serum titer level of RP/Fr. The least amount of specific antibodies in the serum was obtained as a result of animal immunization with RP/OG. We found that sera obtained by immunization with all RP pattern had the high value of IA (Table 2). Thus, the low level of antibodies against recombinant porin obtained by immunization of mice with RP/OG did not affect the avidity of these antibodies. A similar result was observed earlier in (Vermot et al, 2002), where the avidity of the serum obtained by animal immunization with *Neisseria* porin was shown to be virtually independent of the level of specific antibodies in this serum.

Sample	AT (-lg)	AI (%)
RP	2,5	85
RP/Fr	3,55	89
RP/Zw	2,8	82
RP/OG	1,9	79

Table 2. Antibody titers (AT) and avidity index (AI) in the antisera obtained by immunization of mice with different patterns of RP.

2.3.2 Stimulation of murine macrophages by recombinant porin

One of the most important indicators of the host's immune system is the level of functional activity of mononuclear phagocytic cells. Macrophages are the first cells interacting with alien antigens during the infection development and playing an important role in antimicrobial host defense. Activation of macrophages is accompanied by oxygen-dependent metabolic "explosion" with the production of highly unstable products of oxygen reduction including hydrogen peroxide. Hydrogen peroxide is the main substrate for the enzyme myeloperoxidase - an important component of the antimicrobial activity of the phagocytic system. Myeloperoxidase catalyzes the reaction of the formation of hydrogen peroxide in the presence of chloride anions (Ruleva et al, 2007).. Thus, the change in the amount of myeloperoxidase is a measure of the functional status of phagocytic cells (Menshikova et al, 1994).

Y. pseudotuberculosis is known to interact with macrophages and inhibit the activity of oxygen-dependent microbicidal system by supressing enzyme activity during natural infection (Somov et al, 1990). Increase of activity of enzymes involved in synthesis of active oxygen metabolites, including myeloperoxidase, was observed in peritoneal neutrophils infected by *Y. pseudotuberculosis* cells *in vitro*. It was the evidence of the development of cell protective reaction in response to the bacterial invasion. In our work we studied the effect of RP on the functional state of macrophages from peritoneal exudate of mice (intact and immunized with RP) *in vivo* and *in vitro* and estimated the amount of myeloperoxidase synthesized by phagocytes in response to stimulation by *Y.pseudotuberculosis* cells.

Cells of peritoneal exudate were obtained by washing the abdominal cavity of mice with 5 ml of chilled Hanks balanced solution containing 2 ml of heparin. The amount of cells was counted and their viability was determined by trypan blue test (Merck, Germany). Cell suspension (50 μl) was added into the 96-well plate wells and incubated for 2 h in an atmosphere of 5% CO_2 at 37°C, the medium was then removed and the wells were washed with Hanks solution to remove the not adherent cells. To determine the effect of RP on macrophages *in vitro*, cells were pre-incubated with various concentrations of RP and antigen solution was removed after 1 h. To determine the induced production (IP) of myeloperoxidase we added 20 µl (per a well) of suspension containing a different amount of *Y. pseudotuberculosis* cells (strain 512, serovar IB) killed by autoclaving. To determine the spontaneous enzyme production (SP), saline solution (20 µl) was added as control. The plates were incubated for 1 h at 37° C, washed three times with Hanks solution, and 100 µl (per a well) of phosphate-citrate buffer (pH 5.0) containing 0.04% of *o*-phenilendiamin and 0.003% of H_2O_2 were added. After 10 min the reaction was stopped by adding 100 µl of 10% H_2SO_4. The amount of peroxidase was estimated by the optical density (OD) at 492 nm. Stimulation index (IS) was calculated as the ratio of induced and spontaneous production of peroxidase: IS = PI / SP.

It was established that immunization of mice with RP caused an increased production of myeloperoxidase (Fig. 7a). Increase of myeloperoxidase level indirectly characterizes oxygen-dependent killing of bacteria in phagocyte (complete phagocytosis), therefore it shows that the three-time immunization of mice with RP (100 µg/mouse) leads not only to the synthesis of specific antibodies but stimulates the enhancement of induced bactericidal activity of peritoneal macrophages as well. This result coincides with previous data that increased activity of macrophages is a result of experimental pseudotuberculosis infection (Timchenko et al, 1990) and immunization with the porin isolated (Portnyagina et al, 1999).

Experiment *in vitro* also showed that the addition of RP into system intact macrophage/*Y. pseudotuberculosis* cells enhanced the synthesis of myeloperoxidase in the monolayer of peritoneal macrophages and the amount of the enzyme depended on the dose of RP (Fig. 7b).

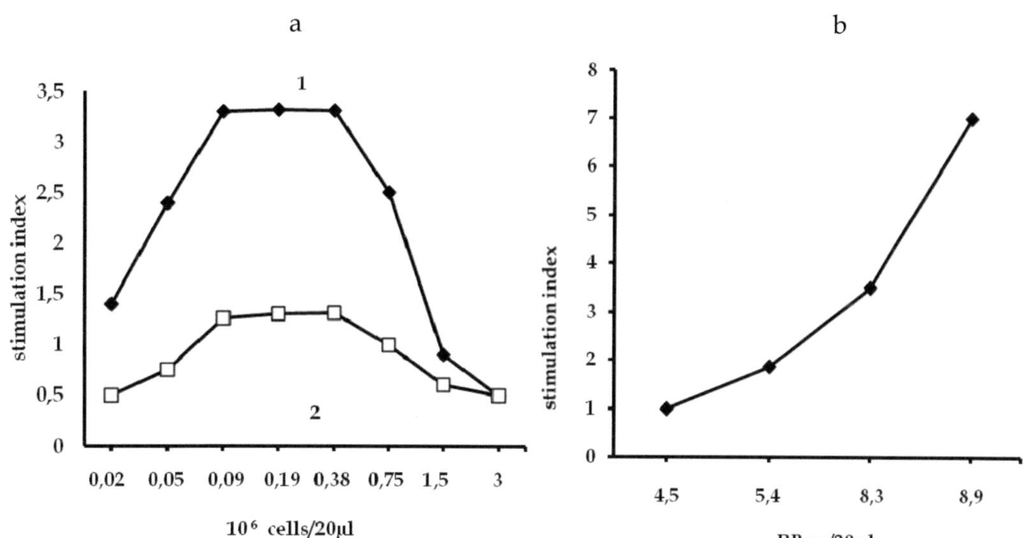

Fig. 7. Synthesis of myeloperoxidase in macrophages of immune (1) and non-immune (2) mice (a). The effect of RP on the synthesis of myeloperoxidase in non-immune macrophages of mice (b).

In the cause of addition the antibodies against RP to the system of non-immune macrophages/*Y. pseudotuberculosis* cell, (Fig. 8) decrease of myeloperoxidase production by the phagocytes was observed. Probably, this is the consequence of interaction of the surface antigens of Y. *pseudotuberculosis* with the opsonic factors of serum (Somov et al, 1990), this effect is most typical for mice. In addition, specific antibodies to RP are supposed to block the adhesion receptors on the surface of bacterial cells since these receptors are the regions of the outer loops of the porin molecule (Plekhova et al, 2007). This leads to the decrease of the stimulatory effect of bacteria in relation to macrophages.

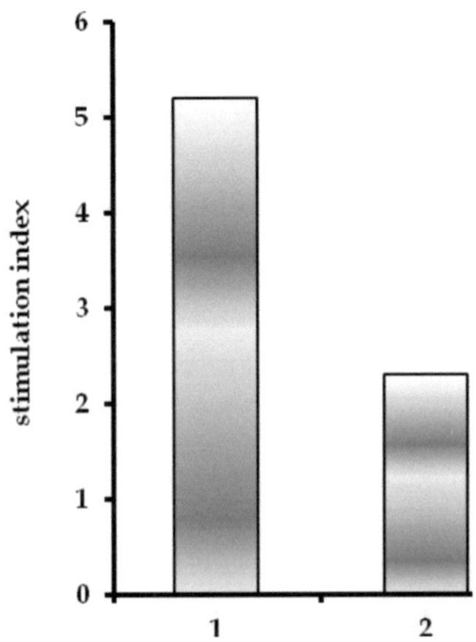

Fig. 8. Amount of peroxidase produced by macrophages of non-immune mice in the absence (1) and presence (2) antibodies to RP.

Thus, immunization with *Y. pseudotuberculosis* RP was found to stimulate the host's immediate protection factors by activating the oxygen-dependent bactericidal activity of phagocytes and initiating the development of humoral immune response. Consequently, the recombinant porin can be used as a component of vaccine preparations for effective protection against infection caused by *Y. pseudotuberculosis*.

2.4 Recombinant porin as diagnostic antigen

It is widely known that the use of recombinant proteins or synthetic peptides as components of diagnostic test systems can increase the sensitivity of the latter and exclude non-specific hyperdiagnostics. Using RP in ELISA kit developed by us earlier (Gordeets et al, 2000), sera of patients with acute intestinal pseudotuberculosis infection were analyzed. It was shown that specific antibodies in patients' sera (dilution 1:800) were detected by RP. Activity of RP as diagnostic antigen was found to be comparable to that of OmpF-m used in ELISA kit (Fig. 9a). A similar result confirming the specificity of this reaction was obtained by inhibiting the interaction of antigen (RP or OmpF-m) with the sera obtained from sick childs with an acute form of pseudotuberculosis. It was found that RP inhibits the binding reaction in 1.43 times more efficient compared to OmpF-m (the data are not shown).

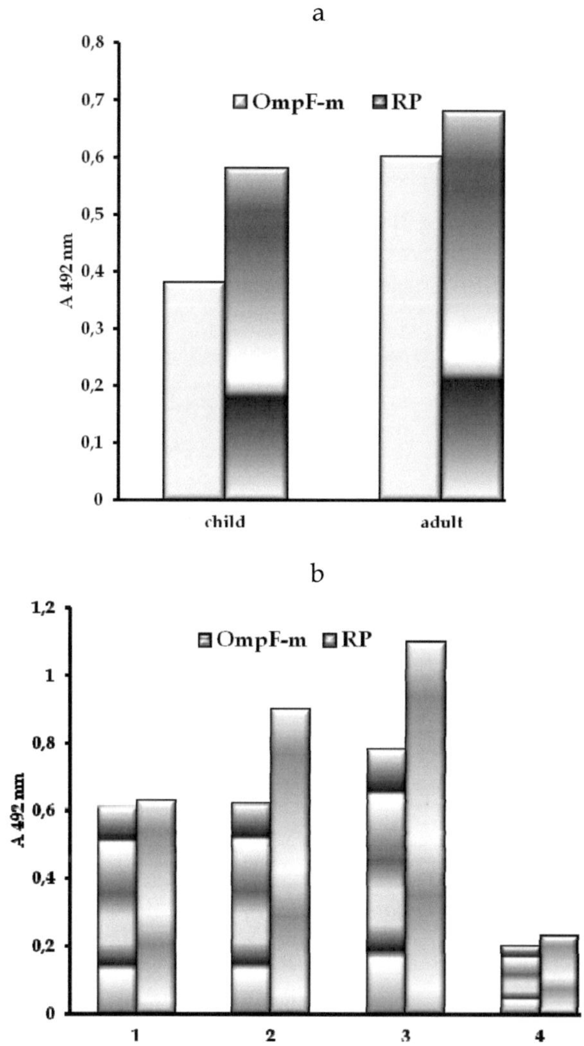

Fig. 9. ELISA of interaction of RP and OmpF-m antigens with specific antibodies in sera of: patients with acute intestinal pseudotuberculosis (a) and patients with secondary forms of pseudotuberculosis (b). 1, 2 - sera of patients with symptoms of lesions of the peripheral nervous system, 3 - sera of patients with symptoms of lesions of the musculoskeletal apparatus, 4 – sera of healthy donors.

It is known that the secondary pseudotuberculosis forms are often accompanied by disorders of the cardiovascular and nervous systems, musculoskeletal system, urinary system, and gastrointestinal tract (Tseneva, 2006). To identify the yersiniosis etiology of diseases in patients with similar symptoms, the sera of patients with lesions of musculoskeletal system and peripheral nervous system were also analyzed. The specific antibodies to *Y. rseudotuberculosis* RP were detected in significant number of sera of both groups of patients, 40 and 17%, respectively (Fig. 9b). RP was found to reveal the specific antibodies on the average 1.3 times more effective than OmpF-m. Perhaps, the greater efficiency of RP as a diagnostic antigen is a result of more correct assembly of porin spatial structure during RP refolding. Therefore, antigenic epitopes of RP are more corresponding to the conformational determinants of native protein structure than that of OmpF-m due to loss of a part of conformational determinants of OmpF-m during the isolation procedure (Haltia & Freire, 1995).

In addition, recombinant porins with the external loops deletions were also found to interact with the antibodies in the serum of the patients with acute intestinal and second-hearth forms of pseudotuberculosis. However, their activity in case of acute pseudotuberculosis was much lower compared to the OmpF-m (Fig. 10).

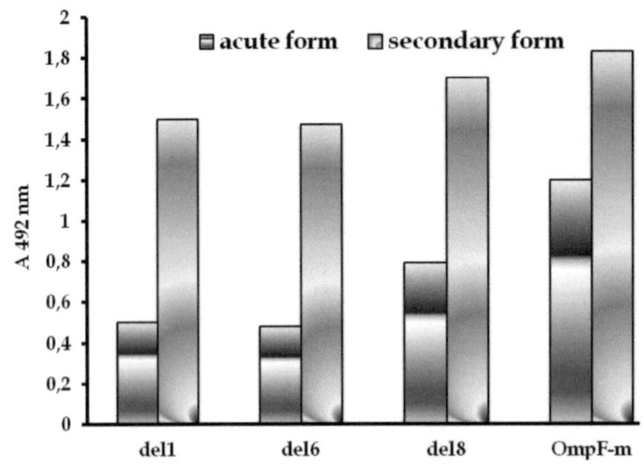

Fig. 10. ELISA of interaction of OmpF-m and mutant porins with specific antibodies in sera of patients with acute intestinal and second-hearth forms of pseudotuberculosis.

3. Conclusion

The recombinant porin (RP) of *Y. pseudotuberculosis* was obtained as a result of expression in *E. coli* cells. RP antigenic structure was shown to be partly similar to the structure of isolated OmpF in monomeric form (OmpF-m). RP was immunogenic for mice. Immunization of mice resulted in production of high-avidity antibodies to porin and stimulated bactericidal activity of peritoneal macrophages. Using site-directing mutagenesis, mutant porins with external loops deletions were also obtained. The external loops L1, L6, and L8 were not found to involve in the formation of antigenic determinants of RP. Nevertheless, the absence of L8 reduced the efficiency of interaction of del8 with antiserum to OmpF-m by 30-40%. Probably, L8 is the part of the conformational determinants of OmpF-m formed at the level of tertiary and quaternary structure of porin.

Studies on antigenic properties and immunochemical activity of RP showed that the protein could be successfully used as diagnostic antigen to detect specific antibodies in the sera of patients with acute and secondary forms of pseudotuberculosis. In future, we plan to continue our work to create new vaccine preparations for animals and human on the basis of RP.

4. Acknowledgement

The authors are grateful to Mrs. Nataly Shepetova to helpful discussions and kind assistance in correcting the English version.

5. References

Achouak,W., Heulin, T., & Pages, J.M. (2001) Multiple facets of bacterial porins. *FEMSMicrobiology Letters.* Vol.99, pp.1-7.

Antonets, D.V., Bakulina, A.Y., Portnyagina, O.Y., Sidorova, O.V., Novikova, O.D., & Maksyutov, A.Z. (2007) Prediction of antigenically active regions in the OmpF-like porin of Yersinia pseudotuberculosis. *Dokl. Acad. Sci.* (section Biochem Biophys). Vol.414, pp.124-6.

Arockiasamy, A., Kumar, P.D., Sundara Baalaji, N.,Rukmini, M.R., and Krishnaswamy, S.(2004) Folding and structural stability of OmpC from Salmonella typhi: Role of LPS and environment *Curr. Science.*Vol. 87, pp. 197–202.

Elkins,C., Barkley, K.B., Carbonetti, N.H., Coimbre, H.J., & Sparling, P.F. (1994) Immunobiology of purified recombinant outer membrane porin protein I of *Neisseria gonorrhoeae. Mol. Microbiol.* Vol. 14, pp. 1059-1075.

Gordeets, A.V., Portnyagina, O.Yu., Vostrikova, O.P., Malashenkova, V.G., Beniova, S.N,, Novikova, O.D., & Solov'eva, T.F. (2000) The method of diagnosis of pseudotuberculosis. *Patent.* 2153172 Russian Federation № 98122085/14, Bull. No 20. p. 8.

Guzev, K.V., Isaeva, M.P., Novikova, O.D., Solov'eva, T.F., & Rasskazov, V.A. (2005) Molecular characteristics of OmpF-like porins from pathogenic Yersinia. *Biochemistry* (Mosc).Vol.70, No.10, pp.1104-1110.

Haltia,T., & Freire, E. (1995) Forces and factors that contribute to the structural stability of membrane proteins. *Biochim. Biophys. Acta,* Vol. 1241, pp. 295–322.

Issaeva, M.P., Guzev, K.V., Novikova, O.D., Solovjeva, T.F., Degtyarev, S., & Rasskazov, V.A. (2003) Porin from Yersinia pseudotuberculosis: cloning and analysis of primary structure. *Adv Exp Med Biol.* Vol. 529, pp. 257-260.

Likhatskaya, G.N., Solov'eva, T.F., Novikova, O.D., Issaeva, M.P., Gusev, K.V., Kryzhko, I.B., Trifonov, E.V., & Nurminski, E.A. (2005) Homology models of the Yersinia pseudotuberculosis and Yersinia pestis general porins and comparative analysis of their functional and antigenic regions. *J Biomol Struct Dyn.* Vol. 23, No. 2, pp. 163-174.

Lupi, N., Bourgois, A., Bemadac, A., Laboucari, S., & Pages J.-M. (1989) Immunological analysis of porin polymorphism in *Escherichia coli* outer membrane. *Mol. Immunol,* Vol. 26, pp. 1027-1036.

Menshikova, E.B., Zenkova, N.K., & Shergin, S.M. (1994) *Biochemistry of oxidative stress,* SB RAMS, Novosibirsk.

Novikova, O.D., Frolova, G.M., Vakorina, T.I., Tarankova, Z.A., Glazunov, V.P., Solov'eva, T.F., and Ovodov, Yu.S. (1989) Conformational stability and immunochemical properties of yersinin--a basic protein of the outer membrane of the Pseudotuberculosis microbe *Bioorg. Khim.,* 1989, vol. 15, pp. 763–772.

Peeters, C.C.A.M., Claassen, I.J.T.M., Schuller, M., Kersten, G.F.A., van der Voort, E.V.R., & Poolman, J.T. (1999) Immunogenicity of various presentation forms of PorA outer membrane protein of *Neisseria meningitidis* in mice. *Vaccine,* Vol. 27, pp. 2702-2712.

Plekhova, N.G., Luba, L.M., Okhotin, S.V., Drobot, E.I., & Goncharuk, Y.N. (2006) Metabolic activity of neutrophils at pseudotuberculosis infection. *Zhurn. Microbiology,* Vol. 3 (Appendix), pp. 43-47.

Portnyagina, O.Y., Novikova, O.D., Vostrikova, O.P., & Solov'eva T.F. (1999) Dynamics of immune response to porin from outer membrane of Yersinia pseudotuberculosis. *Bull. exp. Biol. med.* Vol. 128, No. 10, pp. 437-440.

Portnyagina, O.Y., Sidorova, O.V., Khomenko, V.A., Novikova, O.D., Vostrikova, O.P., & Solovjeva, T.F. (2009) Immunogenic characteristics of recombinant OMPF-like porin from Yersinia pseudotuberculosis outer membrane. *Bull Exp Biol Med.* Vol. 148, No. 1, pp. 72-74.

Portnyagina, O.Y., Sidorova, O.V., Novikova, O.D., Vostrikova, O.P., Khomenko, V.A., & Solov'eva, T.F. (2010) Immunochemical Characteristics of Synthetic Peptides with T_cellular and B_cellular Epitopes of Nonspecific Porins of Pathogenic *Yersinia. Russian Journal of Bioorganic Chemistry.* Vol. 36, No. 6, pp. 713–721.

Ranling, E.G., Martin, N.L., & Hancock, R.E.W. (1995) Epitope mapping of the *Pseudomonas aeruginosa* major outer membrane porin protein OmpF. *Infect. Immunol,* Vol. 63, No. 1, pp. 38-42.

Ruleva, N.Y., Zvyagintsev, M.A., & Dugin, S.F. (2007) Myeloperoxidase: biological functions and clinical implications. *Modern high technologies.* Vol. 8. pp.11-15.

Shaw, J., Grund, V., Durling, L., Crane, D., & Caldwell H.D. (2002) Outer membrane protein antigen elicit a $CD4^+$-type 2 rather than type 1 immune response that is not protective. *Infect. Immun,* Vol. 70, No. 3, pp. 1097-1105.

Singh, S.P., Williams, Y.U., Benjamin, W.H., Klebba, P.E., & Boyd D. (1996) Immunoprotection by monoclonal antibodies to the porins and lipopolysaccharide of *Salmonella typhimurium. Microbial. Pathogenesis,* Vol. 21, No. 4, pp. 249-263.

Somov, G.P., Pokrovsky, V.I., & Besednova, N.N. (1990) *Pseudotuberculosis,* Meditsina, Moscow.

Supotnitsky, M. (1996) Protective properties of pore-forming proteins pathogenic bacteria. *Bulletin of the Russian Academy of Medical Sciences,* No. 8, pp. 18 – 22.

Timchenko, N.F., Novikova, O.D., Pavlov, G., Venediktov, V.S., & Solov'eva, T.F. (1990) Protective properties of porin from the outer membrane of Yersinia pseudotuberculosis. *Zhurn. Microbiology,* Vol. 11, pp. 48-50.

Tseneva G.Y. (2006) *Yersinia and yersiniosi,* Medmassmedia, SPb.

Vermont, C. L., van Dijken, H.H., van Limpt, C. J., de Groot, R., van Alphen, L., & van den Dobbelsteen G.P.J.M. (2002) Antibody avidity and immunoglobulin G isotipe distribution following immunization with a monovalent meningococcal B outer membrane vesicle vaccine. *Infect. Immune,* Vol. 70, pp. 584-590.

Vostrikova, O.P., Malashenkova, V.G., Novikova, O.D., Gordeets, A.V., & Solov'eva, T.F. (2009) The outer membrane porin from *Yersinia enterocolitica* in yersiniosis diagnostics. *Biochemistry* (Moscow), Supplement Series A: Membrane and Cell Biology, Vol. 3, No. 4, pp. 438–446.

Vostrikova, O.P., Novikova, O.P., Drobkov, I.V., Darmov, I.V., Marakulin, I.V., & Solov'eva, T.F. (2000) The immune response to the main pore-forming outer membrane protein Yersinia pseudotuberculosis in humans and laboratory animals. *Immunology,* No 795-V, pp. 15.

Wang, W., & Malcolm, B. (1999) Two-Stage PCR Protocol Allowing Introduction of Multiple Mutations, Deletions and Insertions Using Quik Change Site-Directed Mutagenesis. *BioTechniques,* Vol. 26, pp. 680-682.

Wright, J.C., Williams, J.N., Christodoulides, M., & Heckels, J.E. (2002) Immunization with the recombinant PorB outer membrane protein induced a bactericidal immune response against *Neisseria meningitidisS. Infect. Immun.* Vol. 70, No. 8, pp. 4028-4034.

16

Wash-LOCI – A Semi-Heterogeneous Version of the LOCI Technology Allowing Removal of Unbound Material After Each Assay Step

Fritz Poulsen
Novo Nordisk,
Denmark

1. Introduction

Pharmacokinetic (PK) studies are a crucial part of drug discovery. These studies require analysis of high numbers of plasma or serum samples from animals and humans to measure concentrations of peptide-/protein-drugs. The demands to assays are that they have a high capacity, only need low sample volumes, have a broad working range to avoid testing too many dilutions of samples, and have a good sensitivity. They have to be fast to develop and preferentially be more or less ready "on the shelf". When new drug candidates like peptides, proteins or peptide-/protein-analogues are developed it is important that assays are available to all relevant peptide-/protein-drugs in due time.

Immunoassays will often be the method of choice for this kind of testing. Especially the luminescent oxygen channeling immunoassay (LOCI) fulfill most requirements to PK testing of peptide and protein drugs (Poulsen & Jensen, 2007). LOCI™ is a trade name of Siemens. Perkin Elmer is using the name AlphaLISA for the technology. This superior technology also has its limitations. To release the full potential of LOCI sandwich assays monoclonal antibodies (MCA) are needed due to the high percentage (100%) of specific antibody.

It may take long time and it may be difficult to generate antibodies against relevant parts of a drug molecule and to obtain monoclonal antibodies which will cooperate in a sandwich. Developing polyclonal antibodies is much faster than developing monoclonal antibodies thus allowing faster establishment of assays. Furthermore polyclonal antibodies may contain many antibody specificities against an analyte molecule and may allow using many different species for antibody generation which may give more specificity options.

The LOCI sandwich assay requires high concentration and high density of antibodies on beads. Since the fraction of specific antibodies in a polyclonal antibody (PCA) is low (1-5%) (Lipman et al., 2005) the density of specific antibodies on the A beads will with PCAs be reduced to 5% or less compared to MCAs. The binding capacity of SA-D beads and limitations of the SA-D bead concentrations means that high concentrations of biotin-antibody is not tolerated. This means that use of PCA in LOCI which will require high concentrations of biotin-PCA to have enough specific antibody is not feasible or suboptimal. Immunopurification will thus be required to have enough specific antibodies in the assay. The immunopurification is time and resource consuming. It results in loss of antibody and potential loss of high avidity antibodies. Finally the antibodies may be partially denatured resulting in increased non-specific binding of the purified antibodies. To avoid this we have developed the wash-LOCI, a semi-heterogeneous LOCI version allowing direct use of high concentrations of PCA, and giving binding of a high amount of specific antibodies.

The new assay is based on the LOCI technology and is able to run with the same reagents, readers and robotic system as the normal LOCI and is only slightly more cumbersome to run than LOCI.

The wash-LOCI version allows removing non-bound biotin-PCA before addition of SA-D beads. A separation could be done by binding antibody-A beads to the well bottom, by a filtration step or by using magnetic beads (Hall et al., 1999; Koskinen et al., 2004; Kulmala et al., 2002; McCrindle et al., 1985; Namba et al., 2000; Obenauer-Kutner et al., 1997; Okano et al., 1992; Sardesai et al., 2009; Sin et al., 2006; Soukka et al., 2001). All the described methods are based on particulate labels. Since it turned out to be impossible to find 384-well filter plates with a pore size trapping the beads without being clogged by plasma this approach was given up. The LOCI A beads are not magnetic so to use magnets it would be necessary to couple the A beads to magnetic beads. The magnetic beads might give optical shielding problems and the process would be more complicated. We therefore decided to go for the version with A beads coupled directly to the well bottom.

This work was done with human insulin as a model system. Chicken plasma was used since chicken insulin cannot be measured in the assays and endogenous insulin will thus not blur the results.

The LOCI technology is based on two types of latex beads. One type, the D beads, contains a photosensitizer. The other type, the A beads, are chemiluminescent beads (Ullman et al., 1994; Ullman et al., 1996). Pairs of D beads and A beads are formed in the assay through specific binding interactions by combining sample and the two bead types. Irradiation causes photosensitized formation of singlet oxygen which migrates to and activates bound chemiluminescent beads thereby initiating a delayed luminescence emission. The basic technology is homogeneous requiring no separation and no washing. It lends itself for miniaturization to 384 allowing low sample volumes and for high capacity measurements. Run as a double antibody sandwich assay it has a very good sensitivity and a very broad working range.

The goal was to obtain usable LOCI assays based on a monoclonal and a polyclonal antibody or on a PCA pair. The PCAs must be used without immunopurification. Furthermore, the homogeneous LOCI is vulnerable to strong hemolysis or to inner filter effects or singlet oxygen quenchers in general and to hook effect at very high analyte concentrations. These limitations were tried avoided by modification of the LOCI assay. The core of this modification is anchoring the antibody-coated A-beads to the well bottom allowing wash/separation in the assay.

2. Materials and methods

2.1 Plates and plate equipment

Plates, AlphaPlate-384 High Binding (light grey) were from Perkin Elmer. Plate centrifuge, Multifuge 3 S-R Hereus. Plate washer, Tecan Power Washer 384 using wash program "cell wash 384_51". Plate shaker, Titramax 100 from Heidolph using speed 6. Plate reader, Envision Turbo Alpha from Perkin Elmer.

2.2 Reagents

Unconjugated Eu-acceptor beads (A beads) and streptavidin-coated donor beads (SA-D beads) were from Perkin Elmer.

The monoclonal antihuman insulin antibodies HUI018, HUI001, and OXI005 were from Novo Nordisk. The polyclonal guinea pig anti-insulin antisera were from Fitzgerald, Millipore, Peninsula, and Novo Nordisk. The IgG fraction from these antisera was isolated by protein A chromatography and is then referred to as Fz, Mill, Pen, and 4078E respectively.

Antibodies were coupled to A beads as described by the manufacturer except that the antibody was in 0.1 M phosphate (sodium), pH 8.0, and the amount of antibody used was 0.6 mg/mg beads. The resulting product is antibody-A beads.

Biotinylation of antibodies was done as described by Poulsen & Jensen (2007).

Human insulin was from Novo Nordisk.

Normal chicken, rat and pig EDTA plasma pools were from Bioreclamation.

2.3 Plate coating

Plates were coated with antibody-A beads, 35 µl/well, 5 µg/ml in PBS pH 7.2. After addition of beads the plates were centrifuged for 2 h at 3452xg followed by incubation for 20h at 4°C. Before use the wells were washed with wash buffer and afterwards completely emptied from liquid.

2.4 Assays

2.4.1 LOCI

LOCI was performed as described previously (Poulsen & Jensen, 2007). In brief the assay was performed in 384-well plates. Five µl of test samples were added to the wells followed by 15 µl of a mixture of antibody-A beads and biotin-antibody. The plates were incubated for 1 hour at 22 °C. Then 30 µl of SA-D beads were added. After 30 minutes of incubation at 22 °C the plates were measured on an Envision reader.

2.4.2 Wash-LOCI

The assay was performed in AlphaPlate-384 High Binding (light grey) 384-well plates.

The assay buffer contained 25 mM Hepes, 50 mM NaCl, 10 mM EDTA (tripotassium salt), 2 mg/mL Dextran T500 (Pharmacosmos, Holbaek, Denmark), 0.5% bovine serum albumin (A-7888; Sigma-Aldrich, St. Louis, MO), 0.1% bovine gamma globulin (G-5009; Sigma-Aldrich), 0.2 mg/mL mouse immunoglobulin (HBR1; Scantibodies Laboratories, Santee, CA), 0.1% (w/v) Tween 20, 0.01% Proclin 300 (Sigma-Aldrich), and 0.01% gentamycin sulphate (Biological Industries, Israel) and was adjusted to pH 7.4.

Biotin-antibody buffer was assay buffer + 0.2 M Na-Citrate + 1% guinea pig serum, pH 7.40.

Sample dilution buffer: Assay buffer with 0.015% (w/v) Triton X-100 and 0.05% (w/v) SDS.

Wash buffer: PBS pH 7.20 with 0.05% (w/v) Tween 20.

The test samples and standards were diluted 1+2 in sample dilution buffer and 10 µl of this (3.3 µl plasma) were added to the wells. The plates were covered and incubated at 22 °C for 1 hour with shaking. The plates were washed on the plate washer 2x with wash buffer. Biotin-antibody in biotin-antibody buffer (10 µL) was then added to the wells and the plates incubated and washed as described above. Finally 10 µl SA-D beads were added and the plates incubated as described above (except that it was in the dark). Immediately after this incubation the plates were read on an Envision without wash separation of unbound material utilizing the homogeneous nature of the LOCI technology.

The concentrations in wells were as follows:

Plasma sample 33%, biotin-antibody 4.5 nM for MCA and 80 nM for PCA, and SA-D beads 100µg/ml.

The results were measured on an Envision Turbo Alpha (Perkin Elmer) with 1 detector, 70 ms excitation time and 140 ms detection time i.e. same adjustment for LOCI and wash-LOCI. The total processing time per 384-well plate was about 2.75 minutes, and the time for measuring from the 1st to the last well was about 2.33 minutes.

If nothing else mentioned the standard conditions described above are used in the experiments.

3. Results and discussion

3.1 Wash-LOCI principle

The principle of the wash-LOCI is illustrated in Figure 1. Accordingly the A beads coated with antibody are attached to the bottom of the microtiter plate. After binding of insulin unbound insulin is washed away.

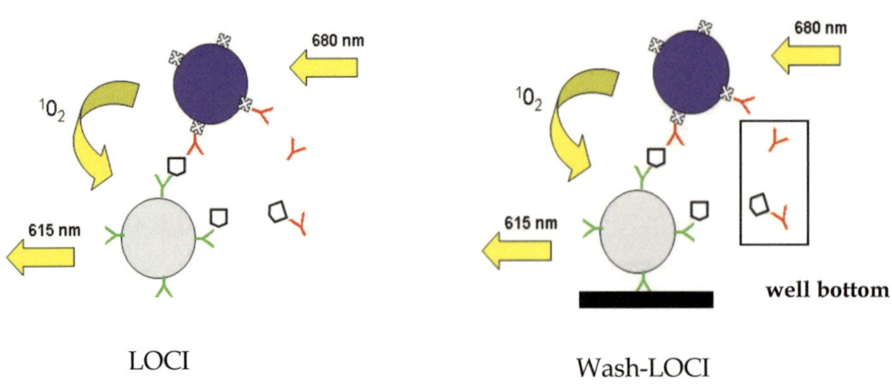

Fig. 1. Principle of wash-LOCI and LOCI.

This is followed by binding of biotin-antibody and again unbound molecules are washed away. The last step is addition of SA-D beads and after incubation the wells are measured in the Envision reader without washing utilizing the proximity principle of LOCI.

In this study wash-LOCI and normal LOCI are compared and from the figure it can be seen that the assays are identical except that the A beads are anchored in the wash-LOCI allowing for removal of unbound material by washing. The bead pairs are formed on the well bottom and not in suspension. This means that reading is surface reading in stead of suspension reading. To have the optimal surface to volume ratio the beads are bound to the well bottom only and not to the walls. This will also, with small sample and reagent volumes, result in faster assays. The Envision reader collects the signal from only a small part of the well bottom surface. This means that analyte bound to the bottom will be measured whereas analyte bound to the well walls will not be detected. Uniformity of the bead-coating on the bottom is crucial for this surface reading. Uniform and reproducible distribution of sample and reagents over the bottom are also important for that. The assay is run as a sequential procedure. This procedure has been found to be beneficial when a MCA/PCA sandwich is used (Obenauer-Kutner, 1997). The procedure removes analyte as well as interfering components before the biotin-antibody is added which gives a system different from and complementary to the LOCI assay.

3.2 Coating of plates with antibody-A beads

Coating was performed by centrifugation to secure that beads were coming into contact with the well bottom allowing them to bind.

The volume of beads for coating must have a size securing an even distribution over the well bottom. Too small bead volumes for coating will result in uneven coating. During reading the laser light from the Envision will hit the bottom and excite the D beads bound resulting in light output from the A beads. An uneven layer of coated A beads will thus be detrimental to the assay. Furthermore, since Envision is only exciting on the well bottom it is important that analyte and reagents are bound on the bottom.

Centrifugation is important for binding of beads by increasing the amount of beads bound and the speed of bead binding. It is important to have a high density of antibody beads on the bottom to have high antigen binding capacity. Centrifugation gave a more reproducible coating and a more uniform coating within a plate and an extra 20 h incubation following the centrifugation increased this positive effect. The centrifugation also prohibited or reduced the binding of beads to the walls.

For all results in this work 35 µl have been used for coating but 15 µl seem to work equally well. Lower volumes than 15 µl should not be used since this may result in inconsistent coating. The optimal amount of beads added per well was found to be 185-370 ng/well.

Since the beads are only passively bound to the bottom the stability of this binding was tested. After coating with beads the coated plates were pretreated by incubating with assay buffer for 20 hours. The coated plates were washed before and after the incubation. Then an assay was run. No effect of this extra treatment was observed showing that the binding of the beads was strong (data not shown).

The bead-coated plates may be stored for at least 5 days at 4°C. Plate coating is thus not considered part of the assay.

3.3 Wash-LOCI and LOCI with MCA and PCA

LOCI and wash-LOCI with MCA and PCA were developed and compared.

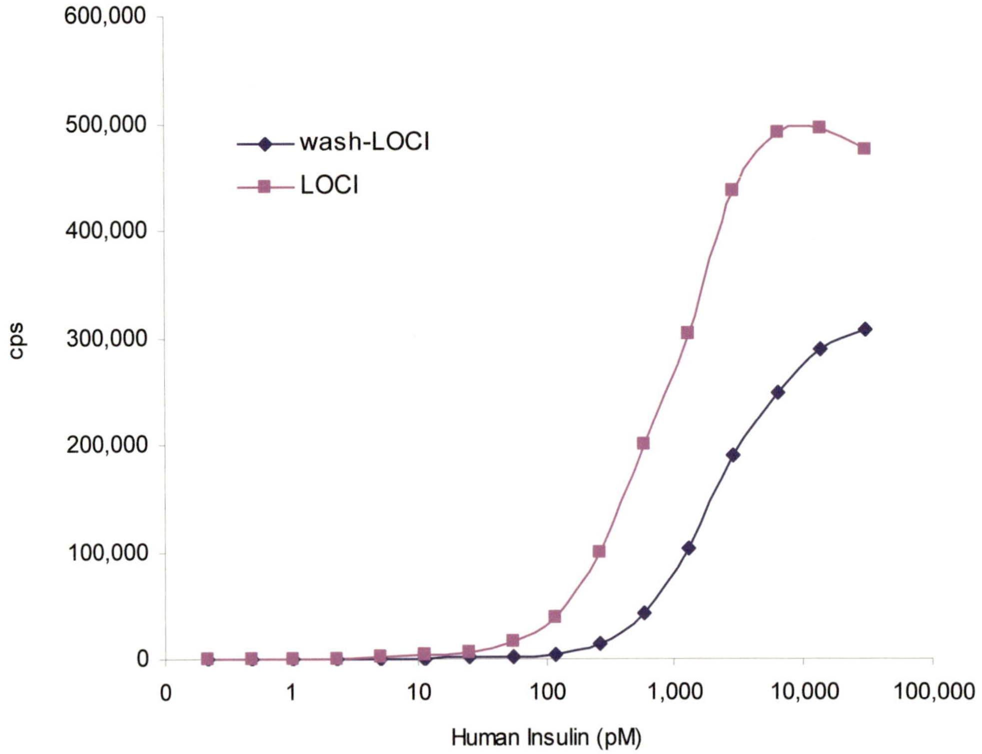

Fig. 2. Comparison of wash-LOCI and LOCI with HUI018-A beads and biotin-OXI005 in both assays.

The first characterization of the wash-LOCI was done by running LOCI and wash-LOCI with the same two MCAs (HUI018 and OXI005) used by Poulsen & Jensen (2007). From Figure 2 it is clear that the wash-LOCI concept is working but that the LOCI assay is superior with respect to sensitivity and working range and the signal is also higher. The lower signal with wash-LOCI is probably related to the amount of HUI018-A beads per well which is higher in LOCI. On the other hand the assay performance of the wash-LOCI shows that the wash-LOCI concept is working well.

A number of sandwich combinations with MCA and PCA have been investigated in the wash-LOCI and normal LOCI. The results are illustrated in Figure 3. The MCA pair gave obviously the best LOCI assay (Fig. 3 C). It can be seen that MCA on the A-beads generally gave the best assays (Fig. 3 A and C). In both assay versions PCA coupled to the A beads gave assays with lower signal, reduced sensitivity, and reduced working range (Fig. 3 B and D). This is ascribed to the low amount of specific antibodies in PCA which results in a lower binding capacity on the A beads. With respect to the biotin-antibody then the PCA gave lower sensitivity and range in LOCI (Fig. 3 C). This again must be due to a low concentration of specific antibody which can not be compensated by increasing the concentration of biotin-IgG because of a limited amount of SA-D beads (see also Fig. 9).

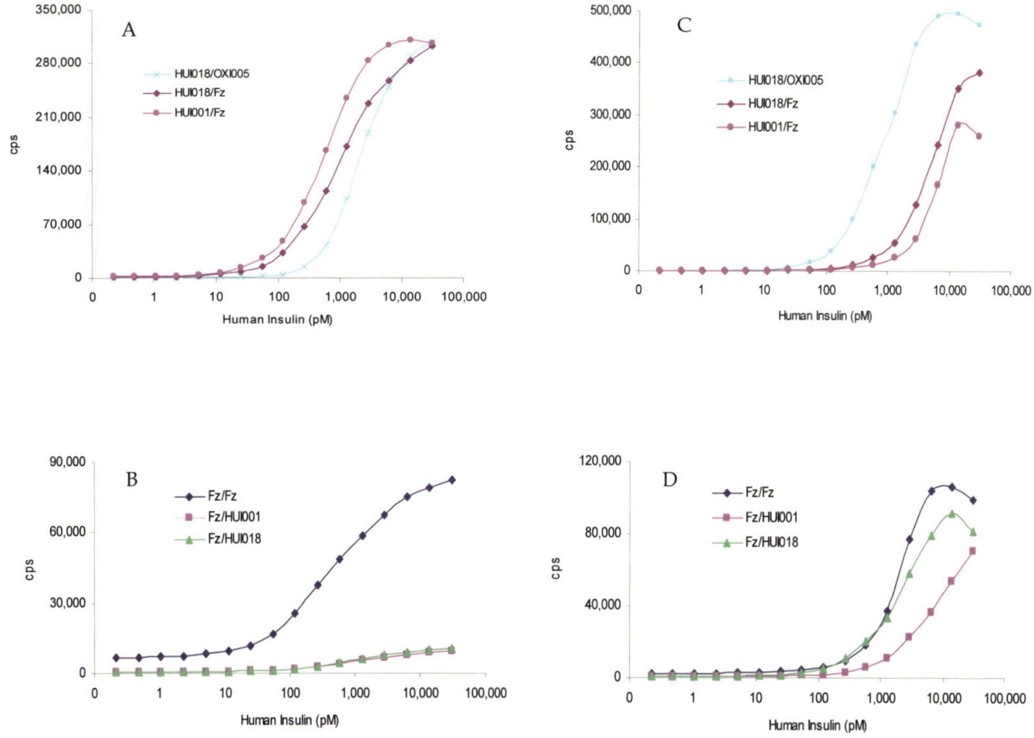

Fig. 3. Comparison of wash-LOCI (A and B) and LOCI (C and D) with various MCA and PCA combinations. The antibody pairs are shown as antibody-A bead/biotin-antibody. The same antibodies are used in the two assays for direct comparison.

The SA-D bead amount has to be limited in LOCI probably because of optical problems with too high concentrations of SA-D beads. This means that increase of the amount of biotin PCA will not be possible since it will be counter-productive (see also Fig. 9). In LOCI the excess biotin-MCA cannot be removed meaning that excess biotin-PCA will not be bound to the SA-D beads. In wash-LOCI biotin-antibody is bound only to antibody immobilized insulin which is what has to be detected. In the wash-LOCI good assays were obtained with biotin-PCA (Fig. 3 A and B). This is because a higher concentration of biotin PCA can be used since biotin-(non-specific)-IgG not bound to the solid phase is washed away before addition of the SA-D beads. This result in a high amount of specific antibodies bound to insulin on antibody-A beads. The assays based on a PCA-A/biotin-MCA pair were better with LOCI than with wash-LOCI (Fig. 3 B and D). This can be explained by competition between PCA and MCA for an epitope since the sequential procedure in the wash-LOCI allows the PCA to bind before the MCA is added. LOCI functioned optimally with the two MCAs whereas in the wash-LOCI the MCA-A beads with biotin-Fz gave the best results (Fig. 3 A and C).

These data confirm that without the wash separation, immunopurification of PCAs was necessary for their use in LOCI. Otherwise the signal level will be too low, the detection limit too high and the working range too narrow. Omitting this purification step makes it much easier especially when many different antibodies have to be used. The wash-LOCI thus makes the use of PCAs in the LOCI technology much more feasible.

Fz was the best PCA in as well LOCI as in wash-LOCI. The LOCI assay performs well with this antibody but wash-LOCI still shows the best sensitivity with this antibody.

Comparison of wash-LOCI and LOCI with other polyclonal antibodies showed that wash-LOCI had a more dramatic effect with these PCAs resulting in nice wash-LOCI assays but very low sensitivity assays in LOCI (Fig. 4).

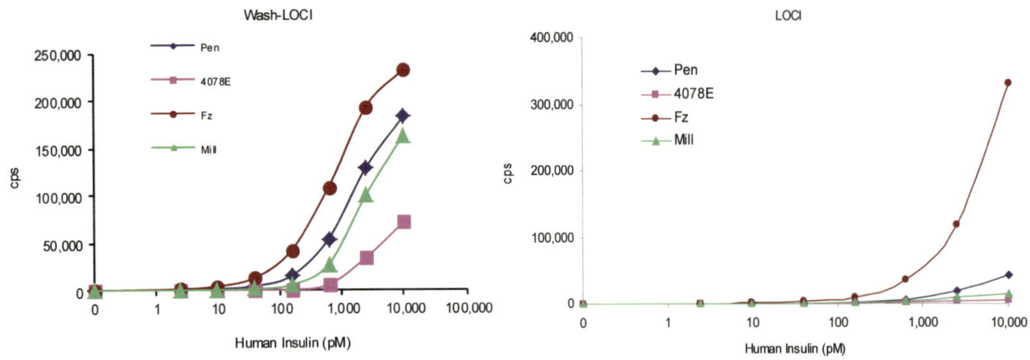

Fig. 4. Comparison of wash-LOCI and LOCI with various biotin-PCAs (Fz, Mill, Pen, and 4078E) combined with HUI018-A beads. The same antibodies are used in the two assays for direct comparison.

It can be seen that the difference between PCAs becomes smaller in wash-LOCI probably because the low PCA titre i.e. lower concentration or avidity of specific antibodies was compensated by using higher concentrations of PCA.

In Table 1 the performance of two different PCAs are shown in wash-LOCI and LOCI. It can be seen that the signal-to-noise ratio was higher with Fz in both assays. The wash-LOCI had higher ratios in the low concentration range whereas the LOCI had higher ratios in the high concentration range. For Mill the wash-LOCI had generally the best S/N ratios. The data indicated that the wash-LOCI had the best sensitivity with both antibodies and the broadest working range with Mill. The LOCI had the broadest working range with the best of the two PCAs i.e. Fz.

It was possible to obtain human insulin dose-response curves in LOCI with Fz with good but not necessarily acceptable sensitivity. Fz was used in this study to illustrate that it is possible to develop good LOCI assays with PCAs with high avidity/high concentration specific antibodies. The advantage of wash-LOCI was much bigger with low-titer anti-insulin PCA and with such PCAs only the wash-LOCI is working with PCA (Fig. 4).

Figure 5 (A and B) shows the best assays obtained with the two LOCI versions. It shows that with the right choice of PCA in the wash-LOCI an assay which performs comparable to our best MCA based LOCI was obtained. It was possible to run the wash-LOCI assay with PCA without immunopurification of the specific antibodies. Sensitivity and working range being comparable to the MCA based LOCI. The variation is smaller for the LOCI assay.

	S/N			
Analyte concentration	Wash-LOCI		LOCI	
	Fz	Mill	Fz	Mill
10000	299	217	737	49
2500	249	134	263	33
625	138	36	78	14
156	54	8	22	5
39	17	3	6	2
10	6	1	2	1
2	3	1	1	1
0	1	1	1	1

Table 1. Signal-to-noise (S/N) ratios calculated as the ratio between a signal and the 0-concentration signal. The assays are based on HUI018-A beads and biotin-Fz or biotin-Mill.

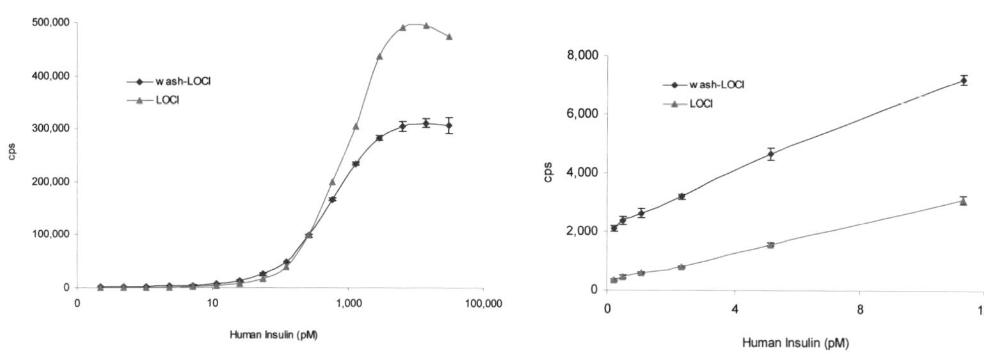

Fig. 5. Comparing optimal wash-LOCI and LOCI assays. Wash-LOCI with HUI001-A and biotin Fz and LOCI with HUI018-A and biotin-OXI005. Full concentration range, log-lin plot (left) and low concentration range, lin-lin plot (right). Data represent the mean of replicate measurements (n=4) of each calibrator ± 1 SD (error bars).

3.4 Kinetics

The kinetics of the wash-LOCI is due to diffusion distance in the semi-heterogeneous procedure different from the kinetics of the homogeneous LOCI. The reason for that is the diffusion distance to the immobilized beads on the bottom of the wells and the sequential nature of the wash-LOCI. However the low volume of sample and reagents in wash-LOCI and a favorable surface-to-volume ratio gave a shorter distance to diffuse; resulting in relative short assay times.

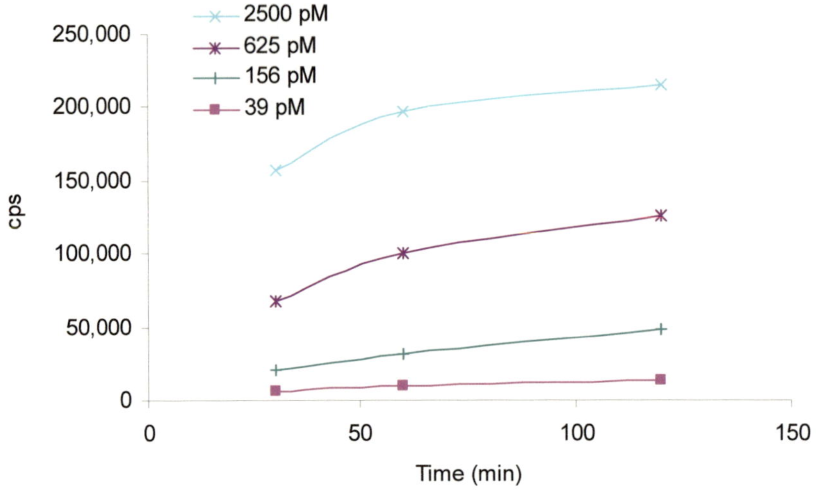

Fig. 6. Kinetics of analyte binding in wash-LOCI with the four insulin concentrations shown. The antibody pair used was HUI018-A beads/biotin-OXI005.

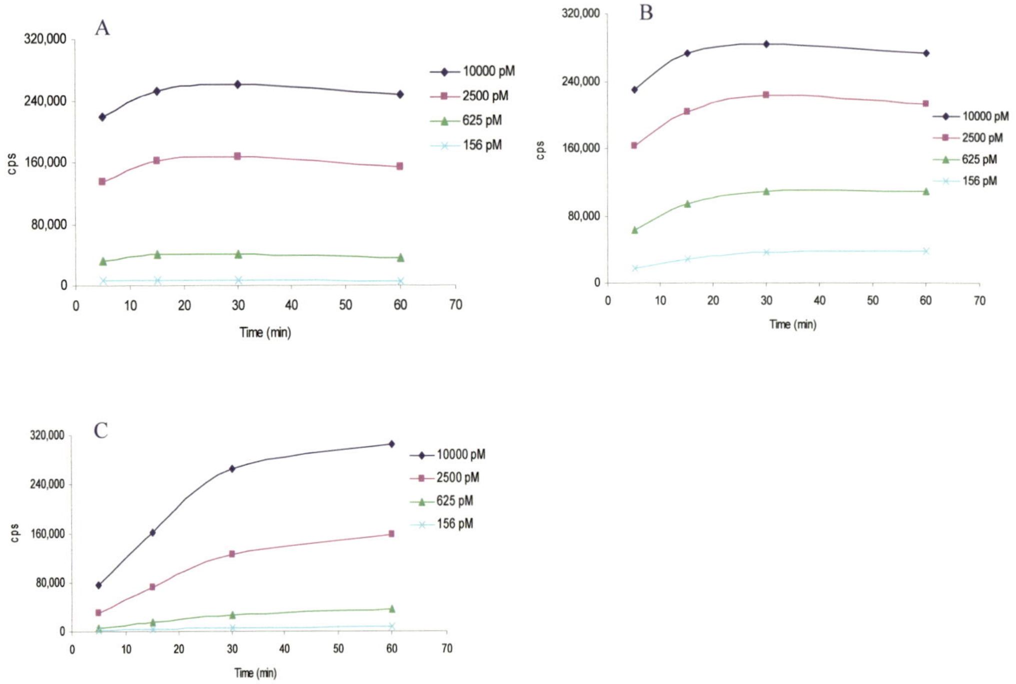

Fig. 7. Kinetics of biotin-antibody binding in wash-LOCI. HUI018-A beads with biotin-OXI005 (A), biotin-Fz (B), and biotin-Mill (C). The four insulin concentrations used were as shown.

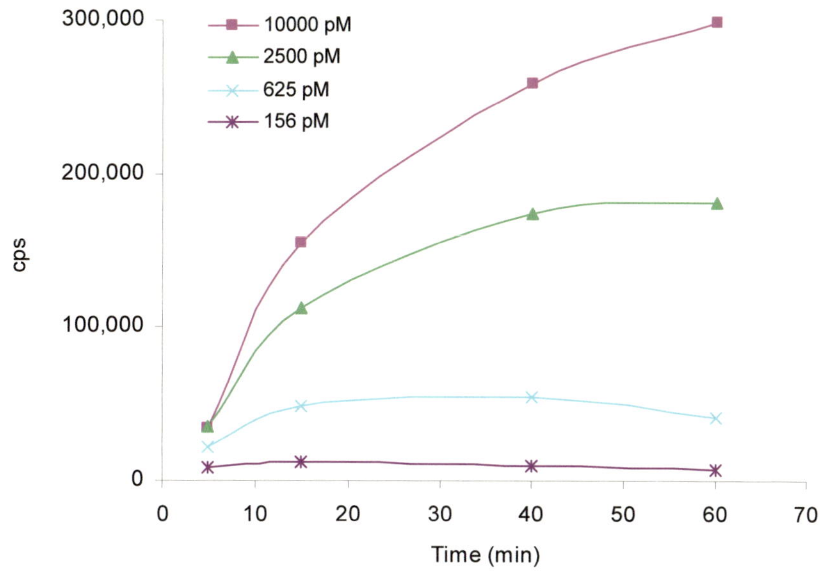

Fig. 8. Kinetics of binding of SA-D beads in wash-LOCI. The antibody pair used was HUI018-A beads/biotin-OXI005 and the four insulin concentrations used are shown.

The results of the investigation of the analyte binding are shown in Figure 6. The curves show that the analyte reaction had moved forward after 30 minutes and was still developing at 2 hours incubation. Longer incubation will give further increase in signal and improvement of sensitivity for some assays. However for practical reasons an incubation time of 1 hour was chosen. The fact that 1 hour of incubation may be needed in spite of the short diffusion distance to the bottom and in spite of the large surface-to-volume ratio may be explained by a relatively low antibody density on the bottom.

The reaction was faster at higher insulin concentrations. The antibody density was lower than in LOCI because beads bound to the well bottoms only expose part of the coupled antibodies. Furthermore fewer beads were used per well in wash-LOCI compared to normal LOCI.

Binding of biotin-OXI005 and biotin-Fz reached its maximum after 30 minutes; probably due to the high concentration of specific antibodies (Fig. 7 A and B). The biotin-Mill was obviously much slower in accordance with lower titer of this antibody (Fig. 7 C). As a compromise for the different antibodies a reaction time of 60 minutes was chosen as the standard condition, though after 15 minutes good assays were obtained.

The kinetics of the SA-D beads was expected to be hampered by the size of the beads. The data show hat the binding of SA-D beads continued to increase from 5 minutes and to 40 minutes (Fig. 9). The reaction did not develop further between 40 and 120 minutes (data not shown). For practical reasons and since the sensitivity of the assay was better after 60 minutes, this time has been chosen as standard condition but good assays could also be obtained after 40 minutes incubation in this step.

Based on the kinetics studies it can be seen that the assay, which presently run as a 3 hours assay, can be run with a total assay time of 1.5 hours (sample 35 minutes, biotin antibody 15 minutes and SA-D beads 45 minutes).

3.5 Reagent concentrations and amounts

A sample volume of 10 µl was found to be the smallest volume able to cover the well bottom.

Lower volumes will result in an uneven coating of the bottom. Higher volumes of sample will increase the reaction time. An amount of SA-D beads of 1 µg/well was found to give maximum signal in wash-LOCI (data not shown). Higher concentrations of SA-D beads did not increase the signal. The maximum amount of SA-D beads in LOCI is 2 µg.

The effect of concentration (final) of biotin-antibodies on wash-LOCI and LOCI is shown in Figure 9. The results show that a higher concentration was required for the biotin-PCAs than for biotin-OXI005 to get maximum signal in the wash-LOCI. There was a slight increase in signal with increasing biotin-Fz concentration from 20 nM with maximum signal and sensitivity at 80 nM. With biotin-OXI005 the maximum signal was obtained between 6.65 and 13.3 nM. With biotin-Mill the signal continued to increase up to at least 160 nM. The higher concentration needed for PCA is in accordance with the fact that only a smaller percentage of the IgG in PCA is specific antibodies. For both antibodies (Fz and Mill) 12 µg/ml seemed to be suitable.

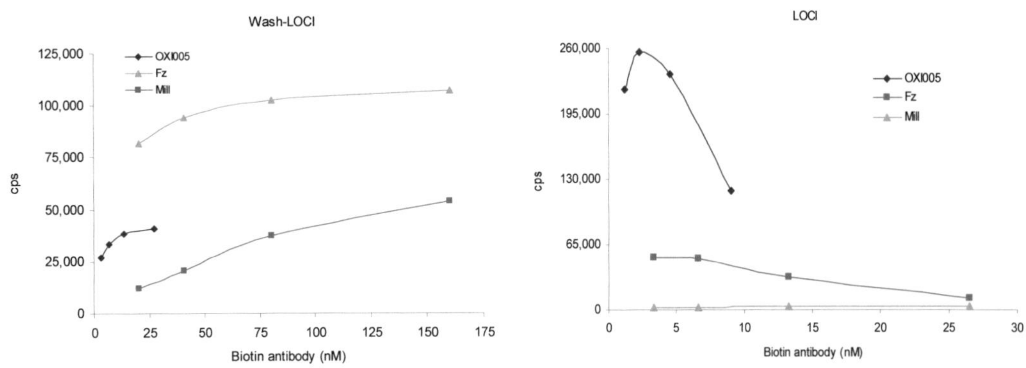

Fig. 9. Biotin-antibody concentrations in wash-LOCI and LOCI both with HUI018-A beads. The biotin-antibody concentration is shown as final concentration in a well. The insulin concentration was, in all cases, 625 pM.

It is clear that the wash-LOCI tolerated much higher concentrations of biotin-IgG than LOCI. With LOCI the signal was going down with higher concentrations of biotin-IgG.

From Figure 9 it is clear that there was an upper limit for the concentration of the biotin-antibody concentration in LOCI. The reason is a limiting amount of SA-D beads. The SA-D beads can not be increased to above 2 µg/well without signal reduction; probably due to optical effects. With this maximum concentration of SA-D the biotin-ab concentration should not be higher than 4.5 nM. Higher concentrations will reduce the signal. The decrease in signal was seen at the same concentration of biotin-OXI005, biotin-Fz and biotin-Mill. This decrease limits the application of biotin-PCA in LOCI

3.6 Hook effect and interference

The sequential incubations in the wash-LOCI reduced interference from plasma samples and removed the risk of hook effect at high analyte concentrations. Figure 10 shows the results of testing very high concentrations of insulin in wash-LOCI and LOCI. As expected there was no hook effect up to at least 100,000 pM with the wash-LOCI since excess unbound analyte was washed away prior to addition of biotin-antibody. The hook effect in the normal LOCI assays is seen at 30,000 pM. This hook effect was caused by excess insulin preventing sandwich formation. The difference between wash-LOCI and LOCI was not dramatic since LOCI has a very broad working range. However with even higher insulin concentrations the wash-LOCI has an advantage by not showing drop in signal at very high insulin concentrations.

The plasma was affecting the antigen-antibody reactions and/or the signal. This effect is shown for wash-LOCI and LOCI with chicken plasma, rat plasma pig plasma compared to assay buffer (Fig. 11). In LOCI the effect of plasma compared to assay buffer was much more pronounced. Also there was more difference between calibration curves in plasma from different species. This difference in wash-LOCI between assay buffer and plasma may be due to the effect on the antigen-antibody reaction.

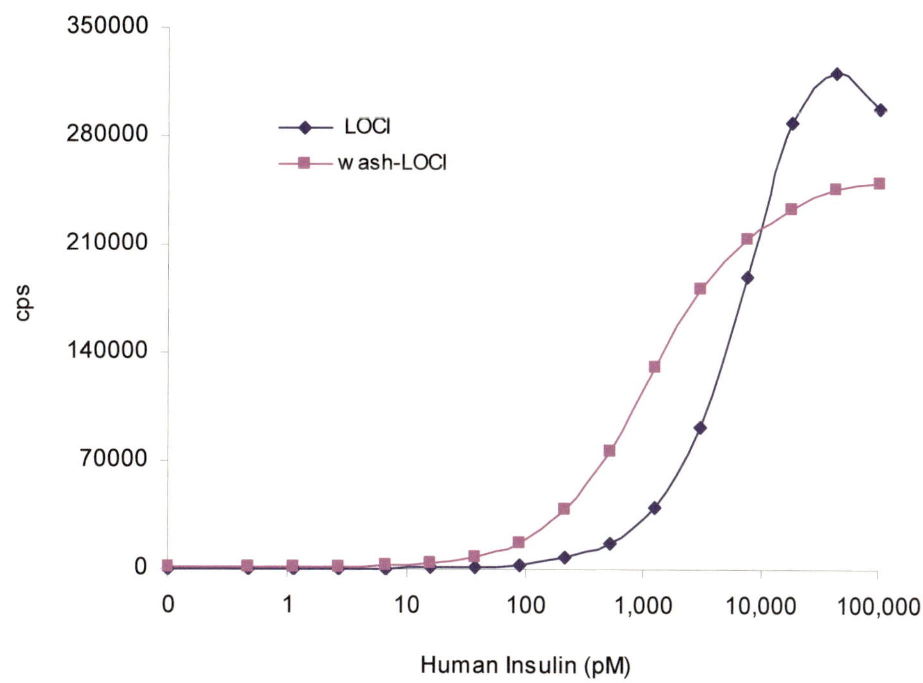

Fig. 10. Hook effect for wash-LOCI and LOCI. Antibody pairs were HUI001-A beads/biotin-Fz in wash-LOCI and HUI018-A beads/biotin OXI005 in LOCI.

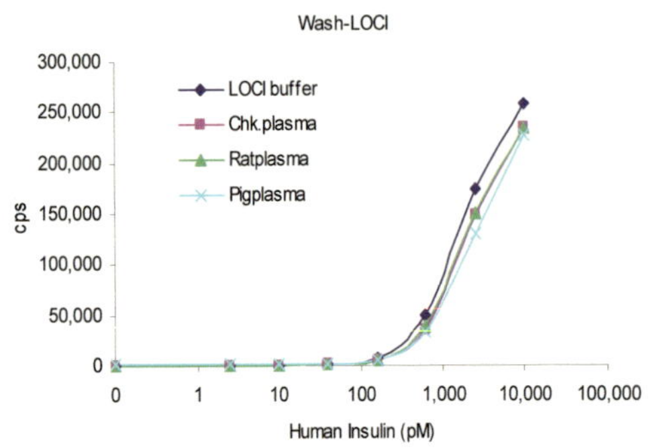

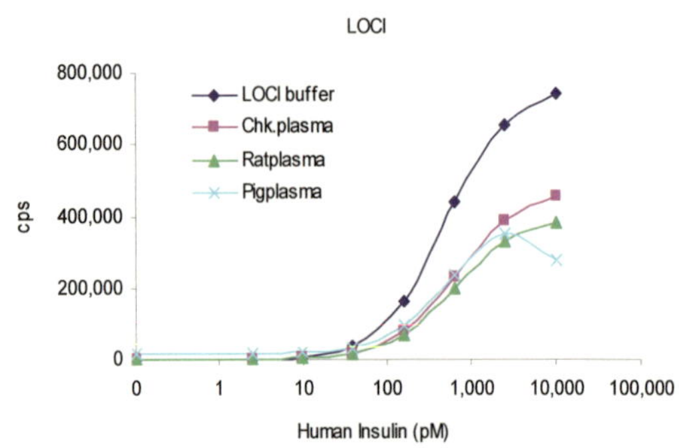

Fig. 11. Interference/matrix effects in wash-LOCI and LOCI both with HUI018-A beads/OXI005. Calibrators in assay buffer, chicken plasma, rat plasma, and pig plasma.

The effect of hemolysis is caused by quenching of singlet oxygen and is thus affecting the signal output. This is in accordance with the limited effect in wash-LOCI compared to LOCI (Table 2).

Wash-LOCI		LOCI	
Hemoglobin(mg/dl)	% Recovery	Hemoglobin(mg/dl)	% Recovery
0	100	0	100
94	94	94	92
187	97	187	82
375	97	375	80
750	87	750	74
1500	82	1500	61
3000	75	3000	46

Table 2. Interference from hemoglobin in plasma. The assays were run with HUI018-A beads and biotin-OXI005. A chicken plasma sample spiked with 800 pM human insulin and with hemolysate of human erythrocytes to give the hemoglobin concentrations shown.

It can be seen that the wash-LOCI tolerated up to 1500 mg hemoglobin/dl compared to 375 mg/dl for the LOCI assay. The results with removal of hemolysate interference by washing show that the wash-LOCI may be used for samples containing interfering components. The wash-LOCI was more robust to plasma effect, singlet oxygen quenchers and inner filter effects. Only one of the antigen-antibody reactions was directly affected since plasma was washed away before the biotin-antibody was added and all plasma components were washed away before measurement.

3.7 Plate uniformity

Reproducibility studies were performed by running a plate with the same sample (1000 pM of human insulin in chicken plasma) in all wells except for the two calibrator columns 11 and 12. The variation in signal was 3.8% and there were no marked patterns on the plate. The wash-LOCI is more prone to variation than the homogenous version due to the plate coating and washing steps. It is important that the plate washer is washing all wells exactly the same way and that no or very little wash fluid is left in the wells.

4. Conclusion

This study has shown that the traditional homogeneous LOCI assay can be converted into a new semi-heterogeneous wash-LOCI which includes wash separation. Human insulin was used as a model analyte. LOCI and wash-LOCI were based on the same reagents and equipment. The only difference being that the antibody coated A-beads were anchored to the bottom of the plate wells in wash-LOCI. This anchoring allows introducing wash steps which will render the LOCI technology even more versatile. The assay worked (due to wash after biotin-antibody incubation) with not-immunopurified PCA. It was performed with the two antigen-antibody reactions as separate steps followed by addition of SA-D bead i.e. a sequential assay. Due to wash after sample incubation this assay was less prone to sample interferants. The signal was measured directly from the bottom of the well.

Wash-LOCI assays showed very good sensitivity and a broad working range. It worked with low plasma sample volume (3 µl per well). The assay has a high capacity and may be run with the same equipment and on the same robotic lines as LOCI. With PCA and wash-LOCI it may be possible to measure molecules which can not be measured in existing MCA/MCA assays.

Wash-LOCI should be seen as a supplement to LOCI. It is very easy to switch from the no wash version to the wash version. However the normal LOCI is much easier to run and is a better assay so the wash-LOCI should only be considered for special purposes.

The LOCI technology thus has the potential for non-separation-based (no-wash) and separation-based (wash) immunoassays.

5. Acknowledgements

The author thanks Kirsten Borres Jensen for excellent technical assistance and valuable discussions.

6. References

Hall, M.; Kazakova, I. & Yao, Y.-M. (1999). High Sensitivity Immunoassays Using Particulate Fluorescent Labels. *Analytical Biochemistry*, Vol. 272, pp.165-170, ISSN 0003-2697

Koskinen, J.O.; Vaarno, J.; Meltola, N.J.; Soini, J.T.; Hänninen, P.E.; Luotola, J; Waris, M.E.& Soini, A.E. (2004). Fluorescent nanoparticles as labels for immunometric assay of C-reactive protein using two-photon excitation assay technology. *Analytical Biochemistry*, Vol. 328, pp.210-218, ISSN 0003-2697

Kulmala, S.; Håkonson, M.; Spehar, A.-M.; Nyman, A.; Kankare, J; Loikas, K.; Ala-Kleme, T. & Eskola, J. (2002). Homogeneous and heterogeneous electrochemiluminescence assays of TSH at Disposable Oxide-Covered aluminum electrodes. *Analytica Chimica Acta*, Vol. 458, 271-280, ISSN 0003-2670

Lipman, N.S.; Jackson, L.R.; Trudel, L.J. & Weis-Garcia, F. (2005). Monoclonal versus polyclonal antibodies: Distinguishing Characteristics, Applications, and Information Resources. *Institute for Laboratory Animal Research Journal*, Vol.46, 3, pp. 258-268, ISSN 1084-2020

McCrindle, C.; Schwenzer, K. & Jolley, M.E. (1985). Particle Concentration Fluorescence Immunoassay: A New Immunoassay Technique for Quantification of Human Immunoglobulins in serum. *Clinical Chemistry*. Vol 31, (9), pp.1487-1490, ISSN 0009-9147

Namba, N.; Sawada, T. & Suzuki, O. (2000). Development of High Sensitivity Ru-Chelate Based ECL Immunoassay 2: Electrochemical and Immunochemical Studies on Homogeneous and Heterogeneous ECL Excitation. *Analytical Sciences*, Vol.16, pp.757-763, ISSN 0910-6340

Obenauer-Kutner, L.J.; Jacobs, S.J.; Kolz, K.; Tobias, L.M. & Bordens, R.W. (1997). A Highly Sensitive Electrochemiluminescence Immunoassay for Interferon alpha-2b in human serum. *Journal of Immunological Methods*, Vol. 206, 25-33, ISSN 0022-1759

Okano, K.; Takahashi, S.; Yasuda, K.; Tokinaga, D.; Imai, K. & Koga, M. (1992). Using Microparticle Labelling and Counting for Attomole-Level Detection in Heterogeneous Immunoassay. *Analytical Biochemistry*, Vol 202, 120-125, ISSN 0003-2697

Poulsen, F & Jensen, K. B. (2007). A Luminescent Oxygen Channeling Immunoassay for the Determination of Insulin in Human Plasma. *Journal of Biomolecular Screening*, 12, (2), 240-247, ISSN 1087-0571

Sardesai, N.; Pan, S. & Rusling, J. (2009). Electrochemiluminescent immunosensor for detection of protein cancer biomarkers using carbon nanotube forests and [Ru-(bpy)$_3$]-doped silica nanoparticles. *Chemical Communication (Cambridge)*. Vol 7, (33), 4968-4970, ISSN 0959-9428

Sin, K.-K.; Chan, C.P.-Y.; Pang, T.-H.; Seydack, M. & Renneberg, R. (2006). A highly sensitive fluorescent immunoassy based on avidin-labelled nanocrystals. *Analytical and Bioanalytical Chemistry*. Vol. 384, 638-644, ISSN 1618-2642

Soukka, T; Antonen, K.; Härmä, H.; Pelkkikangas, A.-M.; Huhtinen, P. & Lövgren, T. (2003). Highly sensitive immunoassay of free prostate-specific antigen in serum using europium(III) nanoparticle label technology. *Clinica Chimica Acta*,Vol. 328, 45-58, ISSN 0009-8981

Ullman, E.F.; Kirakossian, H.; Singh, S.; Wu, Z.P.; Irvin, B.R.; Pease, J.S.; Switchenko, J.D.; Irvine J.D.; Dafforn, A.; Skold, C.N. & Wagner D.B. (1994). Luminescent oxygen channelling immunoassay : measurement of particle binding kinetics by chemiluminescence. *Proceedings of the National Academy of Sciences USA*. Vol. 91, 5426-5430, ISSN 0027-8424

Ullman, E.F.; Kirakossian, H.; Switchenko, A.C.; Ishkanian, J.; Ericson, M.; Wartchow, C.A.; Pirio, M.; Pease,J.; Irvin, B.R.; Singh, S.; Singh, R.; Patel, R.; Dafforn, A.; Davalian, D.; Skold, C.; Kurn, N. & Wagner, D.B. (1996). Luminescent oxygen channelling assay (LOCI): Sensitive, broadly applicable homogeneous immunoassay method. *Clinical Chemistry*. Vol. 42, (9), 1518-1526, ISSN 0009-9147

17

Immunoassay – A Standard Method to Study the Concentration of Peptide Hormones in Reproductive Tissues *in vitro*

Agnieszka Rak-Mardyła, Anna Ptak and Ewa Łucja Gregoraszczuk
Department of Physiology and Toxicology of Reproduction,
Jagiellonian University,
Poland

1. Introduction

Immunoassay analysis has been widely used in many important areas of pharmaceutical analysis, such as in diagnosing diseases, monitoring therapeutic drugs, and studying clinical pharmacokinetics and bioequivalence in drug discovery and pharmaceutical industries (Findlay et al., 2000). Immunoassays are standard biochemical tests that are used to measure concentrations of various hormones, including peptide hormones, in biological fluids, such as serum/plasma, urine, follicular fluid or culture medium. In addition, immunoassays are also used to determine the level of peptide hormones in various tissues, including reproductive tissues, such as ovary, placenta, or testis.

The female reproductive system and status, such as puberty and later regular estrus cycle, are regulated by the hypothalamic-pituitary-ovary axis, which produces many hormones. In addition, the ovary produces steroid hormones, growth factors and peptides that regulate ovarian follicle development, the onset of puberty and/or ovulation. In the last decade, studies have shown that ghrelin, leptin, or resistin, which are produced and secreted mainly by the stomach or adipose tissue, are also expressed and concentrated in reproductive tissues, suggesting an autocrine or paracrine role in female reproduction.

This article focuses on one of the methods used for measuring concentrations of protein hormones, such as ghrelin, leptin, and resistin, in reproductive tissues.

2. Biological function of ghrelin, leptin and resistin

2.1 Ghrelin

Ghrelin is a 28-amino-acid peptide that is produced predominantly by the stomach, although its expression has also been demonstrated in other tissues, including the bowel, pancreas, kidneys, lung, placenta, gonads, pituitary, and hypothalamus (van der Lely et al., 2004). In its acylated form, ghrelin displays strong GH (growth hormone)-releasing activity, which is mediated by the activation of the GH secretagogue (GHS) receptor (GHS-R) type

1a. Two GHSR subtypes generated by alternative splicing of a single gene have been identified: the full-length type 1a receptor and the truncated type 1b. GHS-R1a is the functionally active, signal transduction form of the receptor. In contrast, GHS-R1b lacks transmembrane domains 6 and 7 and is unable to bind a ligand or transduce a signal. GHS-Rs are primarily expressed in the hypothalamus-pituitary unit but are also found in other central and peripheral tissues (Gnanapavan et al., 2002). Moreover, ghrelin has other endocrine and nonendocrine actions, such as stimulating lactotroph and corticotroph secretion; inhibiting the gonadal axis; controlling energy expenditure with orexigenic effects coupled; controlling gastric motility and acid secretion; and influencing endocrine and exocrine pancreatic functions, glucose metabolism, cardiovascular actions, behavior and sleep, cell proliferation, and apoptosis (Figure 1). Circulating ghrelin is primarily found in the unacylated form. Although only the acylated form of ghrelin mediates endocrine actions, the unacylated form influences gastric secretion; in fact, unacylated ghrelin is reduced by 70% after gastrectomy and gastric bypass in humans. One of the hydroxyl groups located on a serine residue of ghrelin is uniquely acylated by n-octanoic acid. Of the two circulating ghrelin forms, acylated (Ac) and unacylated (UnAc), the acylated form is essential for ghrelin biological activity (Kojima et. al., 1999). Plasma ghrelin levels are elevated after fasting and are reduced after eating. In normal-weight humans, the fasting plasma level of ghrelin is approximately 250 pg/ml (Rigamonti et al., 2002).

Circulating ghrelin levels are also increased by fasting and energy restriction and are decreased by food intake. Moreover, ghrelin secretion is negatively correlated with the body mass index (BMI). In fact, circulating ghrelin levels are increased by anorexia and cachexia, reduced by obesity with or without type 2 diabetes, and restored by weight recovery. Interestingly, these changes are the opposite of those observed with leptin, and it has been suggested that both ghrelin and leptin signal a metabolic balance and manage the neuroendocrine and metabolic response to starvation.

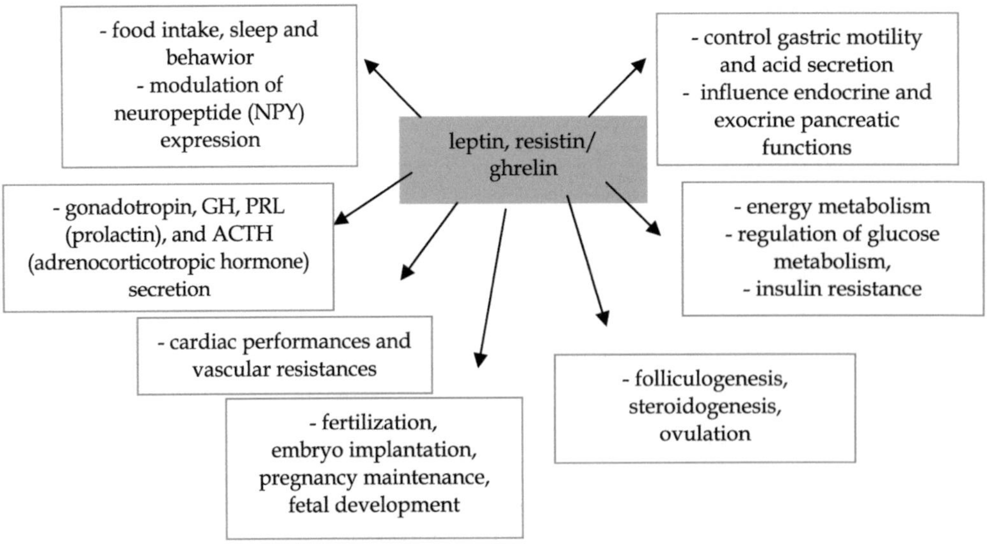

Fig. 1. Biological function of the peptide hormones.

2.2 Leptin

Leptin, the obese (ob) gene product, is a 16-kDa protein that is primarily synthesized by white adipose tissue. The secretion of this hormone is pulsatile and shows a circadian rhythm with a nocturnal rise that peaks between 1 and 2 h. Circulating levels of free/unbound leptin have been strongly correlated with both the BMI and the total amount of body fat. Plasma leptin levels were increased in overweight/obese women (37.7 ng/ml) as compared with normal-weight women (3.92-16.9 ng/ml) (Havel et al., 1996). However, in some obese individuals, the leptin levels are as high as 100 ng/ml (Knerr et al., 2006). With anorexia nervosa, severe undernutrition is associated with low plasma and cerebrospinal fluid leptin levels below 1.85 ng/ml (Mantzoros et al., 1997).

Leptin regulates energy homeostasis primarily in the brain where it might be transported by a receptor-mediated saturable transport mechanism across the blood–brain barrier. Leptin promotes weight loss by reducing appetite and increasing energy expenditure by stimulating sympathetic nerve activity in the thermogenic brown adipose tissue. Leptin induces sympathetic activation to other organs that are not usually considered thermogenic, such as the kidney, hindlimb, adrenal gland, and bone. Moreover, leptin action in the hypothalamus participates in the control of cardiovascular function, bone formation, glucose metabolism, sexual maturation and reproduction, the hypothalamic-pituitary-adrenal system, and fatty acid oxidation. The pleiotropic nature of leptin is supported by the universal distribution of OB-R leptin receptors. Leptin acts via transmembrane receptors, which show structural similarity to the class I cytokine receptor family. Ob-R has a single membrane-spanning domain and exists in different isoforms (Ob-Ra, Ob-Rb, Ob-Rc, Ob-Rd and Ob-Re) that are derived from the alternative splicing of mRNA. Although the white adipocytes mainly produce and secrete leptin into the bloodstream, there are other potential sources of the hormone. The placenta, gastric mucosa, bone marrow, mammary epithelium, skeletal muscle, pituitary, hypothalamus and bone also produce small amounts of leptin under certain circumstances.

2.3 Resistin

Resistin is a novel 12.5-kDa adipokine that belongs to a family of cysteine-rich C-terminal domain proteins called resistin-like molecules (RELMs) (Steppan & Lazar, 2004). The human peptide consists of 114 amino acids, which include a signal peptide of 17 amino acids, a variable region of 37 amino acids, and a conserved C-terminus. Splice variant of human resistin was characterized by the complete loss of exon 2, leading to protein truncation (Steppan et al., 2001) but this effect has not yet received further attention.

In human studies, resistin gene expression is detected in the adipocytes, and its levels are increased in morbidly obese humans as compared with lean control subjects. Whether resistin is involved in energy homeostasis is still unclear; however, its expression patterns are similar to leptin expression. Fasting reduces leptin and resistin expression, and both hormones were increased after eating. Some studies have reported a significant association between resistin and the development of obesity and insulin resistance (Ukkola, 2002). In animal experiments resistin induces insulin resistance. The human physiological effect of this cytokine is less pronounced. Increased serum resistin levels were found in obese individuals, but some controversies exist concerning its role in type II diabetes, insulin resistance and hypertension in humans. Despite much research concerning the mechanism of role and action of resistin, the receptor mediating its biological effects has not yet been identified, and little is known about the intracellular signaling pathways that are activated by this peptide hormone.

3. Characteristics of the methods

3.1 Immunoassay

The immunoassay is based on the reaction of an antigen with a selective antibody to generate a useful product. Several types of labels have been used in immunoassay:

- Radioactivity is used in radioimmunoassay (RIA), a highly sensitive and specific assay method in which the radiolabeled and unlabeled substances compete in an antigen-antibody reaction to determine the concentration of the unlabeled substance.
- Enzymes are used in the enzyme-linked immunosorbent assay (ELISA), which is also known as an enzyme immunoassay (EIA).
- Fluorescence, luminescence or phosphorescence has also been used.

The most common label for clinical and biological analysis is the use of enzymes and colorimetric substrates.

- In capture enzyme-linked immunosorbent method, a capture antibody (Y) is passively adsorbed on a solid phase (Figure 2, Shan et al., 2002 with modification).
- The target protein contained in the sample and the enzyme-labeled reported antibody (Y-E) is added.
- Both the capture antibody and the enzyme-labeled reporter antibody bind to the target protein at different sites, thereby "sandwiching" the protein between the two antibodies.
- After a washing step, the substrate (◊) is added, and colored product (♦) is formed after reaction.
- The amount of colored product generated is directly proportional to the amount of target protein captured.

3.1.1 Sample collection and preparation

In our experiments, we used reproductive tissue, including the ovarian follicles, corpus luteum, placenta or human ovarian cell line (OVCAR-3) or breast cancer cell line (MCF-7). Independently on the sample used, tissue or cells are homogenize and then sonificated twice in appropriate ice-cold lysis buffer. For tissue sample lysis buffer I is used, why for cell line sample lysis buffer II. The lysates are clarified by centrifugation at 15,000 g at 4°C for 30 min, and supernatants are subsequently transferred to separate tubes. The protein content in the lysates are determined with Bradford reagent (Bio-Rad Protein Assay; Bio Rad Laboratories, Munchen, Germany) using bovine serum albumin (BSA) as a standard. After homogenization, the supernatants will be collected and stored at -20°C until further use in the ELISA analysis.

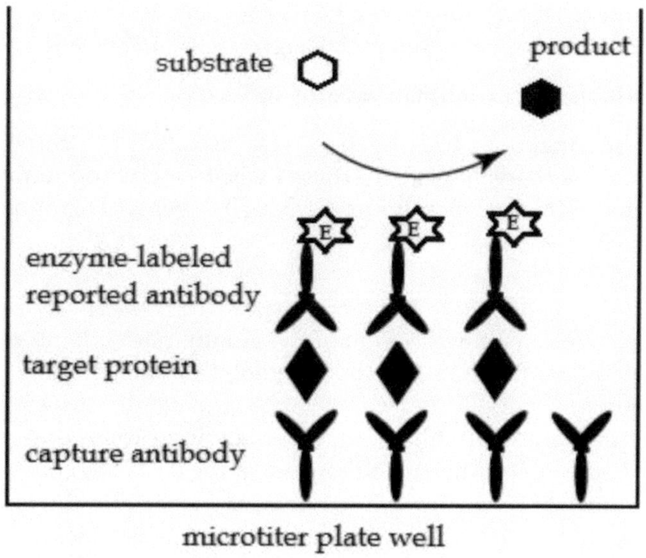

Fig. 2. Enzyme-linked immunosorbent assay (ELISA) (Shan et al., 2002 with modification).

- Lysis buffer I: 50 mM Tris-HCl, pH 7.5, 100 mM NaCl, 0.5 % Na-deoxycholate, 0.5 % NP-40, 0.5 % SDS and EDTA-free protease inhibitors
- Lysis buffer II: PBS, pH 7.2, 0.5 % Tween-20, 1 nM EDTA and 1 nM phenylmethylsulfonyl fluoride (PMSF)

3.1.2 Protocol of peptide determination

It is possible prepare entire procedure described by Fujinami et al., (2004) (1) or use commercially available kits (2) to determine the peptide hormone concentration:

1. Enzyme-linked immunosorbent assay (ELISA) using polyclonal antibodies for measurement concentration of human resistin (Fujinami et al., 2004).

Preparation of the anti-human resistin antibody

In their study, Fujinami et al. (2004) used a synthetic peptide that corresponded to residues 17–44 of human resistin as deduced from the nucleotide sequence of the human resistin gene, which was generated with an additional cysteine-residue located at its N-terminus (Biologica, Nagoya, Japan).

- Following purification by reverse-phase HPLC, the synthetic peptide (purity >85 %) was coupled to a keyhole limpet hemocyanin by an N-(q-maleimidocaproyloxy) succinimide (Sigma, St. Louis, MO).
- The carrier-conjugated peptide was subsequently emulsified with Freund's complete adjuvant (Difco Laboratories, Detroit, MI), and rabbits were subcutaneously injected (0.5 mg/injection) a total of 6 times at 10-day intervals.
- Blood samples were collected at 10 days after the last injection.
- The specific antibody in the sera was purified using a resistin peptide-coupled CNBr-activated Sepharose affinity column.

- Anti-resistin antiserum was raised in a similar manner by injecting a rabbit with 50 μg of recombinant human resistin (Research Diagnostic, Flanders, NJ) into a rabbit.

Preparation of biotinylated anti-human resistin antibody

The human resistin antibody IgG fraction was isolated by chromatography on a recombinant human resistin-coupled CNBr-activated sepharose affinity column and biotinylated with 5-(N-succinimidyl-oxycarbonyl) pentyl-D-biotinamide (Dojindo, Kumamoto, Japan) (Fujinami et al., 2004).

Assay procedure

- Microtiter plates are coated with 100 μl of the affinity purified anti-resistin IgG against human (1.5 μg/ml) that is diluted with 10-mmol/l-carbonate buffer, pH 9.3, for 1 h at room temperature.
- After washing the plate twice, the nonspecific binding sites in each well were blocked with 200 μl of 10-mmol/l-carbonate buffer containing 0.5 % BSA.
- Standard solution (0.5–100 ng/ml of recombinant human resistin) and samples diluted in sample buffer are added to the wells, and then plate are incubated for 1 h at room temperature.
- After 1 h of incubation, plates are washings with BSA-free sample buffer and 100 μl biotinylated anti-recombinant human resistin IgG (5 ng/ml) was added to each well for the next 1 h of incubation.
- Next, after three more washing times, the plate are incubated for 1 h at room temperature with 100 μl of streptavidin-horseradish peroxidase diluted 10,000-fold.
- After three final washes, the plates are treated for 20 min with 100 μl of substrate solution containing 3, 3V, 5, 5V-tetramethylbenzidine (TMB) and H_2O_2.
- The reaction is stopped by the addition of 100 μl of 1 mol/l phosphoric acid, and subsequently, the absorbance is recorded at 450 nm using an ELISA plate reader.
- All washings and incubations were carried out with gentle shaking.

Sample buffer: 50 mmol/l Tris–HCl buffer, pH 7.0, containing 200 mmol/l NaCl, 10 mmol/l CaCl2, 0.1% Triton X-100 and 1% BSA

2. Much simpler and faster methods of peptide hormone determination are commercially available. Currently, many competitors provide a wide range of kits for the determination of various peptides hormones in many animal species and various biological materials.

In our study, the concentration of ghrelin, leptin or resistin in reproductive tissue was measured by ELISA using a commercially available kit (Table 1).

Standard procedure

In this assay, the immunoplate is pre-coated with anti-human peptide hormone capture antibodies, and the nonspecific binding sites are blocked. The peptides hormones in the sample or in the standard solution bind to the capture antibody immobilized in the wells. After washing, the biotinylated anti-peptide hormone detection antibody, which can bind to the peptide hormones trapped in the wells, is added. After washing, the streptavidin-horseradish peroxidase (SA-HRP), which catalyzes the substrate solution (TMB), is added (Figure 3).

	Cat. no/company	*Sensitivity*	*Inter- /intra-run precision*	*Standard curve*
Ac ghrelin	RD194062400R/ BioVendor GmbH, Heidelberg, Germany	0.3 pg/ml	8.3 %/8.1 %	0-250 pg/ml
UnAc ghrelin	RD194063400R/ BioVendor GmbH, Heidelberg, Germany	0.2 pg/ml	3.80 %/3.20 %	0-250 pg/ml
Leptin	RD191001100/ BioVendor GmbH, Heidelberg, Germany	0.2 ng/ml	4.4-6.7 %/ 4.2-7.6 %	0–50 ng/ml
Resistin	4945/DRG International Inc., USA	0.016 ng/ml	15 % / 10 %	0-10 ng/ml

Table 1. Commercially available kits used to determine the concentration of peptide hormones in reproductive tissue.

Summary of commercially available kit protocol

Add the freshly prepared standard solutions, positive controls and samples into immunoplate

↓

Immunoplate incubate at room temperature for 2 h

↓

Wash immunoplate with assay buffer

↓

Add biotinylated anti-peptide detection antibody into immunoplate

↓

Immunoplate incubate at room temperature for 2 h

↓

Wash immunoplate with assay buffer

↓

Add Streptavidin-Horseradish Peroxidase (SA-HRP) into immunoplate

↓

Immunoplate incubate at room temperature for 30 minutes

↓

Wash immunoplate with assay buffer

↓

Add substrate solution (TMB) into immunoplate

↓

Immunoplate incubate at room temperature for 30 minutes

↓

Terminate the reaction with stop solution

↓

Measure absorbance values at 450 nm using an ELISA plate reader

Fig. 3. Summary of commercially available ELISA assay procedure (according to the enclosed assay instructions).

The enzyme-substrate reaction is terminated by the addition of a stop solution. The intensity of the color is directly proportional to the amount of peptide hormones present in the standard solutions or samples. The standard curve is produced from the data obtained using the serial dilutions of the standards with the concentration plotted on the x-axis (log scale) versus absorbance on the y-axis (linear) (Figure 4). The absorbance values were measured at 450 nm using an ELISA plate reader.

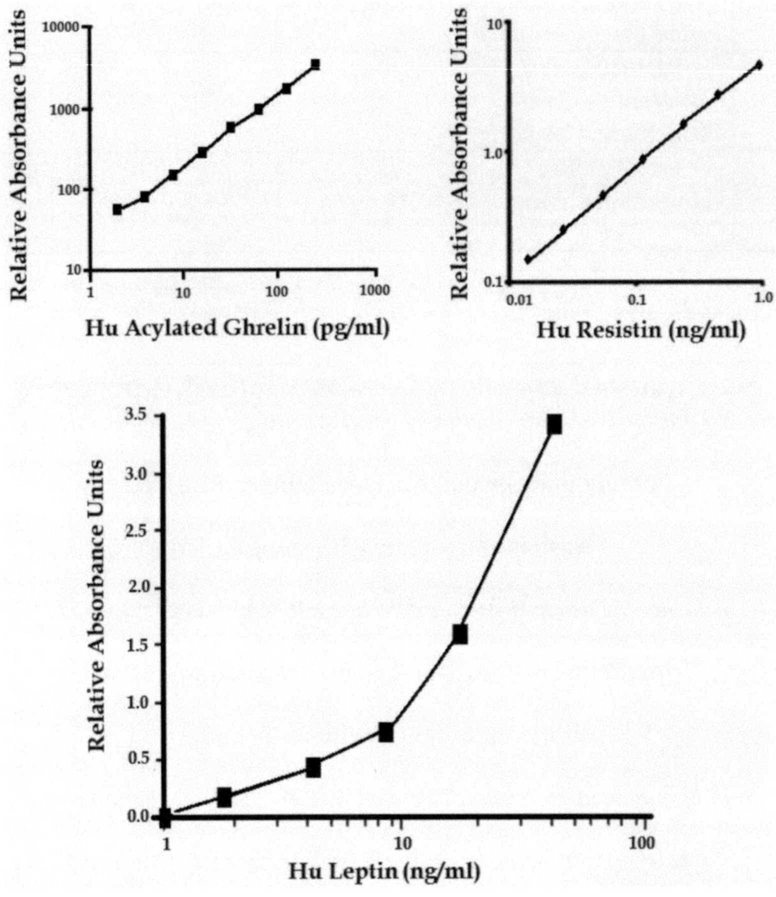

Fig. 4. Typical standard curve for peptide hormones determined by ELISA. The absorbance values were measured at 450 nm for leptin and resistin and at 414 nm for Acylated Ghrelin.

3.2 Western immunoblot assay

The Western immunoblot assay is an alternative detection method to ELISA and is used to confirm our immunoassay results. Western immunoblott is based on the detection of proteins using specific antibodies. This assay utilizes specific antibodies to proteins that have been separated according to size (molecular weight) by gel electrophoresis. The blot is a membrane, which is commonly composed of nitrocellulose or PVDF (polyvinylidene fluoride). The gel is placed next to the membrane, and an electrical current is used to transfer the proteins from the gel to the membrane where they adhere. As a result, the membrane becomes a replica of the protein gel, which can subsequently be stained with an antibody.

3.2.1 Sample collection and preparation

To prepare samples for electrophoresis, the tissues and cells are lysed to release the proteins of interest. This lysis solubilizes the proteins for their individual migration through the separating gel. There are many recipes for lysis buffers, but only a few are appropriate for Western blotting. In brief, they differ in their ability to solubilize proteins. Those containing sodium dodecyl sulfate and other ionic detergents are considered to be the harshest and are therefore most likely to generate the highest yield. In our experiments, the reproductive tissues were homogenized twice in ice-cold lysis buffer. Subsequent to sonication for 10–15 seconds to complete cell lysis, the DNA was sheared to reduce sample viscosity and centrifuged at 10000 x g for 10 minutes at 4°C. The lysate protein concentrations were determined using the Bradford assay. Equal amounts of protein were added to an equal volume of 2X sample buffer and boiled at 95-100°C for 5 minutes.

- Sample buffer: 125 mM Tris-HCl (pH 6.8 at 25°C), 4 % w/v SDS, 25 % glycerol, 20 mM DTT, 0.01 % w/v bromophenol blue or phenol red

3.2.2 Electrophoresis

Electrophoresis is a standard technique for separating proteins according to their molecular weight. Samples (10 µl) are separated by SDS-PAGE (sodium dodecyl sulfate polyacrylamide gel electrophoresis; 10 cm x 10 cm; BioRad Mini-Protean II Electrophoresis Cell), and the proteins are transferred to nitrocellulose membranes (BioRad Mini Trans-Blott apparatus). The separation of molecules is determined by the relative size of the pores formed within the gel. We used electrophoresis control markers for qualitative molecular mass determinations: tubulin (55 kDa) or β-actin (42 kDa).

- Electrophoresis buffer: 25 mM Tris base, 0.2 M glycine, 0.1 % SDS
- Transfer buffer: 25 mM Tris base, 0.2 M glycine, 20 % methanol

	Molecular weight (kDa)	*SDS-PAGE gel (%)*	*Loading control*	*PVDF membranes*	*Wet transfer conditions*
Ghrelin	3-4	20 %	tubulin	0.2 µm	1A/45 min
Ghrelin receptor (GHSR-1a)	41	10 %	tubulin	0.45 µm	1A/60 min
Leptin	16	15 %	β-actin	0.2 µm	1A/45 min
Leptin receptor (Ob-R)	100-125	7 %	β-actin	0.45 µm	1A/ 60 min
Resistin	12.5	12 %	β-actin	0.2 µm	1A/45 min

Table 2. Characteristic parameters in electrophoresis.

3.2.3 Immunoblotting

After the transfer procedure, the membranes are washed, and nonspecific binding sites are blocked with 5 % no fat milk and TBS/T (Tris-buffered saline/Tween) buffer in at room temperature for 2 h. Then, the membranes were washed three times for 5 min each with TBS/T. The membranes are incubated overnight with diluted primary antibody in 10 ml of

TBS/T/milk buffer with gentle shaking at 4°C. After incubating the membranes with the primary antibody, the membranes are washed with TBS/T and incubated for 1 hour with horseradish peroxidase-conjugated secondary antibody diluted at 1:500 in TBS/T. The signals are detected by chemiluminescence (ECL) using Western Blotting Luminol Reagent (sc-2048, Santa Cruz Biotechnology) and visualized using a ChemidocTM Reader. All data bands visualized by chemiluminescence are quantified using a densitometer.

- TBS/T buffer: 0.2% Tween-20 in 0.02 M TBS

	Primary antibody	*Secondary antibody*
Ghrelin	Goat polyclonal antibody raised againstA peptide mapping within an internal region of ghrelin of human origin	Horseradish peroxidase-conjugated antibody
Ghrelin receptor (GHSR-1a)	Goat polyclonal antibody raised againstA peptide mapping near the C-terminus of GHS-R1a of human origin	Horseradish peroxidase-conjugated antibody
Leptin	Mouse monoclonal anti-leptin (Ob) clone LEP-13 reacts specifically with human leptin	Polyclonal goat anti-mouse/HRP
Leptin receptor (Ob-R)	Mouse monoclonal Ob-R (B-3) antibody detection of short and long forms of Ob-R of mouse, rat and human	Polyclonal goat anti-mouse/HRP
Resistin	Goat polyclonal antibody raised againstA peptide mapping within an internal region of resistin of human origin	Horseradish peroxidase-conjugated antibody

Table 3. Antibodies used in immunoblotting procedure.

4. Effect and concentration of peptide hormones in reproduction

Proper nutrition has a significant influence on fertility. In both animals and humans, appropriate weight determines the transition from puberty into maturity. Appropriate nutrition also influences the adequate amount of adipose tissue and thus the levels of hormones secreted by the adipose cells. The nutritional status is connected with reproductive efficiency; therefore, researchers have focused on the role of peptide hormones in the regulation of reproductive function and its concentration in reproductive tissue.

4.1 Ghrelin

The expression of ghrelin and its receptor has been detected in the reproductive tissues of humans, and many species such as rats, pigs, sheep and chickens (Gnanapavan et al., 2002, Caminos et al., 2003, Sirotkin et al., 2006), and in other tissues, such as the hypothalamus, pituitary, and placenta (Zhang et al., 2008, Gualillo et al., 2001). Ghrelin gene expression was consistently detected in the rat ovary throughout the estrous cycle and pregnancy, with higher levels present in the corpus luteum and during the first days of gestation (Caminos et al., 2003). The highest ghrelin gene expression levels in the pig ovary occur during the diestrous phase and that the lowest levels occur during the proestrous phase was observed by Zhang et al., (2008). Data concerning the role of ghrelin in ovarian function are conflicting. In rats, the systematic administration of ghrelin reduces the gonadotropin-releasing hormone pulse frequency in vivo. Moreover, in the rat and human pituitary, ghrelin can suppress luteinizing hormone (LH) and follicle-stimulating hormone (FSH) secretion. However, in women, the administration of ghrelin did not affect basal and GnRH-induced LH and FSH secretion during the menstrual cycle.

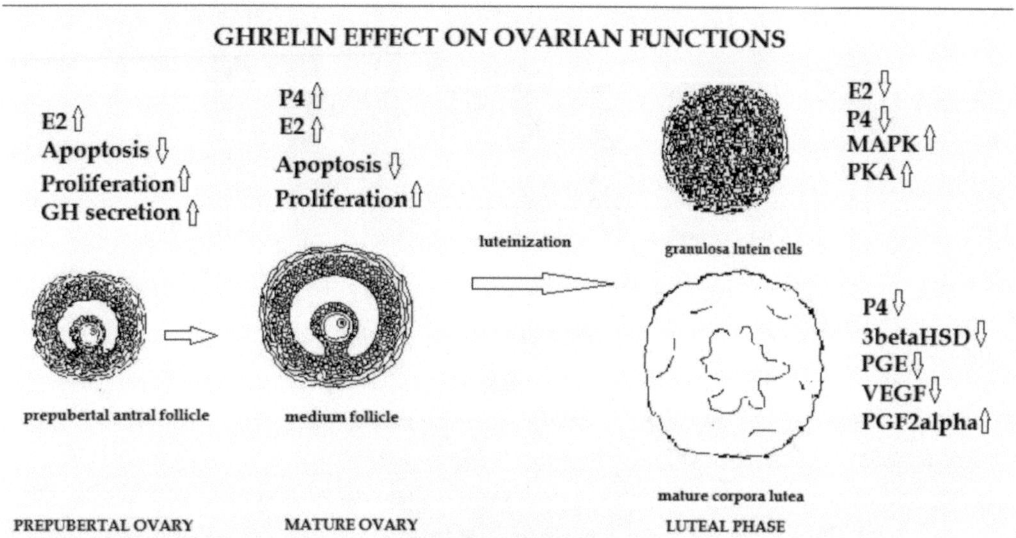

Fig. 5. Effect of ghrelin in reproduction. (↑) stimulatory and (↓) inhibitory effect, (Sirotkin et al., 2006, Rak & Gregoraszczuk, 2008, 2009, Viani et al., 2008).

Our data demonstrated that porcine ovarian follicles collected from prepubertal animals secreted ghrelin and stimulated estradiol secretion through aromatase activity (Figure 5) (Rak & Gregoraszczuk 2008, 2009). Ghrelin stimulates the secretion of progesterone, estradiol, IGF-I and arginine vasotocin in an in vitro study of chicken ovarian tissues (Sirotkin et al., 2008). However, ghrelin had an inhibitory effect on steroid synthesis in cultured human granulosa luteinizing cells (Viani et al., 2010).

An immunoassay method using a double-antibody sandwich enzyme immunoassay was used to study the levels of acylated and unacylated ghrelin throughout the normal menstrual cycle. The concentration of both forms of ghrelin remained unchanged during the entire cycle (Dafopoulos et al., 2009). Only sporadic significant correlations were found between acylated and unacylated ghrelin and E2 levels, suggesting that the magnitude of physiological changes of the sex steroids during the menstrual cycle had no major effect on ghrelin secretion from the stomach.

Using commercially available kits, our experiments showed that ghrelin was present in the porcine ovarian follicles (the follicular fluid and in follicular wall), and it is hormone that is secreted into the culture medium during the first 24 h of ovarian follicle incubation (Rak & Gregoraszczuk, 2009). Moreover, the results clearly showed that the level of ghrelin in the follicular fluid was the sum of the amounts found in the follicular wall and the culture medium (Table 4).

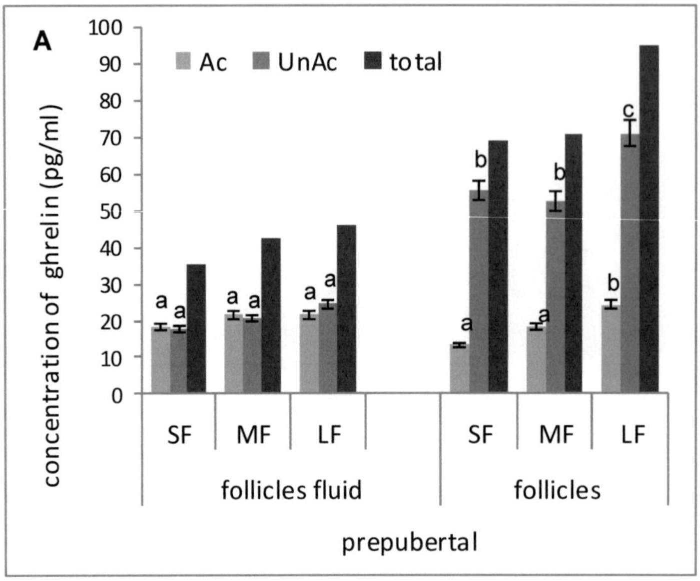

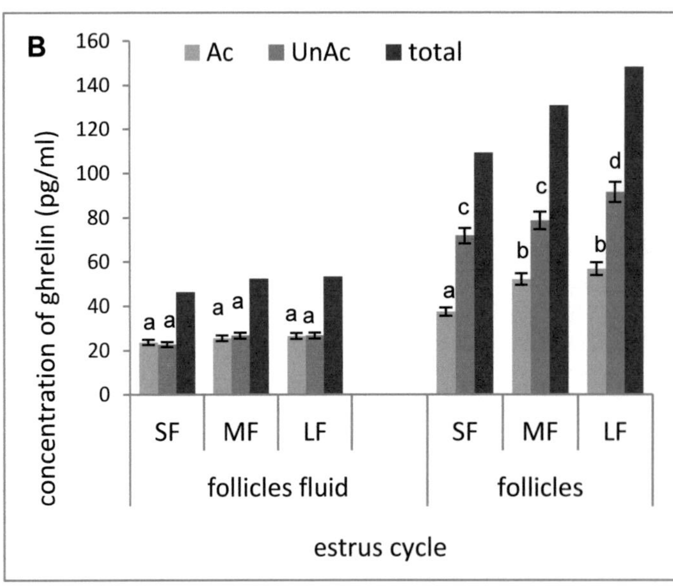

Fig. 6. Concentrations of both Ac and UnAc ghrelin in the follicular fluid of small (SF), medium (MF) and large (LF) ovarian follicles collected from (A) prepubertal animals and (B) ovarian follicles from cycling animals measured by ELISA assay. All samples were performed in triplicate in the same assay. All data are expressed as the mean ± SEM. Different letters indicate statistically significant differences among groups ($p<0.05$). (Rak-Mardyła & Gregoraszczuk, 2011, unpublished results).

	Follicular fluid	*Follicular wall*	*Medium from culture*
Ghrelin (pg/ml)	18.638 ± 5.9	13.750 ± 1.5	4.672 ± 2.0

Table. 4. Ghrelin levels in prepubertal pig ovary measured by ELISA assay (Rak & Gregoraszczuk, 2009).

Additional experiments using the ELISA method showed the concentrations of ghrelin Ac, UnAc and total (Ac plus UnAc) in ovarian follicles and the follicular fluid. In prepubertal animals, the total concentration of ghrelin was higher in the ovarian follicles than in the follicular fluid. The highest concentrations of both forms of ghrelin were observed in the large follicles. As in the case of the prepubertal animals, the total concentration of ghrelin in cycling animals was higher in the ovarian follicles than in the follicular fluid (Rak-Mardyła & Gregoraszczuk, 2011, unpublished results) (Figure 6).

The corpus luteum (CL) plays a central role in regulating the estrous cycle and in maintaining pregnancy. In addition to gonadotropins, locally produced hormones, proteins, growth factors and cytokines play crucial roles in regulating CL function. Results of our date showed, that concentration measurement by ELISA method of Ac ghrelin was unchanged during luteal phase, why levels of UnAc ghrelin significantly increased from early luteal phase to middle luteal phase (Figure 7) and was on the same levels in late luteal phase (Rak-Mardyła et al., 2012, in press). Although, first UnAc was considered an inactive form of ghrelin, accumulating evidence indicates that UnAc can modulate metabolic activities of the ghrelin system either independently or in opposition to those of Ac. Examples of UnAc actions include improvement of pancreatic β-cell function and survival and a beneficial role in cardiovascular function.

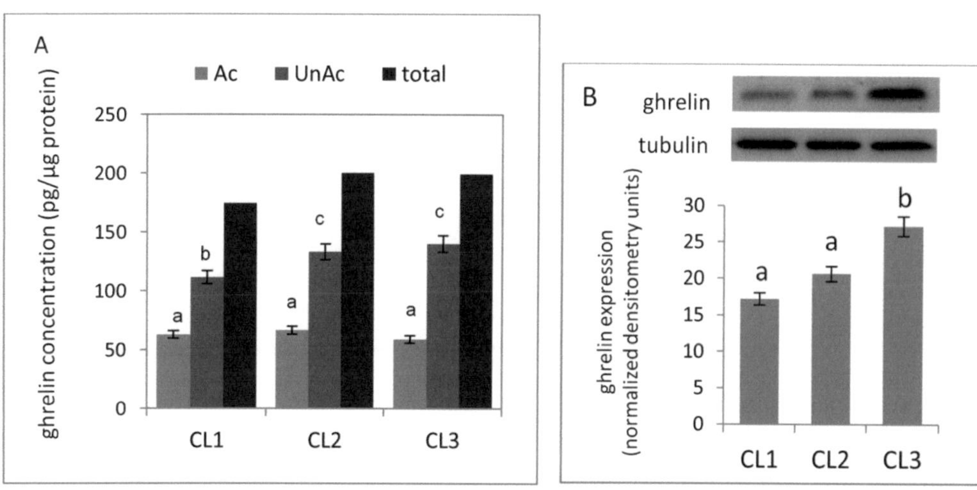

Fig. 7. Concentrations of both Ac and UnAc ghrelin in in different stages of corpus luteum development measured by ELISA assay (A) and protein expression of ghrelin measured by Western immunoblotting procedure (B). All samples were performed in triplicate in the same assay. All data are expressed as the mean ± SEM. Different letters indicate statistically significant differences among groups ($p<0.05$) (Rak-Mardyła et al., 2012, in press).

The presence of ghrelin and ghrelin receptors in the placenta clearly demonstrates that this hormone has a role in placental physiology. In humans, high placental ghrelin peptide levels are observed in the first trimester of pregnancy, primarily in cytotrophoblasts, whereas such high levels are not observed in the third trimester placental tissues (Gualillo et al., 2001). Only a few studies have reported the course of circulating ghrelin levels as measured by immunoassay during pregnancy in humans. The longitudinal changes in serum ghrelin levels during pregnancy in 11 pregnant women showed that normal nondiabetic women have maximum serum values during mid-pregnancy (Fuglsang et al., 2005). However, the serum levels declined to the lowest levels in pregnancy at the end of the third trimester with a 28 % decrease on average as compared with the mid-pregnancy values. Similar observations have been reported in a cross-sectional study measuring acylated ghrelin. The lowest circulating ghrelin levels are observed in late pregnancy and may be even lower than in nonpregnant subjects. Ghrelin is involved in the decidualization of human endometrial stromal cells. During pregnancy, ghrelin levels are at their maximum at mid-pregnancy and are at their lowest in the third trimester (at the time of increased body weight), suggesting that ghrelin is an important autocrine/paracrine factor for the growth and maintenance of the placenta during pregnancy (Fuglsang et al., 2005).

4.2 Leptin

Mice lacking leptin or the leptin receptor (Ob-R, db/db) exhibit low gonadotropin levels, incomplete development of reproductive organs and do not reach sexual maturation (Zhang et al., 1994). Leptin administration to ob/ob mice induces puberty, maturation of the gonads, gonadotropin secretion and restores fertility. Humans with congenital leptin deficiencies or leptin receptor mutations recapitulate most of the leptin-deficient reproductive phenotypes observed in the mouse models. Moreover, in young women that do not undergo puberty, leptin treatment can induce pubertal development. Plasma leptin concentrations are low after weaning in the female and progressively increase during the prepubertal and pubertal period.

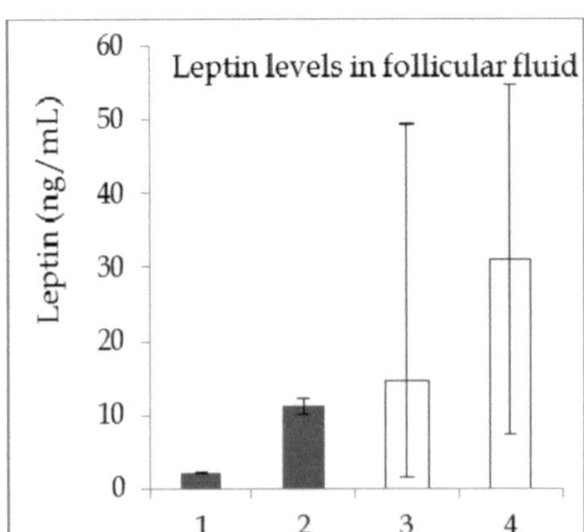

Fig. 8. Mean leptin levels in the porcine (1) and human (2-4) follicular fluid (black columns - RIA, white columns - ELISA) (1) Gregoraszczuk et al., 2004; (2) Welt et al., 2003; (3) Wunder et al., 2005, (4) Hill et al., 2007.

Leptin acts at various levels of the hypothalamic-pituitary-gonadal axis, involving different biochemical pathways. Leptin has stimulatory effects on the hypothalamic-pituitary-gonadal axis at normal serum concentrations but can have inhibitory effects when its levels are elevated, such as with obese individuals. Leptin and its receptors are expressed in the hypothalamus and pituitary, and leptin acts indirectly on the gonadotrophin-releasing hormone secreting cells (Quennell et al., 2003). Leptin also has activity at an ovarian level, and the leptin receptor expression has also been demonstrated by immunoassay in theca and granulosa cells as well as oocytes (Table 5). Moreover, the effects of leptin on ovarian cells are inhibitory and can be attributed to attenuation of gonadotropin, insulin, insulin-like growth factor 1 (IGF-I) and/or glucocorticoid-mediated steroidogenesis (Gregoraszczuk et al., 2003, 2004, 2006).

	Species/cell type	*Measure*	*References*
Ovarian follicles 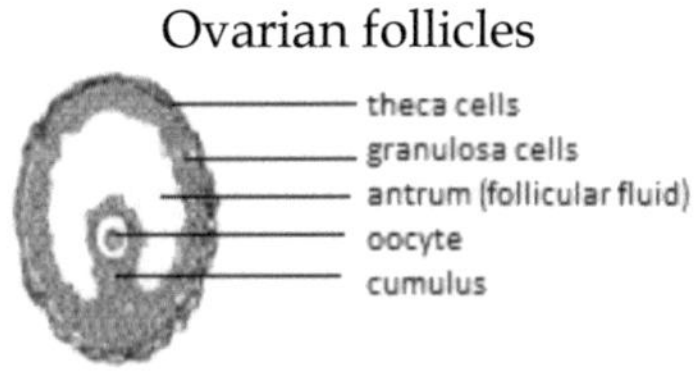	Human/gc/c/o	Leptin/ immunofluorescence staining	Cioffi et al. 1997
	Human/ff	Leptin/RIA	
	Human/gc/th/o	Leptin/ immunohistochemistry staining	Loffler et al. 2001
	Human/ff	Leptin/RIA Ob-R/ELISA	Welt et al. 2003
	Porcine/ff	Leptin/RIA	Gregoraszczuk et al. 2004
	Rat/th/o	Ob-R/ immunohistochemistry staining	Ryan et al. 2003
	Rat/th/o	Leptin/ immunohistochemical staining	Archanco et al. 2003
Corpus luteum (CL)	Human	Leptin/ immunohistochemistry staining	Loffler et al. 2001
	Porcine	Ob-R/ immunoblot	Ruiz-Cortes et al. 2000
	Porcine	Leptin/ immunoblot	Smolinska et al 2010
	Rat	Ob-R/ immunohistochemistry staining	Ryan et al. 2003
	Rat	Leptin/ immunohistochemistry staining	Archanco et al. 2003

Table 5. Location of leptin and (or) leptin receptor in the ovarian tissues of several species. gc: granulosa cells, tc: theca cells, ff: follicular fluid, o: oocyte, c: cumulus.

Consistent with these findings, our data indicated that in large porcine follicles, leptin inhibited basal and GH- or IGF-I-stimulated estradiol secretion. In contrast, leptin augmented two and four times the respective stimulatory effect of basal, IGF-I and GH on progesterone secretion. Our observations indicate that leptin's action on steroidogenesis depended on the stage of follicular development (Gregoraszczuk et al., 2003, 2004) (Fig. 9). We conclude that in preovulatory follicles, leptin is involved in the process of luteinization, which starts just before ovulation. Furthermore, the role of leptin in CL is restricted to the period of the luteal phase. Leptin protects luteal cells from excessive apoptosis and supports an appropriate cell number, which is necessary for maintenance of homeostasis in developing CL (Gregoraszczuk & Ptak, 2005).

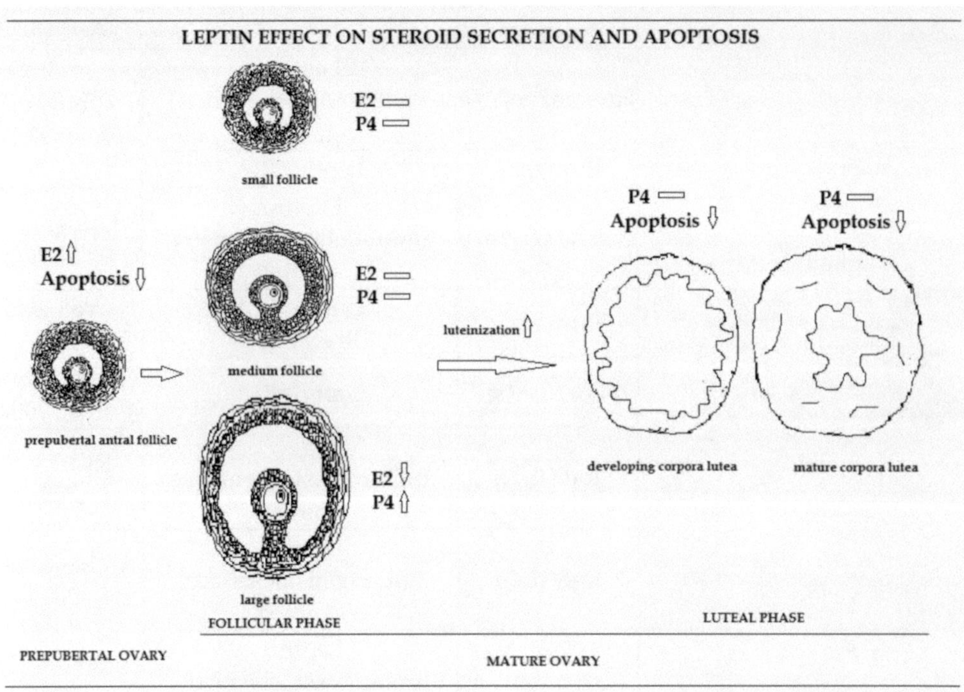

Fig. 9. Schematic summarizing leptin effect on steroid secretion in porcine ovary. (—) no effect, (↑) stimulatory effect, and (↓) inhibitory effect (Gregoraszczuk et al., 2004, 2005, 2006)

Evidence has also emerged indicating a potential direct role for leptin in the regulation of mammalian oocyte and preimplantation embryo development. Leptin and its receptor have been observed by immunoblotting and immunohistochemistry methods to be present in the secretory endometrium and preimplantation embryos. The expression of leptin and its functional receptor in the endometrium and regulation of endometrial leptin secretion by the human embryo suggests that the leptin system may be implicated in the human implantation process. Supplementation of culture medium with leptin promotes the development of preimplantation embryos from the 2-cell stage to the blastocysts, fully expanded blastocysts and hatched blastocysts (Kawamura et al., 2003). As such, perturbations in the leptin system, as observed with obese individuals, may disturb endometrial receptivity and implantation, leading to impaired fecundity. Patients with endometriosis had significantly less serum leptin (15.6 ng/ml) than the controls (30.3 ng/ml). Perhaps, as suggested for the placenta and other tissues, leptin may regulate uterine angiogenesis and cytokine production (Matarese et al., 2000).

Thus, normal leptin secretion is necessary for normal reproductive function to proceed. In women, serum leptin levels are increased during puberty development and during pregnancy. In addition, some studies have reported higher leptin levels in the luteal phase of the cycle, while others have found no difference in leptin levels during normal menstrual cycle as measured by ELISA and or RIA assay (Table 6).

	Follicular phase	*Luteal phase*	*Methods*	*References*
Leptin (ng/ml)	25.7±3.1-28.1±3.0	28.5±3.3	RIA	Yamada et al., 2000
	14.9±2.9	20.4±4.2 *	RIA	Riad-Gabriel et al., 1998
	10.2±7.1	11.8±6.9	RIA	Teirmaa et al., 1998
	13.15±1.60	16.57±1.68 8*	ELISA	Einollahi et al., 2010
	18.14±0.28	23.75±0.64 **	ELISA	Asimakopoulos et al., 2009
Resistin (ng/ml)	4.68±0.07	5.30±0.23	ELISA	Asimakopoulos et al., 2009

Table 6. Mean serum leptin and resistin concentrations in women (normal menstrual group) (* p<0.01, ***p<0.001 *vs.* follicular phase).

Relative leptin deficiency is an emerging clinical syndrome that is associated with several clinical conditions, including exercise-induced energy deficiency, hypothalamic amenorrhea and anorexia nervosa (AN). Leptin levels in AN were first measured in 1995 using an enzyme-linked immunosorbent assay. In most anorexic patients, low leptin serum levels were detected compatible with their underweight and were associated with amenorrhea. In women with hypothalamic amenorrhea, resulting from a negative energy balance, leptin treatment increased pulse frequency and mean levels of LH, ovarian volume, the number of dominant follicles and estradiol levels.

	Human	Pig	Rat
Ovary	+, *	+, #	*
Uterus	#, *	#	no data
Placenta	+, *	#	#

Table 7. Expression of leptin protein in reproductive tissue: + ELISA or RIA detection, # Western Immunoblotting detection, * Immunohistochemical detection

Interestingly, recent studies have demonstrated that leptin stimulates growth, migration, invasion, and angiogenesis in tumor cell models, suggesting that leptin is able to promote an aggressive cancer phenotype. Several studies have indicated that serum leptin levels are positively associated with endometrial cancer, breast cancer, and ovarian cancer. Interestingly, both leptin and the leptin receptor (ObR) appear to be significantly overexpressed in the epithelium, breast and ovarian cancer tissue (Garafalo and Surmacz, 2006) as compared with noncancerous tissues.

Our data indicated that leptin, at physiological relevant concentrations, has no effect on ovarian cancer cell proliferation. Notably, leptin in obese women stimulated cell growth by the up-regulation of genes that are responsible for inducing cell proliferation and the down-regulation of genes that are involved in the inhibition of cell proliferation. The antiapoptotic action of leptin on ovarian cancer cells was due to overexpressing anti-apoptotic factors of both extrinsic and intrinsic caspase-dependent pathways (Ptak et al., 2011, unpublished data).

4.3 Resistin

There are a few studies that indicate a connection between resistin and reproduction function. Resistin dose dependently increases both basal and human chorionic gonadotropin (hCG)-stimulated in vitro testosterone secretion from rat testicular tissue (Nogueiras et al., 2004). Additionally, the pituitary hormones LH and FSH regulate the mRNA expression of resistin in the testis. There are some data concerning resistin and female reproduction. A recent paper by Maillard et al., (2011) demonstrated that resistin is expressed in whole bovine and rat ovaries and that it can modulate ovarian steroidogenesis and proliferation. Ovarian gene expression of resistin was found throughout the estrous cycle in rats. Moreover, resistin mRNA expression in adipose tissue increases during puberty in 45-day old female rats. A recent work demonstrates that resistin mRNA is expressed in the mouse brain and pituitary gland (Morash et al., 2002). Pituitary expression of resistin is regulated in a nutritional-, age- and gender-specific manner. Furthermore, resistin gene expression increases to a peak level in the pituitary of prepubertal mice (Morash et al., 2004). In cultured theca cells, resistin enhanced 17α-hydroxylase activity, which is a marker of ovarian hyperandrogenism in polycystic ovarian syndrome (PCOS) women (Figure 10). This result suggests that resistin may play a local role in stimulating androgen production by theca cells (Munir et al., 2005). Furthermore, resistin mRNA expression in the adipocytes from PCOS women is 2-fold higher than that in the controls. However, used the ELISA method demonstrate that serum resistin levels remain unchanged in normally cycling women, suggesting that physiological changes of sex steroid levels have no effect on resistin secretion from adipocytes (Dafopoulus et al., 2009).

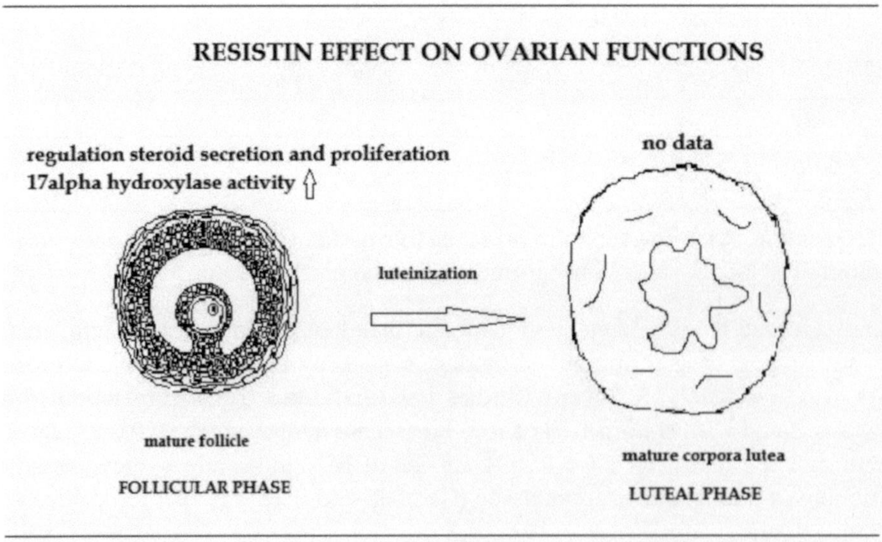

Fig. 10. Effect of resistin in ovarian reproduction. (↑) stimulatory effect, (Maillard et al., 2011, Munir et al., 2005).

Using commercially available ELISA kits, our experiments showed that the concentration of resistin increases during follicular growth, with the highest level in large follicles collected from prepubertal animals (Rak-Mardyła & Gregoraszczuk, 2011, unpublished results). We found no difference in resistin concentration in the ovarian follicles collected from animals during the estrous cycle). These results were confirmed by Western immunoblotting (Figure 11).

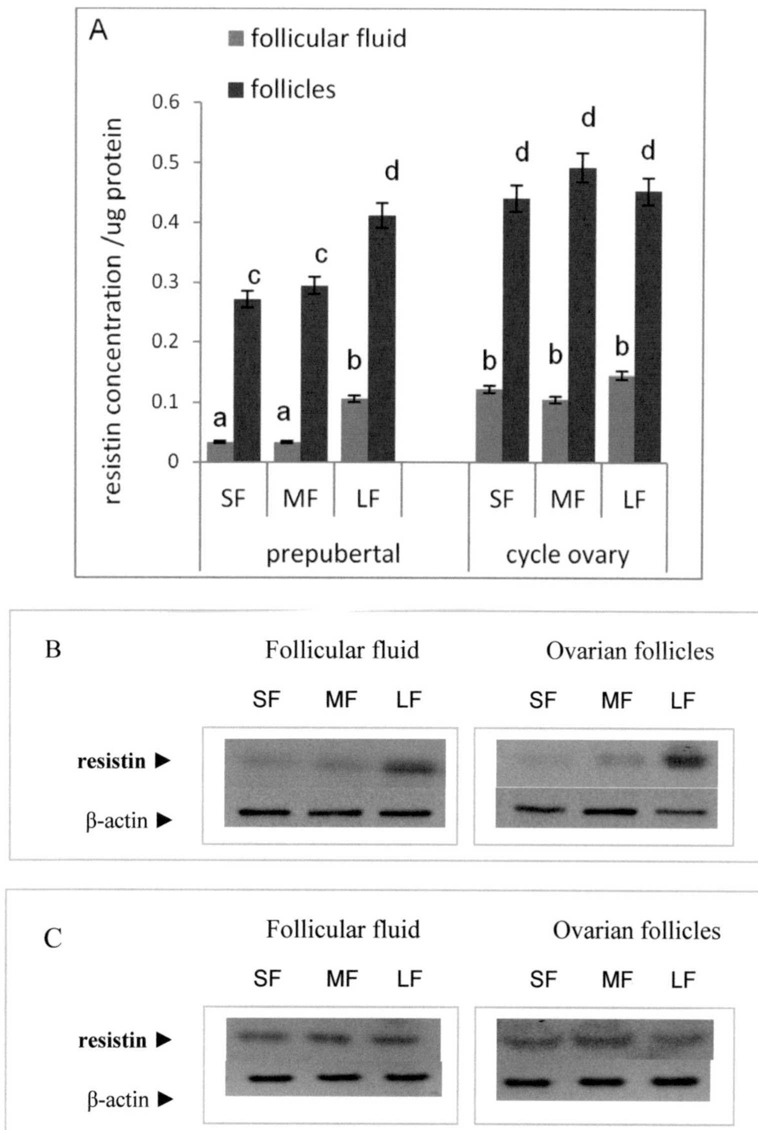

Fig. 11. (A) Concentrations of resistin in follicular fluid and ovarian tissue collected from prepubertal animals measurement by ELISA assay and (B and C) Western blotting. All samples were performed in triplicate in the same assay. All data are expressed as the mean ± SEM. Different letters indicate statistically significant differences among groups ($p<0.05$) (Rak-Mardyła & Gregoraszczuk, 2011, unpublished results).

5. Conclusion

Immunoassay methods are widely used in many studies to measure the concentration of peptide hormones, such as ghrelin, leptin or resistin in reproductive tissue. These methods are suitable for measuring a number of locally secreted peptides, such as growth hormone, insulin-like growth factor-I, insulin or the peptides hormones, ghrelin, leptin and resistin, which influence follicular development during different physiological stages.

6. Acknowledgment

This research was supported by the Polish Committee for Scientific Research "Iuventus Plus" from 2010 to 2011 as project number 0343/POI/2010/70 a part of K/ZDS/001945, DS/MND/WBiNoZ/IZ/6/2011 and from 2010 to 2013 as project 0050/B/PO1/2010/38. Dr. Agnieszka Rak-Mardyła was awarded the *Polish Science Foundation* Award in 2009 and 2010.

7. References

Archanco, M., Muruzábal, FJ., Llopiz, D., Garayoa, M., Gómez-Ambrosi, J., & Frühbeck, G. (2003). Leptin expression in the rat ovary depends on estrous cycle. *The journal of histochemistry and cytochemistry*,Vol.51, No.10, (October 2003), pp.1269-1277, ISSN 0022-1554

Asimakopoulos, B., Milousis, A., Gioka, T., Kabouromiti, G., Gianisslis, G., Troussa, A., Simopoulou, M., Katergari, S., Tripsianis, G., & Nikolettos, N. (2009). Serum pattern of circulating adipokines throughout the physiological menstrual cycle. *Endocrine journal*, Vol.56, No.3, (February 2009), pp.425-433, ISSN 0918-8959

Caminos, J., Tena-Sempere, M., Gaytán, F., Sanchez-Criado, J., Barreiro, M., Nogueiras, R., Casanueva, F., Aguilar, E. & Diéguez C. (2003). Expression of ghrelin in the cyclic and pregnant rat ovary. *Endocrinology,* Vol.144, No.4, (April 2003), pp.1594-15602, ISSN 0013-7227

Cioffi, JA., Van Blerkom, J., Antczak, M., Shafer, A., Wittmer, S., & Snodgrass, HR. (1997). The expression of leptin and its receptors in pre-ovulatory human follicles. *Molecular human reproduction,* Vol.3, No.6, (June 1997), pp. 467-472, ISSN1360-9947

Dafopoulos, K., Sourlas, D., Kallitsaris, A., Pournaras, S. & Messinis IE. (2009). Blood ghrelin, resistin, and adiponectin concentrations during the normal menstrual cycle. *Fertility and sterility*. Vol.92, No.4, (October 2009), pp.389-394, ISSN 0015-0282

Einollahi, N., Dashti, N., & Nabatchian, F. (2010). Serum leptin concentrations during the menstrual cycle in Iranian healthy women. *Acta medica Iranica,* Vol.48, No.5, (September-October 2010), pp.300-303, ISSN 0044-6025

Findlay, J., Smith, W., Lee, J., Nordblom, G., Das, I., De Silva, B., Khan, M. & Bowsher, R. (2000). Validation of immunoassays for bioanalysis: a pharmaceutical industry perspective. *Journal of Pharmaceutical and Biomedical Analysis,* Vol.21, No.6, (January 2000), pp. 1249-1273, ISSN 0731-7085

Fuglsang, J., Skjaerbaek, C., Espelund, U., Frystyk, J., Fisker, S., Flyvbjerg, A. & Ovesen, P. (2005). Ghrelin and its relationship to growth hormones during normal pregnancy. *Clinical Endocrinology,* Vol.62, No.5, (May 2005), pp. 554-559, ISSN 0300-0664

Fujinami, A., Obayashi, H., Ohta, K., Ichimura, T., Nishimura, M., Matsui, H., Kawahara, Y., Yamazaki, M., Ogata, M., Hasegawa, G., Nakamura, N., Yoshikawa, T., Nakano, K.

& Ohta M. (2004). Enzyme-linked immunosorbent assay for circulating human resistin: resistin concentrations in normal subjects and patients with type 2 diabetes. *Clinica chimica acta; international journal of clinical chemistry,*Vol.339, No.(1-2), (January 2004), pp. 57-63, ISSN 0009-8981

Garofalo, C. & Surmacz, E. (2006). Leptin and cancer. *Journal of cellular physiology,* Vol.207, No.1, (April 2006), pp.12-22, ISSN0021-9541

Gnanapavan, S., Kola, B., Bustin, SA., Morris, D., McGee, P., Fairclough, P., Bhattacharya, S., Carpenter, R., Grossman, AB. & Korbonits, M. (2002). The tissue distribution of the mRNA of ghrelin and subtypes of its receptor, GHS-R, in humans. *Journal of clinical endocrinology & metabolism,* Vol. 87, No. 6, (June 2002), pp. 2988, ISSN 0021-972X

Gregoraszczuk, EŁ. & Ptak, A. (2005). In vitro effect of leptin on growth hormone (GH)- and insulin-like growth factor-I (IGF-I)-stimulated progesterone secretion and apoptosis in developing and mature corpora lutea of pig ovaries. *The Journal of reproduction and development,* Vol.51, No.6, (December 2005), pp.727-733, ISSN 0916-8818

Gregoraszczuk, EL., Ptak, A., Wojtowicz, AK., Gorska, T. & Nowak, KW. (2004). Estrus cycle-dependent action of leptin on basal and GH or IGF-I stimulated steroid secretion by whole porcine follicles. *Endocrine regulations,* Vol. 38 No.1, (March 2004), pp.15-21, ISSN 1210-0668

Gregoraszczuk, EL., Rak, A., Wójtowicz, A., Ptak, A., Wojciechowicz, T. & Nowak, KW. (2006). Gh and IGF-I increase leptin receptor expression in prepubertal pig ovaries: the role of leptin in steroid secretion and cell apoptosis. *Acta veterinaria Hungarica,* Vol.54, No.3, (September 2006), pp.413-426, ISSN 0236-6290

Gregoraszczuk, EL., Wójtowicz, AK., Ptak, A. & Nowak, K. (2003). In vitro effect of leptin on steroids' secretion by FSH- and LH-treated porcine small, medium and large preovulatory follicles. *Reproductive biology,* Vol.3, No.3, (November 2003), pp.227-239, ISSN1642-431X

Gualillo, O., Caminos, J., Blanco, M., Garcìa-Caballero, T., Kojima, M., Kangawa, K., Dieguez, C. & Casanueva F. (2001). Ghrelin, a novel placental-derived hormone. *Endocrinology,* Vol. 42, No.2 (February 2001), pp.788–794, ISSN 0013-7227

Havel, PJ. Kasim-Karakas, S., Mueller, W., Johnson, PR., Gingerich, RL. & Stern, JS. (1996). Relationship of plasma leptin to plasma insulin and adiposity in normal weight and overweight women: effects of dietary fat content and sustained weight loss. *The Journal of Clinical Endocrinology & Metabolism,* Vol.81, No.12, (December 1996), pp. 4406-4413, ISSN0021-972X

Hill, MJ., Uyehara, CF,, Hashiro, GM. & Frattarelli, JL. (2007). The utility of serum leptin and follicular fluid leptin, estradiol, and progesterone levels during an in vitro fertilization cycle. *Journal of assisted reproduction and genetics,* Vol.24, No.5, (May 2007), pp.183-188, ISSN 1058-0468

Kawamura, K., Sato, N., Fukuda, J., Kodama, H., Kumagai, J., Tanikawa, H., Murata, M., & Tanaka, T. (2003). The role of leptin during the development of mouse preimplantation embryos. *Molecular and cellular endocrinology,* Vol.28, No.202, (April 2003), pp.185-189, ISSN0303-7207

Knerr, I., Herzog, D., Rauh, M., Rascher, W. & Horbach, T. (2006). Leptin and ghrelin expression in adipose tissues and serum levels in gastric banding patients. *European Journal of Clinical Investigation,* Vol.36, No.6, (June 2006), pp. 389-394, ISSN0014-2972

Kojima, M., Hosada, Y., Date, M., Nakazato, H., Matsuo, H. & Kangawa, K. (1999). Ghrelin a growth hormone releasing acylated peptide from stomach. *Nature,* Vol.402, No.6762, (December 1999), pp. 656-660, ISSN 0028-0836

Löffler, S., Aust, G., Köhler, U. & Spanel-Borowski, K. (2001). Evidence of leptin expression in normal and polycystic human ovaries. *Molecular human reproduction,* Vol.7, No.12, (December 2001), pp. 1143-1149, ISSN 1360-9947

Maillard, V., Froment, P., Ramé, C., Uzbekova, S., Elis, S. & Dupont J. (2011). Expression and effect of resistin on bovine and rat granulosa cell steroidogenesis and proliferation. *Reproduction,* Vol.141, No.4, (April 2011), pp. 467-749, ISSN 470-1626

Mantzoros, C., Flier, JS., Lesem, MD. & Brewerton, TD. (1997). Jimerson DC Cerebrospinal fluid leptin in anorexia nervosa: correlation with nutritional status and potential role in resistance to weight gain. *The Journal of clinical endocrinology and metabolism,* Vol.82, No.6, (June 1997), pp. 1845-1851, ISSN0021-972X

Matarese, G., Alviggi, C., Sanna, V., Howard, JK., Lord, GM., Carravetta, C., Fontana, S., Lechler, RI., Bloom, SR., & De Placido, G. (2000). Increased leptin levels in serum and peritoneal fluid of patients with pelvic endometriosis. The Journal of clinical endocrinology and metabolism, Vol.85, No.7, (July 2000), pp.2483-2487, ISSN0021-972X

Morash, BA., Ur, E., Wiesner, G., Roy, J. & Willkinson M. (2004). Pituitary resistin gene expression: effects of age, gender and obesity. *Neuroendocrinology,* Vol.79, No.3, (March 2004), pp.149–156, ISSN 0028-3835

Morash, BA., Willkinson, D., Ur, E. & Willkinson M. (2002). Resistin expression and regulation in mouse pituitary. FEBS Letters, Vol.526, No.1-3 (August 2002), pp.26–30, ISSN 0014-5793

Munir, I., Yen, HW., Baruth, T., Tarkowski, R., Azziz, R., Magoffin, DA. & Jakimiuk AJ. (2005). Resistin stimulation of 17alpha-hydroxylase activity in ovarian theca cells in vitro: relevance to polycystic ovary syndrome. *The Journal of clinical endocrinology and metabolism,* Vol.90, No.8, (August 2005), pp.4852-4857, ISSN 0021-972X

Nogueiras, R., Barreiro, ML., Caminos, JE., Gaytán, F., Suominen, JS., Navarro, VM., Casanueva, FF., Aguilar, E., Toppari, J., Diéguez, C. & Tena-Sempere M. (2004). Novel expression of resistin in rat testis: functional role and regulation by nutritional status and hormonal factors. *Journal of cell science,* Vol.117, No. 2004; (July 2004), pp.3247–3257, ISSN 0021-9533

Quennell, JH., Mulligan, AC., Tups, A., Liu, X., Phipps, SJ., Kemp, CJ., Herbison, AE., Grattan, DR., & Anderson, GM. (2009). Leptin indirectly regulates gonadotropin-releasing hormone neuronal function. Endocrinology, Vol,150, No.6, (June 2009), pp.2805-2812, ISSN0013-7227

Rak, A. & Gregoraszczuk, EL. (2009). Ghrelin levels in prepubertal pig ovarian follicles. *Acta veterinaria Hungarica,* Vol. 57, No.1, (March 2009), pp. 109-113, ISSN 0236-6290

Rak, A. & Gregoraszczuk, EL. (2008). Modulatory effect of ghrelin in prepubertal porcine ovarian follicles. *Journal of Physiology and Pharmacology,* Vol.59, No.4, (December 2008), pp. 781-793, ISSN 0867-5910

Rak, A., Szczepankiewicz, D. & Gregoraszczuk, EL. (2009). Expression of ghrelin receptor, GHSR-1a, and its functional role in the porcine ovarian follicles. *Growth hormone & IGF Research,* Vol.19, No.1, (February 2009), pp. 68-76, ISSN 1096-6374

Riad-Gabriel, MG., Jinagouda, SD., Sharma, A., Boyadjian, R., & Saad, MF. (1998). Changes in plasma leptin during the menstrual cycle. *European journal of endocrinology*, Vol.139, No.5, (November 1998), pp.528-531, ISSN 0804-4643

Rigamonti, A., Pincelli, A., Corra, B., Viarengo, R., Bonomo, S., Galimberti, D., Scacchi, M., Scarpini, E., Cavagnini, F. & Muller, E. (2002). Plasma ghrelin concentrations in elderly subjects: comparison with anorexic and obese patients. *The Journal of endocrinology*, Vol.175, No.1, (October 2002), pp. 1-5, ISSN 0022-0795

Ruiz-Cortés, ZT., Martel-Kennes, Y., Gévry, NY., Downey, BR., Palin, MF. & Murphy, BD. (2003). Biphasic effects of leptin in porcine granulosa cells. *Biology of reproduction*, Vol.68, No.3, (March 2003), pp.789-796, ISSN 0006-3363

Ruiz-Cortés, ZT., Men, T., Palin, MF., Downey, BR., Lacroix, DA. & Murphy, BD. (2000). Porcine leptin receptor: molecular structure and expression in the ovary. *Molecular reproduction and development*, Vol.56, No.4, (August 2000), pp.465-474, ISSN 1040-452X

Ryan, NK., Van der Hoek, KH., Robertson, SA. & Norman, RJ. (2003). Leptin and leptin receptor expression in the rat ovary. *Endocrinology*, Vol.144, No.11, (November 2003), pp. 5006-5013, ISSN 0013-7227

Shan, G., Lipton, C., Gee, S. & Hammock, B. (2002). Immunoassay, biosensors and other nonchromatographic methods. *Handbook of Residue Analytical Methods for Agrochemicals*, Philip W. Lee, pp. 623–679, ISBN 0471 49194 2, Chichester

Sirotkin, AV. & Grossmann R. (2008). Effects of ghrelin and its analogues on chicken ovarian granulosa cells. *Domestic animal endocrinology*, Vol.34, No.2 (February 2008), pp.125-134, ISSN 0739-7240

Sirotkin, A.; Grossmann, R.; María-Peon, M.; Roa, J.; Tena-Sempere, M. & Klein, S. (2006). Novel expression and functional role of ghrelin in chicken ovary. *Molecular and cellular endocrinology*, Vol.26, No.257-258, (September 2006), pp.15-25, ISSN 0303-7207

Smolinska, N., Kaminski, T., Siawrys, G. & Przala, J. (2010). Leptin gene and protein expression in the ovary during the oestrous cycle and early pregnancy in pigs. *Reproduction in domestic animals*, Vol.45, No.5, (October 2010), pp.174-183, ISSN0936-6768

Steppan, C. & Lazar, M. (2004). The current biology of resistin. Journal of internal medicine, Vol.255, No.4, (March 2004), pp.439-447, ISSN 0954-6820

Steppan, C., Brown, E., Wright, C., Bhat, S., Banerjee, R., Dai, C., Enders, G., Silberg, D., Wen, X., Wu, G. & Lazar MA. (2001). A family of tissue-specific resistin-like molecules. *Proceedings of the National Academy of Sciences of the United States of America*, Vol.98(2), No.16, (January 2001), pp.502-506, ISSN 0027-8424

Teirmaa, T., Luukkaa, V., Rouru, J., Koulu, M. & Huupponen, R. (1998). Correlation between circulating leptin and luteinizing hormone during the menstrual cycle in normal-weight women. *European journal of endocrinology*, Vol.139, No.2, (August 1998), pp.190-194, ISSN 0804-4643

Ukkola, O. (2002). Resistin – a mediator of obesity-associated insulin resistance or an innocent bystander? *European Journal of Endocrinology*, Vol.147, No.5 (November 2002), pp.571–574, ISSN 0804-4643 van der Lely, AJ., Tschop, M., Heiman, ML. & Ghigo, E. (2004). Biological, physiological, pathophysiological, and pharmacological aspects of ghrelin. *Endocrine reviews*, Vol.25, No.3, (October 2004), pp.426–457, ISSN 0163-769X

Viani, I., Vottero, A., Tassi, F., Cremonini, G., Sartori, C., Bernasconi, S., Ferrari, B. &, Ghizzoni L. (2008). Ghrelin inhibits steroid biosynthesis by cultured granulosa-lutein cells. *The Journal of clinical endocrinology and metabolism,* Vol. 93, No.4, (April 2008), pp.1476-1481, ISSN 0021-972X

Welt, C.K., Schneyer, AL., Heist, K. & Mantzoros, CS. (2003). Leptin and soluble leptin receptor in follicular fluid. *Journal of assisted reproduction and genetics*, Vol.20, No.12, (December 2003), pp. 495-501, ISSN1058-0468

Wunder, DM., Kretschmer, R. & Bersinger, NA. (2005). Concentrations of leptin and C-reactive protein in serum and follicular fluid during assisted reproductive cycles. *Human reproduction*, Vol.20, No.5, (May 2005), pp.1266-1271, ISSN 0268-1161

Yamada, M., Irahara, M., Tezuka, M., Murakami, T., Shima, K. & Aono, T. (2000). Serum leptin profiles in the normal menstrual cycles and gonadotropin treatment cycles. *Gynecologic and obstetric investigation,* Vol.49 No.2, pp.119-123, ISSN 0378-7346

Zhang, W.; Lei, Z., Su, J. & Chen, S. (2008). Expression of ghrelin in the porcine hypothalamo-pituitary-ovary axis during the estrous cycle. *Animal Reproductive Science*, Vol.109, No.1-4, (December 2008),pp. 356-367, ISSN 0378-4320

Zhang, Y., Proenca, R., Maffei, M., Barone, M., Leopold, L. & Friedman, JM. (1994). Positional cloning of the mouse obese gene and its human homologue. *Nature,* Vol.372, No.6505, (December 1994), pp. 425-432, ISSN 0028-0836

18

Detection Curb

Hiroshi Saiki
School of Bioscience and Biotechnology, Tokyo University of Technology, Japan

1. Introduction

Immunoassay is an analytical method based on antigen-antibody reaction. The antigen-antibody reaction is specific for substrate, and provides tight bondage between them. Though the characteristics of the bondage has not been understood completely, it is considered as morphological interaction between them. It has resemblance to enzymatic reactions which has the interaction like between key and key hole. Beside the morphological interaction it include some interactions such as hydrophilic and hydrophobic interactions. Hydrogen bond is frequently included in the interaction. Such weak interactions are accumulated to form strong bondage. The accuracy of the method is based on the quality of the antibodies. A good antibody has a high specificity for antigen and tight bondage for antigen, resulting good sensitivities. Enzyme-Linked Immunosolvent assay (ELISA) has been developed. Because of its convenient and simple operation, it has been widely spread as commercial reagents or kits to detect chemicals of various field, pesticide, herbicide, endocrine disruptor, antibiotics, and human hormones. While ELISA is a batch system of immunoassay, flow systems have been developed such as Surface Plasmon Resonance (SPR) and Kinexa (will be mentioned in this chapter). In the flow system, the signal for immunoassay directly reflects equilibrium state between antigen and antibody. Theoretically it enables the analysis of the equilibrium between antigens and antibodies In this chapter, based on data obtained by an instrument, Kinexa 3000 from Sapidyne Instruments Inc.(Boise, ID), fundamental issues, such as shape of detection curbs, detection range, detection limit, and inherent error are theoretically mentioned.

2. Detection range and limit with monoclonal antibody

Calibration curbs for detection of analyte was provided with various concentration of antibody and antigen(analyte) where antibody-antigen reaction is at equilibrium. Usually, the concentration of analyte is decided by measuring the concentration of free-antibodies which is not bound for analyte. When total concentration of antibody is known and free-antibody concentration is decided, the analyte binding antibody concentration can be decided. The free analyte concentration can be decided with the concentration of free-antibody, the concentration of analyte binding antibody, and dissociation constant (Kd). Then, the total analyte concentration is decided as sum of free and antibody-bound analyte. A calibration curb provide the relationship between free antibody concentration and total analyte concentration.

Calibration curbs are usually demonstrated on semi log graph. X axe is percentage of free antibody concentration for total antibody concentration, Y axe is logarithmic scale of total antigen concentration. In immunoassay, calibration curbs are available for the 10^{2-3} order of analyte concentration. Then, the logarithmic scale is used. With the curb, total analyte concentration is easily decided from the ratio of free-antibody concentration by total antibody concentration.

2.1 Detection range

The model calibration curb are demonstrated in Figure 1, where antibody is monoclonal one, its concentration is 1 Mol, and antibody has dissociation constant, Kd value of 2M. The curb is drawn with various analyte concentrations. The calculation was carried out under the assumption that an antibody has only one site for binding antigen, though actual antibody has two. Then, free antibody concentration is given for total antigen. The ideal calibration curb shows a sigmoid curb as shown in Fig.1, The steep part of the sigmoid is the detection range, since the other part gave more errors for detection of the concentration.

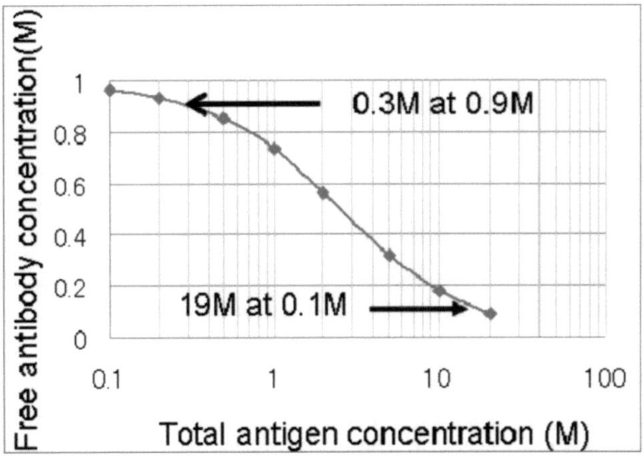

Fig. 1. A model detection curb with a model antibody. The antibody is monoclonal one, and its concentration is 1M. The dissociation constant of the antibody is 2M.

If detection range is assumed by the range from 0.1M(10%) to 0.9M(90%) of free-antibody concentration, the detection concentration will be from 0.3 to 19 Mol. This range shows that the detection range will be about 10^2 in the model detection curb. If we want to make a calibration curb with more high concentration of analyte, more concentration of antibody is required. When a half of antibody reacts with antigen, the point of half antibody reaction is the center of detection curb. The antibody concentration affects the detection range of the curb. The comparable amount of antibody is used to detect the high concentration of analyte. The detection curbs with high concentration of the antibody are summarized in Fig.2 where X axe is normalized as percentage to compare the detection curbs of various concentration of antibody each other. With the high concentration of antibodies, the detection curbs become steep, For 100 M antibody concentration, detection rage is from 10 to 95 M, this range is within 10 times. When compared with 1M detection curb, 100 M detection curb is almost one tenth of detection range.

The detection range can be calculated from equation (1)., (2), and (3). Dissociation constant is expressed by the equilibrium state between free antibody concentration, free antigen concentration, and complex concentration of antibody and antigen.

$$Kd = [Ab] \times [Ag] / [AbAg] \tag{1}$$

$$[Ab_0] = [Ab] + [AbAg] \tag{2}$$

$$[Ag_0] = [Ag] + [AbAg] \tag{3}$$

[Ab]: free antibody concentration, [Ag]: free antigen concentration, [AbAg]: complex between antigen and antibody, $[Ab_0]$: total concentration of antibody, $[Ag_0]$: total concentration of antigen.

When free antibody is 10% of total antibody, complex formation is 90% from equation 2. In this condition, equation 1 can be written as follow.

$$Kd = 10 \times [Ag]/90 = 1/9 \times [Ag] \tag{4}$$

Then, the [Ag] and $[Ag_0]$ can be presented for 10% antibody complex formation as follow

$$[Ag] = 9Kd \tag{5}$$

$$[Ag_0] = 9Kd + [AbAg] \tag{6}$$

The [AbAg] is 90% of total antibody, then the analyte concentration(total antigen concentration) can be expressed as the function of total antibody concentration, Ab_0,

$$[Ag_0] = 9Kd + 0.9[Ab_0] \tag{7}$$

For the condition 90% free antibody and 10% complex formation. Similar calculation give equation 8.

$$[Ag_0] = 1/9Kd + 0.1[Ab_0] \tag{8}$$

From equation 7 and 8, the detection range is defined for the assumption of the range from 90% free antibody to 10% free antibody. If we use a low concentration of antibody, term $[Ab_0]$ will be negligible, the detection range will be from 1/9Kd to 9 Kd. The width is 81, ca. 10^2 order. On the other hand, when we use a high concentration of antibody, Kd value will be negligible. Then, the detection range will be from $0.1[Ab_0]$ to $0.9\ [Ab_0]$. This width is 9, and steeper curb than the low concentration antibody.

2.2 Detection limit

As shown in Fig.2, for the high concentration of antigen, we can provide the detection curbs with high concentration of antibodies. On the other hand for the low concentration of antigen, we can observe that the detection curbs are superimposed at antibody concentration of 0.01 and 0.1M. The detection curb would not shift to lower concentration any more. It shows that there are limits of detection value. This value is controlled by Kd values.

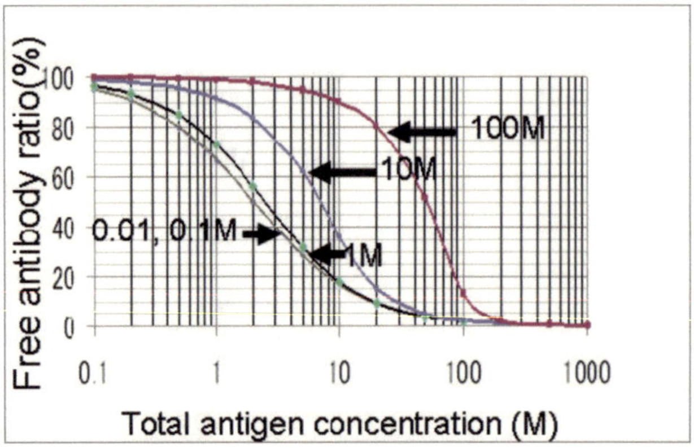

Fig. 2. Theoretical detection curbs for various antibody concentration. A model antibody has Kd values of 2M, Antibody concentration is changed from 0.01 to 100M.

If the 50% of antibody is bound to antigen, free antibody concentration is equal to Antibody-antigen complex concentration. Equation 2 can be written as follow.

$$[Ab_0] = [Ab] + [AbAg] = 2[Ab] = 2[AbAg] \tag{9}$$

Then, equation 1 becomes more simple one.

$$Kd = [Ag] \tag{10}$$

In this condition, equation 3 becomes as follow

$$[Ag_0] = [Ag] + [AbAg] = Kd + 1/2[Ab_0] \tag{11}$$

Equation 11 shows that at the center of the detection curb, where 50% of antibody is free,

analyte concentration (Ag_0) is expressed as the function of Kd values and initial antibody concentration (Ab_0). From equation 11, it is also observed that by dilution of antibody, the detection curb shift toward lower concentration of analyte. However, the detection curbs would not shift to beyond Kd value at the center of the curb. This is experimentally proved by Ohmura et al in 2001. In fig. 3, detection curb of estradiol is prepared with a estradiol antibody. The measurement was done in solution phase with KinExa 3000. The Kd value of the antibody is 28 pM. The detection curbs would not shift to lower concentration of estradiol, when the antibody is less than 10 pM (Fig. 3A, symbol of solid circle). If the center points of detection curbs (50% of free antibody) are plotted versus antibody concentration, the value of the center point approaches to Kd value (solid line in Fig.3B), by the decrease concentration of antibody (Fig.3B). This is a detection limit of immunoassay using monoclonal antibodies. If the 90% of free antibody concentration is the detection limit of immunoassay, 1/9 Kd is the limit as shown in equation 8.

3. Detection curb with multiple antibodies

In the previous paragraph, it is shown that antigen-antibody reactions are governed by affinity of antibody (Kd values). As every antibodies have their own affinities, in the mixture of multiple antibodies and antigens, it is expected that each antigen-antibody

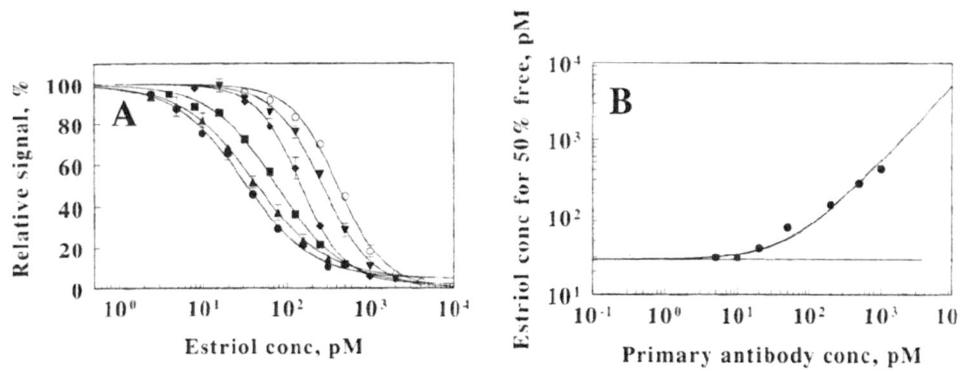

Fig. 3. Detection limit of antibody controlled by dissociation constant, Kd. A; response plotted as a function of estriol concentration. The concentration of antibody are 10(●), 20(▲), 50(■), 200(◆), 500(▼), and 1000(○) pM. B; detection limit of the assay. The y axis shows estriol concentration at 50% of free antibody, while the x axis total antibody concentration. All plots are derived from Fig.A. (cited from Analytical Chemistry vol.73, pp3392-3393,(2001))

reactions occur simultaneously. If these multiple antigen-antibody reactions are mutually independent, we can use multiple antibodies with variety in single immunoassay. It can be applied to detect multiple analyte in an immunoassay or to expand dynamic range of immunoassay, using a mixture of antibodies. In this paragraph, expansion of dynamic range is focused on.

3.1 Combination of plural antibodies

In an ideal antigen-antibody reaction, detection range is within an order of 100. If we use more than two antibodies, we can expand the detection range. The example is shown in Fig.4. Two kinds of antibodies are used to provide individual and combined detection curbs. The measurements were done in solution phase with KinExa 3000 instrument from Sapidyne Instruments Inc.(Boise, ID). A detection curb was made with an anti-estrogen antibody of 10 pM, which has a dissociation constant of 22 pM. It is expressed dashed line with symbol of ○. Another detection curb was made with the antibody of 40pM, dissociation constant of 89pM, shown with symbol △. Then, the two antibodies were mixed and detection curb was made as solid line with symbol of □. Signal % is as the same as the ratio of free antibody. When two antibodies were used independently, the half maximum signals were obtained at 55 pM and 140 pM, respectively. When, these antibodies were used together, the half signal was obtained at 115pM. This shift indicates that two antibodies to same antigen works independently, and the affinity of each antibody is reserved even in a mixture. Because of similar affinities of two antibodies, the overlap of two detection curbs result in little change in dynamic range. Then, the mixture of two antibodies which have large different affinities would give the larger dynamic range. A high affinity of antibodies would bind to low concentration of antigen, whereas a low affinity of antibodies would give a good detection curb at high concentration of antigen. In Fig. 4B, the antibody which has Kd of 3 nM, is used instead of the antibody with Kd of 89pM. It is expressed dashed line with symbol of △. This antibody is sensitive to the antigen in the range between 1nM and

1 μM, whereas the other antibody is sensitive between 10pM and 1nM. Then, the mixture of the two antibodies give the expansion of dynamic range. This detection curb is shown as a solid line with symbol of ○ (Fig. 4B). The dynamic range is the sum of two antibodies. To achieve the expansion of dynamic range, the overlap of two detection curb is necessary. If the overlap does not exist, the mixture of the antibody would not give a continuous change in the detection curb as sum of two detection curbs. Though there are no commercial kits that use more than two antibodies simultaneously, it will be possible to give the expansion of dynamic range. The combinational use of antibody can be also applied for the detection of multiple analyte., This application is not mentioned n this chapter.

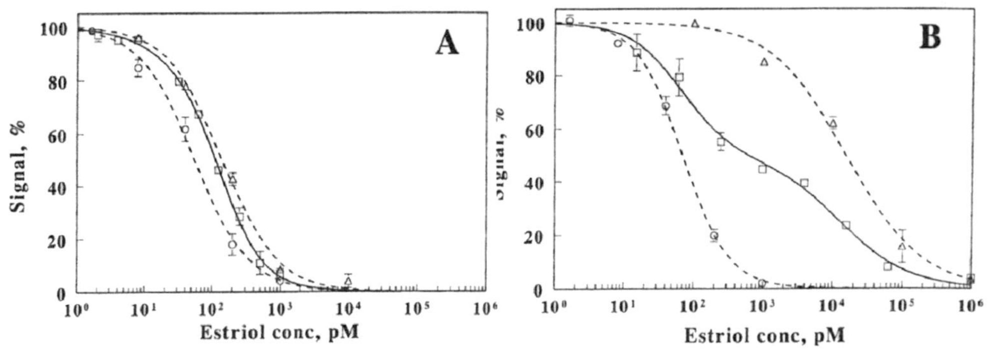

Fig. 4. Coordinative work of two antibodies, A. Two dashed lines are curb with antibody of Kd 22 pM (lefts side, ○, concentration of 10pM) and with antibody of Kd 89 pM (right side, △, concentration of 40 pM). Solid line is a detection curb made by a mixture of them. B. Dashed lines are with antibody of Kd 22 pM (lefts side, ○, concentration of 10pM) and antibody of Kd 3.1 nM (right side, △, concentration of 100 pM). Solid line is a mixture of them. (cited from Analytical Chemistry vol.75, pp104-110,(2003))

3.2 Polyclonal antibody

Polyclonal antibodies can be regarded as a mixture of huge amount of monoclonal antibodies which have different specificity and dissociation constant. If, so, the detection curb would become a straight line in a semi-log graph like a dashed line in Figure 5. This is a speculated detection curb of polyclonal antibody based on an assumption that the distribution of Kd consisted of Bolzman distribution. As shown in previous paragraph, mixing monoclonal antibodies which have different Kd's will give the extension of detection range. The shape and slope of the detection curb depends on the distribution of Kd's of polyclonal antibody. However, actual polyclonal antibodies, which we can obtain from reagent companies, gave the detection curb that was identical to those of monoclonal antibodies. As shown in Figure 5, solid line is a detection curb obtained from a polyclonal antibody. It was identical to the monoclonal antibody which has kd values of 0.1 nM. Probably, this is because of their use in a purified form. Polyclonal antibodies are usually sold after being purified by affinity column chromatography. After that process, the broad range of Kd values of polyclonal antibody may become narrower, though the distribution of kds of polyclonal antibody has not been investigated.

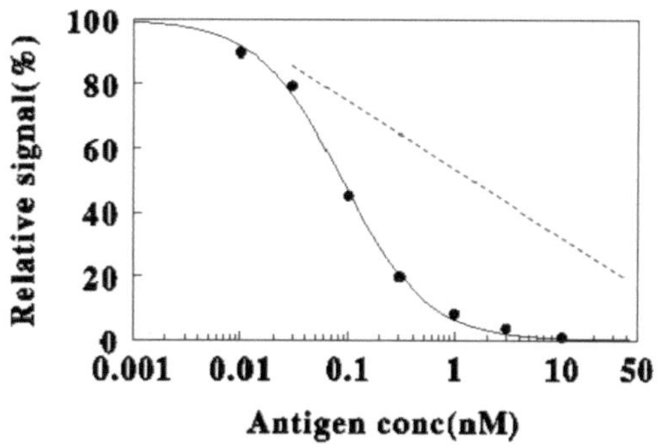

Fig. 5. Detection curb with polyclonal antibody. Dashed line; speculative detection curb under the assumption of that Kd distribution is Bolzman distribution. Solid line: Antibody is Cy5-conjugated AffiniPure Goat Anti-Mouse IgG (Jacson Immuno Research Laboratories, INC.) Code Number:115-175-008, The data was taken with Kinexa 3000 by Dr. Ohmura of Central Research Institute of Electric Power Industry.

4. Inherent error of immunoassay with antibody

For usually immunoassay, an antibody is used as detection prove. In most cases, free antibody concentration is decided by capture with an antigen which are usually fixed on a solid phase. Antibody has two binding sites. We used it under the assumption that they have equal binding affinity, and that each one site does not affect the other when binding with the antigen. Then, we use antibodies in the condition that the concentration of binding site is twice of antibody concentration.

Under these assumptions, the fraction of the binding site which binds to an antigen is demonstrated as F. F can be changed from 0 to 1. The fraction of a free binding site will be 1-F. Since the right side binding site reacts with an antigen as the left side, both site occupied antibody has the fraction of left side times right, i.e. F^2 from a mathematical independence. Therefore, all fractions will be presented both free antibody, right filled antibody, left filled antibody, and both filled antibody as $(1-F)^2$, (1-F)F, F(1-F), and F^2, respectively. The sum of all fractions will be total fraction and 1. From these values, the fraction of the antibodies which is half occupied by antigen, will be calculated by the following two equations, that should give same solution.

Both free and occupied fractions are subtracted from total fraction to give the half occupied fraction/

$$1 - (1-F)^2 - F^2 = 2F - 2F^2 \qquad (12)$$

The sum of fractions of either right or left occupied fraction is

$$F(1-F) + (1-F)F = 2F - 2F^2 \qquad (13)$$

In an immunoassay, the detection signal is directly reflected to the fraction of free antibodies, the antibodies of half binding site occupied will captured on the solid phase of the detection system by the 50% possibilities when compared with both free antibodies, to give the 50% strength of signal for detection. The ideal condition can be stated as

$$P_{c2} = 2P_{c1} \quad (14)$$

Where P_{c2} presents the probability of capture of antibodies with two binding sites, and P_{c1} the probabilities of capture of half-occupied antibodies.

The above equation shows an ideal probability. This probability, Pc2 can be calculated for divalent antibody in the other way. The probability of capture of a single binding site to the solid phase is defined as P. In this case, the probability of not capturing a site is 1-P. For a bivalent antibody where both sites are not captured, the probability of not capturing can be calculated as left side possibility times right side possibility, i.e., (1-P) x (1-P), or $(1-P)^2$. The probability of bivalent antibody capturing is expressed by subtraction of the possibility of not capturing from total probability:

$$1 - (1-P)^2 = 2P - P^2 \quad (15)$$

In the equation 15, P is regarded as probability of capturing half-occupied antibody. The probability of capturing antibody with two free sites can be written as follows.

$$P_{c2} = 2P_{c1} - (P_{c1})^2 \quad (16)$$

When compared with equation 14, equation 16 shows the difference from ideal antibody behavior. The term $(P_{c1})^2$ is inherent error on bivalent antibody. This error demonstrates that the probability of antibody is detected at lower level than an actual concentration by possibilities, $(P_{c1})^2$. The meaning of error, $(P_{c1})^2$ is the probability that both sites are captured on the solid phase. To reduce the error, it is necessary that absolute value of Pc1 is small. To reduce P_{c1}, flow detection systems are desired such as SPR and Kinexa. In the flow systems, the contact time of antibodies to the solid phase is limited to less than one second , then the probability of capturing on a solid phase will be decreased to less than 10%. For these systems, the contribution of $(P_{c1})^2$ will be less than 1%. On the other hand, in batch system such as competitive ELISA, the error is inevitable and becomes large. In this case, the detection curb will be far from ideal curb. This error is inherent to bivalent antibodies. On the other hand, monovalent receptors such as receptors of chemicals or fragment of antibody which have only one site for binding are free from the inherent errors.

5. Kinetic exclusion assay

Immunoassay is based on the equilibrium between antibody and antigen. Analyte concentration is usually determined from the concentration of free antibodies which is in equilibrium with antigen. To determine the free antibody concentration, another antigen is used, it is usually fixed on a solid phase. Free antibodies are trapped by the antigens on a solid phase, and then, the concentration of trapped antibody is determined by a secondary antibody which is labeled with dyes for spectroscopy or enzymatic reaction. In this scheme, a simple equilibrium does not exist any more, since there are two kinds of equilibrium. One is based on equilibrium between solution phase antigen and antibody. The other is based on solid phase antigen and solution phase antibody. As a result, a mixture of two kinds of reaction for the same antibody can occur. The ligand exchange can also occur. In this case, the shape and range of detection curb would not become that of an ideal curb.

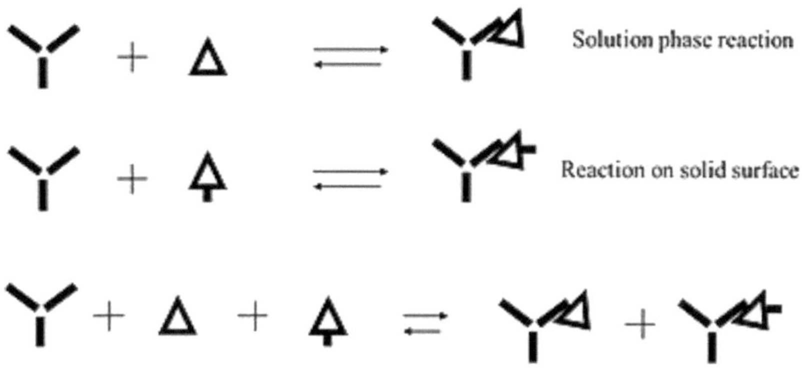

Y:antibody, Δ : antigen, Δ:antigen on solid phase

To avoid the influence of the reaction between antibody and solid phase antigen, it is necessary that flow system is adopted. In the flow system, the mixture of antigen and antibody which is in equilibrium state is drawn to the solid phase where another antigen is fixed on solid phase. The mixture will be exposed on the solid phase antigen in very limited time, so that the influence of the reaction between antibody and solid phase antigen is limited on the solution phase antigen-antibody reaction. Steve, inventor of machine, KinExa, named it Kinetic Exclusion Assay. In the flow system, influence of the reaction between antibody and solid phase antigen would be kinetically exclusive. Then, the equilibrium of original antibody-antigen reaction would be kept.

One of the flow systems is KinExa series (Sapidyne Instruments Inc., ID). The schematic diagram is shown in Fig. 6. The system consists of a capillary flow cell fitted with a microporous screen, which is integrated into an epi-illumination filter fluorometer system and through which flowed selected solutions under negative pressure created by a syringe pump. The beads were packed into the flow cell by drawing a beads' suspension through the cell, washing it by phosphate buffer solution(PBS, pH7) , and allowing it to settle for 15 seconds, thus creating a uniform bed. On a bead, antigens were immobilized to capture antibodies which were present in equilibrated mixtures of antibody, antigen, and antibody-antigen complexes. The mixture was drawn though the beads to accumulate unbound antibody. Excess antibody, antigen, and antibody-antigen complexes were washed out of the flow cell by drawing PBS though the cell. After the wash, Cy5-conjugated secondary antibody solution was drawn though the beads pack to label the captured primary antibody. Unbound secondary antibody was removed by washing the pack with PBS. All steps, including beads preparation, were accomplished though the combined function of a variety of pumps and valves within a computer controlled system. Throughout the experiments, fluorescence was sampled at a rate of one measurement per second, and the data were stored as voltages on a computer.

Typical fluorescence signals, along with schematic diagrams of the binding events occurring during each assay step, are illustrated in Figure 7. In the first step, the binding mixture was drawn through the beads pack, capturing unbound antibody, and then excess primary antibody and antigen were removed by a buffer wash. The fluorescence signal recorded during this period provided the base line fluorescence response of the beads pack prior to the addition of fluorescent tracer. In the second step, the steepest portion of fluorescence trace was elicited when Cy5-conjugated secondary antibody was drawn into the flow cell. This signal reflects the presence of both unbound secondary antibody filling the interstitial regions

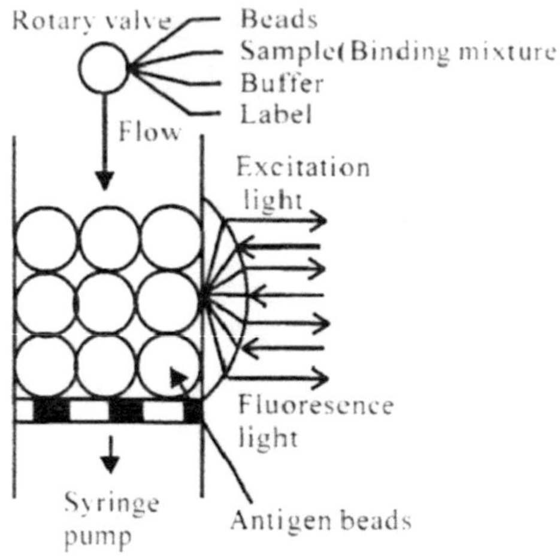

Fig. 6. Schematic diagram of an automatied immunoassay instrument. The system consist of capillary flow cell fitted with a micro porous screen, where micro beads are packed. Flow cell is illuminated by excitation light. Fluorescence light is used to detect free antibody which is tapped on a beads surface and labeled by secondary sntibody. (cited from Analytical Chemistry vol.75, pp104-110,(2003))

between the beads and that bound to the primary antibody. In the third step, unbound secondary antibody was washed out of the cell with PBS, thus enabling quantification of remaining antibody bound in the beads pack. The difference in fluorescence intensity between the base line and the plateau phase was considered to present the bound signal.

With Kinexa 3000, the kinetically exclusive assay was investigated. effects of reaction of solid phase were investigated on the equilibrium between antigen and antibody. For the theoretical detection curb, binding of the free antibody to the immobilized ligand does not lead to a shift in the equilibrium between the antibody and antigen during the detection, and the binding of the immobilized antigen and soluble one should be mutually exclusive. The beads pack provided high ligand capacity, which lead to that the same percentage of antibody is captured on the ligand of the beads regardless of absolute concentration of free antibody. As shown in Fig7, when antibody concentration became higher, the captured amount of antibody became larger. However, the percentage of the antibody captured remained constant. The average amount of the captured was 1.4%. The binding of free antibody to the immobilized ligand during the limit contact was a pseudo-first-order process as a result of excess solid phase ligand. The small percentage of capturing free antibody ensured that the perturbation of capturing the free antibody on the equilibrium between antibody and antigen would be negligible. The equilibrium dissociation constant(Kd) is expressed as dissociation rate constant by association rate constant. If dissociation constant (Kd) is 10^6, it means that the dissociation rate is 10^6 times slower than the association rate. The small percentage of capturing free antibody also indicates that any shift based on the very slow dissociation of antigen-antibody complex would not occur in the equilibrium in a brief contact time, the contact time was 480 ms for the lowest flow rate with KinExa 3000. This brief contact time and kinetic slower rate also inhibits competition reactions. This measurement method provided that the perturbation reactions are kinetically exclusive, and that immunoassay based on theoretical equilibrium can be carried out.

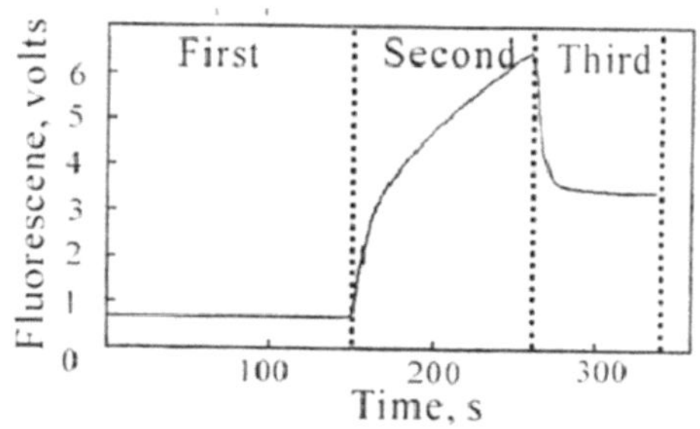

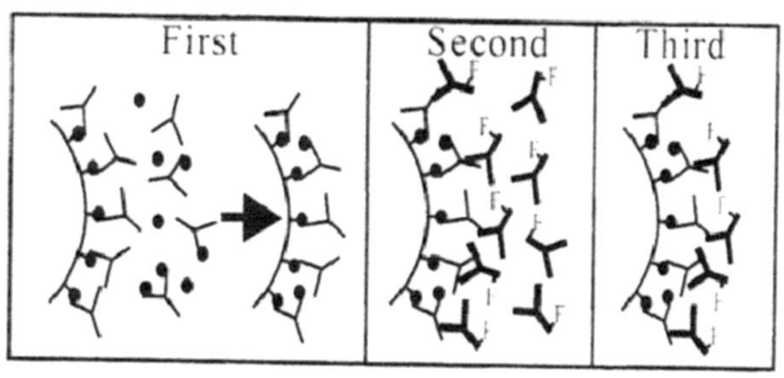

Fig. 7. signal transformation in immunoassay. Upper: change of fluorescence intensity during the three assay steps; step1, an equilibrated mixture of antigen and primary antibody is drawn through the beads pack, followed by buffer wash; step2, Cy5-labelled secondary antibody fills the beads pack and binds to the primary antibody bounds to the beads; step3, excess secondary antibody is removed by buffer wash, and remaining fluorescence intensity is recorded as the response signal. Lower: schematic images depicting events at each step. (cited from Analytical Chemistry vol.75, pp104-110,(2003))

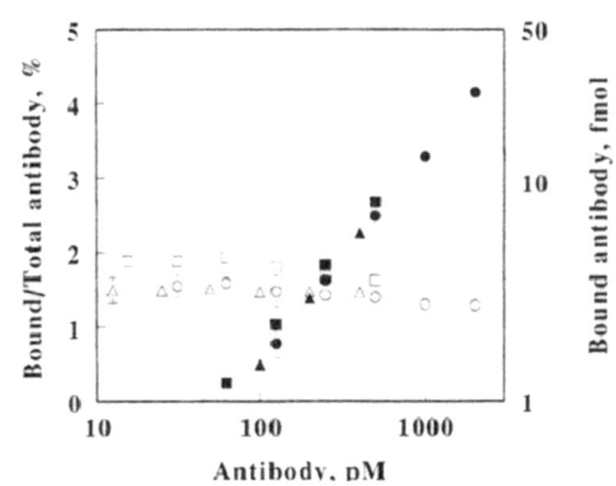

Fig. 8. small ratio of captured free antibodies. Cy5-labelled anti-estriol antibodies (1ml, each) at various concentrations were drawn through the flow cell containing beads coated with BSA-conjugated estriol at 0.25mL/min. Closed and open symbols were shown as a portion of the bound antibody in the entire beads pack and the percentage of antibody bound, respectively. Two different Cy5-labelled antibodies were used. They were shown as triangle and square. (cited from Analytical Chemistry vol.75, pp104-110,(2003))

6. Summary

In this chapter, an ideal detection curb was mentioned. The ideal curb was identical to the curb based on the equilibrium between antibody and antigen. From a view point of analysis, ideal detection curb is not always necessary. For instance, ELISA system always provide the detection curbs which is far from ideal one. Though the detection curb is far from ideal one, the curbs is practically usefull for an analysis and the reproductivities of the analytical data are always obtained. The system fulfilled the elemental requirements of chemical analysis. The ideal curb is especially important for kinetic analysis of antigen-antibody reaction, or determination of dissociation constants. For immunoassay, ideal detection curb is desirable for the accurate detection and for the detection low antibody levels. On the other hand, when unexpected side reaction such as matrix effects or cross reaction is involved in an immunoassay, it will appear as the change of shape with the detection curb from the ideal curb. Ideal detection curbs are important not only for theoretical analysis of antibody-antigen equilibrium, but also for accurate detection of analyte in an immunoassay.

7. Acknowledgement

This chapter is based on results of cooperative research with Dr. Naoya Ohmura of Central Research Institute of Electric Power Industry, Steve J. Lackie of Sapidyne Instrument co, and Tohomas R. Glass of Sapidyne Instrument co.. The author appreciates their co-operation, efforts and passion.

8. References

[1] George Pinchuk, Antibodies and antigens, Immunology, McGraw-Hills New York, 2003

[2] Conners, K.A. Binding constant: The measurments of molecular complex stability, Willey: New York, 1987

[3] Naoya Ohmura, Steve J. Lackie, and Hiroshi Saiki, Analytical Chemistry, 73(14), 3392-3399(2001)

[4] Naoya Ohmura, Yukiko Tsukidate, Hiraku Shinozaki, Steve J. Lackie, and Hiroshi Saiki, Analytical Chemistry, 75(1), 104-110(2003)

[5] Thomas R. Glass, Naoya Ohmura, Keiichi Morita, Kazuhiro Sasaki, Hiroshi Saiki, Yoko Takagi, Chiwa Kataoka, and Akikazu Ando, Analytical Chemistry, 78(20), 7240-7247(2006)

19

Carbon Nanoparticles as Detection Label for Diagnostic Antibody Microarrays

Aart van Amerongen[1,2,*], Geert A.J. Besselink[3], Martina Blazkova[4], Geertruida A. Posthuma-Trumpie[1], Marjo Koets[1] and Brigit Beelen-Thomissen[1]

[1]*Wageningen University and Research Centre, Food and Biobased Research – Biomolecular Sensing and Diagnostics,*
[2]*Laboratory of Organic Chemistry, Wageningen University,*
[3]*MESA+ Institute for Nanotechnology, University of Twente,*
[4]*Institute of Chemical Technology, University of Prague,*
[1,2,3]*The Netherlands,*
[4]*Czech Republic*

1. Introduction

The presence of harmful pathogenic microorganisms is a growing problem in healthcare, food, feed and the environment. In addition, the increasing appearance of antibiotic resistant microorganisms adversely affects this situation. In the current standard detection methods time-consuming and expensive enrichment protocols are being used. Generally, these methods need to be performed in highly equipped laboratories by trained personnel. Often the time needed to confirm the presence of a particular pathogen using standard methods averages 2 to 7 days, which is too long to timely take actions. In human health for example this lack of speed can result in lost working hours, hospitalization or even death. The recent outbreak of food-borne *Escherichia coli* in Germany and other European countries (May 2011) has shown the dramatic consequences of pathogen contaminated food (Askar et al. 2011; Frank et al. 2011). Apart from *E. coli* there are several other pathogenic microorganisms that have to be monitored intensively in the food chain. Amongst those are *Bacillus cereus, Listeria monocytogenes and Salmonella typhimurium.* As different strains of these species may have various degrees of pathogenicity it is very informative to be able to discriminate between harmless and harmful strains. In food production good manufacturing programs were set up to ensure food safety. To comply with these safety rules it would be advantageous to have a versatile, fast, low-cost and on-site assay format available for (on-line) monitoring of food-borne pathogens with a suitable number of target organisms. In the majority of diagnostic questions this number is 5 to maximally 10.

Many efforts have been made to speed up the detection of harmful microorganisms, the focus of these developments being on faster, more sensitive and more convenient methods (Mandal et al. 2011). Especially when handling large amounts of samples it is a great asset if a detection method allows for medium- to high-throughput screening. In these cases it is also valuable if the steps from sample processing to read-out of the results have been maximally automated.

In drug discovery and life sciences research both DNA and, increasingly, protein microarrays are crucial tools (Timlin 2006), whereas the application of microarrays as diagnostics is very promising (Venkatasubbarao 2004). Pathogen detection in food by DNA microarrays has been reported by various groups (D'Agostino et al. 2004; Glynn et al. 2006; Kostrzynska & Bachand 2006; Volokhov et al. 2002). However, despite its high potential the microarray platform is still not an emerging tool in the regular diagnostic field, especially in the case of protein microarrays (Dieterle & Marrer 2008). Several reasons may be responsible for this limited presence of protein microarrays such as the lack of sufficient biological recognition elements (e.g., antibodies) and/or their sensitivity and specificity and the inferior conformational stability that some proteins may have. Many problems have still to be overcome for validated in vitro diagnostics using protein microarrays (Hartmann et al. 2009).

To increase the applicability and to reduce the costs of protein microarrays we investigated the use of carbon nanoparticles as signal labels and a conventional flatbed scanner to digitize the image. A nucleic acid detection format was used employing double-tagged amplicons that can be sandwiched between array-immobilised anti-tag antibodies and neutravidin coated carbon nanoparticles. The image was processed using image analysis software to produce the pixel grey volume of the spots generated by the label. As an alternative label to gold and latex, carbon nanoparticles have been used to develop lateral flow immunoassays (LFIA) for over 15 years (Aldus et al. 2003; Capps et al. 2004; Kalogianni et al. 2011; Koets et al. 2006; Koets et al. 2011; Lonnberg et al. 2008; Noguera et al. 2011; Posthuma-Trumpie et al. 2008; van Amerongen et al. 1993; van Amerongen & Koets 2005; van Dam et al. 2004). The possibility to use the pixel grey volume of the carbon particles in data processing following digitization by a CCD camera and image analysis was already shown in 1994 in a comparison between a simple one-step lateral flow immunoassay and a radioimmunoassay specific for the human choriogonadotropin hormone (van Amerongen et al. 1994). Excellent agreement was achieved among these two techniques with a correlation coefficient of 0.999. The use of a conventional flatbed scanner to digitize carbon lines was described (Lonnberg & Carlsson 2001), which by that time was 300 times more sensitive than the CCD camera used in 1994 (van Amerongen et al. 1994). In a recent PubMed literature survey conducted by FIND Diagnostics and published in Clinical Chemistry on the sensitivity of lateral flow immunoassays (Gordon & Michel 2008) the sensitivity of the carbon label was calculated to be in the low picomolar range for LFIAs specific for a *Schistosomiasis* carbohydrate antigen and fungal alpha-amylase, respectively, even when the assays were judged by visual inspection (Koets et al. 2006; van Dam et al. 2004). The position occupied by carbon nanoparticles in the sensitivity ranking list of nanoparticles (Gordon & Michel 2008) holds great promise for the application of these particles as signal labels in microarrays too. Recently, a review about the carbon label in diagnostics has been published (Posthuma-Trumpie et al. 2012).

In this chapter we describe the multi-analyte detection of amplified DNA using an antibody microarray. The nucleic acid detection is based on the use of tagged primers in a PCR resulting in double-tagged amplicons that can be sandwiched between immobilised anti-tag antibodies and neutravidin. Reverse primers were tagged by using biotin and forward primers by discriminating tags such as digoxigenin (DIG), dinitrophenol (DNP), fluorescein (FL), and Texas Red (TxR). In this one-step format, the labelled amplicons were mixed with the conjugate of neutravidin and carbon nanoparticles in incubation buffer, immediately applied and detected after one to several hours. Such mixed immuno-DNA formats have been used in lateral flow and microfluidic detection assays (Baeumner 2004; Blazkova et al. 2009; Blazkova et al. 2011; Corstjens et al. 2001; Koets et al. 2009; Kozwich et al. 2000; Mens et al. 2008; Noguera et al. 2011; van Amerongen & Koets 2005; Wang et al. 2006). To get proof of concept for the use of carbon nanoparticles as signal labels in antibody microarrays we studied two applications in which the antigens consisted of double-tagged DNA amplicons: the detection of *L. monocytogenes* and the detection of three antibiotic resistance genes from *Salmonella* spp. (D'Agostino et al. 2004; van Hoek et al. 2005).

2. Materials and methods

2.1 Chemicals

NeutrAvidin Biotin-Binding Protein (neutravidin) and biotin-labelled bovine serum albumin were from Pierce Biotechnology (Perbio Science Nederland BV, Etten-Leur, The Netherlands); anti-digoxigenin antibody (α-DIG) and $MgCl_2$ were from Roche (Almere, The Netherlands); anti-texas red antibody (α-TxR) and goat anti-human immunoglobulin G (α-hIgG) were from Molecular Probes (Paisly, UK); anti-fluorescein antibody (α-FL) was obtained from Biomeda (Foster City, California, USA) and anti-dinitrophenol antibody (α-DNP) was from USBiological (Swampscott, USA). Human IgG, mouse IgG, Bovine serum albumin (BSA), essentially IgG free, and fluorescein isothiocyanate were from Sigma (Sigma-Aldrich Chemie B.V., Zwijndrecht, The Netherlands). Primers were from Eurogentec (Eurogentec Nederland bv, Maastricht, The Netherlands); dNTPs were from Pharmacia Biotech (GE Healthcare Europe GMBH, Branch office Benelux, Diegem, Belgium). Other chemicals were of the highest purity available and purchased from Merck (Amsterdam, The Netherlands).

2.2 Polymerase Chain Reaction

All PCRs were performed in the GeneAmp 9700 96 well thermal cycler (Applied Biosystems, Foster City, CA, USA). The resulting PCR products were analysed with an Agilent 2100 Bioanalyzer (Agilent Technologies, Santa Clara, CA, USA) using the DNA 1000 kit.

Bacillus cereus: A set of primers was used to amplify part of the *gyrB*1 gene sequence. The reverse primer was 5′-tagged with DIG and the forward primer with biotin. Primer sequences are shown in Table 1. The reaction mixture consisted of 1 μL *B. cereus* genomic DNA, 25 μL redTaq mastermix (Sigma), 10 pmol Rprimer, 10 pmol Fprimer, in a final reaction volume of 50 μL. The amplification reaction consisted of an initial denaturation step of 5 min at 94 °C, and 30 cycles of each 30 s 94 °C, 30 s 55 °C and 1 min 72 °C, followed by the final polymerisation at 74 °C for 5 min. In Fig. 1 a scheme of the technique is depicted.

Listeria spp.: A set of primers specific for *L. monocytogenes* was used to amplify a part (274 bp) of the *prfA* gene encoding the central virulence gene regulator as described (Blazkova et al. 2009). One of these primers was 5′-tagged with DIG and the other with biotin. To detect all *Listeria* species, a generic primer set for amplification of *Listeria* spp. has been selected (Herman et al. 1995), this primer set has been labelled with fluorescein/biotin.

Primer	Sequences	Tag	Specificity	Ref.
gyrB Bc1	5′-ATTGGTGACACCGATCAAACA-3′	Biotin	*B. cereus*	(Chen & Tsen 2002)
gyrB Bc2r	5′-TCATACGTATGGATGTTATTC-3′	DIG	*B. cereus*	(Chen & Tsen 2002)
prfA LIP1	5′-GAT ACA GAA ACA TCG GTT GGC-3′	Biotin	*L. monocytogenes*	(D'Agostino et al. 2004)
prfA LIP2	5′-GTG TAA TCT TGA TGC CAT CAG G-3′	DIG	*L. monocytogenes*	(D'Agostino et al. 2004)
16S rRNA C	5′-AGG TTG ACC CTA CCG ACTTC-3′	Biotin	*Listeria* spp.	(Herman et al. 1995)
16S rRNA D	5′-CAA GGA TAA GAG TAA CTG C-3′	FL	*Listeria* spp.	(Herman et al. 1995)
tet(G)-F	5′-AAA GCC GGT TCG CAT CAA AC-3′	DNP	tetracycline resistance gene	Van Hoek, pers. comm.
tet(G)-R	5′-GGA AGA TCG CAT GTG TTG CC-3′	Biotin	tetracycline resistance gene	Van Hoek, pers. comm.
*aad*A2-F	5′-GCA GCG CAA TGA CAT TCT TG-3′	TxR	streptomycin resistance gene	(van Hoek et al. 2005)
*aad*A2-R	5′-CAT CCT TCG GCG CGA TTT TG-3′	Biotin	streptomycin resistance gene	(van Hoek et al. 2005)
bla$_{PSE-1}$-F	5′-CGC TAT CTG AAA TGA ACC AG-3′	DIG	β-lactam resistance gene	(van Hoek et al. 2005)
bla$_{PSE-1}$-R	5′-TTT CGC TCT GCC ATT GAA GC-3′	Biotin	β -lactam resistance gene	(van Hoek et al. 2005)

Table 1. Primer sequences used to amplify target microorganisms

S. typhimurium antibiotic resistance genes: The three resistance gene specific forward primers were 5'-tagged with a distinguishing tag: tetracycline with a DNP-tag, streptomycin with a TxR-tag and β-lactam with a DIG-tag. The reverse primers were labelled with a common biotin tag (Table 1). The amplification was performed using the Accu Prime PCR reaction kit (Invitrogen, Breda, The Netherlands). The reaction mixture consisted of 5 µL 10x Accu Prime PCR buffer II, 10 pmol primer for the single analyte assay, 20 pmol primers for the multiplexed assay, 2.5 U Accu Prime Taq polymerase, 40 ng genomic DNA in a final volume of 50 µL. Amplification was performed as follows: 30 s at 94 °C, 30 cycles of 30 s at 94 °C, 30 s at 55.8 °C and 1 min at 68 °C. After 30 cycles, the mixture was kept at 72 °C for 7 min.

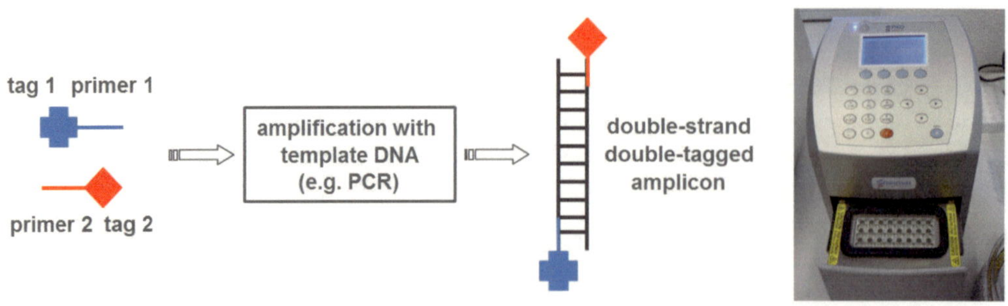

Fig. 1. Scheme of the amplification technique incorporating tags during amplification and a photograph of a low-cost and fast thermocycler to perform the amplification.

Primer sequences are shown in Table 1. The reaction mixture consisted of 2.5 mM $MgCl_2$, 0.15 mM dNTP, 0.1 μM primers LIP1 and LIP2, 0.2 μM of primers C and D, 2 U FastStart Taq DNA Polymerase (Roche, Almere, The Netherlands), 2 μL genomic DNA in a final volume of 25 μL. The amplification program consisted of an initial denaturation step at 95 °C for 4 min, 25 cycles each having a denaturation step at 94 °C for 30 s, annealing at 55 °C for 30 s and polymerisation at 74 °C for 1 min, followed by the final polymerisation at 74 °C for 5 min.

2.3 Preparation of carbon nanoparticles – NeutrAvidin conjugate

Neutravidin was conjugated to colloidal nanoparticles as described in several patents by van Doorn et al. (van Doorn et al. 1987, 1996, 1997). Briefly, a colloidal carbon suspension (Spezial Schwartz 4, Evonik Degussa Industries AG, Essen Germany) was prepared as a stock at 1% (w/v) in demineralised water. The suspension was sonicated for 5-10 min on ice using a Branson model 250 sonifier (output control 3~27 W, 20 KHz). This carbon suspension was diluted five times with 5 mM borate buffer pH 8.8 to give a carbon concentration of 0.2% (w/v), and sonicated for a second time as above. Neutravidin dissolved in 5 mM borate buffer pH 8.8 was added to the diluted colloidal carbon suspension at a concentration of 350 μg of protein per mL of suspension. The pH was readjusted to pH 8.8 and the mixture was incubated overnight by end-over-end mixing at 4 °C. Neutravidin-carbon conjugate was washed two times in a 5 mM borate buffer, pH 8.8, containing 1% (w/v) BSA, and re-suspended and stored in a 100 mM borate buffer, pH 8.8, containing 1% (w/v) BSA, 0.02% (w/v) NaN_3 as a 0.2% (w/v) carbon suspension.

2.4 Preparation of microarrays

Antibodies and other proteins were spotted on microscope glass slides by means of a TopSpot device (BioFluidix GmbH, Freiburg, Germany) (de Heij et al. 2004), which is a non-contact printing method. A 24-channel print head was employed for delivering ≈1 nL droplets onto a substrate from which immobilisation of anti-tag antibody and other proteins was allowed to take place (Fig. 2). This resulted in an array of 4×6 protein spots with a pitch of 500 μm. Spot diameters are variable and depend on the type of protein, type of substrate, and printing buffer composition and viscosity. In between printing runs the print head was cleaned by ultrasonic treatment for 10 minutes in a 0.12 M NaOH/1% (v/v) Triton X-100 cleaning solution.

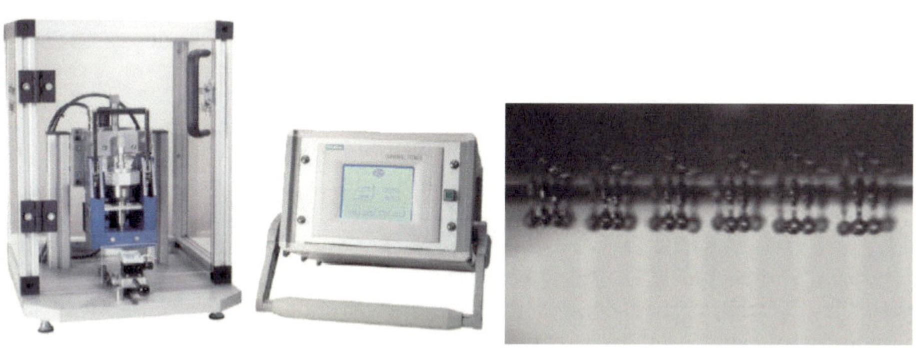

Fig. 2. The Topspot/E (left) and the formation of droplets from the print head (right).

Three different, commercially obtained, types of glass substrates were used. Antibody arrays of α-DIG, α-FL, α-TxR, and α-DNP were prepared on these very types of substrate as follows:

1. UltraStick slides (Ted Pella Inc., Redding, CA, USA): 3-aminopropyl-triethoxysilane (APTES)-modified glass consisting of a monolayer functionalized with primary amino groups useful for adsorption of proteins. Printing was performed using different concentrations of human IgG, anti-DIG antibody and FL-labelled mouse IgG in PBS. Immediately after arraying, the slides were placed in a humidity chamber and incubated at room temperature for 30 min in order to allow protein adsorption to proceed. Care was taken to prevent any drying of the spotted droplets. After incubation, the slides were flushed extensively with washing solution (10% (w/v) BSA in Phosphate Buffered Saline (PBS)) and arrays were kept covered with fresh washing solution for 10 minutes. Usage of this high protein containing washing solution is essential in order to prevent the smearing of the surplus IgG that had not adsorbed in the first step. Slides containing human IgG spots were incubated with FL-labelled anti-human IgG. Finally, the slides were rinsed quickly with PBS and MilliQ before being dried under a gentle stream of nitrogen gas.
   After completion of the procedure, the arrays containing the FL-labelled IgGs were observed by fluorescence microscopy employing an inverted Olympus IX51 microscope equipped with a mercury arc in combination with an Olympus U-MWB2 filter. Images were taken with a digital ColorViewII CCD camera (Soft Imaging Systems, Münster, Germany).
2. SL HCX slides (XanTec bioanalytics GmbH, Düsseldorf, Germany): contain an attached layer of N-hydroxysuccinimide-activated carboxylated hydrogel (<5 μm thick), attached to borosilicate glass, that can be used for covalent coupling of proteins. Printing was done with different concentrations of anti-DIG and anti-FL antibody in PBS. Directly after printing the array was incubated for 4 h in a humidity chamber at room temperature. After immobilization, any residual activated groups on the slide surface were quenched by reaction for 10 min with ethanolamine (1 M, pH 8.0) at room temperature. After quenching, the slides were rinsed quickly with MilliQ and, finally, the slides were dried by applying a gentle stream of nitrogen gas.
3. FAST™ 16 slides (Whatman Nederland BV, 's-Hertogenbosch, The Netherlands): on a standard microscope slide are positioned two rows of eight pads (5x5 mm) of an 11 μm thick microporous (0.2 μm pore size) nitrocellulose film for irreversible adsorption of proteins. Arrays of different concentrations and combinations of anti-DIG, anti-FL, anti-TxR, and anti-DNP antibodies were spotted on FAST16 slides. Printing buffer was 5 mM borate buffer, pH 8.8. Immediately after printing the slides were put in an incubator at 37 °C for 3 hours. No blocking step was used.

2.5 Amplicon detection assay

Incubations were performed in a dedicated slide holder with varying amounts (0.5-2 μL) (0.2% w/v) of colloidal carbon nanoparticles with immobilised neutravidin (Fig. 3a) and varying amounts (25, 50 or 75 μL) of incubation buffer (100 mM borate, 1% (w/v) BSA, 0.05% (v/v) Tween20, 0.02% (w/v) NaN_3, pH 8.8). Following the incubation, positive spots could be easily detected (Fig. 3b) when amplicons were sandwiched between anti-tag antibodies and (black) carbon-neutravidin particles as shown Fig. 3b,c. Control spots (no antibody printed) were used as negative controls. Arrays were recorded by conventional flatbed scanning using an Epson 3200 Photo scanner (Seiko Epson, Nagano, Japan). The

Pixel Grey Volume of positive spots were obtained using image analysis software (TotalLab, Nonlinear Dynamics, Newcastle upon Tyne, UK). Microsoft Excel and SigmaPlot 11 (Systat Software, Inc., San Jose, CA, USA) were used for subsequent data analysis and visualisation of the results.

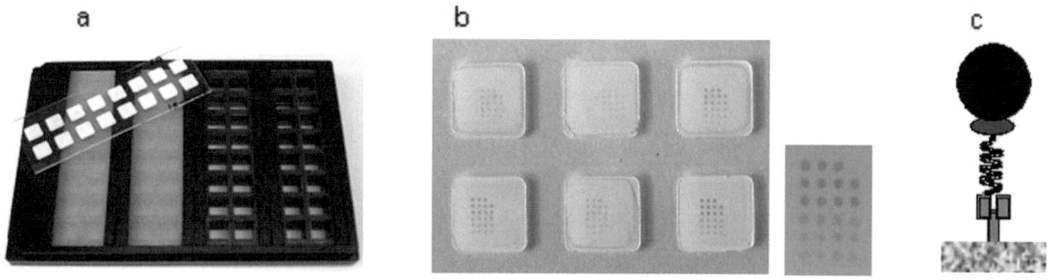

Fig. 3. Overview of antibody microarray tools and the test layout: a) holder for 4 slides with incubation chamber set-up (16 per slide); b) example of six membranes with 24 spot arrays; c) drawing of part of the nitrocellulose membrane with anti-tag antibody, 2-tagged amplicon and neutravidin-coated carbon nanoparticle (not to scale).

3. Results and discussion

3.1 Antibody microarray printing and quality

One of the advantages of non-contact as compared to contact (pin based and other) printing methods is the inherently lower risk of damaging the substrate surface, which is especially relevant in the case of more fragile structures. This added property is expected to benefit the quality, functionality and reproducibility of the fabricated microarrays.

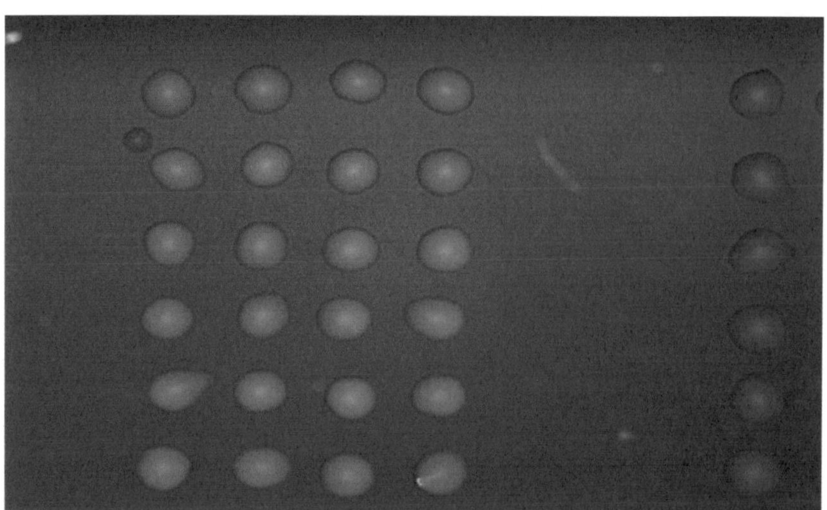

Fig. 4. Droplet microarray obtained after printing of 40% (v/v) glycerol/water onto bare unmodified glass as observed by light microscopy.

Unmodified, clean glass has a very hydrophilic nature leading to a tendency for droplets to spread out on the surface and, as a result, to touch each other and to coalesce. This can be overcome by using higher viscosity printing media, for example, 40% (v/v) glycerol in water. Printing of this solution onto bare glass delivers a nice regular droplet array as shown by the light microscopic image of Fig. 4.

UltraStick slides, on the other hand, are useful substrates for printing of low viscosity solutions, even pure water, with no drop coalescence occurring and thereby yielding a proper array structure. The same is valid, to some lesser degree, for the SL HCX slides.

Interestingly, IgG, BSA and other proteins (e.g., fosforylase B, cytochrome C, streptavidin and neutravidin) tend to adsorb spontaneously onto the UltraStick slide surface. This adsorption is rather strong stemming from the observation that ultrasonic treatment (for 20 min) and long soaking (for up to 2 days) in detergent solution (5% Tween-20 in PBS) did not lead to a significant extent of protein desorption.

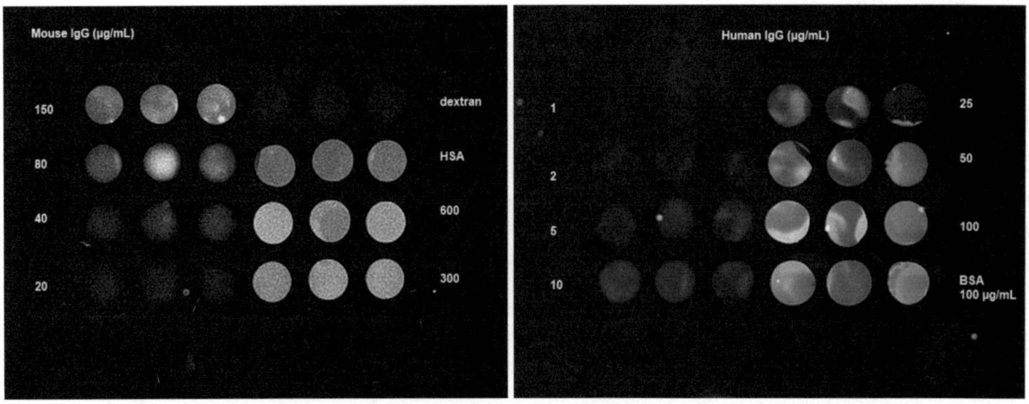

Fig. 5. Fluorescence micrographs of antibody microarrays obtained after printing (in triplicate) of different antibody concentrations on UltraStick slides. Left panel: fluorescein-labelled Mouse IgG; Right panel: array obtained after printing with human IgG and consecutive incubation of the printed array with fluorescein-labelled goat anti-human IgG. Fluorescein-labelled HSA, BSA and dextran were used as references.

The fluorescence images obtained with arrays of fluorescein-labelled mouse IgG are shown in Fig. 5, left panel. Spot fluorescence intensity increased with increasing printing concentration, in the range from 20 to 300 µg/mL.

However, immobilised protein already appeared to be present after printing and incubation at much lower printing concentrations (down to 1 µg/mL). This was deduced from an amplified detection test in which mouse IgG arrays were incubated with fluorescein-labelled detecting antibody (anti-mouse IgG) (Fig. 5, right panel).

The reproducibility of printing on the UltraStick slides, as judged by fluorescence microscopy on a large number of arrays, seemed to be low. A lot of variation was seen in brightness and brightness pattern when comparing spots.

3.2 Amplicon detection assay

3.2.1 Introduction

A series of experiments was performed with *Bacillus cereus* amplicons to evaluate the signal on three types of microscope slides: UltraStick slides, SL HCX slides and nitrocellulose-coated FAST16 slides.

On nitrocellulose FAST16 slides the detection of *Listeria monocytogenes* and *Listeria* 16S rRNA amplicons was optimised for critical parameters such as stirring speed, incubation volume and time, amount of carbon suspension, amount of antibody printed and amount of PCR product added. On the same slides incubations were performed to detect several antibiotic resistance genes from *Salmonella* spp. The specific amplicons were discriminated by using various tags and the antibodies to those tags were spotted in a distinguishing pattern.

3.2.2 Choice of target substrate

A comparison was made between the final yields obtained with UltraStick slides (APTES surface), XanTec slides (pre-activated hydrogel coating) and Whatman FAST16 slides (coated with nitrocellulose). Different amounts of tagged amplicons of *B. cereus* were mixed with various volumes of 0.2% (w/v) colloidal carbon nanoparticles-neutravidin conjugate in a total volume of 70 µL and incubated at room temperature for 7.5 min to several hours. Initial results indicated that approximately 0.5 to 2 µL of PCR material, 1 µL carbon conjugate and incubation for 15 min to 1 hour is sufficient to obtain significant results by flatbed scanning and image analysis (Fig. 6). Although these results with UltraStick seemed fine in first instance, they were not very reproducible and the response faded very soon after incubation.

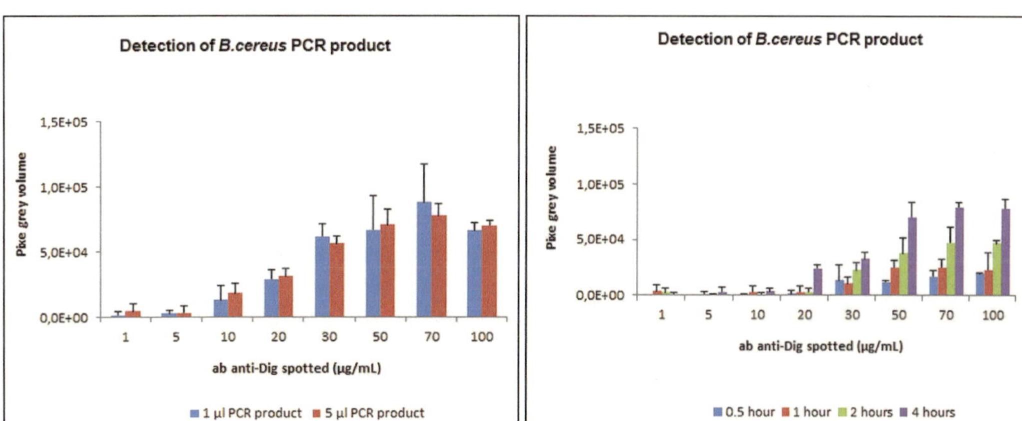

Fig. 6. Antibody microarray with serial dilutions of printed antibodies on UltraStick target. Left panel: influence of amount of amplicon added and antibody concentration, 1 µL carbon conjugate, 4 hours incubation time; Right panel influence of antibody concentration and incubation time, 1 µL of carbon conjugate and 1 µL of amplicon.

The SL HCX hydrogel slides did not deliver much signal in the amplicon detection assay even when larger printing concentrations of IgG (up to 4000 µg/mL) were applied during the preliminary step of array fabrication. Spots became increasingly visible in the concentration range of 400 up to 3000 μg/mL, but even then the response remained modest.

The results with the activated hydrogel SL HCX slides were very disappointing, since it was expected that due to its larger loading capacity and presumed lower non-specific binding, the use of such a gel layer could be advantageous compared to a planar sensor surface. Unfortunately, it was not possible to assess the level of porosity of the gel layer and, therefore, it cannot be excluded that it may have limited accessibility for carbon nanoparticles (∅ 100-200 nm). This is supported by our report of a restricted accessibility of sensor hydrogel surfaces toward latex beads (Besselink et al. 2004) that have a size comparable to that of the carbon nanoparticles used in the present study.

Results with Whatman FAST16 slides were promising (Fig. 3b). This was a little bit unexpected considering its behaviour during antibody printing. The hydrophilic coating on the FAST16 slides showed very fast absorption and migration of the liquid from spotted droplets always leading to an extensive overlap of fluid area between neighbouring spots. Nevertheless, in the end, well defined spots were obtained with the colloidal carbon/amplicon test. Apparently, adsorption of antibody (proteins) to the nitrocellulose substrate is an instantaneous process. FAST16 slides were used in all further experiments.

3.2.3 Single - analyte detection using the antibody microarray

Increasing the stirring speed from 100 to 500 min^{-1} revealed that the influence of stirring speed on the final signal is only marginal, at least for the speeds applied (Fig. 7). The stirring speed of 300 min^{-1} was used in all further experiments. It is shown here that the response is increasing with increasing antibody concentration up to a concentration of 333 μg/mL.

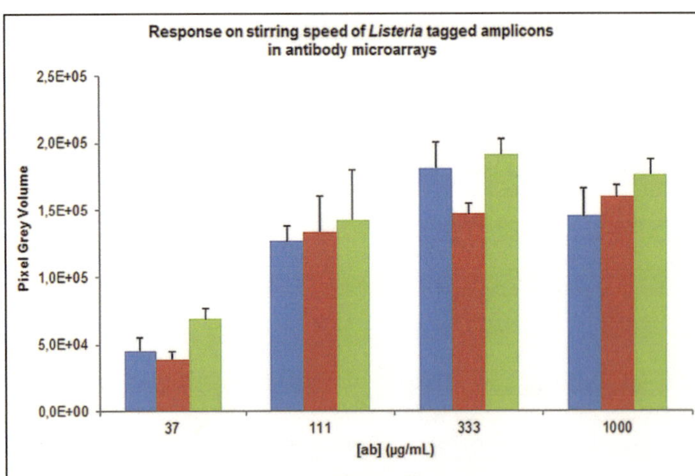

Fig. 7. Influence of stirring speed on pixel grey level, shown for different antibody concentrations, 1 μL of carbon-neutravidin conjugate, 1 μL of DIG-tagged *Listeria* amplicons, 25 μL total incubation volume and 30 min incubation time.

A series of incubation times of 7.5 to 60 min revealed that 30 min was sufficient to statistically discriminate between different spots if 1 μL of amplicon was added (Fig. 8). As measured with the Bioanalyzer this volume corresponded to 31.5 ng DNA in the *Listeria monocytogenes* amplicon solution and to 41 ng in the *Listeria* spp. amplicon solution.

In another experiment the incubation buffer amount varied from 25, 50 to 75 µL, which revealed that 25 µL is enough for a good and reproducible response, although 75 µL is advised by the supplier and, indeed, more convenient. In addition, nitrocellulose pads were better wetted with 75 µL as compared to 25 µL total volume.

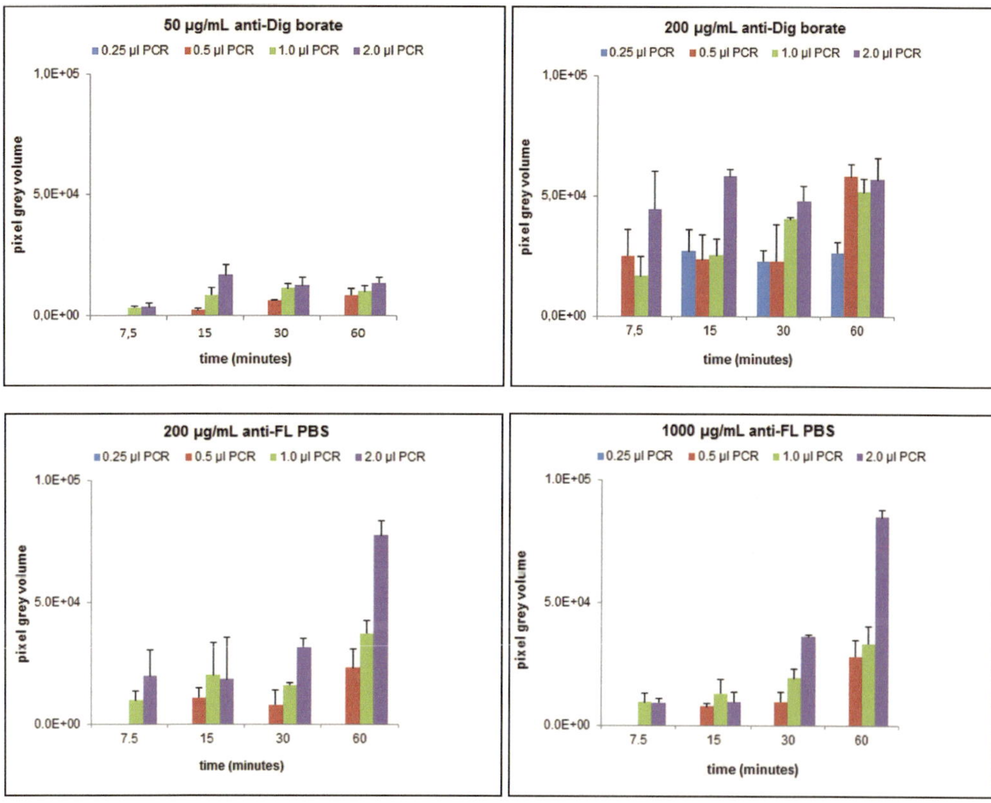

Fig. 8. Influence of incubation time and amount of added amplicon *Listeria monocytogenes* with DIG as label and *Listeria* spp. with FL as label. Two concentrations of antibody were spotted with two different printing buffers.

The amount of amplicon added varied from 0.5, 1 to 2 µL, where 1 µL was sufficient to give a good signal, corresponding to an amount of 20-300 fmol sample DNA with similar concentrations of DNA in both samples (31.5 vs. 41 ng DNA/µL for *Listeria monocytogenes* amplicon solution and the *Listeria* spp., respectively). Increasing the concentration of the printed antibody showed an optimum for 333 µg/mL for this combination of labelled amplicon and antibody.

A summary of the influence of buffer volume, antibody concentration and incubation time is shown in Fig. 9 for digoxigenin and in Fig. 10 for fluorescein as a tag. In the case of the anti-DIG antibody signal intensity increased upon printing more antibody molecules per spot up to a concentration of 333 µg/mL. For the influence of the anti-FL antibody concentration no clear conclusions could be drawn. In addition, the total incubation volume was not of much influence, which was similar in the anti-DIG incubations. Whereas in the incubations with the anti-DIG antibody the signal intensity was higher in the 30 minutes as compared to the 10 minutes incubation, no differences could be seen in the case of the anti-FL antibody.

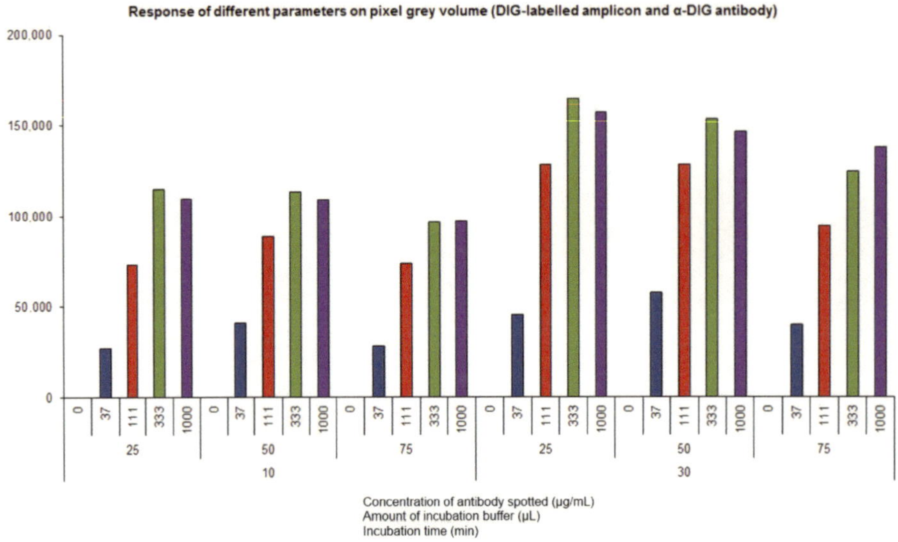

Fig. 9. Influence of the α-DIG antibody concentration (37, 111, 333, or 1000 µg mL^{-1}), incubation time (10 or 30 min) and volume (25, 50 or 75 µL from left to right) using 1 µL of the amplicon of *L. monocytogenes* labelled with biotin and DIG, 1 µL of carbon-neutravidin conjugate, a stirring speed of 300 min^{-1}, and two incubation times: 10 min or 30 min.

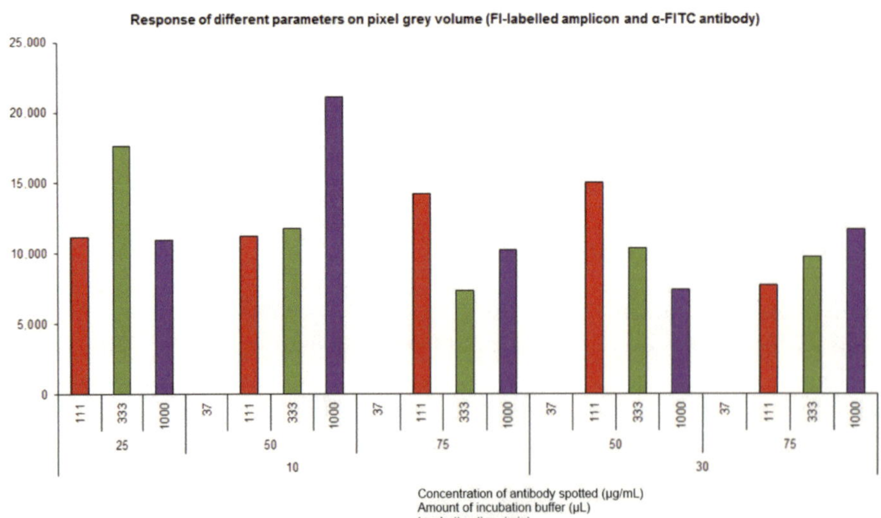

Fig. 10. Influence of the α-FL antibody concentration (37, 111, 333, or 1000 µg mL^{-1}); conditions as described under Figure 9 except for the amplicon: 1 µL of the amplicon of *Listeria* 16S RNA labelled with biotin and fluorescein.

Obviously, optimisation of a microarray immunoassay is dependent on the particular antibodies used and, hence, should be a compromise to enable acceptable sensitivity of all targets involved.

In addition, only PBS was used as a printing buffer, since from the preceding and other (not shown) experiments it was concluded that the results in PBS and in 100 mM borate pH8.8 were very similar. Since commercial antibodies are often shipped in or lyophilized from PBS it was decided to use this buffer in all further experiments.

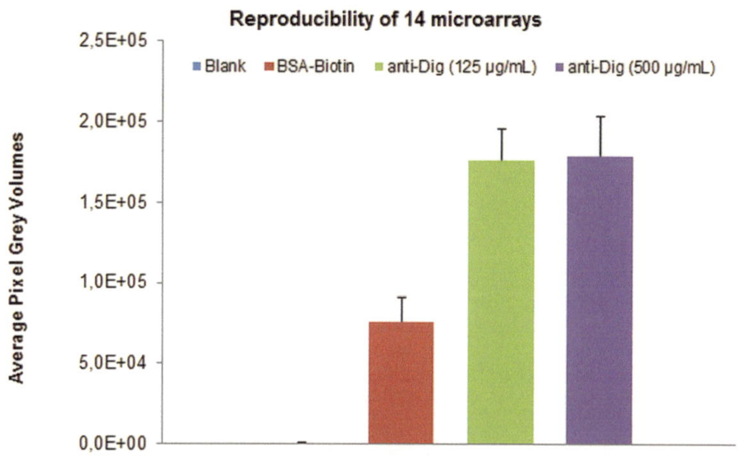

Fig. 11. Reproducibility of a FAST16 slide microarray with 1 µL of a *L. monocytogenes* amplicon using biotin and DIG as the tags, 14 arrays with 9 spots each of BSA-biotin, α-DIG 125 µg mL^{-1}, α-DIG 500 µg mL^{-1} and 1 µL of carbon conjugate. The total volume was 25 µL and samples were incubated for 30 min at a stirring speed of 300 min^{-1}.

The reproducibility of the assay using the above-mentioned optimized parameters was evaluated using 14 individual microarrays with nine spots each of BSA-biotin (500 µg mL^{-1}), α-DIG (125 µg mL^{-1}) and α-DIG (500 µg mL^{-1}). Amplicons used were 1 µL of the DIG-labelled *L. monocytogenes* type, 1 µL of the carbon-conjugate suspension in a total volume of 25 µL. Incubation time was 30 min. Blanks were evaluated using empty spots. Results are shown in Fig. 11. An intra-assay standard error of less than 10% was achieved and an inter-assay standard error of less than 20% was calculated. These results clearly show the reproducibility of the test.

Optimisation of several parameters in the three-analyte approach was performed using the amplified products of *S. typhimurium* antibiotic resistance genes (Table 1). Serial dilutions of α-TxR, α-DIG or α-DNP antibody (1000, 500, 250, 125, 62.5 or 31.25 µg mL^{-1}) were printed. Judged from a fixed amount of carbon-neutravidin conjugate (1 µL) and serial dilutions of amplicon (0.125, 0.5, 1, or 2 µL), 1 µL of each of the amplicons proved to be optimal for a good response (Fig. 12), although 0.125 µL could be positively scored in all cases as well. Based on a fixed amount of amplicon (i.e., 1 µL) and serial dilutions of carbon-neutravidin conjugate (0.5, 1, 2, 4 µL) the optimal amount of the carbon-neutravidin conjugate suspension was 1-2 µL at antibody concentrations of 125-250 µg mL^{-1} (Fig 12).

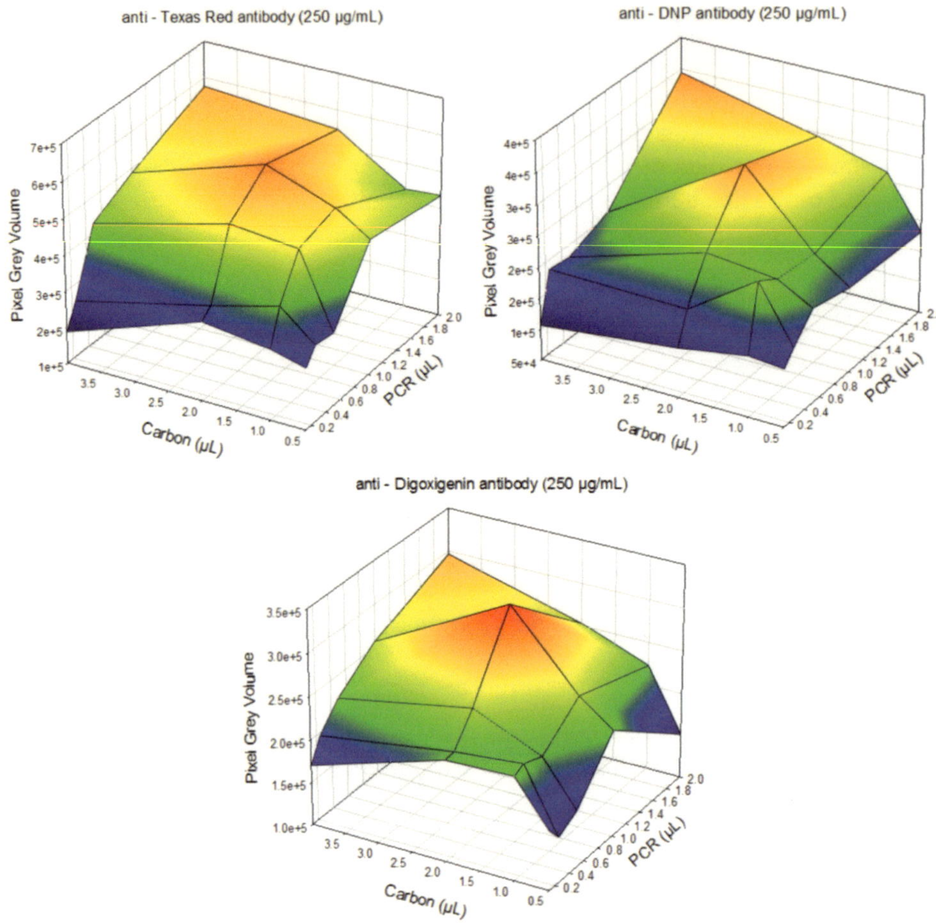

Fig. 12. Contour plots of the influence of addition of amount of amplicon and carbon-neutravidin conjugate. Initial results of individual additions of the tagged amplicons of some of the *Salmonella* antibiotic resistance genes. Shown here are the products tagged with texas red (left upper panel), dinitrophenol (right upper panel) and digoxigenin (lower panel).

3.2.4 Three - analyte detection using the antibody microarray

The response of the addition of a mixture of the individually amplified and labelled antibiotic resistance genes is shown in Fig. 13. No quantification of the DNA content of the amplicons was made, and 0.5 µL of each amplicon was added to each well. Serial dilutions of antibodies printed showed a concentration-dependent response for every amplicon-antibody pair. The total volume was 25 µL and the samples were incubated for 30 min, however, in this case 2 µL of the carbon conjugate suspension was used.

Signals with the anti-DNP antibodies were twice as high as those with the other anti-tag antibodies and the optimal antibody concentration appeared to be 125 to 250 µg/mL.

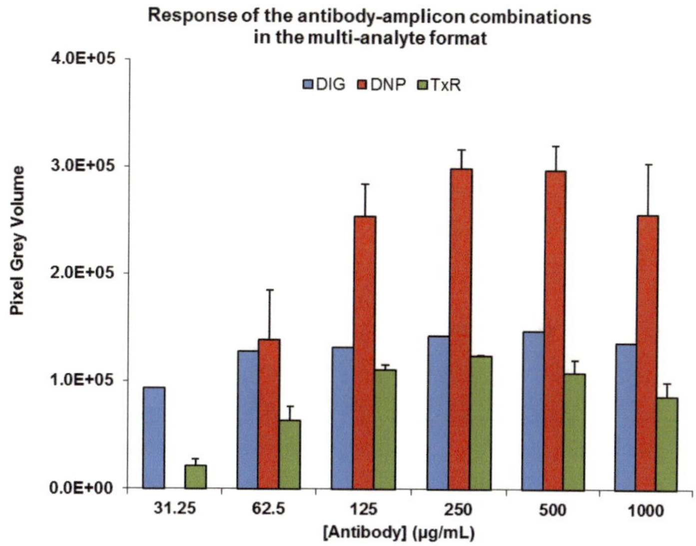

Fig. 13. Response of the multi-analyte format when serial dilutions of the three antibodies were spotted. Incubation was done with addition of 0.5 µL of each of the *Salmonella* amplicons of the antibiotic resistance genes, 2 µL of carbon conjugate suspension in 25 µL of incubation volume. Incubation time was 30 min.

Tagged amplicons added				Pixel Grey Volume		
Dig	DNP	TxR		α-Dig	α-DNP	α-TxR
-	-	-		0	0	0
+	+	+		1.3×10^5	2.5×10^5	1.1×10^5
+	-	-		1.6×10^5	0	0
-	+	-		0	3.4×10^5	0
-	-	+		0	0	1.5×10^5
+	+	-		1.7×10^5	3.0×10^5	0
+	-	+		1.6×10^5	0	1.5×10^5
-	+	+		0	3.2×10^5	1.1×10^5

Table 2. Specificity in the three-analyte test (PGV average of 2 tests).

To study whether the simultaneous presence of various targets could be detected in the microarray an experiment was done in which the amplicons, each having a specific DNP, DIG, or TxR tag, were incubated in different combinations. Fixed amounts of anti-tag antibodies were used (125 µg/mL for each of the antibodies). The results are presented in Table 2. In all cases the presence of a particular amplicon resulted in a high-intensity spot with PGV > 1×10^5. In the absence of a particular amplicon no PGV was detected. Hence, all scores correctly indicated the composition of the various samples.

The most optimal parameters in this format are summarised in Table 3. With minimal volume of 1 µL of amplicon (containing 20 to 30 fmol DNA after amplification), a printing volume of 1 nL containing 125-250 pg of antibody (absolute amount) and low-cost resources it is possible to discriminate between three antibiotic resistance genes from *Salmonella* spp.

Stirring speed	300 min^{-1}
Incubation time	30 min
Volume	25 to 50 µL
Antibody spotted	125-250 µg mL^{-1}
Carbon nanoparticles	2 µL
PCR amplicon (20 to 30 fmol; 20 to 300 nmol L^{-1})	1 µL

Table 3. Most optimal parameters in the 3-analyte format.

3.3 Costs

Assuming the end-user obtains printed antibody microarrays several costs have to be taken into account. Kits for DNA extraction should be purchased, although recent advances allow for direct PCR on samples if very robust polymerases are being used. Furthermore, some hard- and software is obligatory. These consist of a thermocycler, a personal computer with flatbed scanner or CCD camera and image analysis software. The price of the chemicals (conjugate, PCR reagents) is less than 1 euro per slide. However, one should realize that applications as outlined above, when applied in resource-poor settings, at least need the availability of electricity.

4. Conclusions and future research

Carbon nanoparticles with adsorbed neutravidin are suitable as label in nitrocellulose-based antibody microarrays. The versatility has been shown using different types of microorganisms. The format is generic; the only discriminating factor is the sequence of the primers used in the amplification step and the use of the discriminating tag/antibody combination. Although much more space is available on the nitrocellulose pads (5x5 mm) we used 4x6 arrays with spots of about 200 µm in diameter to study the applicability of the carbon nanoparticles. Unfortunately, there is a paucity in tags and/or their corresponding antibodies that can be used to discriminate between all kinds of food pathogens. Increasing the availability of label/antibody combinations will be a significant improvement in the multi-analyte character of the microarray test procedure as described here.

The best surface for the microarrays as developed in this study is the FAST16 slide with 16 nitrocellulose membranes. We did not have to block the membranes in advance, as is generally done (Jonkheijm et al. 2008). Nevertheless, this one-step procedure resulted in a complete absence of background signal (Fig. 11).

The sensitivity of the proposed microarray procedure with carbon nanoparticles can be improved when a fusion product of neutravidin and enzyme is adsorbed onto the nanoparticles. To this end, neutravidin - alkaline phosphatase and - horseradish peroxidase products are commercially available. Carbon nanoparticles can be labelled with these protein fusion products and specific interaction of these conjugates with biotin-labelled targets results in the presence of a large number of enzyme molecules at the spot. A short, additional incubation step with a precipitating substrate (10 min) substantially increases the signal due to the formation of a precipitable dye on the spot. Preliminary experiments in our laboratory indicate that the sensitivity (PGV) can be increased by a factor 5 to 10.

Nowadays, various nanoparticles are used in diagnostics, i.e. quantum dots, dye-doped silica, noble metals, and magnetic particles as reviewed (Gomez-Hens et al. 2008). Lönnberg and Carlsson were the first to combine carbon nanoparticles with flatbed scanning (Lonnberg & Carlsson 2001). Some other authors also mentioned the use of flatbed scanning using gold nanoparticles (Han et al. 2003; Sun et al. 2007; Taton et al. 2000) or enzyme (Petersen et al. 2007). Inexpensive flatbed scanners and CCD-based detectors open new opportunities to develop microarray applications, even for low-facility laboratories and under field conditions (Rasooly & Herold 2008). Even a visual read-out of the signal is possible when coloured nanoparticles are being used as is valid for the carbon nanoparticles in this study. On the other hand, battery-powered hand-held microarray readers for evaluation of the signal are readily available as well. Since shaking can even be omitted (results not shown) the method can easily be made available to resource-poor settings.

Antibody microarrays are especially applicable when intermediate numbers of samples have to be assayed, application at point of care/need is required, when costs play an important role and highly trained personnel is not available. The presented procedure with signal generation by carbon nanoparticles meets these characteristics.

5. Acknowledgement

The generous gift of *Salmonella* template from Dr A.H.A.M. van Hoek and Dr H.J.M. Aarts (RIKILT, Institute of Food Safety, Wageningen University and Research Centre, The Netherlands) is gratefully acknowledged.

6. References

Aldus, C.F., et al. (2003). Principles of some novel rapid dipstick methods for detection and characterization of verotoxigenic *Escherichia coli*. *Journal of Applied Microbiology*, Vol. 95, No. 2, (August 2003), pp, 380-389, ISSN 1364-5072

Askar, M., et al. (2011). Update on the ongoing outbreak of haemolytic uraemic syndrome due to Shiga toxin-producing *Escherichia coli* (STEC) serotype O104, Germany, May 2011. *Eurosurveillance*, Vol. 16, No. 22, (May 2011), pp, pii=19883, ISSN 1560-7917

Baeumner, A.J. (2004). Nanosensors identify pathogens in food. *Food Technology*, Vol. 58, No. 8, (August 2004), pp, 51-55, ISSN 0015-6639

Besselink, G.A.J., et al. (2004). Signal amplification on planar and gel-type sensor surfaces in surface plasmon resonance-based detection of prostate-specific antigen. *Analytical Biochemistry*, Vol. 333, No. 1, (October 2004), pp, 165-173, ISSN 0003-2697

Blazkova, M., et al. (2009). Development of a nucleic acid lateral flow immunoassay for simultaneous detection of *Listeria* spp. and *Listeria monocytogenes* in food. *European Food Research and Technology*, Vol. 229, No. 6, (October 2009), pp, 867-874, ISSN 1438-2377

Blazkova, M., et al. (2011). Immunochromatographic strip test for detection of genus *Cronobacter*. *Biosensors and Bioelectronics*, Vol. 26, No. 6, (February 2011), pp, 2828-2834, ISSN 0956-5663

Capps, K.L., et al. (2004). Validation of three rapid screening methods for detection of Verotoxin-producing *Escherichia coli* in foods: Interlaboratory study. *Journal AOAC International*, Vol. 87, No. 1, (January 2004), pp, 68-77, ISSN 1060-3271

Chen, M.L. & Tsen, H.Y. (2002). Discrimination of *Bacillus cereus* and *Bacillus thuringiensis* with 16S rRNA and *gyrB* gene based PCR primers and sequencing of their annealing sites. *Journal of Applied Microbiology*, Vol. 92, No. 5, (May 2002), pp, 912-919, ISSN 1365-2672

Corstjens, P., et al. (2001). Use of up-converting phosphor reporters in lateral-flow assays to detect specific nucleic acid sequences: A rapid, sensitive DNA test to identify human papillomavirus type 16 infection. *Clinical Chemistry*, Vol. 47, No. 10, (October 1, 2001), pp, 1885-1893, ISSN 0009-9147

D'Agostino, M., et al. (2004). A validated PCR-based method to detect *Listeria monocytogenes* using raw milk as a food model-towards an international standard. *Journal of Food Protection*, Vol. 67, No. 8, (August 2004), pp, 1646-1655, ISSN 0362-028X

de Heij, B., et al. (2004). Highly parallel dispensing of chemical and biological reagents. *Analytical and Bioanalytical Chemistry*, Vol. 378, No. 1, (August 2004), pp, 119-122, ISSN 1618-2642

Dieterle, F. & Marrer, E. (2008). New technologies around biomarkers and their interplay with drug development. *Analytical and Bioanalytical Chemistry*, Vol. 390, No. 1, (January 2008), pp, 141-154, ISSN 1618-2642

Frank, C., et al. (2011). Large and ongoing outbreak of haemolytic uraemic syndrome, Germany, May 2011. *Eurosurveillance*, Vol. 16, No. 21, (May 2011), pp, pii=19878, ISSN 1560-7917

Glynn, B., et al. (2006). Current and emerging molecular diagnostic technologies applicable to bacterial food safety. *International Journal of Dairy Technology*, Vol. 59, No. 2, (May 2006), pp, 126-139, ISSN 1471-0307

Gomez-Hens, A., et al. (2008). Nanostructures as analytical tools in bioassays. *Trends in Analytical Chemistry*, Vol. 27, No. 5, (May 2008), pp, 394-406, ISSN 0165-9936

Gordon, J. & Michel, G. (2008). Analytical sensitivity limits for lateral flow immunoassays. *Clinical Chemistry*, Vol. 54, No. 7, (July 2008), pp, 1250-1251, ISSN 0009-9147

Han, A., et al. (2003). Detection of analyte binding to microarrays using gold nanoparticle labels and a desktop scanner. *Lab on a Chip*, Vol. 3, No. 4, (September 2003), pp, 329-332, ISSN 1473-0197

Hartmann, M., et al. (2009). Protein microarrays for diagnostic assays. *Analytical and Bioanalytical Chemistry*, Vol. 393, No. 5, (March 2009), pp, 1407-1416, ISSN 1618-2642

Herman, L.M.F., et al. (1995). A multiplex PCR method for the identification of *Listeria* spp. and *Listeria monocytogenes* in dairy samples. *Journal of Food Protection*, Vol. 58, No. 8, (August 1995), pp, 867-872, ISSN 0362-028X

Jonkheijm, P., et al. (2008). Chemical strategies for generating protein biochips. *Angewandte Chemie International Edition*, Vol. 47, No. 50, (December 2008), pp, 9618-9647, ISSN 1521-3773

Kalogianni, D.P., et al. (2011). Carbon nano-strings as reporters in lateral flow devices for DNA sensing by hybridization. *Analytical and Bioanalytical Chemistry*, Vol. 400, No. 4, (May 2011), pp, 1145-1152, ISSN 1618-2642

Koets, M., et al. (2006). A rapid lateral flow immunoassay for the detection of fungal alpha-amylase at the workplace. *Journal of Environmental Monitoring*, Vol. 8, No. 9, (July 2006), pp, 942-946, ISSN 1464-0325

Koets, M., et al. (2009). Rapid DNA multi-analyte immunoassay on a magneto-resistance biosensor. *Biosensors and Bioelectronics*, Vol. 24, No. 7, (March 2009), pp, 1893-1898, ISSN 0956-5663

Koets, M., et al. (2011). Rapid one-step assays for on-site monitoring of mouse and rat urinary allergens. *Journal of Environmental Monitoring*, Vol. 13, No. 12, (November 2011), pp, 3475-3480, ISSN 1464-0325

Kostrzynska, M. & Bachand, A. (2006). Application of DNA microarray technology for detection, identification, and characterization of food-borne pathogens. *Canadian Journal of Microbiology*, Vol. 52, No. 1, (January 2006), pp, 1-8, ISSN 0008-4166

Kozwich, D., et al. (2000). Development of a novel, rapid integrated *Cryptosporidium parvum* detection assay. *Applied and Environmental Microbiology*, Vol. 66, No. 7, (July 1, 2000), pp, 2711-2717, ISSN 0099-2240

Lonnberg, M. & Carlsson, J. (2001). Quantitative detection in the attomole range for immunochromatographic tests by means of a flatbed scanner. *Analytical Biochemistry*, Vol. 293, No. 2, (May 2001), pp, 224-231, ISSN 0003-2697

Lonnberg, M., et al. (2008). Ultra-sensitive immunochromatographic assay for quantitative determination of erythropoietin. *Journal of Immunological Methods*, Vol. 339, No. 2, (December 2008), pp, 236-244, ISSN 0022-1759

Mandal, P.K., et al. (2011). Methods for rapid detection of foodborne pathogens: An overview. *American Journal of Food Technology*, Vol. 6, No. 2, (July, 2010), pp, 87-102, ISSN 1557-4571

Mens, P.F., et al. (2008). Molecular diagnosis of malaria in the field: development of a novel 1-step nucleic acid lateral flow immunoassay for the detection of all 4 human *Plasmodium* spp. and its evaluation in Mbita, Kenya. *Diagnostic Microbiology and Infectious Disease*, Vol. 61, No. 4, (May 2008), pp, 421-427, ISSN 0732-8893

Noguera, P., et al. (2011). Carbon nanoparticles in lateral flow methods to detect genes encoding virulence factors of Shiga toxin-producing *Escherichia coli*. *Analytical and Bioanalytical Chemistry*, Vol. 399, No. 2, (October 2010), pp, 831-838, ISSN 1618-2642

Petersen, J., et al. (2007). Detection of mutations in the [beta]-globin gene by colorimetric staining of DNA microarrays visualized by a flatbed scanner. *Analytical Biochemistry*, Vol. 360, No. 1, (January 2007), pp, 169-171, ISSN 0003-2697

Posthuma-Trumpie, G.A., et al. (2008). On the development of a competitive Lateral Flow ImmunoAssay for progesterone: Influence of coating conjugates and buffer components. *Analytical and Bioanalytical Chemistry*, Vol. 392, No. 6, (November 2008), pp, 1215-1223, ISSN 1618-2642

Posthuma-Trumpie, G.A., et al. (2012). Amorphous carbon nanoparticles: a versatile label for rapid diagnostic (immuno)assays. *Analytical and Bioanalytical Chemistry*, Vol. 402, No. 2, (January 2012), pp, 593-600, ISSN 1618-2642

Rasooly, A. & Herold, K.E. (2008). Food microbial pathogen detection and analysis using DNA microarray technologies. *Foodborne Pathogens and Disease*, Vol. 5, No. 4, (August 2008), pp, 531-550, ISSN 1535-3141

Sun, Y., et al. (2007). Label-free detection of biomolecules on microarrays using surface-colloid interaction. *Analytical Biochemistry*, Vol. 361, No. 2, (February 2007), pp, 244-252, ISSN 0003-2697

Taton, T.A., et al. (2000). Scanometric DNA Array Detection with nanoparticle probes. *Science*, Vol. 289, No. 5485, (September 2000), pp, 1757-1760, ISSN 00368075

Timlin, J.A. (2006). Scanning microarrays: Current methods and future directions, In: *Methods in Enzymology*, O. Alan Kimmel and Brian, (Ed), 79-98, Academic Press, ISBN 978-0-12-182816-5, Amsterdam, The Netherlands

van Amerongen, A., et al. (1993). Colloidal carbon particles as a new label for rapid immunochemical test methods: Quantitative computer image analysis of results. *Journal of Biotechnology*, Vol. 30, No. 2, (August 1993), pp, 185-195, ISSN 0168-1656

van Amerongen, A., et al. (1994). Quantitative computer image analysis of a human chorionic gonadotropin colloidal carbon dipstick assay. *Clinica Chimica Acta*, Vol. 229, No. 1-2, (September 1994), pp, 67-75, ISSN 0009-8981

van Amerongen, A. & Koets, M. (2005). Simple and rapid bacterial protein and DNA diagnostic methods based on signal generation with colloidal carbon particles, In: *Rapid Methods for Biological and Chemical Contaminants in Food and Feed*, A. van Amerongen, D. Barug, M. Lauwaars, (Ed), 105-126, Wageningen Academic Publishers, ISBN 9076998531, Wageningen

van Dam, G.J., et al. (2004). Diagnosis of schistosomiasis by reagent strip test for detection of circulating cathodic antigen. *Journal of Clinical Microbiology*, Vol. 42, No. 12, (December 1, 2004), pp, 5458-5461, ISSN 0095-1137

van Doorn, A.W.J., et al. (1987). Immunodetermination using non-metallic labels. International Patent Number: 0321008 B1, European Union

van Doorn, A.W.J., et al. (1996). Method for determining the presence of analyte using a stable colloidal carbon sol. International Patent Number: 5,529,901, United States of America

van Doorn, A.W.J., et al. (1997). Stable aqueous carbon sol composition for determining analyte. International Patent Number: 5641689, United States of America

van Hoek, A.H.A.M., et al. (2005). Detection of antibiotic resistance genes in different *Salmonella* serovars by oligonucleotide microarray analysis. *Journal of Microbiological Methods*, Vol. 62, No. 1, (July 2005), pp, 13-23, ISSN 0167-7012

Venkatasubbarao, S. (2004). Microarrays - status and prospects. *Trends in Biotechnology*, Vol. 22, No. 12, (December 2004), pp, 630-637, ISSN 0167-7799

Volokhov, D., et al. (2002). Identification of *Listeria* species by microarray-based assay. *Journal of Clinical Microbiology*, Vol. 40, No. 12, (December 2002), pp, 4720-4728, ISSN 0095-1137

Wang, J., et al. (2006). A disposable microfluidic cassette for DNA amplification and detection. *Lab on a Chip*, Vol. 6, No. 1, (December 2005), pp, 46 - 53, ISSN 1473-0197

Section 2

Review Articles

20

Utilization of the *Staphylococcus aureus* Protein 'A' and the *Streptococcus* spp. Protein 'G' in Immunolabelled Techniques

Eltayb Abuelzein
Department of Internal Medicine, Faculty of Medicine,
King Abdul-Aziz University, Jeddah,
Saudi Arabia

1. Introduction

Immuno-labelled techniques (ILTs) depend on linking of a specific antibody to a labelling material. The so-produced conjugate is utilized to detect or assay a specific reactant against which the antibody, in the conjugate, is directed. Many labelling materials have been conjugated to specific antibodies. The most commonly used labels included enzymes, avidin-biotin, radioactive materials, fluoriscin dyes, ferritin, gold and possibly others.

The specific conjugates could be used to:

a. Detect antibodies in sera of humans or different animal species.
b. Detect antigens such as viruses, bacteria, parasites ..etc.
c. Detect physiological materials such enzymes, hormones, cytokines etc..
d. Detect other materials from plants and insects.
e. Detect pharmaceutical products.

For antibody detection in a specific animal species, the conjugate to be used for that purpose, usually consists of the labelling material (e.g. an enzyme) linked to antibodies against the immunoglobulins of that particular animal species. This necessitates the use of a conjugate against each animal species. However, when for example conducting a serological survey, against a specific disease, in various species of animals including man, the ideal situation, in this case , is to use a single conjugate against all the animal species to be tested. This dilemma was resolved, to a greater extent, by employment of the *Staphylococcus aureus* Protein 'A' and the *Streptococcus* spp. Protein 'G' in conjugates used in ILTs.

2. PA in Immuno-labelled techniques

Protein 'A' (PA) is a novel cell wall protein of the *S. aureus* that binds the Fc portion, of most mammalian IgG molecules (Forsgren & Sjoquist 1966). This binding is not an antigen-antibody reaction, because it does not involve the antigen binding fraction (FAB) of the IgG molecule. This property gave PA special novelty in being a natural universal reagent. So, it is now widely utilized in ILTs.

PA is 40-60 KD. It can bind four molecules of IgG . Optimum binding occurs at pH 8.2. It is stable in the pH range of 1.0 - 12.0. *In vivo* PA disrupts opsonization and phagocytosis in blood of an infected host by the *S.aureus* bacteria. So, it is regarded as a potential microbial surface component recognizing adhesive matrix molecules (MSCRAMM).

By virtue of its ability to bind to the Fc portion of most mammalian IgG molecules, PA has been extensively utilized in the different fields of ILTs. It was linked to enzymes such as horse radish peroxidase (Engval 1978) and alkaline phosphatase (e.g. Alnaeem & Abuelzein 2008; Dubois-Dalcq et al 1977; Crowther & Abuelzein 1980), to fluorescin dye (e.g. Ghetie et al 1974), to radioactive materials (e.g. Langone 1978; Colombatti & Hilgers 1979; Crowther & Abuelzein 1980), to gold (e.g. Faulk & Taylor 1971), to avidin-biotin (e.g. Hsu & Raine 1981). Accordingly, PA conjugates have been exploited in various areas of ILTs such as ELISA, Radioimmunoassay (RIA), Immuno-histochemistry (IHC), Immuno-electron microscopy (IEM), as an immunological probe to identify cell surface markers (e.g. markers on T and B lymphocytes), to precipitate antigen-antibody complexes without the use of antispecies antibodies, and in other areas of research.

The major value of the use of PA in ILTs is that, it replaced the use of antispecies conjugates against each mammalian species.

2.1 PA – ELISA

ELISA, in which antispecies conjugates had been used, was applied with great success in many vital fields of biological sciences such as medicine, veterinary medicine, plant research, entomology, biotechnology, general microbiology and possibly in other fields where ILTs are applicable. Commercial antispecies conjugates are available in the market. However, a problem is always faced when there is a need to examine several animal species, especially those in the wild(e.g. antelopes, skunks, mongoose, hedgehogs, bats etc..). Usually no commercial conjugates are available for these animal species. So, the requirement for one conjugate to cover these species would be ideal. To overcome this obstacle, scientists thought of the use of PA & PG conjugated to enzymes to examine a wide range of IgGs of domestic and wild mammals. As a result, PA - ELISA has found its way in various applications of research. Presently, commercial Kits utilizing PA conjugates in ELISA systems are readily available; and can be employed in the different fields of biological research.

2.1.1 PA – ELISA in the medical field

In the medical field PA-ELISA has been applied in laboratory diagnosis and research. It was applied for the detection of antibodies, against viral (e.g. Madore & Baumgarten 1979; AL-Nakib 1981; Schountz et al 2007) , bacterial (e.g. Ansorg et al 1984; Fuquay et al 1986; Chaud et al 1988; Considine et al 1986; Jagannath & Sehgal 1989; Stobel et al 2002; Nielsen et al 2004) and parasitic diseases (e.g. Mohammed et al 1985; Gandhi et al 1987; Felix de Lima et al 2005) in humans and other mammals. These mammals may act as reservoirs of human diseases or may show overt clinical signs of a zoonotic disease e.g. Rift Valley Fever (RVF); (Madani 2005) or Brucella infection (e.g. Chaud et al 1988; Jagannath & Sehgal 1989).

2.1.1.1 PA - ELISA in veterinary research

PA - ELISA found wide application in veterinary research because of the multiple species of mammals dealt with in the veterinary profession. The technique was applied for the detection of antibodies against viral (Crowther & Abuelzein 1980; Du Plessis et al 1990; Inoshima et al 1999; Smith et al 2004; Schountz et al 2007), bacterial (e.g. Lawman et al 1984; Chand et al 1988; Nielsen et al 2004) and parasitic (e.g. Lima et al 2004) diseases.

2.1.1.2 PA-ELISA in other areas of research

PA-ELISA was applied in plant virology to detect Bacaulovirus (Brown et al 1982). Beside its application in immunodiagnosis, PA has potential applications in immunotherapy and affinity purification of monoclonal antibodies (MABs) (e.g. Considine et al 1986).

2.2 PA – Radioimmunoassay (PA-RIA)

PA-RIA was applied in the different fields of biological sciences (e.g. Dorval et al 1975; Langone 1978; Enzmann 1978; Crowther & Abuelzein 1980). However, its uses in many laboratories was; and so predominantly replaced by the handy ELISA technique.

2.3 PA in immuno-histochemisty

PA has been utilized with great success and versatility in IHC. It was readily conjugated to enzymes such as peroxidase (e.g. Dubois-Dalcq et al 1977;) to avidin- biotin (e.g. Su Ming & Raine 1981) to ferritin (e.g. Templeton & Douglas 1978) to gold (e.g. Roth & Heitz 1989), to fluorescein isothiocyanate (e.g. Notani et al 1979); and used to detect various antigens in tissues (e.g. Alnaeem & Abuelzein 2008; Abuelzein & Elnaeem 2009) either under light or electron microscopes. The advantages of using PA in IHC over other analogous techniques have been well documented (e.g. Dubois-Dalcq et al 1977; Su Ming & Raine 1981; Roth & Heitz 1989). Beside its versatility in being used against a wide range of animal species, the non-specific reaction experienced with other analogous techniques was not a problem when using PA- IHC . So, PA-IHC was found to be a valuable tool for localization of antigens in tissues.

2.4 PA in Immuno-Electron Microscopy (PA – IEM)

PA conjugated to enzymes (e.g.Dubois-Dalcq 1977), ferritin (e.g. Bachi et al 1977), colloidal gold (e.g. Horisberger & Clerc 1985), avidin-biotin (e.g. Hsu & Raine 1981) has been used with great success in immuno-election microscopy. The technique found successful applications in diagnosis and research in virology (e.g. Wendelschafer et al 1976; Shukla & Gough 1979) , bacteriology (e.g.Van Laere et al 1985) and other areas of research such as histopathology (e.g. Roth & Heitz 1989), andrology (e.g. Schrader et al 2005) and haematology (e.g. Bachi et al 2006).

3. *Streptococcus* spp. protein G in immuno-labelled techniques

Streptococcus spp. Protein G is a cell wall protein from *Streptococcus* spp. (Kronvall 1973; Bjorck & Kronvall 1984). Its gene structure and protein binding properties were described by Sjobring et al (1991). Like PA it binds to the Fc portion of IgGs from many mammalian species over a wide range of pH from 4.0-8.0. However, it has a broader range of reactivity than PA. A novel property of PG, is its ability to react with human IgG_3. The significance of this, is that IgG_3 is over expressed in several autoimmune diseases, representing up to 45% of the autoimmune antibodies. This property has nominated PG to be a candidate of choice for applications in autoimmunity studies and diagnosis.

Due to binding of the native PG molecule to albumin, which is a major component of serum, PG application was rather limited as compared to PA. However, by removal of the binding site from the recombinant forms, PG is now applied with success to various areas of research.

Like PA, PG has been linked to enzymes (e.g. Inoshima et al 1999; Kramsky et al 2003; Stobel et al 2002; Vansnick et al 2005) & gold (e.g.Taatjes et al 1987) and used in analogous techniques similar to those employed for PA conjugates such as ELISA, IHC & IEM; but to a limited extent.

4. Discussion

The aim of this overview was to through some light for researchers, to consider the use of PA & PG conjugates where-ever feasible. The merits of using these two types of conjugates over the antispecies ones were discussed above. However, with the emergence of new pathogens in the different geographical regions of the world, researchers find themselves in a situation whereby they should examine various wild mammals for presence of antibodies against the emerging disease. In such situations they need sensitive immunolabelled methods. For these methods antispecies conjugates are required. Such conjugates against these wild mammals are not usually available in the market. So, the need for PA & PG conjugates becomes vital. On the other hand, the use of PG conjugates, for example, can be vital also in some diagnostic situations, such as in the case of autoimmune diseases.

Before using PA or PG conjugates in wild mammals, the reaction of their IgGs against PA & PG conjugates should be assessed, (Inoshima et al 1999).

The choice of using either type of conjugate, PA or PG, depends on the species of animal(s) to be tested. This is because the intensity of reactions of PA & PG with the different species of mammals vary (Inoshima et al 1999; Crowther & Abuelzein 1980). To over come this, some authors used a conjugate combination of both PA & PG (Nielsen et al 2004).

Of the merits of using PA &PG conjugates in ILTs is that the non-specific reactions in the tests are greatly reduced or completely cut down (Crowther & Abuelzein 1980; Alnaeem & Abuelzein 2008; Abuelzein & Alnaeem 2009).

In conclusion, and because of the above mentioned merits, it is recommended that PA & PG are to be used where -ever feasible.

5. References

Abu Elzein E.M. and Al-Naeem A. (2009). Utilization of protein -A in immune-histochemical techniques for detection of Peste des Petits Ruminants (PPR) virus antigens in tissues of experimentally infected goats. Trop. Anim. Health Prod. 41, (1), 1-4.

Al-Naeem A. and Abu-Elzein E.M.E. (2008). In situ detection of PPR virus antigen in skin papules around the mouth of sheep experimentally infected with PPR virus. Trop. Anim. Health Prod. 40, (4), 239-241.

Al-Nakib W. (1981). Trypsinised human O erythrocytes in the detection of rubella-specific IgM by sera fractionation on sucrose density gradient and absorption with staphylococcal protein A. J Clin Pathol 34, 670-673.

Ansorg R.A. Heine S. and Kraus C.J. (1984). Substitution of anti-human globulin by Protein A - bearing staphylococci in the detection of Brucella antibodies. Med. Microbiol. Immunol. 173, 233-240.

Bachi T., Dorval G. and Wigzell H. et al (1977). Stahpylococcal Protein A in Immunoferritin Techniques. Scandinavian Journal of Immunology 6, 241-246.

Wendelschafer-Crabb G., Erlandsen S.L. and Walker, JR D.H. (1976). Ultrastructural Localization of Viral Antigens Using The Unlabeled Antibody-Enzyme Method. The Journal of Histochemistry and Cytochemistry 24, (3), 517-526.

Bjorck L. and Kronvall G. (1984). Purification and some properties of streptococcal protein G, a novel IgG-binding reagent. The Journal of Immunology 133, (2), 969-974.

Brown D.A., Allen C.J. and Bignell G.N. (1982).The Use of Protein A Conjugate in an Indirect Enzyme-linked Immunosorbent Assay (ELISA) of Four Closely Related Baculoviruses from Spodoptera Species. J. gen. Virol. 62, 375-378.

Chand P., Batra H.V. and Sadana J.R. (1988). Detection of brucella-specific Protein A - reactive antibodies in buffaloes by dotenzyme-linked immunosorbent assay. Vet. Rec. 122, 162-163.

Considine P.J., Duggan P. and Eadie A. (1986).Enzyme Linked Immunosorbent Assay (ELISA) for the Determination of Protein-A. Bioscience Reports 6, (11).

Crowther J.R. and Abu-Elzein E.M.E. (1980).Detection of Antibodies Against Foot-And-Mouth Disease Virus Using Purified Staphylococcus A Protein Conjugated with Alkaline Phosphatase. Journal of Immunological Methods 34, 261-267.

Dorval G., Welsh K.I. and Wigzell H. (1975). A radioimmunoassay of cellular surface antigens on living cells using iodinated soluble protein A from *Staphylococcus aureus*. J. Immunol. Meth. 7, 237.

Dubois-Dalcq M., McFarland H. and McFarlin D. (1977).Protein A-peroxidase: a valuable tool for the localization of antigens. Journal of Histochemistry & Cytochemistry 25, (11), 1201-1206.

Du Plessis D.H., van Wyngaardt W and Bremer C.W. (1990).An indirect sandwich ELISA utilizing F (ab')2 fragments for the detection of African horsesickness virus. J. Virol Methods 29, (3), 279-89.

Engvall E. (1978).Preparation of Enzyme-labelled Staphylococcal Protein A. and its Use for Detection of Antibodies. Scand. J. Immunol. 8,(7), 25-31.

Faulk W.P. and Tayler G.M. (1971). 'An immunocolloid method for the electron microscope" Immunochemistry 8, (11), 1081-3.

De Lima V.M.F., Biazzona L. and Silva A. C. et al (2005).Serological diagnosis of visceral leishmaniasis by enzyme immunoassay using protein A in naturally infected dogs. Pesq. Vet. Bras. 25, (4) , 215-218.

Forsgren A. and Sjoquist J. (1966)."Protein A" from S. Aureus, Pseudo-Immune Reaction with Human {gamma} - Globulin. The Journal of Immunology 97, 822-827.

Fuquay J.I. , Deryk T. L. and Barnes D.W. (1986). Binding of *Staphylococcus aureus* by Human Serum Spreading Factor in an In Vitro Assay. Infection and Immunity 714-717.

Gandhi B.M., Irshad M. and Chawla T.C. et al (1987).Enzyme linked protein-A: an ELISA for detection of amoebic antibody.Transactions of the Royal Society of Tropical Medicine and Hygiene 81, (2), 183-185.

Ghetie V., Fabricus H.A. and Nilsson K. et al (1974). Movement of IgG receptors on the Iymphocyte surface induced by Protein A of *Staphylococcus aureus*. Immunology 26, 1081.

HSU SU-Ming and Raine L. (1981).Protein A, Avidin, and Biotin in Immunohistochemistry. The Journal of Histochemistry and Cytochemistry 29, (11), 1349-1353.

Inoshima Y., Shimizu S. and Minamoto N. et al (1999). Use of Protein AG in an Enzyme-Linked Immunosorbent Assay for Screening for Antibodies against Parapoxvirus in Wild Animals in Japan. Clinical and Diagnostic Laboratory Immunology 6, (3), 388-391.

Jagannath C. and Sehgal S. (1989). Enhancement of the antigen - binding capacity of incomplete IgG antibodies to Brucella melitensis through Fc region interactions with staphylococcal Protein A. J. Immunol. Meth. 30, 251-257.

Krawmsky J.A., Manning E.J. and Collins M.T., et al (2003). Protein G binding to enriched serum immunoglobulin from nondomestic hoofstock species. Journal of Veterinary Diagnostics Investigation 15, 253-261.

Kronvall G. (1973). A Surface Component in Group A, C, and G Streptococci with Non-Immune Reactivity for Immunoglobulin G. The Journal of Immunology 111, (5), 1401-1406.

Langone J.J. (1978).J. Immunol. Methods 24, 269.

Lawman M.J. Thurmond M.C. and Reis K.J. et al (1984). Solid – phase radioimmunoassay for the detection of immunoglobulins against bovine Brucella abortus. Vet. Immunol. Immunopathol. 6, 291-305.

Madore H.P and Baumgarten A. (1979). Enzyme-Linked Protein A: an Enzyme-Linked Immunosorbent Assay Reagent for Detection of Human Immunoglobulin G and Virus-Specific Antibody. Journal of Clinical Microbiology 10, (4), 529-532.

Horisberger M. and Clerc M.F. (1985). Labelling of colloidal gold with Protein A. Histochemistry and Cell Biology 82, (3), 219-223.

Nielsen K., Smith P. and Yu W. et al (2004). Enzyme immunoassay for the diagnosis of brucellosis: chimeric Protein A-Protein G as a common enzyme labeled detection reagent for sera for different animal species. Veterinary Microbiology 101, 123-129.

Notani G.W., Parsons J.A. and Erlandsen S.L. et al (1979).Versatility of *Staphylococcus aureus* protein A in immunocytochemistry. J. Histochem Cytochem 27, 1438.

Roth J. and Heitz P.U. (1989). Immunolabeling with the protein A-gold technique: an overview. Ultrastruct. Pathol. 13, (5-6), 467-84.

Schountz T., Calisher C.H. and Richens T.R. et al (2007). Rapid Field Immunoassay for Detecting Antibody to Sin Nombre Virus in Deer Mice. Emerging Infectious Diseases 13, (10).

Schrader S.M. , Eng. L.A. and Metz C.B. (2005). Immunoferritin labeling of rabbit spermatozoa. Gamete Research 4, 379-386.

Shukla D.D. and Gough K.H. (1979). The Use of Protein A. from *Staphylococcus aureus*, in Immune Electron Microscopy for Detecting Plant Virus Particles. J. gen. Virol. 45, 533-536.

Sjobring U., Bjorck L. and Kastern W. (1991). Streptococcal Protein G, Gene Structure And Protein Binding Properties. The Journal of Biological Chemistry 266, (1), 399-405.

Nielsen K., Smith P. Yu W. et al (2004). Enzyme Immunoassay for the diagnosis of brucellosis: chimeric Protein A-Protein G as a common enzyme labeled detection reagent for sera for different animal species. Veterinary Microbiology 101, 123-129.

Stobel K., Schonberg A. and Staal C. et al (2002).Anew non species dependent ELISA for detection of antibodies to Borrelia burgdor-feri s.l. in zoo animals. International Journal of Medical Microbiology 291, (33), 88-99.

Su-Ming HSU and Raine L. (1981). Protein A, Avidin, and Biotin in Immunohistochemistry. The Journal of Histochemistry and Cytochemistry 29, (11), 1349-1353.

Taatjes D.J., Chen T.H. and Ackerstrom B. (1987). Streptococcal protein G-gold complex: comparison with staphylococcal protein A-gold complex for spot blotting and immunolabeling. Eur J Cell Biol. 45, (1), 151-9.

Templeton C.L. and Douglas R.J. (1978). Ferritin-conjugated protein A. A new immunocytochemical reagent for electron microscopy. FEBS Lett 85, (1), 95-8.

Van Laere O., De Wael L. and De Mey J. (1985). '' Immuno gold staining (IGS) and immune gold silver staining (IGSS) for the identification of the plant pathogenic bacterium Erwinia amylovora (Burril) Winslow et al''. Histochemistry 83, (5), 397-9.

Vansnick E., Vercammen F. and Bauwens L. (2005). A survey for Mycobacterium avium subspecies paratuberculosis in the Royal Zoological Society of Antwerp. The Veterinary 170, 249-256.

21

An Overview of the Laboratory Assay Systems and Reactives Used in the Diagnosis of Hepatitis C Virus (HCV) Infections

Recep Kesli
Konya Education and Research Hospital, Department of Microbiology and Clinical Microbiology, Konya, Turkey

1. Introduction

In the mid-1970s, a new disease entity termed 'non-A, non-B' (NANB) hepatitis was first described and, in the following years, led to discovery of the causative virus, post-transfusion, and to community-acquired NANB hepatitis increasingly becoming recognized as a potentially serious disease that results in liver cirrhosis and/or hepatocellular carcinoma.[16, 26] Hepatitis C virus (HCV) was first identified in 1989 using molecular methods at the Chiron Corporation, but to date, the virus has never been visualized or grown in cell culture.[37] Hepatitis C virus (HCV) is a single-stranded RNA virus with a genome of about 10 000 nucleotides containing a single large, continuous open reading frame and with organization most closely resembling the *Flaviviridae*.[11] HCV is a global healthcare problem and the World Health Organization (WHO) estimates that at least 170 million people (3 % of the world's population) are infected with HCV worldwide and most of the patients are concentrated in developing countries. [48]

HCV Proteins. HCV proteins may be divided in two groups: Structural proteins and nonstructural proteins. Structural Proteins: The nucleocapsid proteins (core), two envelope glycoproteins (E1 and E2), and a small transmembrane protein p7. E2 likely mediates cell entry by binding to one ore more specific cellular receptors or coreceptors, and has also been suggested to interact with and inhibit interferon-inducible protein kinase R (PKR).[26] P7 may function as a viroporin. Non-structural proteins (NS): NS2, NS3, NS4 (A, B), NS 5 (A, B). NS2 may exist an E2p7NS2 processing intermediate due to inefficient signal peptidase cleavages at the E2-p7 and p7-NS2 junctions. NS2 has also been reported to coimmunoprecipitate. Other functions of NS2 are uncertain. NS3 has serine protease/helicase activity and a multifunctional protein. NS4A is associated with membranes. NS4B is important for RNA replication. It has a GTPase acitivity that is important RNA in replication. NS5B has RNA-depndent RNA polymerase activity resulting in initiating in-vitro RNA synthesis both primer dependent and independent. Anti-HCV reactives manufactured from these group of proteins. [4, 15, 35]

Organization of the HCV genome and polyprotein processing presented in **Figure 1.** [26]

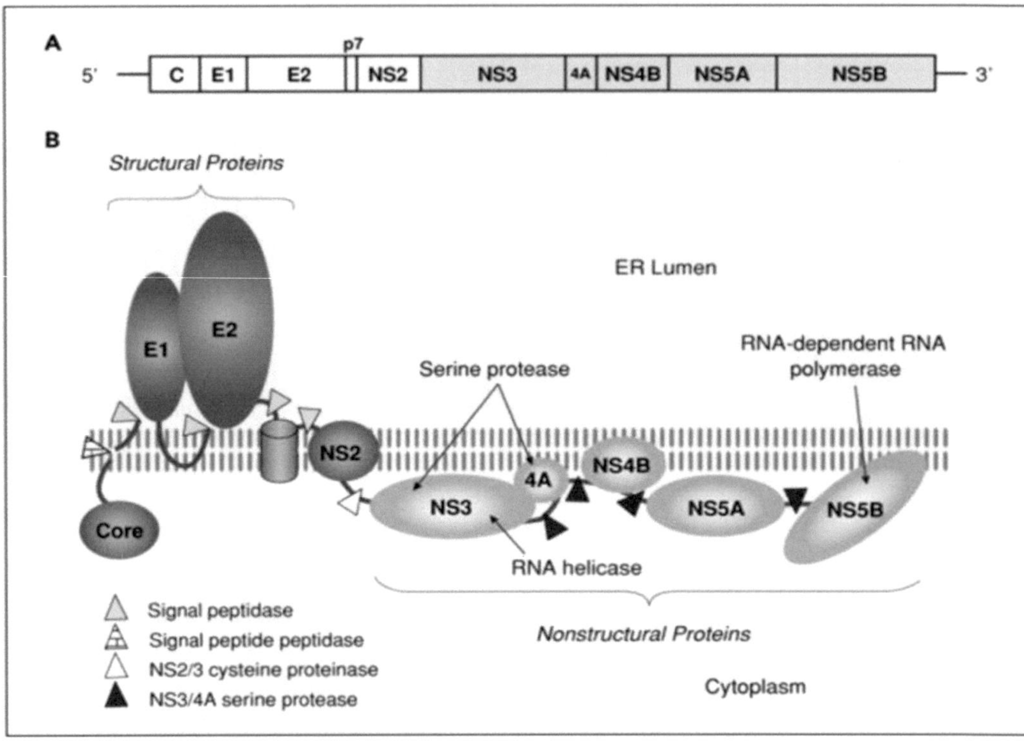

Fig. 1. Organization of the HCV genome and polyprotein.[26]

2. Classification of laboratory assay systems and reactives used in the diagnosis of hepatitis C virus infection.

Immunoasssay systems used in the diagnosis of hepatitis C virus infections may be divided into four groups.

- **2.1.** Anti-HCV assay.
- **2.2.** Strip immunblott assay (SIA).
- **2.3.** Hepatitis C virus core antigen assay.
- **2.4.** HCV RNA assay.

Diagnostic tests used for the diagnosis of HCV infections may be divided into three groups according to aim of use. [22]

1. Screening test (Anti-HCV tests based on EIA or CIA)
2. Supplemental test (Strip immunoblot assay-SIA)
3. Confirmatory test (HCV RNA) (HCV Core Ag as a pre-confirmative test.).

Detection or quantification of HCV RNA an important molecular assay based on the principle of target amplification used for confirming test results of immunoassay reactives. Reactives used in order to diagnose HCV infections also may be divided in to two groups according to identification method of the test. [32]

1. Indirect tests: (Anti-HCV and Strip immunoblot assays).

2. Direct tests: (HCV RNA, HCV Ag, HCV genotyping assays and sequencing of HCV genome).

2.1 Anti-HCV assay

Diagnostic procedures of hepatitis C virus infection in laboratories are principally based on the detection of antibodies (IgG) against recombinant HCV polypeptides by two main methods: Enzyme immunoassay (EIA) and Chemiluminescence immunoassay (CIA). The anti-HCV assay is used as a screening test. Non-structural and recombinant antigens have been used in the production of immunoassay reactives. Serologic and virologic markers of past or present HCV infection include IgG antibodies (anti-HCV). An assay for Ig M anti-HCV is available, but it does not distinguish between acute and chronic HCV infection.[25]

Three different generations of anti-HCV test kits have been developed to date. The first-generation HCV enzyme immunoassay (EIA) detected only antibodies against the non-structural region 4 (NS4) with recombinant antigen c100-3.[25] With the development of second-generation tests, additional antigens from the core region (c22-3), the NS3 region (c33c) and a part of c100-3 (named 5-1-1) from the NS4 region were used.[17] The third-generation EIA anti-HCV test used today includes an additional antigen from the NS5 region and a reconfiguration of the core and NS3 antigens.[46] Anti-HCV assays have several disadvantages, such as a high rate of false positivity, a lack of sensitivity of detection in the early window periods of 45 to 68 days after infection, the inability to distinguish between acute (ongoing active, viremic), past (recovered) and persistent (chronic) infections and a possibility of false negativity with samples from immmunocompromised patients who may not have an adequate antibody response.[19, 30, 33, 36] Inorder to shorten the duration of the diagnosis of heaptitis C virus infection especially in preseroconversion period being capable of the detection of antibodies against NS 5 proteins means that a third generation reactive is very important for anti-HCV assays. Because there remains a window period, estimated at 82 days with the second-generation assays, at 66 days with the third generation assays, between the infection and the detection of HCV antibodies [12]. NS5, enables the detection of HCV antibodies on an average of 26 days earlier in individuals with transfusion-transmitted HCV infection. Furthermore, sensitivity is also improved (approaching 97%), specifically in a high-prevalence population.[14]

Summarized properties of the fully automated CIA based systems and anti-HCV reacitves shown in **Table 1.**

2.2 Strip immunblot assay (SIA)

SIA rectives used as supplementary test, involving recombinant immunblot assay (RIBA) HCV 3.0 strip immunoassay (SIA) (Chiron Corporation, Emeryville, CA, USA), which contained recombinant antigens (c33c, NS5) and synthetic peptides (5-1-1, c100 and c22); and INNO-LIA™ HCV Score (Innogenetics N. V. Ghent, Belgium) is a 3rd generation line immunoassay which incorporates HCV antigens derived from the core region, the E2 hypervariable region (HVR), the NS3 helicase region, the NS4A, NS4B, and NS5A regions. Both SIA's are based on the principle of an enzyme immunoassay. Recombinant immunoblot assays are used as supplementary test of anti-HCV assays. As types of EIA, recombinant immunoblot assays also have several disadvantages, such as being difficult to perform, a high percentage of 'indeterminate' results and a high cost. Therefore, these anti-HCV assays are not often used in developing countries or in routine diagnostic laboratory procedures. [23]

Immunoassay Sytem	Analytic method	Test speed	Anti-HCV reactive
Abbott Arcihtect USA	Chemiluminescent Microparticle Immunoassay (CMIA)	200 Test/h	NS3, NS4.
Abbott Axsyme Plus USA	Microparticle Enzyme Immunoasay (MEIA)	100 Test/h	NS3, NS4, NS5.
SeimensAdvia Centaur XP Germany	Chemiluminescence (CHEM)	240 Test/h	NS3, NS4, NS5.
Seimens Advia Centaur CP Germany	Chemiluminescence (CHEM)	180 Test/h	NS3, NS4, NS5.
Roche Cobas e601 Switzerland	Electrochemiluminesans (ECLIA)	170 Test/h	NS3, NS4.
Roche Cobas e411 Switzerland	Electrochemiluminescence (ECLIA)	86 Test/h	NS3, NS4.
Beckman Coulter UniCel DxI 600/800 USA	Chemiluminescence (CHEM)	200/400 Test/h	NS3, NS4.
Beckman Coulter Access 2 USA	Chemiluminescence (CHEM)	100 Test/h	NS3,NS4.
Ortho-Clinical Diagnostics Vitros 3600 USA	Enhanced Chemiluminescence (ECHEM)	189 Test/h	NS3, NS4, NS5
Ortho Clinical Diagnostics Vitros ECi/ECiQ USA	Enhanced Chemiluminescence (ECHEM)	90 Test/h	NS3, NS4, NS5
Diasorin Laison Italy	Chemiluminescence (CHEM)	180 Test/h	NS3, NS4, NS5

Table 1. Summarized properties of CLIA based basic assay systems and reactives.

2.3 Hepatitis C virus core antigen (HCV Ag) assay

Total serum HCV core antigen, a surrogate marker of HCV replication, can also be detected and quantified. A commercial assay kit for it is available. HCV core antigen can be detected on average, 1 to 2 days after HCV RNA during the pre-seroconversion period. HCV Ag test is presented as a "Direct marker for diagnosis of HCV infection". Sensitivity of HCV core antigen test is slightly lower than HCV RNA assay but many studies carried out with HCV core Ag test compared with HCV RNA, proved that the HCV Ag test is specific, reproducible, highly sensitive and clinically applicable assay. HCV antigen test also showing good correlation comparing with HCV RNA. HCV core antigen test may be used as a second line confirmatory test alternative to HCV RNA.[23, 28, 29] It is also needed as a pre-confirmatory test for anti-HCV results and to distinguish false positives from the accurate ones. This is because it is easy to perform, reliable, has a high specificity and sensitivity rate, is cost effective, is able to shorten the duration of the diagnosis of patients during the window period and has a lower risk of laboratory contamination than assays based on nucleic acid amplification technology. [45, 50]

During the past decade, several HCV Ag tests have been developed as potential alternatives to HCV RNA assay. [5] The first was developed by Tanaka et al.[45] 1995, and then Aeyogi et al.[1] developed a new and 100-fold more sensitive test. In previous studies, the HCV Ag was detected one day after the HCV RNA in patients undergoing seroconversion. [12, 13, 34] The Architect HCV Ag assay (Abbott Laboratories, Diagnostics Division, Abbot Park, IL, USA) is highly specific, sensitive, reliable, easy to perform, reproducible, cost-effective and applicable as a screening, and pre-confirming test for anti-HCV assays in the laboratory procedures used for the diagnosis of hepatitis C virus infection. The Architect HCV Ag assay was performed using the automated Architect® i2000SR CIA system (Abbott Laboratories, Diagnostics Division, Abbot Park, IL, USA). The Architect HCV Ag assay is a two-step chemiluminescent microparticle immunoassay technology for the quantification of the HCV Ag in human serum or plasma samples. The sample volume required is 110 µl, and the total assay time is 36-40 min. The cutoff value is 3.00 fmol/liter (0.06 pg/mL); thus, values <3.00 fmol/l are considered nonreactive, values ≥3.00 fmol/l are considered reactive and values ≥3.00 fmol/l and <10.00 fmol/l are retested in duplicate. If both retest values are nonreactive, the specimen is considered nonreactive for HCV Ag. If one or both of the duplicates have a value ≥3.00 fmol/l, the specimen is considered repeatedly reactive. [29, 38]

2.4 Molecular diagnostic systems, and reactives used for the HCV RNA and HCV genotyping assays

Confirmation test is needed. Although third-generation HCV reactives are more sensitive and specific than older generation assays, they still have a high percentage of false positive reactions, so that it is mandatory to confirm every reactivity, especially with low titers, by anti-HCV CIA or EIA with HCV RNA assay (reactives with a lower limit of detection of 50 IU/mL or less) to avoid false positive results. To minimize the likelihood of false-positive anti-HCV results, the CDC has recommended the confirmation of all anti-HCV results by either RIBA or HCV RNA assay.[28, 29]

HCV RNA is the earliest marker of infection, and a direct indicator of ongoing viral replication. It appears 1 to 2 weeks after infection before any alterations in liver enzyme levels and appearance of anti-HCV antibodies can be detected. If the nucleic acid testing (NAT) result is positive, active HCV infection is confirmed. If NAT result is negative, the HCV antibody or infection status can not be determined. NAT assays are used to detect and quantify HCV RNA. [8, 18, 40]

HCV RNA assay systems can be divided into two groups: qualitative and quantitative HCV RNA.

Qualitative HCV RNA assay. Target amplification methods used qualitative detection of HCV RNA and have lower limits of detection of 5-50 IU/mL: Reverse Transcriptase-PCR (single enzyme RT-PCR, dual enzyme RT-PCR, nested RT-PCR), TMA (transcription-mediated amplification), NASBA (isothermal RNA amplification). This group includes the qualitative RT-PCR, of which the Amplicor™ HCV 2.0 (Roche Molecular Systems, USA) is an FDA- and CE-approved RT-PCR system for qualitative HCV RNA testing that allows detection of HCV RNA concentrations down to 50 IU/ml of all HCV genotypes. [31] Transcription-mediated amplification- (TMA)-based qualitative HCV RNA detection has a very high sensitivity (lower limit of detection 5-10 IU/ml). [20, 41] Transcription Mediated Amplification (TMA) Component System, Versant™ HCV RNA Qualitative Assay (Siemens

Healthcare Diagnostics, Germany) is also commercially available which is accredited by FDA and CE and provides an extremely high sensitivity, superior to RT-PCR-based qualitative HCV RNA detection assays. [21, 42, 43]

Quantitative HCV RNA assay. Quantification of HCV RNA can be determined by target amplification techniques Real-Time PCR assays), or by signal amplification methods (branched DNA- bDNA Assay). Several FDA- and CE-approved standardised systems are commercially available. The Cobas Amplicor™ HCV Monitor (Roche Diagnostics) is based on a competitive PCR technique whereas the Versant™ 440 HCV RNA Assay (Siemens Healthcare Diagnostics) is based on a bDNA technique. Both have restricted lower limits of detection (500-615 IU/ml). More recently, the Cobas TaqMan assay and the Abbott RealTime™ HCV test, both based on real-time PCR technology, have been introduced and now replaced the qualitative and quantitative methods. All commercially available HCV RNA assays are calibrated to the WHO standard based on HCV genotype 1. It has been shown that results may vary significantly between assays with different HCV genotypes despite standardisation. [9, 47]

The Abbott RealTime™ HCV Test provides a lower limit of detection of 12 IU/mL, a specificity of more than 99.5 % and a linear amplification range from 12 to 10,000,000 IU/mL independent of the HCV genotype. [27, 39] VERSANT kPCR Molecular System Siemens Healthcare Diagnostics is also avialable as a real time PCR system for quantification of HCV RNA. Rotor Gene Q real time PCR device and Qiagen HCV RNA kits (Qiagen GmbH, Germany) are used for quantification of HCV RNA by real time PCR method with specificity of 99.0 %, a lower limit of detection 34 IU/ml and capable to detect up to 10, 000,000 IU/mL.

In certain situations HCV RNA result can be negative in persons with active HCV infection. As the titre of anti-HCV increases during acute infection, the level of circulating HCV RNA declines; intermittent HCV RNA positivity has been observed among persons with chronic HCV infection. A negative HCV RNA result can also indicate resolved infection. Follow-up HCV RNA testing is indicated only in persons with serologically confirmed anti-HCV positive results. [8, 18]

Detection and quantification of HCV RNA is used as the only one confirmative test of all the anti-HCV, HCV Ag assays and SIA tests. The HCV RNA assay is a reliable method but needs technical skill and may also result in false positivity because of contamination. It is time consuming and expensive. [18, 38] HCV RNA is extensively used to confirm antibody-based screening test results. Amplification methods (target amplification by RT-PCR, transmission-mediated amplification (TMA), and signal amplification by b-DNA-branch-DNA are the most expensive methods (45-50 USD per test for real-time PCR, 10-12 USD per test for HCV Ag CIA, and 5-6 USD per test for anti-HCV CIA) when compared with anti-HCV and HCV Ag tests; and require sophisticated technical equipment and highly trained personnel. One specific problem with the HCV RNA assay is that HCV RNA can be temporarily undetectable because of the transient, partial control of viral replication by the immune response. Patients in a period of non-viremia may be detected as anti-HCV-positive and HCV RNA-negative. In such a situation, the HCV RNA test should be repeated a few weeks later with a new sample. This need for re-testing is a disadvantage of the HCV RNA test. In addition, nucleic acid amplifications are time-consuming methods and have the risk of laboratory contamination. for these reasons, amplification methods are not suitable for wide use in most laboratories, especially in developing countries. [2, 10, 24, 38, 44]

HCV Genotyping assay. HCV has six genotypes represented by digits (1-6) and multiple subtypes represented by letters (a, b, c…) and most recently a seventh HCV genotype have been characterized. HCV genotyping should be carried out in every patient before antiviral therapy.[6] Both direct sequence analysis and reverse hybridisation technology allow HCV genotyping. Reverse-hybridization method and kits (The VERSANT HCV Genotype Assay (LiPA Line Prob Assay) 2.0, Bayer HealthCare LLC, Tarrytown, NY, USA) also exist for hepatitis C virus genotype assay. The test is mainly based on biotinylated DNA, generated by RT-PCR amplification of the 5'untranslated region (5'UTR) of HCV RNA, is hybiridized to immobilized oligonucleotide probes. The VersantTM HCV Genotype 2.0 System (Siemens Healthcare Diagnostics) is suitable for indentifying genotypes 1-6 and more than 15 different subtypes and is currently the preferred assay for HCV genotyping. By simultaneous analyses of the 5'UTR and core region, a high specificity is achieved especially to differentiate the genotype 1 subtypes (1a versus1b). The TruGene direct sequence assay determines the HCV genotype and subtype by direct analysis of the nucleotide sequence of the 5'UTR region. Incorrect genotyping rarely occurs with this assay. However, the accuracy of subtyping is poor. The current Abbott RealTime™ HCV Genotype II assay is based on real-time PCR technology, which is less time-consuming than direct sequencing. Preliminary data reveal a 96% concordance at the genotype level and a 93% concordance on the genotype 1 subtype level when compared to direct sequencing of the NS5B and 5'UTR regions.

Interpretation of HCV and acute hepatitis C test results are presented in **Tables 2** and **3**.

Immunoassay for anti-HCV	**Nucleic acid test for HCV RNA**	**Supplemental test for anti-HCV**	**Interpretation of HCV status**
Negative	Not applicable	Not applicable	Never infected with HCV
Positive	Not done	Not done	Unknown, positive screening test needs confirmation
Positive	Positive	Positive/not done	Active HCV infection
Positive	Negative	Not done	Unknown, single negative HCV RNA result cannot determine infection status; perform RIBA to rule out screening test false-positive
Positive	Negative	Positive	Has been infected with HCV;repeat testing for HCV RNA to rule out active infection as HCV RNA levels may fluctuate
Positive	Not done	Positive	Has been infected with HCV; follow-up testing for HCV RNA, liver enzymes is indicated to determine current infection status
Positive	Not done/ Negative	Negative	Never infected with HCV

Table 2. Interpretation of HCV test results.[26]

Anti HCV[1]	HCV-RNA[2]	Interpretation
Negative	Negative	Not acute hepatitis C
Negative	Positive	Acute hepatitis C
Positive	Negative	Probably not an acute hepatitis C* (retesting needed)
Positive	Positive	Difficult to discriminate from chronic hepatitis C**

[1]Third-generation EIA, [2]HCV RNA assay with a lower limit of detection ≤50 IU/mL.
*Generally seen in patients who have recovered from a past HCV infection. RIBA should be used. A positive RIBA with two or more HCV-RNA positive results suggest that HCV infection resolved. A negative RIBA result indicates the false positivity of the EIA result, in the both no further testing is needed.
**Acutely infected patients can also have HCV RNA and anti-HCV at the time of diagnosis. It is difficult in these cases to distinguish acute hepatitis C from an acute exacerbation of chronic hepatitis or acute hepatitis of another cause in a patient with chronic hepatitis C.

Table 3. Interpretation of acute hepatitis C test results.[8]

3. False positivity problem and reasons of false positive results of anti-HCV immunoassay reactives

Although the present third generation EIA tests have better sensitivity and specifity rates than their predecessors, there still exists a high prevelance of false-positive results, especially among low risk group, immunocompromised patients or populations without liver diseases, leading to unnecessary cost-effective health expenditures and confusing diagnostic challenges. The most common problem in the laboratory screening assay of anti-HCV is the false positivity of low titers.[3, 7]

Among immunocompromised populations (e.g., hemodialysis patients) the average rate of false-positive results is approximately: 15 %. False positive anti-HCV results obtained from both CIA and EIA-based reactives can be explained by the fact that no structural antigens and proteins have been derived from HCV up to now. HCV has not been cultured and natural viral proteins are not available. Confirmatory test should be used in order to discriminate the false positive results from the accurate ones. [49]

3.1 Reasons of false results of anti-HCV immunoassay reactives.

The amino acid sequence and the purity of the HCV antigen used for assay development are significant factors influencing both the specifity and the sensitivity of anti-HCV immunoassays. Because of the high IgG concentration in human blood (>5 mg/ml)-e.g. in paraproteinemia or auto-antibody production or after Ig G denaturation caused by repeated freezing and thawing or by heat-inactivation of serum samples , there is a strong tendency for some of the IgG molecules to be bound to the micro-well surface by direct adsorbtion or by indirect capture via the surface molecules, and then arouse a signal, giving false-positive results. This problem might be more serious when the samples are from patients with systemic lupus erythematosus (SLE), rheumatoid arthritis (RA), portal cirrhosis, and some infectious diseases due to the very complicated, higher concentration of immunoglobulin components in their blood. [49]

4. References

[1] Aoyagi K, Ohue C, Iida K. et al., Development of a simple and highly sensitive enzyme immunoassay for hepatitis C virus core antigen. J Clin Microbiol 1999; 37:1802–8.

[2] Agha S, Tanaka Y, Saudy N. et al. Reliability of Hepatitis C Virus Core Antigen Assay for Detection of Viremia in HCV Genotypes 1, 2, 3, and 4 Infected Blood Donors: A Collaborative Study Between Japan, Egypt, and Uzbekistan. J Med Vir 2004;73: 216-22.

[3] Ansari MHK, Omrani MD. Evalutaions of diagnostic value of ELISA method (EIA) & PCR in diagnosis of hepatitis C virus in hemodialysis patients. Hepatitis Monthly 2006;6:19-23.

[4] Bartenschlager R. The NS3/4A proteinase of the hepatitis C virus: unravelling structure and function of an anusual enzyme and a prime target for antiviral therapy. J Viral Hepat 1999;6:165-81.

[5] Bouvier-Alias M, Patel K, Dahari H. et al., Clinical utility of total HCV Ag quantification:a new indirect marker of HCV replication. Hepatology 2002;36:211–8.

[6] Bowden DS, Berzsenyi MD. Chronic hepatitis C virus infection: genotyping and its clinical role. Future Microbiol 2006;1:103-12.

[7] Centers for Disease Control and Prevention. Guidelines for laboratory testing and result reporting of antibody to hapatitis C virus. MMWR Morbid Mortal Wkly Rep 2003;52:1-13.

[8] Chevaliez S, Pawlotsky JM. Use of virologic assays in the diagnosis and management of hepatitis C virus infection. Clin Liver Dis 2005;9:371-82.

[9] Chevaliez S, Bouvier-Alias M, Brillet R, Pawlotsky JM. Overestimation and underestimation of hepatitis C virus RNA levels in a widely used real-time polymerase chain reaction-based method. Hepatol 2007;46:22-31.

[10] Chevaliez S, Pawlotsky JM. Hepatitis C virus serologic and virologic tests and clinical diagnosis of HCV-related liver disease. Int J Med Sci 2006; 3:35 - 40.

[11] Choo Q-L, Richman KH, Han JH, et al. Genetic organization and diversity of the hepatitis C virus. Proc Natl Acad Sci USA 1991; 88: 2451 -5.

[12] Courouce AM, Marrec NL, Bouchardeau F. Et al. Efficacy of HCV core antşgen detection during the preseroconversion period. Transfusion 2000;40:1198-202.

[13] Daniel HD, Vivekanandan JP, Raghuraman S. et al., Significance of the hepatitis C virus (HCV) core antigen as an alternative plasma marker of active HCV infection. Indian J Med Microbiol 2007;1:37-42.

[14] Denoyel G, Van Helden J , Bauer R, Preisel-Simmons B. Performance of a new hepatitis C assay on the Bayer Advia Centaur® Immunoassay system. Clin Lab 2004;50:75-82.

[15] Einav S, Elazar M, Danieli T, et al. A nucleotide binding motif in hepatitis C virus (HCV) NS4B mediates HCV RNA replication. J Virol 2004;78:11288-95.

[16] Feinstone SM, Kapikian AZ, Purcell RH, et al: Transfusion-associated hepatitis not due to viral hepatitis type A or B. N Eng J Med 1975; 292: 767 - 70.

[17] Feucht HH, Zöllner B, Polywka S, et al: Study on reliability of commercially available hepatitis C virus antibody tests. J Clin Microbiol 1995, 33: 620 – 4.
[18] Fiebelkorn KR, Nolte SH. RNA virus detection. In Persing DH editor in chief. Molecular Microbiology Diagnostic Principles and Practise. ASM Press, Washington DC, USA. 2004, pp.441-474.
[19] Glynn SA, Wright DJ, Kleinman SH, et al. Dynamics of viremia in early hepatitis C virus infection. Transfusion 2005, 45:994-1002.
[20] Hendricks DA, Friesenhahn M, Tanimoto L, et al. Multicenter evaluation of the VERSANT HCV RNA qualitative assay for detection of hepatitis C virus RNA. J Clin Microbiol 2003;41:651-6.
[21] Hofmann WP, Dries V, Herrmann E, et al. Comparison of transcription mediated amplification (TMA) and reverse transcription polymerase chain reaction (RT-PCR) for detection of hepatitis C virus RNA in liver tissue. J Clin Virol 2005;32:289-93.
[22] Kesli R. Evaluation of assay methods and false positive results in the laboratory diagnosis of hepatitis C virus infection. Arch Clin Microbiol 2011, 2:1-4.
[23] Kesli R, Ozdemir M, Kurtoglu MG, Baykan M, Baysal B. Evaluation and comparison of three different anti-HCV reactives based on chemiluminescence and enzyme immunoassay method used in the diagnosis of Hepatitis C infections in Turkey. J Int Med Res 2009; 37: 1420- 9.
[24] Krajden M, Shivji R, Gunadasa K. et al. Evaluation of the core antigen assay as a second-line supplemental test for diagnosis of active hepatitis C virus infection. J Clin Microbiol 2004; 42:4054–9.
[25] Kuo G, Choo QL, ALter HJ, et al: An assay for circulating antibodies to a major etiologic virus of human non-A, non-B hepatitis. Science 1989; 244:362 –4.
[26] Lemon SM, Walker C, Alter MJ, et al: Hepatitis C virus. In: Fields Virology, 5th ed, Vol 1 (Knipe DM, Howley PM, eds). Philadelphia: Wolters Kluwer -Lippincott Williams & Wilkins, 2007; pp 1253-304.
[27] Michelin BD, Muller Z, Stezl E, Marth E et al. Evaluation of the Abbott Real Time HCV assay for quantificative detection of hepatitis C virus RNA. J Clin Virol 2007;38:96-100.
[28] Miedouge M, Saune K, Kamar N, Rieu M, Rostaing L, Izopet J. Analytical evaluation of HCV core antigen and interest for HCV screening in haemodilysis patients. J Clin Virol, 2010;48:18-21.
[29] Morota K, Fujinamia R, Kinukawaa H, Machidab T, Ohnob K, Saegusab H, Takeda K. A new sensitive and automated chemiluminescent microparticle immunoassay for quantitative determination of hepatitis C virus core antigen. J Virol Methods 2009;157:8-14.
[30] National Institutes of Health.. NIH consensus statement on management of hepatitis C: 2002. NIH Consens. State Sci Statements 19:1–46.
[31] Nolte FS, Fried MW, Shiffman ML, et al. Prospective multicenter clinical evaluation of AMPLICOR and COBAS AMPLICOR hepatitis C virus tests. J Clin Microbiol 2001;39:4005-12.
[32] Pawlotsky JM. Use and interpretation of hepattis C virus diagnostic assays. Clin Liver Dis 2003;7:127-37.
[33] Pawlotsky, JM. Diagnostic tests for hepatitis C. J Hepatol 1999; 31:71–9.

[34] Peterson J, Gren G, Iida K, et al. Detection of hepatitis C core antigen in the antibody negative 'window' phase of hepatitis C infection. Vox Sang 2000;78:80-5.

[35] Reed KE, Rice CM. Overview of hepatitis C virus genome structure, polyprotein processing, and protein properties. Curr Top Microbiol Immunol 2000;242:55-84.

[36] Richter SS. Laboratory assays for diagnosis and management of hepatitis C virus infection. J Clin Microbiol 2002;40:4407–12.

[37] Rosen HR, Pawlotsky JM. Scientific advences in hepatitis C virus. Clin Liver Dis 2003; 7:xiii-xv.

[38] Ross RS, Viazov S, Salloum S. et al., Analytical performance characteristics and clinical utility of a novel assay for total hepatitis C virus core antigen quantification. J Clin Microbiol 2010; 48:1161–8.

[39] Sabato MF, Shiffman ML, Langley MR, et al. Comparison of Performance Characteristics of three Real Time Reverse Transcription-PCR test systems for detection and quantification of hepatitis C virus. J Clin Microbiol 2007;45:2529-36.

[40] Saldanha J, Lelie N, Heath A, and WHO Collaborative Study Grouop. Estabilishment of the first international standart for nucleic acid amplification technology (NAT) assays for HCV RNA. Vox Sang 1999;76:149-58.

[41] Sarrazin C. Highly sensitive hepatitis C virus RNA detection methods: molecular backgrounds and clinical significance. J Clin Virol 2002;25:S23-9.

[42] Sarrazin C, Teuber G, Kokka R, et al. Detection of residual hepatitis C virus RNA by transcription-mediated amplification in patients with complete virologic response according to polymerase chain reaction-based assays. Hepatology 2000; 32:818-23.

[43] Sarrazin C, Hendricks DA, Sedarati F, Zeuzem S. Assessment, by transcription-mediated amplification, of virologic response in patients with chronic hepatitis C virus treated with peginterferon alpha-2a. J Clin Microbiol 2001;39:2850-5.

[44] Tanaka E, Ohue C, Aoyagi K, Evalution of a new enzyme immunoassay for hepatitis C virus (HCV) core antigen with clinical sensitivity approximating that of genomic amplification of HCV RNA. Hepatology 2000; 32: 388– 93

[45] Tanaka TJ, Lau Y, Mizokami M, et al. Simple fluorescent EIA for detection and quantification of hepatitis C viremia. J Hepatol 1995; 23: 742–745.

[46] Thomas DL, Ray SC, Lemon SM: Hepatitis C. In: Mandell, Douglas and Bennett's Principles and Practice of Infectious Diseases, 6th ed. (Mandell GL, Bennett JE, Dolin R, eds). Philadelphia: Churchill Livingstone, 2005; pp 1950 – 81.

[47] Vehrmeren J, Kau A, Gärtner B, et al. Differences between two real-time PCR based assays (Abbott RealTime HCV, COBAS AmpliPrep/COBAS TaqMan) and one signal amplification assay (VERSANT HCV RNA 3.0) for HCV RNA detection and quantification. J Clin Microbiol 2008;46:880-91.

[48] Wasley A, Alter MJ. Epidemiology of hepatitis C: geographic differences and temporal trends. Semin Liver Dis 2000; 20:1-16.

[49] Wu FB, Ouyan HQ, Tang XY, Zhou ZX. Double-antigen sandwich time-resolved immunoflourometric assay for the detection of anti-hepatitis C virus total antibodies with improved specifity and sensitivity. J Medical Microbiol 2008; 57:1-7.

[50] Yokosuka O, Kawai S, Suzuki Y, Evaluation of clinical usefulness of secondgeneration HCV Ag assay: comparison with COBAS AMPLICOR HCV MONITOR assay version 2.0. Liver International 2005;25:1136–41.

22

Multiplex Immunoassay and Bead Based Multiplex

Türkan Yiğitbaşı
Izmir Katip Çelebi University
Turkey

1. Introduction

1.1 Background

Protein immunoassays provide information about quantities and forms of endogenous proteins. Uniplex enzyme immunoassays like Elisa have been the workhorse for protein measurement for decades, but they can be laborious and expensive and consume relatively large amounts of specimen. In comparison to the ELISA for a single analyte, multiplex assays offer the possibility of obtaining more reliable quantitative information in a highly parallel analysis. In addition, quantitative multiplexed assays offer the possibility to identify combinations of biomarkers with higher disease specificity than any single established biomarker alone. Because of these reasons, currently one-analysis, many-metabolites, many-diseases approach is receiving more attention than uniplex system with one-analysis, one-metabolite, one-disease.

1.2 Multiplex immunoassay platforms

Presently, antibody-based platforms are the core technology for protein multiplex arrays. Assay formats include suspension arrays (microbead assays) and planar arrays that use traditional immunometric principles.

Planar arrays: MULTI-ARRAY (Meso Scale Discovery), A2 (Beckman Coulter), and FAST Quant (Whatman Schleicher & Schuell BioScience), Searchlight (Aushon Biosystem).

Suspension arrays: Bio-Plex (Bio-Rad Laboratories), FlowCytomix (Bender MedSystems), cytometric bead array (Becton, Dickinson and Company) and the partners of Luminex Corp (XMAP)].

In the first format, different capture antibodies are spotted at defined positions on a 2-dimensional array. In the second, the capture antibodies are conjugated to different populations of microbeads, which can be distinguished by their fluorescence intensity in a flow cytometer.

Optimal assay performance of multiplex immunoassay platforms depend on proprietary information about the antibody pair, the composition of diluents, and the software. The accuracy of quantification for multiplexed immunoassays depends, as with all ELISAs, on the quality of the calibration curves, assay imprecision (CV), recoveries, and assay linearity (the limits of quantification). Therefore, there is not a single assay platform suitable for all analytes. The selection of a platform or kit should depend on assay sensitivity, the relevant biological concentration to be measured

Platform	MesoScale discovery (MULTI-ARRAY/MULTI-SPOT)	Searchlight	FastQuant (FAST Quant System)
Capture antibody binding surface	Carbon	Plastic	Nitrocellulose
Detection system	Electrochemiluminescent	Biotinylated detector with fluorescent detection	Biotinylated detector with fluorescent detection
Analytes/plex	Up to 10	Up to 24	Up to 10
Image System	CCD camera based	CCD camera based	CCD camera based
Customised array	Yes	Yes	Yes
Kits for designing and building your own assay	Yes	No	No
Reagent company	Waterman Scleicher& Schuell Bioscience	Aushon Biosystem	Waterman Scleicher& Schuell Bioscience
Commercial instrument	Waterman Scleicher& Schuell Bioscience	Aushon Biosystem	Waterman Scleicher& Schuell Bioscience

Table 1. The characteristics of some commercial planar microspot array platforms

Platform	Luminex	Cytometric Bead Array (CBA)
Capture antibody binding surface	Fluorescently tagged beads	Fluorescently labeled beads
Detection system	Biotinylated detector with fluorescent detection	Phycoerythrin conjugated detectors
Analytes/plex	Up to 100	Up to 100
Image System	Luminex XMAP based system	Flow cytometer with dual laser
Customised array	Yes	Yes
Kits for designing and building your own assay	Yes	Yes
Reagent company	Luminex Corp and its partners(many others)	BD Becton,Dickinson and others
Commercial instrument	Lumine(XMAP) and its partners	BD Becton,Dickinson and others

Table 2. The characteristics of some commercial suspension bead array platforms

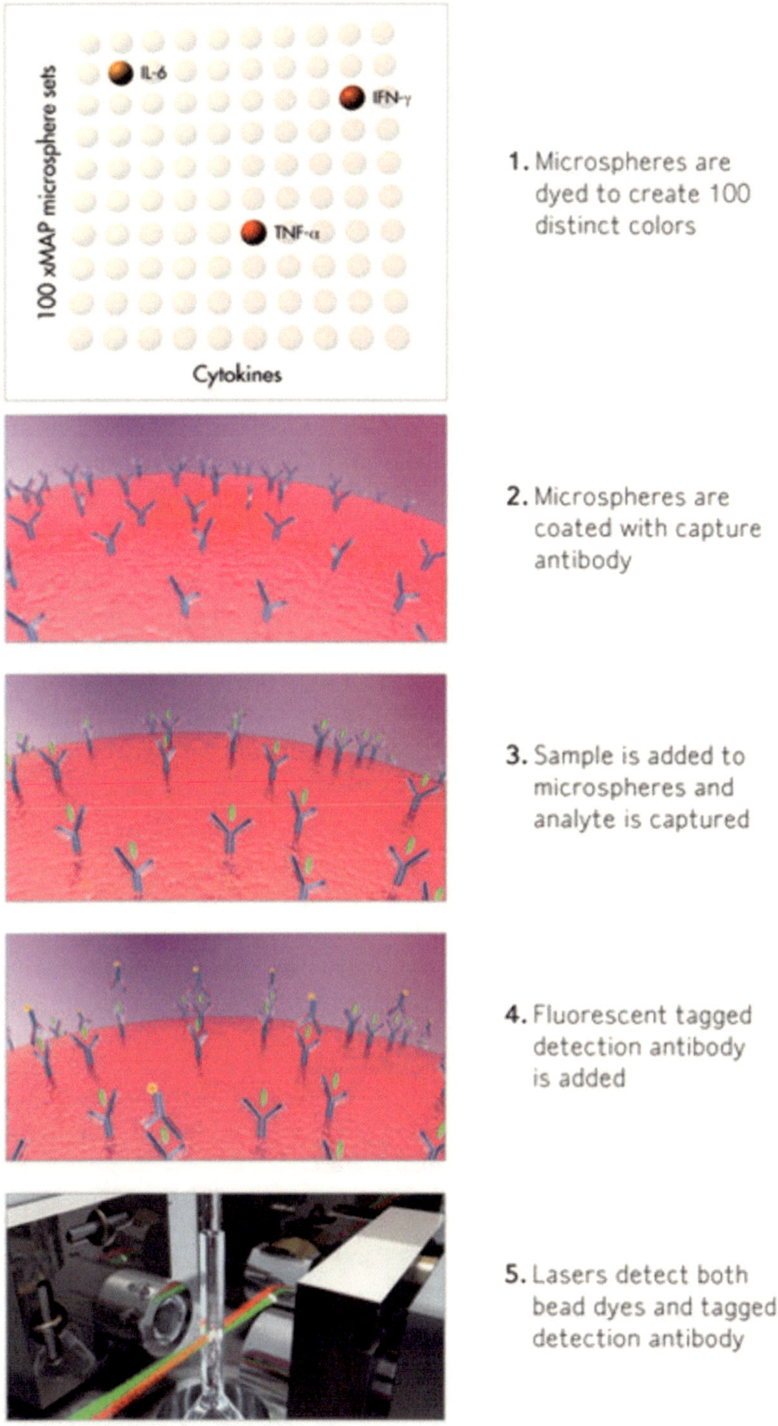

Fig. 1. Process of multiplexed immunodetection using fluorescent-coded beads (www.millipore.com)

2. Bead based multiplex

2.1 Background

In multiplex bead array assays (MBAA), beads of discrete fluorescence intensities and wavelengths provide a capture surface for specific analytes enabling detection of multiple analytes in a single sample. Bead based assays of analyte is an attractive strategy for obtaining large numbers of measurements rapidly. MBAA is an open access system; namely, the parameters to be measured can be determined by the user. The variety of source increases its area of application (nucleic acids, antigens, antibodies, receptors).Since the detection method is based on flow cytometry and this allows repeatability, MBAA performs the quality control of the measurement, simultaneously with the measurement itself.

The MBAA readers allow analysis of up to 100 reactions or assays per well. This remarkable capability allows incorporating a large number of assays, such as DNA, receptor-ligand, Immunoassay and enzyme in life science research, drug discovery as well as diagnostic areas.

2.2 The principle of measurement

These systems depend on measurement of fractional antibody occupancy using two different labels: one labeling the "capture" antibody, the second labeling a "detection antibody", selected to react either with occupied or unoccupied sites on the "capture" antibody. The ratio of signals emitted by the two labeled antibodies reveals the analyte concentration to which the capture antibody has been exposed. An array of capture antibodies, each labeled with the same fluorescent label, is scanned (by a laser), and the fluorescent signal ratio emitted from each discrete antibody couplet in the array is measured.

2.3 Summary of principles

1. Color-coded beads, pre-coated with analyte-specific capture antibody for the molecule of interest are added.
2. Analyte-specific antibodies capture the analyte of interest. Biotinylated detection antibodies specific to the analyte of interest are added and form an antibody-antigen sandwich.
3. Phycoerythrin (PE)-conjugated Streptavidin is added.
4. The beads are read by a dual-laser flow-based detection instrument which excites the internal dyes marking the beads set and a second laser excites PE, the fluorescent dye on the reporter molecule (www.luminexcorp.com).

The system is capable of measuring potentially up to 100 analytes simultaneously in a small sample volume (25–50 μL).

2.4 Advantages of the system

1. **Speed/High Throughput** – Because each microsphere serves as an individual test, a large number of different assays can be performed and analyzed simultaneously
2. **Versatility** – Bead based multiplex system can perform assays in several different formats, including nucleic acids and antigen-antibody binding, along with enzyme, receptor-ligand and other protein interactions

3. **Flexibility** – The technology can be customized for the user's specific needs based upon their analytes of interest
4. **Accuracy** – The technology generates real-time analysis and accurate quantification of the biological interactions (www.luminexcorp.com).

Advantages of this approach also include specimen conservation, limited sample handling, and decreased time and cost. However, it is difficult to optimize assay format for each protein, to select common dilution factors and to establish reliable quality control algorithms.

Characteristics	Antibody-based
Principle	Antibody–antigen interaction
Required reagents/information	Specific antibody pairs
Quantification basis	flowcytometer and others
Multiplexicity	1–100
Clinical diagnostic test	Yes
Sample enrichment	No
Sensitivity	>sub ng/mL–pg/mL
Reproducibility	Excellent
Assay development	Time and resource demanding
Consumable	High demand
Robustness	Yes
Throughput	High
Matrix effect	Yes
Sample manipulation	No
Automation	Yes
History	>15 years

Table 3.The characteristics of MBAA

2.5 Comparison with other technologies and assays

The assay which is most often compared to MBAA is the enzyme-linked immunosorbent assay (ELISA). ELISAs, in general, use a similar immobilized antibody to capture a soluble ligand, with subsequent detection of the captured ligand by a second antibody. There are, however, several substantial differences between MBAA and ELISAs. For example, MBAA uses fluorescence as a detection system where ELISAs use enzyme amplification of a colorimetric substrate. MBAA captures ligands onto spherical beads in suspension while ELISAs generally rely upon flat surfaces in 96-well plates. Most importantly, MBAA techniques, by their very nature, are multiplexed and therefore may be subject to any perturbations that arise from analyzing multiple ligands simultaneously, such as cross-reactivities. By contrast, ELISA methodologies generally study one analyte at a time, and thus avoid any concerns arising from multiplexing.

Multiplex system presents additional Quality control (QC) challenges compared to uniplex analyses. The failure of 1 constituent assay to meet QC specifications results in rejection of results for all assays on the panel. Samples failing QC specifications should be retested using the same measurement system, because substitution of a uniplex assay may introduce bias due to differences in assay format. However, the probability of all assays simultaneously meeting QC specifications is much lower than the probability of a uniplex test passing QC. At present, reference guidelines for multiplex QC programs are under development by the Food and Drug Administration (FDA).

In theory, the MBAA platform may also provide a wider dynamic range than conventional ELISA methods because of the greater linear range of fluorescence intensity compared with absorbance. Detection limits of MBAA (luminex) and ELISA are different. A comparison of detection limits of some test for the Luminex assays and the ELISAs is shown in Table 4. Data Supplement (available at http://www.clinchem.org/content/vol51/issue7/) Disadvantage of MBAA are time consuming in assay development, lacking antibody pairs for new biomarkers and limited commercial multiplex assay kits.

Multiplex panels	Analytes	Luminex	ELISA	ELISA manufacturer
Linco Endocrine	Leptin	0.13 μg/L	1.39 μg/L	Linco
	Insulin	0.31 mIU/L	0.14 mIU/L	Alpco
	C-peptide	0.037 μg/L	0.132 μg/L	Linco
Biosource Chemokine	MCP-1	2.35 ng/L	2.57 ng/L	R&D
	Eotaxin	4.37 ng/L	3.80 ng/L	R&D
Upstate Chemokine	MCP-1	20.5 ng/L	2.57 ng/L	R&D
	Eotaxin	27.72 Eotaxin	3.80 ng/L	R&D
Linco Cytokine	TNF-α	1.61 ng/L	0.092 ng/L	R&D
	IL-8	2.52 ng/L	0.26 ng/L	Biosource
Upstate Cytokine	TNF-α	0.065 ng/L	0.092 ng/L	R&D
	IL-8	0.70 ng/L	0.26 ng/L	Biosource
	IL-6	0.75 ng/L	0.068 ng/L	R&D
R&D Cytokine	TNF-α	1.53 ng/L	0.092 ng/L	R&D
	IL-6	0.977 ng/L	0.068 ng/L	R&D

Table 4. Comparison of detection limits for the Luminex multiplexed assays and the individual ELISAs.

Protein microarray kits, which use capture antibodies and detection antibodies in a multiplex fashion similar to MBAA, should also be considered as a competing technology which is most commonly used for simultaneous determination of multiple proteins in a biological fluid. The technique uses primary antibodies as the immobilized probe on a solid surface, and protein antigens labeled with fluorophores with or without bound secondary antibodies are recognized and detected. However, binding of antibodies and antigens to a solid support can cause denaturation or drying of proteins. MBAA provides multiplexing in a solution phase and thus is particularly flexible and nondestructive for protein analysis. Also protein microarray assay are relatively new, are not widely accepted as a 'gold standard' for clinical use, and also may be of limited sensitivity.

2.6 Areas of application

Since a disease can result from various reasons and it may include functional disorders of multiple genes, a multi analyte analysis is necessary for diagnostic purposes. The technology called omic and multiplex system allows a fast and systematic detection of the effects of micro molecules in different molecular and cellular contexts. In this respect, it can be used for diagnosing multi-reason/multi-gene diseases, performing a comprehensive disease management and investigating complex cellular functions. In addition, it provides a wide range of application area for research area because of its plasticity which allows the researchers to perform various studies.

2.7 Clinical utility

Despite the introduction of hundreds of multiplexed protein immunoassays to the research market in recent years, only a limited number have been cleared by the FDA for clinical use, an observation that illustrates the complexity of constructing robust arrays. Antibody-based multiplexed assay (and commercial instruments and kits) have a relatively long history with over 15 years of development and optimization. However, most commercial multiplex assays are developed for research laboratories and nonclinical tests; only a limited number of multiplex assays are approved by FDA for clinical testing. For example FDA-cleared planar protein multiplex arrays consist primarily of the lateral flow immunoassays used for point-ofcare evaluation . For example, the Triage® Cardio ProfilER® 4-plex measures troponin-I, creatine kinase-MB, myoglobin, and brain natriuretic peptide (BNP) to assist with evaluation of chest pain using a portable lateral flow platform. At present, suspension immunoassay is the prevailing technology for FDA-cleared multiplex protein measurements, especially for testing antibodies in the serum of patients with allergies or autoimmune or infectious diseases in clinical laboratories.

The other platforms for commercial multiplex diagnostic tests include Luminex (www.luminex.com), Triage system (www.Biosite.com), Evidence (www.Randox.com), Vidas (www.biomerieux-diagnostics. com), Planner arrays (www.VBC-genomics),Whatman (www.whatman.com) and bead array (www.bioarrays.com). At present, suspension immunoassay is the prevailing technology for FDA-cleared multiplex protein measurements, especially for testing antibodies in the serum of patients with allergies or autoimmune or infectious diseases in clinical laboratories. Most of the currently available multiplex immunoassays have been designed to quantify the concentrations of various cytokines.The recent development of spectrally-distinguishable fluorescent beads(Luminex) (Kellar and Iannone, 2002) has resulted in the widespread use of antigen-coupled beads for monitoring antibodies in sera by flow cytometry. These bead arrays have been adapted for serologic screening of antigens and have been described for up to ten antigens for HIV (Opalka et al., 2004), HPV (Opalka et al., 2003; Dias et al., 2005), Epstein-Barr virus (Klutts et al., 2004; Binnicker et al., 2008; Gu et al., 2008), B. anthracis (Biagini et al., 2004; Biagini et al., 2005), Influenza (Drummond et al., 2008) and M.tuberculosis (Khan et al.,2008).

The results from a growing number of research studies, demonstrate that multiplex technology may be useful in clinical research to measure a large number of analytes to examine the association with a clinical phenotype and the effects of therapeutic interventions, and that this technology may be particularly useful when sample volume is limited, such as in large epidemiologic studies and clinical trials. Clinical applications must follow establishment of globally accepted calibration standards, performance criteria, and QC programs.

APPLICATION	AVAILABLE KITS*	COMPANY
Allergy Testing	Alternaria (Mold) (h), Bermuda Grass (h), Cat Dander (h), Egg White (h), Milk (h), Mite Pternoyssinus (h), Mountain Cedar (h), Short Ragweed (h), Timothy Grass (h), Wheat (food) (h)	ImTech (h)
Autoimmune	ASCA (h), beta-2 Microglobulin (h,m), Centromere B (h), Chromatin (h), DNA (h),ENA Profile 4 (SSA, SSB, Sm, ENA Profile 5 SSA, SSB, Sm, RNP, Scl-70) (h), ENA Profile 6 (SSA, SSB, Sm, RNP, Scl-70, Jo-1) (h), Gliadin A (h), Gliadin G (h), Histone (h), Histone H1 (h), Histone H2A (h), Histone H2B (h), Histone H3 (h), Histone H4 (h), HSP-27 pS82 (G), HSP-27 Total (G), HSP-32 (h), HSP-65 (h), HSP-71 (h), HSP-90 a (h), HSP-90 b (h), Jo-1 (h), PCNA (h,m), PR3 (h), PR3 (cANCA) (m), RF (h), Ribosomal P (h,m), RNP (h,m), RNP-A (h), RNP-C (h), SCF (h,m), Scl-70 (h,m), Serum Amyloid P (h), SLE Profile 8 (SSA, SSB, Sm, RNP, Scl-70, Jo-1, Ribosome-P, chromatin) (h), Sm (G) (h), Smith (h,m), SSA (h,m), SSB (h,m), Streptolysin O (h), TG (h), TPO (h,m), Transglutaminase A (h), Transglutaminase G (h)	RBM(h,m)
Cancer Markers	Alpha Fetoprotein (h), Cancer Antigen 125 (h), Carcinoembryonic Antigen (h), PSA, Free (h)	RBM(h)
Cardiac Markers	Creatine Kinase-MB (h), Endothelin-1 (m), PAP (h), SGOT (h,m), TIMP-1 (h,m)	RBM(h,m)
Cytokine	Abeta 40 (h), Abeta 42 (h), BDNF (h), DR-5 (h), EGF (h,m), ENA-78 (h), Eotaxin (h,m), Fatty Acid Binding Protein (h), FGF-basic (h,m), G-CSF (h,m), GCP-2 (m), GM-CSF (h,m,rt), GRO alpha (h), GRO-KC (rt), HGF (h,m), I-TAC (h), ICAM-1 (h), IFN-alpha (h), IFN-gamma (h,m,rt), IL-10 (h,m,rt), IL-11 (m), IL-12 (h,m), IL-12 p40 (h,m), IL-12 p40/p70 (m) (rt), IL-12 p70 (h,m,rt), IL-13 (h,m), IL-15 (h,m), IL-16 (h), IL-17 (h,m), IL-18 (rt), IL-1alpha (h,m,rt), IL-1beta (h,m,rt), IL-1ra (h), IL-1ra/IL-1F3 (h), IL-2 (h,m,rt), IL-3 (h,m), IL-4 (h,m,rt), IL-5 (h,m,rt), IL-6 (h,m,rt), IL-7 (h,m), IL-8 (h), IL-9 (m), IP-10 (h,m), JE/MCP-1 (m), KC (m), KC/GROa (m), LIF (m), IL-8 (h), IL-9 (m), IP-10 (h,m), JE/MCP-1 (m), KC (m), KC/GROa (m), LIF (m), MCP-3(h,m), MCP-5 (m)	B-R(m); Bios (h,m,rt); Linco (h,m,rt); RD(h,m); UP(h,m), RBM (h,m)
EndocrineACTH (h), Adiponectin (h,m), Amylin (m) (rt) (h), C-Peptide (h), Calcitonin (h), CRF Linco	ACTH (h), Adiponectin (h,m), Amylin (m) (rt) (h), C-Peptide (h), Calcitonin (h), CRF(h), FGF-9 (m), FSH (h), GH (h), GLP-1 (h,m,rt), Glucagon (m) (rt) (h), Growth Hormone (h,m), Insulin (h,m,rt), Leptin (h,m,rt), LH (h), Lipoprotein (a) (h), PAI-1(active) (h), PAI-1 (total) (h,m), Prolactin (h), Resistin (h,m,rt), T3 (h), T4 (h), TBG (h), Thyroglobulin (h), TSH (h)	Linco (h,m,rt); RBM (h,m)
Gene Expression	IL6R(h), ACTB (h), BAD (h), BAK1 (BAK) (h), BCL2 (h), BCL2L1 (BCL-XL) (h), CDKN1A (CDKN1) (h), CFLAR (CFLIP) (h), CSF2 (h), GAPD (h), IFN-gamma (h), IL-1 beta (h), IL-10 (h), IL-2 (h), IL-6 (h), IL-8 (h), NFKB2 (h), NFKBIA (NFKIA) (h), NKFB1 (h), PPIB (h), Ptk2B (RAFTK) (h), RELA (h), RELB (h), TNF (h), TNFAIP3 (A20) (h), TNFRSF6 (FAS) (h), TNFSF6 (FASL) (h), VEGF (h)	Bios (h); MBio (h)
MMP	MMP-1 (h), MMP-12 (h), MMP-13 (h), MMP-2 (h), MMP-3 (h), MMP-7 (h), MMP-8(h), MMP-9 (h)	RD (h); Bios (h)
Genotyping	FlexMAP™ (G), Mitochondrial DNA Screening (h), Tag-It™ Mutation Detection Kit(G), Y-SNP Identification (h)	Bio (h), Mira(h), TmBio (h)

APPLICATION	AVAILABLE KITS*	COMPANY
Infectious Disease	Adenovirus (h,m), Bordetella pertussis (h), Campylobacter jejuni (h), Chlamydia pneumoniae (h), Chlamydia trachomatis (h), Cholera Toxin (h), Cholera Toxin b (h), Clostridium piliforme (Tyzzer's) (m), Cytomegalovirus (h,m), Diphtheria Toxin (h), Ectromelia virus (m), EDIM (Epidemic diarrhea of infant mice) (m), Encephalitozoon cuniculi (m), Epstein-Barr EA (h), Epstein-Barr NA (h), Epstein-Barr VCA (h), HBV Core (h), HBV Envelope (h), HBV Surface (Ad) (h), HBV Surface (Ay) (h), HCV Core (h), HCV NS3 (h), HCV NS4 (h), HCV NS5 (h), Helicobacter pylori (h), Hepatitis A (h), Hepatitis D (h), HEV orf2 3KD (h), HEV orf2 6KD (h), HEV orf3 3KD (h), HIV-1 gp120 (h), HIV-1 gp41 (h), HIV-1 p24 (h), HPV (h), HSV-1 gD (h), HSV-1/2 (h), HSV-2 gG (h), HTLV-1/2 (h), Influenza A (h), Influenza A H3N2 (h), Influenza B (h), Leishmania donovani (h), Lyme disease (h), Lymphocytic choriomeningitis virus (m), M. pneumoniae (h), M. tuberculosis (h), Minute virus (m), Mumps (h), Mycoplasma pulmonis (m), Parainfluenza 1 (h), Parainfluenza 2 (h), Parainfluenza 3 (h), Parvovirus (m), Pneumonia virus of mice (m)	RBM (h,m)
Isotyping	IgA (h,m), IgE (h,m), IgG1 (m), IgG2alpha (m), IgG2beta (m), IgG3 (m), IgM (h,m), light chain (kappa or gamma) (m)	UP (h,m); RBM(h,m)
Metabolic Markers	Apolipoprotein A-1 (m), Apolipoprotein A-I (h), Apolipoprotein A-II (h), Apolipoprotein B (h), Apolipoprotein C-II (h), Apolipoprotein C-III (h), Apolipoprotein E (h), beta-2 Glycoprotein (h,m), Collagen Type 1 (h), Collagen Type 2(h), Collagen Type 4 (h), Collagen Type 6 (h), Glutathione S-Transferase (h,m), Pancreatic Islet Cells (h), tTG (Celiac Disease) (h)	RBM (h,m), Linco
Tissue Typing	HLA Class I and II (h), HLA Class I Single Antigen Antibody, Group 1 (h), HLA Class I Single Antigen Antibody, Group 2 (h), PRA Class I (h), PRA Class I and II (h), PRA Class II (h), SSO Class I HLA-A (h), SSO Class I HLA-B (h), SSO Class I HLA-C(h), SSO Class II DP (h), SSO Class II DQB1 (h), SSO Class II DRB1 (h), SSO Class II DRB3,4,5 (h)	Lambda (h)
Kinase Phosphorylated Protein	Akt (G), Akt (Ser473) (G), Akt (total) (G), Akt/PKB (total) (G), Akt/PKBpS473 (G), ATF2 (Thr71) (G), ATF2 (total) (G), CREB (pS133) (G), CREB (Total) (G), Erk 1/2(pTpY185/187) (G), Erk 1/2 (Total) (G), Erk-2 (G), Erk1 (Thr202/Tyr204) (G), Erk1/2 (Thr202/Tyr204, Thr185/Tyr187) (G), Erk2 (Thr185/Tyr187) (G), Erk2 (total) (G),GSK 3beta (pS9) (G), GSK-3a/b (Ser21/Ser9) (G), GSK-3beta (G), IGF 1R	UP (G), Bios (G)
Transcription Factors-Nuclear Receptors	AP-2 (G), CREB (G), EGR (h), HIF-1 (h), NF-1 (h), NFAT (h), NFkB Gene Family(h), PPAR (h), SRE (h), YY1 (h)	Bios (h), MBio (h)

* Human (h), mouse (m): rat (rt): general (G), ImmuneTech (ImTech); Rules Based Medicine (RBM); Bio-Rad (B-R); BioSource (Bios); Linco Research (Linco); Qiagen; R&D Systems (RD); and Upstate Group (UP); Marligen Biosciences (MBio), MiraBio (Mira); Tm BioScience (TmBio); One Lambda (LAMBDA).

Table 5. Aplication area and available kits

3. References

[1] Multiplexed Analysis of Biomarkers Related to Obesity and the Metabolic Syndrome in Human Plasma, Using the Luminex-100 System. Liu M.Y, Xydakis A.M, Hoogeveen R.C, Jones P.H, O'Brian Smith E, Nelson K.W, Ballantyn C.M. Clinical Chemistry.2005;51(7):1102–1109 .

[2] Multiplex assays for biomarker research and clinical application: Translational science coming of age. Fu Q, Schoenhoff F.S, Savage W.J, Zhang P, Van Eyk J.E.Proteomics Clin. Appl. 2010;4:271–284.

[3] Comparison of multiplex immunoassay platforms. Fu Q, Zhu J, Van Eyk JE. Clin Chem. 2010;56(2):314-8.

[4] Measurement and Quality Control Issues in Multiplex Protein Assays: A Case Study. Ellington A.A, Kullo I.J, Bailey K.R, Klee G.G. Clin Chem. 2009; 55(6): 1092–1099.

[5] Multi-analyte immunoassay. Ekins RP.Journal of Pharmaceutical and Biomedical Analysis.1989; 7(2):155-168.

[6] US Food and Drug Administration. Guidance for industry and FDA staff: pharmacogenetic tests and genetic tests for heritable markers. (Accessed October 2011].

[7] Multiplexed protein measurement: technologies and applications of protein and antibody arrays. Kingsmore S.F. Nat Rev Drug Discov. 2006; 5(4): 310–3208.

[8] Antibody-Based Protein Multiplex Platforms: Technical and Operational Challenges. Ellington A.A, Kullo IJ, Bailey K.R, Klee G.G. Clin Chem. 2010; 56(2): 186–193.

[10] Rapıd Detectıon of Antıbodıes In Sera Usıng Multıplexed Self-Assemblıng Bead Arrays. Wonga J, Sibanib S, Lokkoa N.N, LaBaerb J, Andersona K. J Immunol Methods. 2009; 31: 171–182.

[11] Multiplex Bead Array Assays: Performance Evaluation and Comparison of Sensitivity to ELISA. Elshal M.F, McCoy J.P. Methods. 2006; 38(4): 317–323.

[12] Obez Hastalarda Büyüme Hormonu, Leptin, Amilin,Glukagon Benzeri Peptid-1 Seviyeleri ile İnsülin Direnci Arasındaki İlişki [Relationship Between The Levels of Growth Hormone, Leptin, Amylin,Glucagon Like Peptide-1 and Insulin Resistance in Obese Patients]. Yiğitbaşı T,Baskın Y, Afacan G, Harmanda A. Turkish Journal of Biochemistry 2010; 35 (3); 177–182.

[13] Eotaxin and Interleukin-4 Levels and Their Relation to Sperm Parameters in Infertile Men. Yiğitbası T,Baskın Y, Afacan G, Karaarslan F, Taheri C, Aslan D. Turkiye Klinikleri J Med Sci 2010;30 (5)1441-1445.